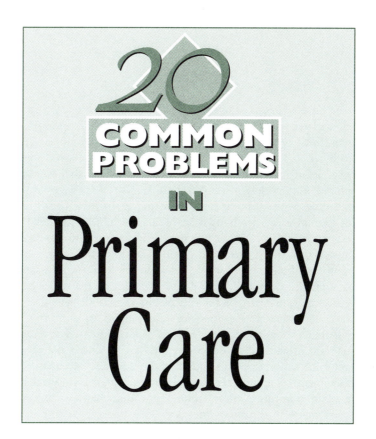

20 COMMON PROBLEMS IN Primary Care

Notice

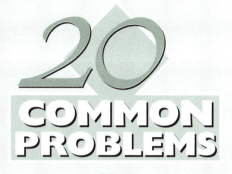

20 COMMON PROBLEMS IN

Primary Care

EDITOR

BARRY D. WEISS, M.D.

Chairman, Department of Family Practice
University of Texas Health Science Center at San Antonio
San Antonio, Texas

McGraw-Hill

Health Professions Division

New York   St. Louis   San Francisco   Auckland   Bogotá   Caracas   Lisbon   London   Madrid
Mexico City   Milan   Montreal   New Delhi   San Juan   Singapore   Sydney   Tokyo   Toronto

McGraw-Hill

A Division of The **McGraw·Hill** *Companies*

20 COMMON PROBLEMS IN PRIMARY CARE

Copyright © 1999 by The McGraw-Hill Companies, Inc. All rights reserved. Printed in the United States of America. Except as permitted under the United States Copyright Act of 1976, no part of this publication may be reproduced or distributed in any form or by any means, or stored in a data base or retrieval system, without prior written permission of the publisher.

1234567890 DOCDOC 998

ISBN 0-07-069609-8

This book was set in Garamond by Better Graphics, Inc.
The editors were Joseph A. Hefta, Susan R. Noujaim, and Lester A. Sheinis.
The production supervisor was Helene G. Landers.
The text was designed by Marsha Cohen/
Parallelogram.
The cover was designed by José R. Fonfrias and Marsha Cohen/
Parallelogram.
Cover: "© TSM/Rob Lewine and Chuck Savage, 1998"
The color inserts were designed by Robert Freese.
The indexer was Irving Conde Tullar.

R.R. Donnelley and Sons Company was the printer and binder.

This book is printed on acid-free paper.

Library of Congress Cataloging-in-Publication Data

20 common problems in primary care. — 1st ed.
      p.   cm.
   Includes bibliographical references.
   ISBN 0-07-069609-8
   1. Primary care (Medicine)   I. Weiss, Barry D.
   [DNLM: 1. Primary Health Care.   WB110 Z2 1999]
RC48.A14   1999
616—dc21
DNLM/DLC
for Library of Congress   98-29864
                              CIP

I dedicate this book to my mother, Ruth,
who always wanted me to be a doctor;
and to my wife, Joyce,
without whose help I never could have been one.

Contents

Contributors

ABDOMINAL PAIN: DYSPEPSIA
(CHAPTER 15)
Alan M. Adelman, M.D.
Professor
Department of Family and Community Medicine
Milton S. Hershey Medical Center
Hershey, Pennsylvania

ANXIETY (CHAPTER 9)
David A. Katerndahl, M.D.
Professor
Department of Family Practice
University of Texas Health Science Center
San Antonio, Texas

BACK PAIN (CHAPTER 12)
Jeff Susman, M.D.
Associate Dean for Primary Care
Department of Family Medicine
University of Nebraska Medical Center
Omaha, Nebraska

BIRTH CONTROL (CHAPTER 20)
Mindy A. Smith, M.D., M.S.
Associate Professor
Department of Family Practice
Michigan State University
Lansing, Michigan

Jill Larkin, M.D.
Clinical Assistant Professor
Department of Family Practice
Michigan State University
Lansing, Michigan

CHEST PAIN (CHAPTER 14)
Michael S. Klinkman, M.D., M.S.
Associate Professor
Department of Family Practice
University of Michigan
Ann Arbor, Michigan

CIGARETTE SMOKING (CHAPTER 1)
William C. Wadland, M.D.
Professor and Chairman
Department of Family Practice
Michigan State University
East Lansing, Michigan

Bertram Stoffelmayr, Ph.D.
Professor
Department of Psychiatry
Michigan State University
East Lansing, Michigan

COUGH (CHAPTER 7)
William J. Hueston, M.D.
Professor and Chairman
Department of Family Medicine
Medical University of South Carolina
Charleston, South Carolina

DERMATITIS-ECZEMA (CHAPTER 16)
Patricia E. Boiko, M.D.
Department of Family Practice
Group Health Cooperative of Puget Sound
Seattle, Washington

Susan Boiko, M.D.
Department of Dermatology
Kaiser Permanente Southern California
San Diego, California

DEPRESSION (CHAPTER 8)
Michael K. Magill, M.D.
Professor and Chairman
Department of Family and Preventive Medicine
University of Utah School of Medicine
Salt Lake City, Utah

DIABETES MELLITUS, TYPE 2
(CHAPTER 4)
Judith Gore Gearhart, M.D.
Associate Professor
Department of Family Medicine
University Medical Center
Jackson, Mississippi

EARACHE (CHAPTER 5)
Evan W. Kligman, M.D.
Director
Northwest Healing Arts
Tucson, Arizona
Clinical Professor
University of Iowa
Iowa City, Iowa

HEADACHE (CHAPTER 10)
Anne D. Walling, M.D.
Associate Dean for Faculty Development
Department of Family and Community Medicine
University of Kansas-Wichita
Wichita, Kansas

HIDDEN PROBLEMS (CHAPTER 17)
Domestic Violence
L. Kevin Hamberger, Ph.D.
Professor
Department of Family and Community Medicine
Medical College of Wisconsin
Racine Family Practice Center
Racine, Wisconsin

The Problem Drinker
Daniel C. Vinson, M.D., M.S.P.H.
Associate Professor
Department of Family and Community Medicine
University of Missouri, Columbia
Columbia, Missouri

Low Literacy
Barry D. Weiss, M.D.
Professor and Chairman
Department of Family Practice
University of Texas Health Science Center
San Antonio, Texas

HYPERTENSION (CHAPTER 3)
Stephen A. Brunton, M.D.
Executive Vice President for Education and Scientific Affairs
Clinical Communications Group
Greenwich, Connecticut

Louis Kuritzky, M.D.
Clinical Associate Professor
Department of Community Health and Medicine
University of Florida
Gainsville, Florida

OBESITY (CHAPTER 2)
David S. Gray, M.D.
Community Hospital Family Practice Residency
Department of Family and Community Medicine
University of California San Francisco
Santa Rosa, California

OSTEOARTHRITIS
(CHAPTER 11)
Jay A. Swedberg, M.D.
Clinical Preceptor
Creighton School of Medicine
Private Practice
Casper, Wyoming

**PREVENTIVE HEALTH
EXAMINATIONS** (CHAPTER 19)
Doug Campos-Outcalt, M.D., M.P.A
Medical Director
Maricopa County Health Department
Phoenix, Arizona

SORE THROAT AND NASAL CONGESTION (CHAPTER 6)

Kay A. Bauman, M.D., M.P.H.
Professor and Cochair
Department of Family Practice
John A. Burns School of Medicine
Mililani, Hawaii

David R. Brown, M.D.
Assistant Professor
Department of Family Practice
John A. Burns School of Medicine
Mililani, Hawaii

SPRAINS AND STRAINS (CHAPTER 13)

James L. Moeller, M.D.
Assistant Director
Family Practice Residency Programs
Director of Sports Medicine
William Beaumont Hospital
Troy, Michigan

Douglas B. McKeag, M.D.
Arthur Rooney Senior Professor
Departments of Medicine and Orthopedic Surgery
University of Pittsburg Medical Center
Pittsburgh, Pennsylvania

URINARY TRACT INFECTION (CHAPTER 18)

Mark H. Ebell, M.D., M.S.
Associate Professor
Department of Family Practice
Michigan State University
East Lansing, Michigan

Henry C. Barry, M.D., M.S.
Associate Professor
Senior Associate Chair
Department of Family Practice
Michigan State University
East Lansing, Michigan

Preface

This book introduces McGraw-Hill's *20 Common Problems* series, a new series devoted to the common clinical problems seen in day-to-day outpatient primary care practice. The concept behind this approach is that primary care clinicians should, above all, have a command of the most-common problems they encounter in their patients. Thus, each chapter gives readers in-depth and up-to-date information needed for diagnosis and management of the most common primary care problems. Each chapter also considers topics such as clinicians' common errors, trends, and innovations that may influence management in the future, patient education, alternative medicine, and a variety of other issues.

Following this first book on the overall most-common problems in primary care, other books planned for the series will concentrate on geriatrics, behavioral health, prevention, women's health, children's health, skin disorders, end-of-life care, sports medicine, the gastrointestinal system, the genitourinary system, cross-cultural medicine, medical ethics, and other topics. These books will deal with the conditions in each area that are most common in primary care practice. It is our intention that the series of books will enhance the learning of trainees in medicine, nursing, and the allied health professions, and serve as a resource for ongoing education of practicing clinicians in a variety of specialties that deal with primary care conditions.

What are the 20 Most-Common Problems in Primary Care Practice?

What are the 20 most-common problems in primary care practice? The answer is not as straightforward as one might think. The National Ambulatory Medical Care Survey (NAMCS), reported periodically by the National Center for Health Statistics, provides data from a nationwide network of office-based, nonfederally employed physicians who collect and report information on their encounters with patients. However, the most-common primary care problems reported by the NAMCS differ substantially from the most-common problems reported by physicians in a variety of primary care settings (Table 1). Furthermore, the

Table 1

Top-Five Reason for Visits to Primary Care Clinicians in Different Settings

RANK	NACMS[1]	MIDWESTERN PRIVATE PRACTICE[2]	FAMILY PRACTICE RESIDENCY CLINIC[3]	SOUTHERN CALIFORNIA HMO[4]
1	Cough	Dermatitis-Eczema	Hypertension	Adult Prevention
2	Sore Throat	Sore Throat	Diabetes	URI
3	Earache	Otitis Media	Abdominal Pain	Cardiovascular Disease
4	Back Problems	Hypertension	Adult Prevention	Hypertension
5	Skin Rash	Urinary Infection	Well-Child Care	Skin Rash

ABBREVIATIONS: HMO, Health Maintenance Organization; NAMCS, National Ambulatory Medical Care Survey; URI, upper respiratory infection.

NAMCS does not include data from nurse practitioners, physician assistants, and a variety of other clinicians that provide primary care services.

In generating the list of 20 common problems to include in this book, a variety of data sources were examined, including those cited in Table 1, attempting to develop a consensus or "average" list from among the many sources of data. After developing the consensus list, however, I found it apparent that a number of extraordinarily common conditions never appear on published lists of common diagnoses, even though they are more common than many of the problems on those lists. These include problems such as cigarette smoking, obesity, and the hidden problems of domestic violence, alcohol abuse, and illiteracy. These common problems were included in this book in lieu of several of the less-common problems that frequently appear on published lists of common diagnoses.

The problems discussed in this book, as outlined in the contents, represent my best estimate of the problems most often encountered by clinicians in primary care practice. If primary care clinicians develop a firm mastery of these problems, those individuals will be able to diagnose and treat most of the conditions for which patients present for care, and follow the evolution of research and knowledge related to those conditions.

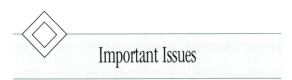

Important Issues

As one reviews each chapter of the book, several issues appear again and again and are worthy of discussion. These include the emerging global problem of antibiotic resistance, the need for clinicians to follow standard guidelines for practice, and the need for research to develop more appropriate practice guidelines for primary care practice.

Antibiotic Resistance

The authors of multiple chapters comment on the growing problem of bacterial resistance to antibiotics. A decade ago, antibiotic resistance was largely a problem of hospitalized patients, frequently those hospitalized in critical care units. Now, however, antibiotic resistance is a major issue in outpatient primary care practice on a global basis.

Each year, primary care clinicians prescribe antibiotics to huge numbers of patients. As noted in the chapter on earache, for example, treatment of otitis media—largely by primary care clinicians—accounts for nearly half of all antibiotics prescribed for children in the United States. Unfortunately, antibiotics are often prescribed inappropriately. Broad-spectrum drugs are used when narrow-spectrum drugs would suffice, and antibiotics are prescribed without indication for pharyngitis, upper respiratory infections, and bronchitis.

Primary care clinicians' widespread use of antibiotics without indication, and their use of broad-spectrum agents in inappropriate situations, places some responsibility for the worldwide bacterial resistance problem squarely on the shoulder of primary care clinicians. Fortunately, there is evidence that the bacterial resistance process can be reversed or lessened by more careful and appropriate prescribing practices.[5] Each of the common infections discussed in this book has clear indications for prescribing and withholding antibiotic treatment, and a specified first-choice drug if antibiotics are indicated. As an essential component of high-quality primary care, clinicians should develop a firm knowledge of these indications and first-line drugs, so as to lessen the unnecessary and inappropriate prescribing of antibiotics.

Practice Guidelines and Standards

In the "errors" section of each chapter, the authors make it clear that as a group, primary care clinicians could do better in complying with current recommendations and standards of medical practice. For example, in addition to inappropriate prescribing of antibiotics, primary care clinicians frequently miss opportunities for immunizations and other preventive care, omit essential components of diabetes cares, use imaging tests inappropriately, and make a variety of other errors of omission or commission that lead to less-than-optimal primary care. By improving compliance with practice standards for the most common problems in practice, as outlined in this book, quality of care could be improved substantially.

Primary Care Research

Concomitantly with the need to follow practice guidelines, there is also a need to develop practice guidelines with better applicability to primary care. Because the predictive value of diagnostic tests varies with the prevalence of the conditions at which the tests are directed, many diagnostic approaches developed in specialty settings are not pertinent to primary care patients who have a lower prevalence of uncommon conditions.

The relatively low prevalence of less common disorders in primary care practice has important implications for care and can lead to both underdiagnosis and overdiagnosis. Underdiagnosis is exemplified by the common problems of depression and anxiety. The standard criteria for diagnosis of major depression and generalized anxiety, developed in specialty and research settings, include constellations of symptoms that may not always apply in primary care practice, because patients frequently present to primary care clinicians with "subsyndromal" symptoms that do not meet the standard diagnostic criteria. Overdiagnosis occurs when primary care clinicians go to great lengths to exclude uncommon conditions out of concern that they might be "missing something" —usually a condition that occurs in specialty practice but is rarely seen in primary care. This approach leads to extensive laboratory testing, false positive results on those tests, further diagnosis and treatment based on test results, and anxiety for patients.

Perhaps the major point of this book is that because of relative differences in the frequency of common and rare conditions, primary care clinicians should place more emphasis on knowledge and diagnosis of common conditions and less emphasis on tracking down unlikely possibilities. Simultaneously, research is needed to establish the best diagnostic and therapeutic approaches to common problems in primary care patient populations.

Thank You

Finally, I must thank the many authors who graciously contributed chapters for this book. Their efforts were impressive and very much appreciated, and the success of this book is attributable largely to their efforts. I also thank the medical editors at McGraw-Hill who provided support and assistance in bringing the book to publication.

REFERENCES

1. Schappert SM: *National Ambulatory Medical Care Survey, 1991*. Hyattsville, MD, National Center for Health Statistics, 1992.
2. Schwiebert LP, Ramsey CN, Davis A: Standardizing the clinical content of a third-year family medicine clerkship. *Fam Med* 25:257,1993.
3. Bethea L, Singh K, Probst JC: Clinical similarities and demographic differences between residency and private practice patients. Fam Med 28:472, 1996.
4. Prislin MD, Fitzpatrick C, Munzing T, et al: Ambulatory primary care medical education in managed care and non-managed care settings. *Fam Med* 28:478, 1996.
5. Seppala H, Klaukka T, Vuopio-Varkila J: The effect of changes in the consumption of macrolide antibiotics on erythromycin resistance in group A streptococci in Finland. *New Eng J Med* 337:441, 1997.

The Major Killers

William C. Wadland
Bertram Stoffelmayr

Chapter

1

Cigarette Smoking

How Common Is Cigarette Smoking?

Cigarette smoking is the number-one preventable cause of morbidity and mortality in the United States. Smoking is responsible for more than 400,000 deaths annually in the United States, or more than one of every six deaths. Approximately 25 percent of adult Americans are cigarette smokers, totaling 46 million people: 24 million men and 22 million women. Over 70 percent of these smoking Americans visit a clinician each year, with only half reporting that they have ever been urged to quit smoking by a clinician. Nonetheless, over 70 percent of smokers say they want to quit and would attempt to do so with support from a health care provider. Therefore, primary care clinicians have an opportunity to prevent the consequences of the number-one killer in the United States: cigarette smoking.

The prevalence of smoking among adults has decreased from 40 percent in 1965 to approximately 25 percent in the 1990s, and nearly half of all living adults who ever smoked have quit. However, several recent research findings and evolving trends are disturbing.

First, there has been very little change in the smoking prevalence among heavy smokers (more than 20 cigarettes per day); about 28 percent of smokers are still classified as heavy smokers. The prevalence of smoking remains higher than in the overall population among African Americans, blue-collar workers, Hispanic males, and less-educated individuals.

Second, it is now clear that smoking primarily begins in childhood and adolescence. The age of initiation of smoking has fallen over time, particularly among women, so that the current average age at which daily smoking begins is now 12 to 14 years (Figs. 1-1 and 1-2). In fact, over 3000

Figure 1-1

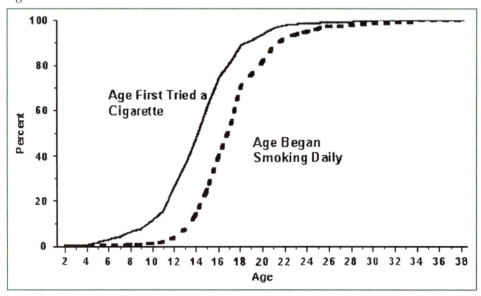

Cumulative age of initiation of cigarette smoking. Data displayed in the graph show that nearly all cigarette smokers begin smoking during their teenage years and nearly all who develop a daily smoking habit do so before their mid-twenties. *(From Centers for Disease Control and Prevention, Tobacco Information and Prevention Sourcepage [http://www.coc.gov/nccdphp/osh/ini.htm.]).*

Figure 1-2

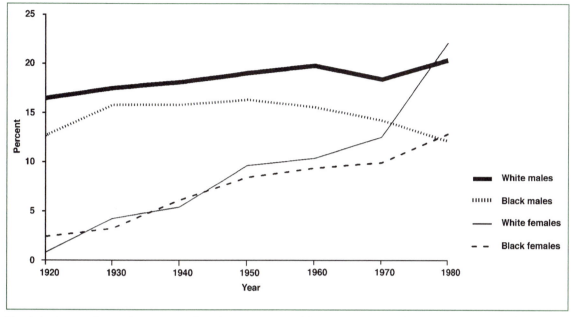

Trends in the prevalence of cigarette smoking by 10 to 19-year-olds. Between 1920 and 1980, the percentage of white male and female, and black female adolescents who smoke has increased. *(Reprinted from Centers for Disease Control and Prevention, Atlanta, 1994.)*

adolescents start smoking each day in the United States, and over 80 percent of smokers report they started to smoke before the age of 18 years. After years of remaining steady, teen smoking rates have been increasing annually since 1992. In 1996, 22 percent of high school seniors smoked daily—up from 17 percent in 1992. Between 1991 and 1996, the percentage of teenagers who reported smoking within the past month increased from 14 to 21 percent among eighth graders and from 21 to 30 percent among tenth graders. In 1998, the Centers for Disease Control and Prevention reported current cigarette use by 36 percent of high school students.

The third disturbing finding is that several studies have revealed nicotine to be addictive much as heroin, cocaine, and alcohol are addictive. Among young smokers, the transition from experimentation to dependence occurs just as frequently with cigarettes as it does with cocaine

and heroin. With the easy availability of cigarettes and the highly addictive nature of nicotine, children and adolescents are highly vulnerable to become smokers. Nearly all experts now recommend that smoking prevention programs in the United States target adolescents and children in addition to heavy smokers, pregnant women, and those traditionally at high risk for smoking, such as minority groups, military personnel, high school dropouts, blue-collar workers, and unemployed persons.

Finally, cigarettes are now heavily marketed around the world, and the tobacco industry enjoys huge profits on the international market. The daily smoking prevalence in many countries is considerably higher than that in the United States with a worldwide prevalence of 47 percent among males and 21 percent among females over the age of 15 years of age (Table 1-1). Smoking cessation and prevention efforts have just begun in many of these countries.

Table 1-1

Daily Smoking Prevalence for Men and Women
Aged 15 and Over

REGIONS	MEN	WOMEN
World Health Organization regions		
African region	29	4
American region	35	22
Eastern Mediterranean region	35	4
Eastern European region	46	26
Southeast Asia region	44	4
Western Pacific region	60	8
More developed countries		
Established market economies	37	23
Former socialist economies of Europe	60	28
Less developed countries		
Middle Eastern nations	41	8
Sub-Saharan Africa	25	3
Latin American and Caribbean	40	21
World	47	12

SOURCE: Adapted from Collishaw.

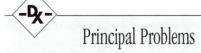

Principal Problems

The risk of illness and death attributable to cigarette smoking far exceeds the risk from other well-known health problems, such as hypertension, hyperlipidemia, and obesity. For example, among men and women less than 65 years of age, smoking accounts for more than 40 percent of cardiovascular deaths, 18 percent of stroke deaths, and 82 percent of deaths from chronic obstructive pulmonary disease (COPD). Because of its importance as a risk factor for death, it has been recommended that clinicians include the identification of smoking as a new "vital sign." In fact, active and past smoking status is more predictive of illness than the results of routine blood pressure, pulse, and weight checks during outpatient visits.

Former smokers live longer than continuing smokers, and the benefits of quitting extend even to those who quit at older ages. For example, persons who quit smoking before the age of 50 have one-half the risk of dying in the next 15 years compared with continuing smokers. The decline in risk of death starts shortly after quitting smoking and continues for 10 to 15 years, at which point the mortality rate from all causes returns nearly to that of persons who never smoked. Helping smokers to become free of tobacco use is, overall, perhaps the most life-extending service that health care providers can offer.

When cigarette smokers inhale, they bring over 4000 compounds, many of which are pharmacologically active, toxic, mutagenic, and carcinogenic, into direct contact with the mucosal membranes of the airways and lung. These compounds, which result from combustion of tobacco, contain carbon monoxide, nicotine, radioactive "tars," and carcinogenic hydrocarbons. Many are rapidly absorbed across the pulmonary alveolar membranes into the bloodstream, inducing systemic effects on blood pressure and pulse, within seconds. Directly or indirectly, these substances are responsible for the variety of adverse effects of cigarette use. In addition to cardiovascular disease, stroke, and chronic lung disease, cigarettes are also responsible for lung cancer, various nonrespiratory cancers, pregnancy complications, nicotine dependence, and ulcers and skin changes.

Cardiovascular and Cerebrovascular Disease

Smoking influences the development of cardiovascular disease through a variety of mechanisms, including effects on vascular endothelium, lipids, platelets, coronary artery musculature, and myocardial oxygen demand.

Smoking has been shown to have a direct toxic effect on vascular endothelium, where it induces degenerative changes. Smoking also has an inverse relationship with high-density lipoprotein (HDL) cholesterol, causing reduction of HDL levels and therefore a reduction in the protective effect of HDL against development of atherosclerosis. Cigarette smoking is highly associated with hypertension, and it increases the adherence of platelets to arterial endothelium, which plays a direct role in acute coronary occlusions. Chronic and acute smoking have also been shown to constrict the coronary arteries. Furthermore, cigarette smoking increases myocardial oxygen demand, which is a critical factor in angina and acute myocardial infarctions. Finally, smoking is related to increased cerebrovascular disease, probably due to the same mechanisms that increase coronary atherosclerosis.

Figure 1-3 illustrates that the beneficial effects of smoking cessation on survival occur even among individuals with documented coronary disease, with significant effects seen within 1 to 2 years. The excess risk of vascular disease caused by smoking is reduced by about half after 1 year of abstinence. After 15 years of abstinence, the risk is similar to that of persons who have never smoked. The risk of stroke returns to the level of persons who have never smoked within 5 to 15 years of abstinence.

Figure 1-3

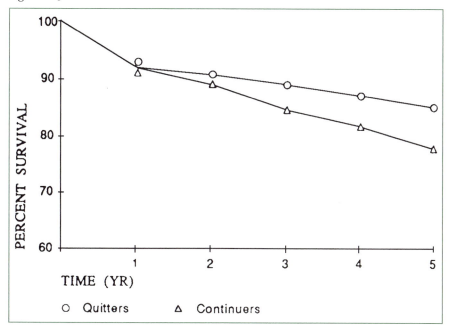

Effect of smoking cessation on survival from coronary atherosclerosis. The graph shows the effect of smoking cessation on survival among men with documented coronary atherosclerosis, demonstrating pooled survival rates among 1490 men who quite smoking and 2675 men who continued to smoke. (*Reprinted from Centers for Disease Control and Prevention, 1990, and RE Vlietstra et al, JAMA. 255:1023–1027, copyright 1986, American Medical Association.*)

Chronic Lung Diseases

Smoking causes several chronic lung diseases. Perhaps the most important is COPD, which consists of chronic bronchitis and emphysema. The sequence of events whereby smoking leads to COPD is hypothesized to be as follows. First, smoking leads to airway and alveolar inflammation (i.e., chronic bronchitis) due to chronic chemical irritation. Second, bronchial narrowing occurs, because cigarette smoking leads to increased levels of bronchial airway "hyperresponsiveness" (i.e., spasm). This airway inflammation and hyperresponsiveness finally leads to breakdown of alveoli and lung parenchyma (i.e., emphysema). In addition to causing direct lung damage in the form of emphysema, smoking is also associated with decreased overall pulmonary function in persons with asthma, and continued smoking adversely affects lung function in those who already have bronchitis and emphysema.

It is encouraging, however, that smoking cessation has beneficial effects on lung function. Smoking cessation reduces respiratory symptoms such as cough, sputum production, and wheezing, and it lowers the frequency of respiratory infections such as bronchitis and pneumonia. In patients who already have COPD, smoking cessation improves pulmonary function by about 5 percent within just a few months after quitting and decreases mortality rates from COPD in comparison to those who continue smoking. Pulmonary function returns to nearly normal levels (i.e., to that of persons who have never smoked) if smoking is stopped before chronic lung changes occur.

Lung Cancer

In 1985, smoking accounted for 87 percent of lung cancer deaths. Studies report that current smokers (of more than 19 cigarettes per day) are 14 times more likely to develop lung cancer than are persons who have never smoked, and the relative risk of lung cancer increases with the duration and intensity of smoking. Thus, largely as a result of the increase in cigarette smoking among women, lung cancer has now surpassed breast cancer as the leading cause of cancer-related deaths in American women.

Forty-three carcinogens have been identified in tobacco smoke. Respiratory tract carcinogenesis from these substances is widely considered to be a multistep process involving sequential changes in cells from the normal to the malignant state. Epithelial changes of the bronchi increase with the amount and length of exposure to cigarette smoking. Patterns of atypical bronchial epithelium have been found in 98 percent of current smokers, 67 percent of ex-smokers, and only 26 percent of never smokers.

The good news, as illustrated in Fig. 1-4, is that the relative risk of lung cancer continues to decrease with time after stopping smoking. In fact, after 10 years of abstinence, the risk of lung cancer is about 30 to 50 percent of the risk in continuing smokers. With further abstinence, the risk continues to decline. The reduced risk of lung cancer resulting from abstinence is independent of the smoker's age and gender and the type of cigarette smoked.

Nonrespiratory Cancers

Smoking has been associated with carcinoma of the oral cavity, esophagus, pancreas, bladder, and cervix. Smoking cessation halves the risks of cancer of the oral cavity and esophagus within 5 years of abstinence. The reduction in pancreatic cancer is measurable only after 10 years of abstinence. Within several years of abstinence, the risk of bladder cancer is reduced over 50 percent. Cervical cancer risk in former smokers is reduced considerably compared to the risk in current smokers, even within 1 to 2 years of abstinence. These changes in cancer prevalence illustrate both the causal associations of smoking and the benefits of smoking cessation.

Figure 1-4

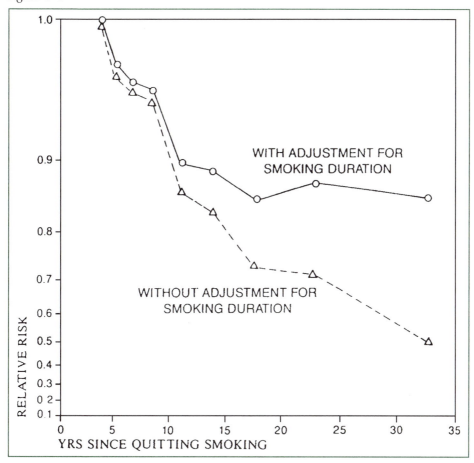

Risk of lung cancer among ex-smokers versus continuing smokers. The risk of lung cancer among ex-smokers decreases with the passage of time after smoking cessation. The magnitude of reduction differs depending on whether adjustments are made for the duration of smoking before cessation. *(Reprinted from J Chron Dis 40(suppl 2), CC Brown, KC Chu. Use of multistage models to infer stage affected by carcinogenic exposure: Example of lung cancer and cigarette smoking, pp 171S–179S, copyright 1987, with permission from Elsevier Science.)*

Poor Pregnancy Outcomes

Smoking is associated with increased rates of spontaneous abortion, infertility, ectopic pregnancy, low birth weight, preterm labor, placental abruption, and placenta previa. Reduced fertility may be due to direct hormonal effects of smoking (smoking increases estrogen metabolism), impaired fallopian tubal motility, impaired im-plantation, and/or altered immunity, leading to more pelvic inflammatory disease. Spontaneous abortion is probably due to nicotine toxicity. Reduced birth weight is thought to result from impaired weight gain due to reduced maternal appetite, nicotine toxicity, carbon monoxide toxicity, and hypoxia either from increased carbon monoxide levels or nicotine-induced vasoconstriction of the umbilical arteries.

Smoking cessation has clear benefits at any time during pregnancy. Women who stop smoking before pregnancy have infants of the same birth weight as those born to never smokers. Pregnant smokers who stop smoking before the thirtieth week of gestation have infants with higher birth weights than do women who continue to smoke. However, reduction (in contrast to cessation) of smoking during pregnancy has virtually no effect on birth weight. Unfortunately, only about 30 percent of women who are smokers quit upon recognizing their pregnancy. It has been estimated that 17 to 24 percent of low birth weight infants in the United States would be of normal weight if smoking during pregnancy were eliminated.

Nicotine Dependence

In 1988, the U.S. Surgeon General's Report established that cigarettes and other forms of tobacco are addictive, largely due to the addictive properties of nicotine. It is surprising that such a statement was not made earlier, since tobacco use has occurred for centuries. In fact, researchers within the tobacco industry were aware of the addictive properties of nicotine and its presence in cigarettes for decades before the Surgeon General's Report. It was known that the addictive threshold for daily smoking was only 5 cigarettes per day, with dose habituation and tolerance increasing with short-term use of 15 to 20 cigarettes per day. This information was withheld from the general public for over 30 years and was released only when nonindustry investigators reported similar findings and "whistle blower" researchers within the tobacco industry disseminated their findings on nicotine addiction and dependency.

The effects of nicotine on the human brain and its neurotransmitters are noted within seconds of inhalation. Nicotine stimulates central nervous system catecholamine activity through release and turnover of both norepinephrine and dopamine. Nicotine works on the dopaminergic pathways similarly to heroin, cocaine, and amphetamines. Nicotine modulates serotonergic neurons, which possibly accounts for the effect of reduced body weight in smokers. These effects of nicotine on neuroreceptors in the brain explain why smokers smoke for multiple reasons, such as craving, relaxation, pleasure, improved attention and cognition, and arousal from depressive moods.

Dependence on nicotine is the reason why smoking cessation is so difficult. In fact, non-nicotine cigarettes marketed in the 1980s were unsuccessful, probably because the product did not satisfy the nicotine addiction of smokers.

The majority of smokers show symptoms of dependence to nicotine. Typical symptoms of nicotine dependence include craving for cigarettes, inability to refrain from use during illness and/or in inappropriate settings, experiencing withdrawal symptoms that are relieved by nicotine, and use of nicotine products within minutes of arising in the morning. These symptoms fit the definition of drug dependence specified in the American Psychiatric Association's *Diagnostic and Statistical Manual for Mental Illness*, fourth edition (DSM IV). The withdrawal syndrome in most nicotine-dependent smokers includes insomnia, anxiety, increased pulse, weight gain, craving for nicotine, hunger, frustration, and decreased alertness and attention.

Persons with depression, adult attention deficit/hyperactivity disorder, and schizophrenia are at higher risk of nicotine dependence. These individuals may find it particularly difficult to quit smoking and may require specialized therapies to become free of nicotine products.

Other Effects

Smokers are at increased risk for developing duodenal and gastric ulcers; both conditions become less frequent with smoking cessation.

The benefit of most ulcer medications is reduced unless smoking cessation occurs. In addition, smoking is associated with prominent facial wrinkles, especially around the eyes, although the pathophysiologic basis for this change is uncertain. Smoking also causes natural menopause to occur 1 to 2 years early.

Passive Smoking

The risk of chronic cardiopulmonary problems is increased in individuals who are passively exposed to smoking by others (environmental tobacco smoke). Passive smoking increases the risk of respiratory infections, asthma, lung cancer, coronary artery disease, and cerebrovascular disease. Childhood exposure to household smoking by adults is associated with reduced pulmonary function, increased respiratory illnesses, middle ear infections, and exacerbated asthma.

Typical Presentation

The most common presentation of cigarette smoking in primary care practice is when a smoker is seen for general medical care not necessarily related to smoking, such as health maintenance visits, preoperative physical examinations, or even injuries. However, since 25 percent of the adult U.S. population smokes cigarettes, it is important to screen every patient for tobacco use. This screening can be performed by the clinician or office staff while documenting routine vital signs by simply asking patients if they have ever smoked and if they are current smokers or former smokers. Current smokers should be identified with the intention of offering assistance with smoking cessation.

Former smokers should be identified to reinforce their success at smoking cessation and to monitor risks related to previous smoking. Nonsmokers (especially children) who are exposed to passive smoke should be identified during routine health maintenance visits, since there is a definite relationship between passive smoke exposure and increased rates of the various medical problems outlined previously.

Smokers also commonly present to primary care clinicians with smoking-related symptoms and conditions, such as respiratory infections, asthma, and dyspepsia. Many smokers, particularly if they are nicotine dependent, will smoke despite these symptoms, even if they are aware that smoking aggravates them. Since smokers generally do not spontaneously reveal their smoking status to a clinician, the clinicians must ask about smoking status to make the association between smoking and the patient's complaints. In particular, all patients with symptoms and signs of vascular disease, cough, or COPD and patients with atypical or dysplastic Pap smear changes should be asked about tobacco use. These medical conditions, all of which are associated with smoking, can frequently serve as motivators to help patients commit to smoking cessation. Primary care clinicians should use these smoking-related symptoms as an opportunity to give advice on cessation to improve immediate health.

In contrast to the presentation in primary care practice, most patients who present to specialists with smoking-related complications (e.g., coronary heart disease) are referred by primary care clinicians. Since less than 5 percent of patients agree to go to special smoking cessation groups or clinics on the advice of a health care provider, specialist physicians should provide counseling about smoking cessation and reinforce smoking cessation advice given by primary care clinicians. However, research indicates that specialist physicians are less likely than primary care clinicians to provide counseling about smoking cessation.

Key History

The U.S. Agency for Health Care Policy and Research (AHCPR) commissioned a multidisciplinary task force to develop guidelines for smoking cessation in primary care. The task force reviewed over 3000 published articles and evaluated them according to strict criteria for assessment of their scientific merit and clinical relevance. The AHCPR task force then fully endorsed the recommendations of the National Cancer Institute for primary care clinicians.

The AHCPR and the National Cancer Institute recommendations involve five A's: all clinicians should *ask* at every visit if a person is a smoker; *advise* identified smokers to set a quit date; *assist* smokers to become tobacco free by both counseling and pharmacotherapy, if indicated; *arrange* follow-up care for all smokers to help counter the possibility of relapse; and *anticipate* that children and adolescents will be exposed to tobacco and enticed to smoke beginning at an earlier age than most clinicians realize—sometimes as early as age 4 years.

Assessing the Ability to Stop Smoking

Once an individual has been identified as a cigarette smoker, primary care clinicians should assess (1) the level of dependence on nicotine, (2) any smoking-related symptoms or conditions, (3) the patient's willingness to quit smoking, (4) personal reasons for quitting, and (5) availability of social support to assist in quitting.

DETERMINING THE PRESENCE OF NICOTINE DEPENDENCE

Nicotine dependence can be assessed by asking five key questions developed by Fagerstrom:

- Do you smoke within 30 min of arising in the morning?

- Do you find it difficult to refrain from smoking in places where smoking is forbidden?
- Do you enjoy the first cigarette of the day?
- Do you smoke more than one pack per day?
- Do smoke even when you are ill?

If the answers to three or more of these questions are "yes," then the diagnosis of nicotine dependence is established. Using additional questions, described later, the degree of dependence can be measured.

DETERMINING THE PRESENCE OF CONDITIONS CAUSED BY OR AGGRAVATED BY SMOKING

As noted, smokers commonly present to the clinician with smoking-related symptoms or conditions such as recurrent bronchitis, frequent upper respiratory infections, or exacerbations of asthma or allergies. The clinician should focus the clinical history on the presence of such symptoms and conditions, and on whether they are exacerbated by smoking. If there are no symptoms directly related to smoking, smokers still may have problems that, in addition to smoking, compound their risk for cardiovascular or pulmonary disease. These conditions include obesity, hyperlipidemia, hypertension, diabetes mellitus, or exposures to air pollutants at home and work. Clinicians should ask about these conditions, as well.

The clinician should also inquire about whether other members of the household smoke and whether other household members, such as children, are exposed to passive smoking. Screening for psychiatric problems, drug use, and alcohol abuse should be done when current smoking status is identified, since smoking is often a marker for these conditions.

All women should be asked if they use oral contraceptives. Cigarette smoking increases the risk of thromboembolic complications in women who use oral contraceptive, a risk that rises substantially in women over the age of 35. The history should also identify women of childbearing age who expect to become pregnant, so that the risks of smoking during pregnancy can be discussed.

Determining Willingness to Quit

The clinician should inquire about willingness to become free of tobacco by asking a straightforward question about the intention to quit. Such a question might be phrased as follows: "Do you have any intentions of quitting smoking in the near future?"

The patient's response can usually be categorized as being in one of three stages of preparation for smoking cessation: (1) precontemplation, (2) contemplation, or (3) action. Smokers in the precontemplation stage have no thoughts of stopping. In fact, they may respond to your inquiry by stating, "I haven't thought of quitting at all and need to smoke to get through my day." Smokers in the contemplation stage are considering quitting but have no clear plans about how to quit, although they may develop such plans over several months. Contemplators may respond by stating, "I have thought about quitting some time this year, but I don't know how to quit, since I have tried several times in the past and failed." Smokers in the action stage are typically ready to set a quitting date and want to know treatment options to assist them in smoking cessation. They may respond to a clinician's inquiry by stating, "I am tired of smoking and want to quit soon. Can you help me?"

Approximately 20 percent of smokers who visit primary care clinicians are in the action stage. Most smokers cycle between the various stages and relapse after they have attempted to quit. The stages can be used by the clinician to help frame counseling and treatment, as discussed below.

Determining the Reason for Wanting to Quit

Clinicians should ask smokers about their personal reasons for wanting to quit, especially if they are in the contemplation or action stage.

Identifying a personal reason for wanting to stop smoking and emphasizing the immediate benefit of doing so has been proven more helpful than just providing general information to smokers on the overall benefits of smoking cessation. Common personal reasons for wanting to quit are health concerns, social pressures, and finances. Adolescents may have concerns about appearance, rejection by friends or potential friends, and inability to perform in sports. If the smoker has a medical condition related to smoking, this condition may have prompted the interest in quitting. Smokers with smoking-related conditions have higher success rates for quitting than smokers who have no such symptoms. Unfortunately, however, in many cases a condition such as lung cancer or myocardial infarction may already have inflicted irreversible damage before a patient considers quitting.

Determining the Availability of Social Support

Clinicians should inquire about other household smokers and friends who are smokers, because it is often more difficult to become free of tobacco use if a spouse or family member smokes. Sometimes the greatest threat to relapse after a smoker has made a commitment to quit is others in the home or work setting who continue to smoke. On the other hand, if a family member and coworkers are also willing to quit or are supportive of the attempt to quit, then the likelihood of success increases.

Other Information on History

Clinicians should ask about the presence of specific symptoms or conditions that might influence the diagnostic workup or choice of treatment. For example, bupropion hydrochloride, a pharmacological agent used in smoking cessation programs, is contraindicated in persons with seizure disorders, anorexia or bulimia, or concurrent use of monoamine oxidase inhibitors.

Recurrent epigastric pain, dyspepsia, or other symptoms of ulcer mandate checking the stool for occult blood and perhaps antiulcer medication and/or endoscopy. Inquiries regarding the possibility of pregnancy are also appropriate, since nicotine replacement therapy in pregnancy is listed as a category C usage by the Food and Drug Administration (category C is an intermediate contraindication, with use of the drug to occur only at the clinician's discretion).

Physical Examination

The key to identification of smoking status is the history. Because cigarette smoking is a major risk factor for many conditions, it merits treatment advice even if no smoking-related findings are present on physical examination. However, common physical examination findings in smokers may warrant direct intervention and may also serve as a motivation to quit smoking.

Assessment of vital signs may show elevated blood pressure, increased pulse rate, or increased respiratory rate, all of which may be related to smoking. Patients may be overweight, which is a co-risk factor, along with smoking, for cardiovascular disease. A patient may have facial wrinkles from smoking, cyanotic changes consistent with chronic lung disease, the odor of cigarette smoke, and/or nicotine staining of fingers and nail beds.

The head and neck examination should be focused on identifying leukoplakic (white premalignant mucosal) changes of the oropharynx and staining of the teeth. The lung examination may reveal findings of COPD, including hyperresonance upon percussion, distant breath sounds, faint wheezes, and rhonchi that clear with coughing. There also may be signs of acute or chronic conditions, such as wheezing from asthma or focal crackles from pulmonary infec-

tions. The findings upon cardiac examination are usually normal, but patients should be assessed for conditions resulting from smoking-related cardiovascular disease, such as early congestive heart failure. The peripheral circulation should be assessed by palpation and auscultation of the carotid arteries. The back examination may reveal kyphosis or lumbar disc disease, both of which are more likely in cigarette smokers.

Specific complaints merit more focused examinations. For instance, recurrent hoarseness warrants examination of the larynx. Epigastric tenderness indicates the need to evaluate the patient for peptic ulcers.

Other findings on physical examination may influence the choice of treatment options. For example, persons with dentures may find it impossible to use nicotine chewing gum for nicotine replacement therapy. Eczema, psoriasis, and extremely hairy skin may make it difficult or impossible to use nicotine patches on the skin. Nicotine nasal sprays may worsen recurrent sinusitis or allergic rhinitis.

Ancillary Tests

There are no laboratory or screening tests for smoking in general clinical use. The major preventive focus with cigarette smokers is not on screening tests to detect disease but on helping smokers become tobacco free.

Screening for Nicotine Dependence

The Fagerstrom tolerance scale (Fig. 1-5) has been used to assess nicotine dependence in a variety of research settings. A score of more than 6 or 7 indicates that the patient is dependent on nicotine and would probably benefit from nicotine replacement therapy. While the full Fagerstrom instrument can be used in clinical practice to

Figure 1-5

1. How many cigarettes do you smoke daily?
   a. 1–15   _____
   b. 16–25   _____
   c. 26 or more _____
2. What is the tar/nicotine rating of the brand you smoke?
   a. Low   _____
   b. Medium   _____
   c. High   _____
3. Do you inhale?
   a. Never   _____
   b. Sometimes _____
   c. Always   _____
4. Do you smoke more in the morning than during the rest of the day?
   a. No   _____
   b. Yes   _____
5. How soon after you wake up do you smoke your first cigarette?
   _____ minutes
6. Which cigarette that you smoke during the day would you most hate to give up?
   _____

7. Do you find it difficult to refrain from smoking in places where it is forbidden (e.g., church, library, movies)?
   a. No   _____
   b. Yes   _____
8. Do you smoke if you are so ill that you are in bed most of the day?
   a. No   _____
   b. Yes   _____

HOW TO SCORE: Higher points are given for answers indicating more addiction. In questions 1, 2, and 3, answers a, b, and c are worth 0, 1, and 2 points, respectively. In question 5, score 1 for smoking within 30 minutes of awakening. In question 6, score 1 if answer is "The first cigarette in the morning." Questions 7 and 8 are scored 0 for no and 1 for yes.

The questionnaire has a range from 0 to 11 points. 0 indicates minimal and 11, maximal physical dependence. Patients whose score is higher than 6 usually benefit from nicotine replacement therapy.

The Fagerstrom nicotine tolerance questionnaire *(Reprinted from Addict Behav 3, K-O Fagerstrom, Measuring degree of physical dependency to tobacco smoking with reference to individualization of treatment, pp 235–241, copyright 1978, with permission from Elsevier Science.)*

determine whether patients are nicotine dependent, dependency can also be assessed with the five simple questions devised by Fagerstrom, discussed above (see "Determining the Presence of Nicotine Dependence").

Screening for Lung Cancer and Chronic Lung Disease

The U.S. Preventive Services Task Force does not recommend routine screening of asymptomatic smokers for lung cancer with chest x-ray because, once lung cancer is visible on a chest x-ray, the average life expectancy is between 3 and 6 months regardless of treatment. For simi-

lar reasons, the task force also recommends against screening sputum cytologicy tests.

Testing with a simple peak flow meter is an inexpensive method of screening smokers for early obstructive lung changes. Screening spirometric testing is not recommended in smokers without symptoms but may be helpful in diagnosing obstructive lung changes in those with symptoms.

Screening for Cardiovascular Disease and Cardiovascular Risk Factors

Routine baseline electrocardiographic assessment is not recommended by the U.S. Preventive

Task Force, even in smokers. In some situations, however, electrocardiographic studies may be helpful in smokers who have multiple other cardiovascular risk factors, such as hypertension, diabetes, hyperlipidemia, or a family history of early coronary heart disease. Smokers with chest pain suggestive of coronary artery disease should, of course, undergo an appropriate evaluation to exclude that diagnosis.

Cigarette smokers should also undergo standard tests for cardiovascular risk factors, such as screening for hyperlipidemia, hypertension, obesity, and diabetes. Smokers with multiple risk factors for cardiovascular disease or with active cardiovascular disease should receive intensive and recurring encouragement and recommendations to become free of tobacco.

Screening for Cigarette Smoking

Carbon monoxide (CO) measurement has been performed in research studies to verify whether an individual smokes. A simple expired breath analysis of CO is performed with a hand-held monitor, which provides a digital readout of expired CO in less than a minute. Levels of CO correlate with the quantity of cigarettes smoked and the blood carboxyhemoglobin (a by-product of cigarette smoking) level. Some studies have reported the successful use of CO test results to motivate smokers to attempt to quit smoking. However, CO measurements have not been used extensively in general medical practice.

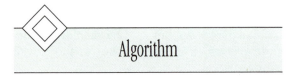

Algorithm

Several algorithmic models for smoking cessation have been proposed. Two of them are discussed here, since they describe different approaches to care. The Hughes algorithm focuses mostly on individual therapy involving the clinician and the patient. The Abrams algorithm puts more emphasis on the role of the health care system in which clinicians work. In using these algorithms, it is important to approach individual patients based on their willingness to attempt smoking cessation, their degree of nicotine dependence, and the health risks they incur from cigarette smoking.

Hughes developed a practical algorithm for the classification of smokers and treatment approaches that can be used by primary care clinicians (Fig. 1-6). Based on the algorithm, smokers who are definitely nicotine dependent should be advised about use of nicotine replacement therapies. Smokers at very high risk for severe outcomes, such as those with active coronary disease, may require more intensive efforts, such as group psychotherapy. However, less than 5 percent of patients in primary care practice will follow through with referrals to intensive smoking cessation programs. Therefore, primary care clinicians must be prepared to follow up on smokers who relapse, and they must be capable of providing various treatment modalities to aid in smoking cessation.

Another comprehensive stepped-care approach to smoking cessation has been proposed by Abrams. In this method, smokers in a health care system are matched to a level of intensity of smoking cessation therapy based on their motivation to make life changes necessary to become free of tobacco. These levels of intensity are (1) minimal care with self-help;, (2) moderate care with brief professional advice, nicotine replacement therapies, and follow-up care; and (3) maximal specialized care in both outpatient and inpatient programs with behavioral treatment specialists, psychiatrists, substance abuse counselors, and medical specialist care. In Abrams's model, the health system would also support smoking cessation with public health campaigns against smoking and would assist clinicians by providing telephone counseling of patients and a tracking system to ensure follow-up care. This comprehensive, integrated practice model for

Figure 1-6

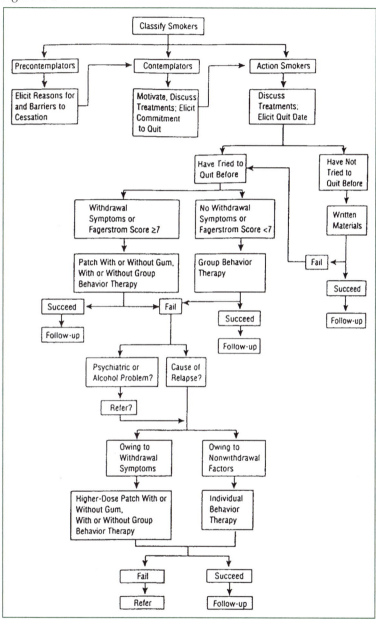

Algorithm for smoking cessation. *(Reprinted from JR Hugh, Arch Fam Med 3:280–285, copyright 1994, American Medical Association.)*

smoking cessation takes a proactive, population-based, primary prevention approach to smoking cessation (Fig. 1-7).

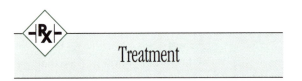

Treatment

In the past 20 years, methods used to evaluate the efficacy of smoking cessation interventions have greatly improved. Our knowledge base, built on past studies that used outcome measures such as short-term quitting rates and decreased smoking, has now been updated with more rigorous research. Many current studies are double-blind, placebo-controlled trials that evaluate long-term (i.e., more than 6 months or 1 year) abstinence that is biochemically verified. These studies show that intensive group therapy with nicotine replacement has the highest overall success, ranging from 30 to 40 percent.

Primary care clinicians must become comfortable talking with smokers about their tobacco use, offering positive advice to become free of tobacco, and advising on treatment, including nicotine replacement therapies that are now available without a prescription. Some patients, particularly those with concomitant psychiatric

Figure 1-7

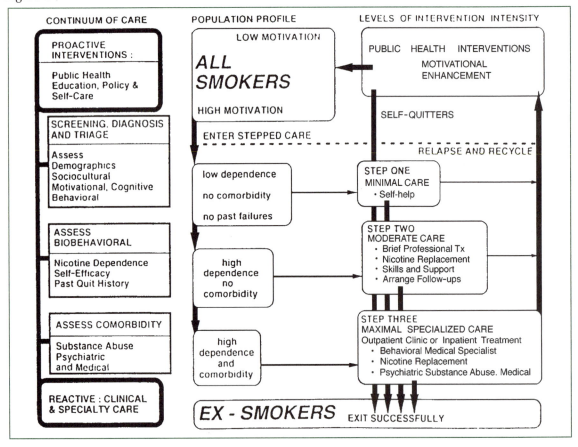

Comprehensive stepped-care model for smoking cessation. (*Adapted from DB Abrams, CT Orlean, RS Niaura, et al, Ann Behav Med 18:290, 1996.*)

conditions or other substance abuse problems, may merit joint management with a primary care clinician and a behavioral health specialist.

Self-Treatment

Most smokers (over 85 percent) attempt to quit smoking on their own without formal treatments or assistance from a health care professional. In addition, 95 percent of smokers who eventually stop smoking do so on their own. However, the majority of smokers who eventually become abstinent have done so only after an average of four serious attempts. In addition, smokers who are able to quit on their own are in all likelihood less dependent on nicotine than those who are unable to do so. Thus, smokers who are unable to quit may need structured approaches to care.

In the past, only 5 percent of smokers used nonprescription or prescription medications as an aid to smoking cessation. However, now that nicotine replacement therapies are available without a prescription, they can be easily obtained by smokers who wish to try stopping on their own. It is important that clinicians, including pharmacists, provide patients with adequate instructions on the proper use of nonprescription nicotine replacement therapies.

Behavioral Treatment

Although there are numerous behavioral interventions for smoking cessation, this discussion focuses on those highlighted by the AHCPR guideline.

BRIEF ADVICE FROM A CLINICIAN

The National Cancer Institute recommends that all smokers be advised by their clinician to quit smoking. A meta-analysis of seven studies that evaluated the effect of such advice found that if a clinician gives less than 3 min of advice to all smokers and encourages smokers to set a quitting date, about 10 percent of patients would be tobacco-free 1 year later. Increasing the

length of counseling to more than 10 min can bring success rates up to about 19 percent, as can scheduling several (5 to 7) follow-up sessions during the first 8 weeks of a patient's attempt to quit. There does not seem to be any added benefit to more than seven sessions, and, in fact, more sessions may be detrimental. Perhaps the most important finding was that patients of clinicians trained in giving smoking cessation advice have twice the long-term success rate of patients of untrained clinicians. Offering self-help materials further enhances smoking cessation success.

Thus, clinicians should advise all smokers to attempt to quit, even if the patient does not seem motivated to do so (but they should not badger patients who are uninterested). Studies have shown that even nonmotivated smokers expect clinicians to give advice about smoking cessation.

On the first visit of a smoking cessation program, patients should receive brief suggestions for how to cope with withdrawal symptoms and situations that trigger the urge to smoke (Table 1-2). For example, many patients experience the urge to smoke after meals. These individuals will require advice on alternative behaviors to substitute for smoking in this situation. Offering a contract or writing out a prescription with the chosen quitting date enhances success. Follow-up contact with the patient should be arranged within 1 to 2 days after the quitting date, since this is the time of greatest risk for relapse.

GROUP COUNSELING

Even though group counseling can double the success rate in comparison to brief advice by clinicians, very few smokers will agree to attend group counseling sessions. In fact, only smokers who are highly motivated to stop will commit to attending a series of scheduled group meetings. The principal method used in group counseling is to have participants develop suggestions and coping strategies, which are then tried out by the participants between sessions. Individuals share their approaches and successes during follow-up

Table 1-2

Strategies for Coping with Situations that Trigger the Urge to Smoke

TRIGGER	COPING STRATEGY
After eating or when drinking coffee	Avoid the situation: drink something besides coffee; get up from the table as soon as the meal is finished.
	Chew on a straw or toothpick.
	Have some other object to play with.
When at a bar	Leave when you have an urge to smoke.
	Tell others you have stopped smoking; ask them not to offer you a cigarette.
	Talk with nonsmokers.
When around others who are smoking	Chew gum or munch on ice, carrots, celery, etc.
	Leave the room.
	Ask the person not to smoke around you while you are in the early stage of stopping.
	Reduce contact temporarily with smoking friends.
	Plan activities where your friend is less likely to smoke (e.g., go to the movies).
When experiencing emotional stress	Talk with a family member of friend.
	Take a walk; exercise.
	Consider that the cigarette will not help the crisis.
	Consider how important it is to keep healthy during this difficult time.
When first getting up in the morning	Brush teeth and notice fresh breath.
	Exercise and take a shower.
	Think about getting through this one day without a cigarette.
	Get enough sleep in order to have the strength to cope with the urge to smoke.
	Review yesterday's success at not smoking.
When there is a need to "do something" with hands	Keep other objects in hands.
	Practice clasping hands together when urge to smoke is present.
	Doodle
When craving for cigarettes is unbearable	Chew gum or munch on ice, celery, carrots, etc.
	Practice relaxation exercises, perform deep breathing, or get some physical exercise.
	Contact a friend who can talk you out of smoking.
	Take a bath or shower.
	Remind yourself that you are a nonsmoker.

sessions. Often the participants reinforce each other's changed behavior.

A number of no-cost and commercial programs are available for group therapies. Schwartz comprehensively reviewed these programs and found reported success rates between 20 and 40 percent. Clinicians should become familiar with the availability, cost, and quality of programs in their region.

OTHER BEHAVIORAL TREATMENT

The AHCPR review did not find sufficient evidence to recommend hypnosis, cueing, or acupuncture for use in smoking cessation regimens. When studied in controlled fashion, none of these methods is consistently better than placebo.

Nicotine Replacement Therapy

The main rationale for nicotine replacement therapy is to counter the symptoms of withdrawal from nicotine, thereby allowing the abstinent smoker to focus on the behavioral triggers for smoking activity. Besides countering withdrawal, replacement therapies are said to work because, by providing round-the-clock nicotine replacement, they make nicotine intake independent of environmental triggers.

NICOTINE GUM

Nicotine polacrilex chewing gum is now available without prescription in doses of 2 and 4 mg. The 1-year success rate of 2-mg nicotine gum is approximately 10 percent when it is given as an adjunct to brief advice from a physician. When given with group therapy, success increases to 27 percent at 6 months.

Nicotine gum must be chewed slowly and intermittently, and parked in the mouth as a lozenge between chewing to enhance absorption. Approximately 10 to 20 sticks should be chewed daily to enhance success. In highly dependent smokers (i.e., those who smoke 1.5 packs of cigarettes or more per day), a minimum of 10 sticks per day is recommended. Use of 10 to 20 4-mg (instead of 2-mg) sticks of gum has greater efficacy in highly dependent smokers.

The main side effects of nicotine gum are gastrointestinal upset, jaw pain, hiccups, diarrhea, and mouth sores. The usual duration of therapy is 10 to 12 weeks. Since nicotine gum is self-administered, there is a potential for abuse in the form of continued use beyond the usual treatment period. This occurs in about 10 to 15 percent of smokers.

TRANSDERMAL NICOTINE

Various transdermal nicotine products are also available without a prescription. Products vary minimally and have similar safety and efficacy profiles. Wholesale costs range from about $4 to $5 per day. Meta-analyses indicate that active patch use is twice as likely to be successful as placebo (22 percent versus 9 percent at 6 months) when given with brief advice from a clinician. Brief advice is as effective as intensive counseling, and the effective length of patch therapy is 8 weeks. There is no difference in success rates when using 24-h versus 16-h patches, nor is there an advantage to tapering the dose (i.e., starting at 21 mg, decreasing to 14 mg, and then decreasing to 7 mg). The most common adverse effects are insomnia and skin irritation. About 1 to 2 percent of patients will continue using the patch beyond the recommended 8-week treatment.

NICOTINE NASAL SPRAYS AND INHALERS

Nicotine is now available by prescription in the form of nasal sprays and bronchial inhalers. Reported long-term success rates range between 15 and 25 percent for both devices. The advantages of nasal sprays and bronchial inhalers are that they mimic smoking and have a rapid effect. The latter occurs because of rapid nicotine absorption across the nasal and bronchial mucosal membranes. The most common difficulty experienced with the spray is nasal irritation. In addition, some persons find it to lack social desirability. Use of the sprays beyond the recommended duration of treatment has been reported in over 43 percent of smokers who use this form of treatment. Prolonged use raises concern that these treatments will sustain nicotine dependence rather than serve as effective smoking cessation tools.

NONNICOTINE PHARMACOTHERAPY

A variety of pharmacologic agents have been recommended and used as adjuncts to smoking cessation programs. These include lobeline (a nicotinic agonist), silver salts, clonidine, buspirone, beta blockers, sedatives/hypnotics, antidepressants, and stimulants. The AHCPR guideline found no substantive evidence that these medications are effective, and did not recommend them for smoking cessation therapy. A recent review by Hughes concurred with the guideline recommendations.

Initial research indicates that there may be a beneficial effect from using agents such as mecamylamine (a nicotinic receptor agonist) and naltrexone (and opioid receptor agonist-antagonist), especially in conjunction with transdermal nicotine. Further studies are needed to substantiate initial trials.

BUPROPION

Bupropion hydrochloride, a nontricyclic antidepressant, has had success rates of 19 percent at 6 months in controlled smoking cessation trials and 20 to 25 percent at 1 year using a sustained-release preparation. The recommended treatment regimen starts at 150 mg/d for 3 days and then increases to 300 mg/d for 12 weeks or longer. With the sustained-release preparation, the dose is 200 to 300 mg/d. Patients should be taking bupropion for 1 week before attempting to discontinue smoking.

Bupropion's most common side effects are agitation and insomnia. Psychotic reactions have occurred in patients taking bupropion simultaneously with fluoxetine or amantadine. Bupropion's most serious side effect is seizures, which occur in about 0.1 percent of patients treated with bupropion for depression; however, seizures have not occurred in patients taking bupropion in smoking cessation trials. Contraindications to bupropion treatment include seizure disorders and eating disorders (which increase the risk of bupropion-induced seizures), and use of amantadine or other psychoactive medications. Further studies are needed in primary care settings to assess the long-term success and safety profile of bupropion.

Relapse Prevention

Preventing relapse (i.e., return to smoking) is a major concern in any treatment program. The majority of smokers (over 85 percent) will relapse after they attempt to quit. Clinicians should be prepared to continue working with smokers who have relapsed. The psychological triggers that led to relapse, such as negative moods or stresses, should be documented and explored. Specific coping strategies should be offered based on the individual smoker's situational triggers (Table 1-2). Smokers who have relapsed while on a treatment regimen that did not include pharmacotherapy should be evaluated for dependency to nicotine. If the smoker is dependent on nicotine, consideration should be given to using nicotine replacement or other appropriate pharmacotherapy with the next attempt at smoking cessation.

Education and Family Approach

Smokers who wish to quit should clear their household environment of all smoking products. They should also ask other smoking family members to participate in the cessation program or at least refrain from smoking in the house. When there are several family members who smoke, scheduling joint sessions for brief advice and follow-up is convenient and may enhance success due to a group commitment. In this regard, primary care clinicians have a special advantage over other clinicians when they provide of care for multiple members of the same family or household. Counseling on the risk of exposure to passive smoke for other household members, especially children, may serve as a motivation for smoking cessation.

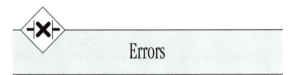

Errors

Although smoking cessation guidelines are advocated by national agencies, surveys of practicing clinicians indicate that many primary care clinicians have not fully endorsed these guidelines, do not follow them in daily practice, and frequently have not even heard of them. Thus, clinicians make a variety of errors in dealing with cigarette smokers and prescribing smoking cessation treatments.

One important error is failure to identify all smokers in one's practice. Because about one-quarter of all patients seen in primary care practice smoke cigarettes, any clinicians identifying substantially fewer smokers are probably failing to recognize patients who smoke. Data from the National Ambulatory Medical Care Survey (NAMCS) indicate that, in about one-third of visits to office-based physicians, the patient's smoking status is not ascertained. Furthermore, counseling about smoking cessation takes place in only about 38 percent of smokers' visits to primary care clinicians.

A second error is failure to arrange adequate follow-up care for smokers who are willing to quit. As noted above, patients are at high risk to relapse in the early days and weeks of a smoking cessation program, and further relapses occur with the passage of time. Clinicians must maintain contact with patients during the early phases of smoking cessation treatment in order to provide support and intervention to decrease the likelihood of relapse, and then monitor and reinforce long-term success. It is not acceptable to simply prescribe nicotine replacement or other therapy and not arrange for periodic follow-up with the patient.

A third error is not prescribing or recommending adequate doses of nicotine replacement therapies for patients who are heavily dependent to nicotine. NAMCS data show that nicotine replacement is prescribed at only about 2 percent of smokers' visits to primary care clinicians. The identification of heavy nicotine dependence and recommended dosing regimens were discussed earlier and are reviewed in detail in package inserts.

A fourth, and unfortunately very common, error is failure to intervene during severe illnesses related to smoking (such as during hospitalization for a myocardial infarction). When patients experience smoking-related complications, especially serious or highly symptomatic complications, they may be more amenable to consider smoking cessation than at any other time. Not encouraging and providing interventions for smoking cessation in this setting is an opportunity lost.

Finally, clinicians often fail to identify co-morbid conditions that make smoking cessation more difficult. These include conditions such as alcohol abuse or psychiatric illness. Once identified, smokers with multiple addictions and psychiatric conditions will most likely require co-management with a psychiatrist and the primary care clinician.

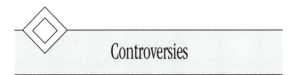

Controversies

One of the major current controversies revolves around the conceptual desirability of nicotine replacement therapy. Other controversies concern the degree to which the health care system should support smoking cessation efforts and the role of political action by clinicians.

Chronic Nicotine Replacement Therapy

Much of the pharmacologic management of smoking cessation involves nicotine replacement therapy (i.e., nicotine patches, gum, and sprays). Currently, nicotine replacement is recommended only for short-term treatment, but it should be recognized that some authors advocate chronic use of such products as an alternative to continued cigarette smoking. The rationale for chronic use of nicotine replacement is that it is less harmful than continued smoking. This is a highly controversial issue, since it puts clinicians and the pharmaceutical industry in the role of maintaining the nicotine addiction of ex-smokers.

Lack of Resources for Smoking Cessation Efforts

The ideal approach to smoking cessation, given the current state of our knowledge, involves an integrated practice approach. This ideal approach would identify all smokers in each practice, arrange for professional personnel to coordinate smoking cessation measures for all smokers identified, and provide tracking systems for follow-up to ensure and encourage participation in treatment programs. Telephone counselors can be trained in relapse prevention and can attend to smokers during times when relapse is most likely (i.e., the initial 12 weeks after beginning a smoking cessation program). A telephone support service would take the burden off individual clinicians and office support staff. In these comprehensive models, nicotine replacement therapies and support services would be completely covered by insurance formularies.

Despite the strength of the recommendation for such a comprehensive, integrated approach, health care plans and insurers are reluctant to invest in smoking cessation measures because of the high cost. However, cost-effectiveness studies show that smoking cessation interventions are by far more cost-saving than other common preventive interventions for which all insurers provide coverage (e.g., hypertension and hyperlipidemia treatment) (Table 1-3). The controversy over whether health insurers should provide coverage for smoking cessation treatments is likely to continue.

The Role of Political Action

Another controversy of sorts involves the extent to which clinicians and their professional organizations should become involved in the sociopolitical processes that determine the availability, cost, and chemical composition of tobacco products. Many "special-interest" health care groups have taken a stand and facilitated legislation on

Table 1-3

Cost Savings per Quality-Adjusted Life Year Saved by Smoking Cessation and Other Medical Strategies

STRATEGY	COST SAVINGS TO HEALTH CARE SYSTEM, $
Smoking cessation (stopping on one's own)	100–500
Smoking cessation (brief counseling by clinician)	1,000–5,000
Smoking cessation (specialty program)	3,000–6,000
Hypertension management	20,000–100,000
Hyperlipidemia management	20,000–150,000

SOURCE: Adapted from Abrams DB, Orleans CT, Niaura RS, et al.

a variety of medical issues ranging from mammogram screening to infant automobile safety seats. Some argue that clinicians and their professional societies have not taken a sufficiently strong stand against the sale and use of cigarettes, despite the fact that cigarettes cause more serious illness and deaths than any of these other problems.

Emerging Concepts

A variety of pharmacologic treatments are now available to aid in smoking cessation. In coming years, some of these treatments may be combined to achieve better results. Likely combination treatments include simultaneous use of nicotine gum and nicotine patch, or bupropion combined with the nicotine patch. It may also be found that certain heavily addicted smokers require sustained pharmacotherapy to prevent relapses. Further research is needed to clarify the role of combined and/or extended treatments.

Genetic Treatments

As understanding of the human genome is expanded, an understanding of the genetic mechanisms of nicotine addiction is likely to develop. This knowledge may provide a basis for new pharmacological interventions or gene therapies aimed at the biochemical basis for nicotine addiction.

Long-Term Nicotine Maintenance Therapy

Numerous "nicotine-delivery devices" are under development and in testing. These include nicotine inhalers, nicotine lozenges and lollipops, and smokeless cigarettes that deliver nicotine as an aerosolized mist. These products are intended to serve as a substitute for chronic cigarette smoking, maintaining smokers' nicotine addiction after they discontinue smoking. Such products may or may not be regulated by the Food and Drug Administration and, if marketed successfully, could be available to large populations of consumers. As noted above, the concept of nicotine maintenance is controversial among health professionals, but clinicians are likely to see increasing use of these products in the future.

Targeted Smoking Cessation Efforts

It is likely that in the future smoking cessation interventions will be targeted at special populations, such as adolescents, children, and individuals with coexisting psychiatric problems. Research is needed to evaluate the effectiveness of pharmacologic and behavioral interventions in these special populations and to determine the effectiveness of brief-advice models in preventing relapse in these and other special-risk groups.

Bibliography

Abrams DB, Orleans CT, Niaura RS, et al: Integrating individual and public health perspectives for treatment of tobacco dependence under managed health care: A combined stepped-care and matching model. *Ann Behav Med* 18:290, 1996.

Anthony JC, Warner LA, Kessler RC: Comparative epidemiology of dependence on tobacco, alcohol, controlled substances and inhalants: Basic findings from the national comorbidity survey. *Exp Clin Psychopharmacol* 2:244, 1994.

Baer JS, Marlatt GA: Maintenance of smoking cessation. *Clin Chest Med* 12:793, 1991.

Centers for Disease Control and Prevention: *The Health Consequences of Smoking: A Report of the Surgeon General.* Atlanta, U.S. Department of Health and Human Services, 1988.

Centers for Disease Control and Prevention: *Reducing the Health Consequences of Smoking: 25 Years of Progress: A Report of the Surgeon General.* Atlanta,

U.S. Department of Health and Human Services, 1989.

Centers for Disease Control and Prevention: *The Health Benefits of Smoking Cessation: A Report of the Surgeon General.* Atlanta, U.S. Department of Health and Human Services, 1990.

Centers for Disease Control and Prevention: *Preventing Tobacco Use among Young People: A Report of the Surgeon General.* Atlanta, U.S. Department of Health and Human Services, 1994.

Centers for Disease Control and Prevention: *Clinical Practice Guideline: Smoking Cessation.* Atlanta, U.S. Department of Health and Human Services, 1996.

Collishaw NE (ed): The tobacco epidemic: A global public health emergency. *Tobacco Alert.* Geneva, World Health Organization, 1996.

Cromwell J, Bartosch WJ, Fiore MC, et al: Cost-effectiveness of the clinical practice recommendations in the AHCPR guideline for smoking cessation. *JAMA* 278:1759, 1997.

Cummings KM, Pechacek T, Shopland D: The illegal sale of cigarettes to U.S. minors: Estimated by state. *Am J Public Health* 84:300, 1994.

Fagerstrom K-O: Measuring degree of physical dependency to tobacco smoking with reference to individualization of treatment. *Addict Behav* 3:235, 1978.

Fiore MC: The new vital sign: Assessing and documenting smoking status. *JAMA* 266:3183, 1991.

Glantz SA, Slade J, Bero L, et al: *The Cigarette Papers.* Berkeley, University of California Press, 1996.

Glassman AH: Cigarette smoking: Implications for psychiatric illness. *Am J Psychiatry* 150:546, 1993.

Hugh JR: An algorithm for smoking cessation. *Arch Fam Med* 3:280, 1994.

Hughes JR: Pharmacotherapy of nicotine dependence, in *Pharmacological Aspects of Drug Dependence: Toward an Integrative Neurobehavioral Approach,* Handbook of Experimental Pharmacology Series. New York, Springer-Verlag, 1996.

Hurt RD, Dale LC, McClain FL, et al: A comprehensive model for the treatment of nicotine dependence in a medical setting. *Med Clin North Am* 76:495, 1992.

Janerich DT, Thompson WD, Varela LR, et al: Lung cancer and exposure to tobacco smoke in the household. *New Engl J Med* 323:632, 1990.

Lando HA, McGovern PG, Kelder SH, et al: Use of carbon monoxide breath validation in assessing exposure to cigarette smoke in a work site population. *Health Psych* 10:296, 1991.

Lichtenstein E, Hollis JF: Patient referral to smoking cessation program: Who follows through? *Fam Pract* 34:739, 1992.

McIlvain H, Susman MD, Davis C, et al: Physician counseling for smoking cessation: Is the glass half empty? *J Fam Pract* 40:148, 1995.

National Center for Chronic Disease Prevention and Health Promotion, Office on Smoking and Health, Epidemiology Branch: Cigarette smoking among adults: United States, 1995. *Morb Mort Week Rep* 46:1217, 1997.

National Center for Chronic Disease Prevention and Health Promotion, Office on Smoking and Health and Division of Adolescent and School Health: Tobacco use among high school students: United States, 1997. *Morb Mort Week Rep* 47:229, 1998.

Ockene JK, Kristeller J, Goldberg R, et al: Increasing the efficacy of physician-delivered interventions: A randomized clinical trial. *J Gen Intern Med* 6:1, 1991.

Pierce JP, Fiore MC, Novotny TE, et al: Trends in cigarette smoking in the United States: Projections to the year 2000. *JAMA* 261:61, 1989.

Schwartz JL, Rider G: Review and evaluation of smoking control methods: The United States and Canada, 1969–1977. Centers for Disease Control, HEW Publication No (COC) 79–8369, 1978.

Thorndike AN, Rigotti NA, Stafford RS, et al: National patterns in the treatment of smokers by physicians. *JAMA* 279:604, 1998.

Wadland WC: Why is smoking cessation so difficult? Rationale for nicotine replacement therapy. *Mod Med* 62:11, 1994.

Warner KE, Slade J, Sweanor DT: The emerging market for long-term nicotine maintenance. *JAMA* 278:1087, 1997.

Werner RM, Pearson TA: What's so passive about passive smoking? Secondhand smoke as a cause of atherosclerotic disease. *JAMA* 279:157, 1998.

David S. Gray

Chapter 2

Obesity

How Common Is Obesity?

Definition

Estimates of the prevalence of obesity vary depending on how obesity is defined. The most basic definition is the presence of an abnormally large amount of adipose tissue. However, no clear distinction exists between normal and abnormal amounts of adipose tissue.

In certain research settings, adipose tissue is measured using methods such as underwater weighing or isotope dilution. However, these methods are expensive and time consuming, making them unsuitable for use in most clinical settings.

In clinical practice, obesity is often defined and diagnosed subjectively. At the high end of the body-weight spectrum, obesity is obvious and most patients and clinicians have no difficulty agreeing that it is present. At moderate weights, however, it may be more difficult to reach consensus about the presence of obesity using subjective judgment alone, because individual patients and clinicians may have a different sense of what constitutes obesity. Thus, an objective, measurable definition of obesity is needed in clinical practice, especially when potentially risky therapies, such as medications or surgery, are being considered.

One objective method of defining obesity involves expressing body weight as a percentage of desirable (or ideal) weight for height, as defined by life insurance tables. Using this method, obesity is usually defined as 120 or 130 percent of desirable body weight because at this level mortality from weight-related disease begins to increase significantly.

The other, more commonly used method is the body mass index (BMI). The BMI is calculated by dividing the body weight (in kilograms) by the square of the person's height (in meters). The BMI has several advantages over simply comparing a patient's weight to his or her desirable body weight. First, the BMI requires determination of only weight and height, parameters commonly measured in practice. The BMI can then be easily calculated or derived from a nomogram (Fig. 2-1). Second, the BMI is not dependent on an arbitrary standard of desirable weight that might change as actuarial insurance data change over time. Third, the BMI definition of obesity for men and women can be the same. The average BMI for American adults is 25 kg/m^2.

The BMI cutoff point used to define obesity, however, has been debated without clear consensus. Obesity has been variously defined as a BMI that exceeds 27 to 30 kg/m^2. The National Center for Health Statistics used 27 kg/m^2 in epidemiologic studies. Others suggest cutoff points of 28 kg/m^2 or higher. Because the slope of the relationship between BMI and mortality is not very steep between 27 and 29 kg/m^2 and it rises more significantly at BMI levels of 30 kg/m^2 or more, many experts recommend 30 kg/m^2 as the definition of obesity. While arbitrary, this level is easy to remember and can be used as an indication of substantially increased risk for morbidity and mortality from cardiovascular and other obesity-related diseases in both men and women.

Prevalence of Obesity in the Population

The National Health and Nutrition Examination Surveys (NHANES) conducted by the U.S. National Center for Health Statistics collected data periodically between 1960 and 1994 on the prevalence of obesity in the United States. The surveys were based on probability samples representative of the U.S. population and included actual measurements of weight, height, and other health and nutrition parameters for thousands of individuals. The NHANES defined obesity as a BMI of 27.8 kg/m^2 or more for men and

Figure 2-1

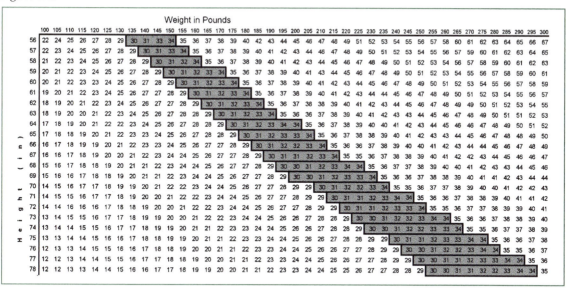

Nomogram for estimating BMI using weight in pounds and height in inches. BMI is read at the intersection of the patient's weight (lb) along the top with the patient's height (in) along the left side of the table. BMI 30 and over = obesity; BMI 35 and over = moderate to severe obesity.

27.3 kg/m^2 or more for women. These represent the eighty-fifth percentile values for BMI for men and women aged 20 through 29 years. They also correspond to 124 and 120 percent, respectively, of actuarially determined desirable body weight for men and women.

Using these definitions, NHANES reported the overall prevalence of obesity for men and women to be 33 percent, based on the data gathered from 1988 to 1991. Obesity prevalence increased with age from 20 percent among men aged 20 to 29 years to 42 percent among men aged 60 to 69 years and then decreased after the age of 70 years. It also increased with age from 20 percent among women aged 20 to 29 years to 52 percent among women aged 50 to 59 years, and, as in men, it decreased at older ages.

Through a repeated series of examinations, although not all performed on the same subjects, NHANES provided estimates of the change in the prevalence of obesity over time. Overall, preva-

lence of obesity remained at about 25 percent from 1960 through 1980. Since then, there has been an increase to the current obesity rate of 33 percent. Other studies from the United States and England also show an increase in the prevalence of obesity over the past two decades, suggesting that the NHANES findings are not due to artifact or differences in subject selection.

As shown in Table 2-1, the prevalence of obesity in NHANES varied considerably by gender and racial or ethnic group. The prevalence was similar for non-Hispanic white and African-American men but was higher for Mexican-American men. Among women, the prevalence was higher for non-Hispanic black or Mexican-American women than for non-Hispanic white women.

International Comparisons

Prevalence of obesity is higher among adults in the United States and Canada than in western

Table 2-1

Age-Adjusted Prevalence of Obesity

POPULATION	PERCENTAGE OF POPULATION	
	MEN	WOMEN
Entire population	31.3	34.7
Non-Hispanic white	31.6	32.1
Non-Hispanic black	31.2	48.5
Mexican American	39.1	47.2

SOURCE: Adapted from Kuczmarski RJ, Flegal KM, Campbell SM, et al.

European countries. Proposed explanations for this difference include more automobile use, differences in diet quality, and less cigarette smoking in the United States and Canada (cigarette smoking increases metabolic rates and, therefore, decreases the rate of obesity). Accurate estimates of the prevalence of obesity in other parts of the world, especially in nonindustrialized nations, are difficult to obtain because of the lack of systematic population studies. Anecdotal evidence indicates that obese individuals exist in most parts of the world, but a statistical comparison to the U.S. prevalence cannot be made until more data are collected.

Prevalence in Primary Care Practice

Because of the high prevalence of obesity in the general population, primary care clinicians see many obese patients. In addition, because patients with chronic medical disorders such as hypertension and diabetes frequently seek care from primary care clinicians and because obesity is associated with these disorders, the likelihood of seeing obese patients in primary care practice is quite high. In fact, in one study in family practice offices, 64 percent of patients seen in the practice met criteria for obesity (defined in that study as a BMI of more than 27 kg/m^2).

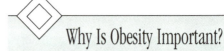

Why Is Obesity Important?

Obesity is a significant contributor to morbidity and mortality rates among adults in the United States. The scope of the problem is large, since an estimated $68 billion is spent each year on medical problems attributable to obesity. The relationship between obesity and health problems was first demonstrated in studies conducted by the life insurance industry. These studies showed that obese individuals died sooner than nonobese individuals of the same age. They also identified the weight (for each given height) that had the lowest mortality rate. The "low-mortality weight" data were used to construct the tables of desirable weight, mentioned above. These early life insurance studies have been criticized for biases, including selection and exclusive study of middle class individuals who purchased life insurance, as well as questionable measurement techniques. However, other studies that used more representative samples and rigorous measurement techniques have generated similar results.

The conclusion that obesity is a significant factor in higher mortality rates led to development of a graph estimating the effects of obesity on mortality rates (Fig. 2-2). The graph reveals a "J-shaped" relationship between degree of obesity and mortality rates, with minimum mortality rates at BMI values between 20 and 25 kg/m^2 and substantial increases above a BMI of 30 kg/m^2. The relationship between body weight and death is greatest for adults between 30 and 74 and somewhat less for older individuals.

A variety of obesity-related disorders contribute to the increased morbidity and mortality rates of overweight individuals. These disorders include hypertension, diabetes, and hyperlipidemia, each of which contributes to an increased incidence of cardiovascular disease. The relationship between obesity and hypertension,

Figure 2-2

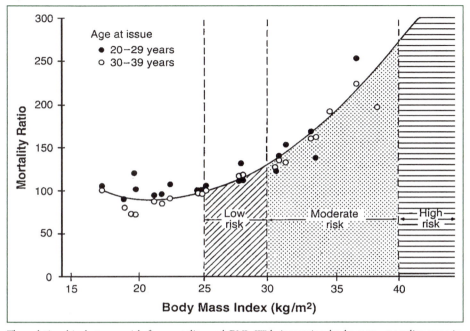

The relationship between risk for mortality and BMI. With increasing body mass, mortality rates increase. Mortality also increases at very low BMI (less than 20 kg/m²). *(Courtesy of George A. Bray, M.D., Baton Rouge, LA, copyright, 1976.)*

diabetes mellitus, hyperlipidemia, and cardiovascular disease is much stronger for abdominal or centrally distributed fat than for fat in the gluteal or hip region or the extremities. Among the obese, all of these conditions are more prevalent in people with centrally distributed fat (abdominal obesity). As discussed below, hyperinsulinemia may underlie each of these obesity-related problems. Other, as yet unrecognized, factors are also probably involved in the higher mortality rates in obese individuals, because the relationship between obesity and cardiovascular death remains significant even after accounting for hypertension, diabetes mellitus, and hyperlipidemia.

In addition, obesity contributes to a higher rate of gallbladder disease, pulmonary problems, osteoarthritis, cancer, and pregnancy complications. Finally, obese individuals may experience discrimination because of their weight. All of these obesity-related disorders result in a large number of visits to primary care physicians.

Hyperinsulinemia and Cardiovascular Disease Risk

Hypertension, diabetes mellitus, and hyperlipidemia are commonly associated with obesity and underlie much of the cardiovascular disease that occurs in obese individuals. Hypertension, diabetes, and hyperlipidemia occur together with obesity so frequently that some authors have suggested they represent a discrete syndrome. Although not proved with certainty, considerable evidence indicates that this syndrome involves elevated serum insulin levels.

HYPERTENSION

While not all patients with hypertension are obese, there is a strong positive relationship between hypertension and obesity. The pathophysiologic process or processes by which obesity might cause hypertension are not known with certainty but, as described above, hyperinsulinemia is a likely mechanism. Insulin resistance and resulting hyperinsulinemia are hypothesized to cause hypertension predominantly through an insulin-induced increase in renal sodium retention (although other mechanisms are also involved). Hypertension, in turn, increases the risk of atherosclerotic vascular disease and other complications outlined in Chap. 3.

Many studies have shown that blood pressure can be lowered with weight loss generated by caloric restriction, drugs, or surgery. In fact, weight loss can be as effective as antihypertensive medication for short-term reduction of blood pressure and may lead to decreased antihypertensive medication requirements for many patients.

DIABETES MELLITUS TYPE 2

Obesity is very common, although not universal, in persons with type 2 (non-insulin-dependent) diabetes mellitus. The many complications of type 2 diabetes are discussed in Chap. 4, but they all contribute to the excess in morbidity and mortality rates for obese diabetic individuals.

The pathophysiologic relationship between obesity and diabetes is still under investigation. Most authorities agree, however, that the insulin resistance accompanying obesity leads to increased pancreatic insulin production in an attempt to maintain normal blood glucose levels. After years of overproduction of insulin to overcome insulin resistance, pancreatic function diminishes, and insulin production falls short of the amount needed to maintain normal blood glucose levels. The process can be viewed as a continuum from obesity to insulin resistance

with hyperinsulinemia and finally to inadequate insulin production and hyperglycemia.

In the early stages of the process, weight loss can induce complete reversal of hyperglycemia in some patients. Complete reversal of the diabetic process is less likely in patients who require insulin to maintain normal blood glucose levels and in those whose diabetes has been present for longer periods of time. However, despite long-established diabetes, weight loss of even modest amounts (5 to 15 percent of body weight) in obese diabetics usually results in decreased medication requirements. Effects are often quite rapid, occurring within the first few weeks of weight loss. No studies have been performed to determine the duration of the beneficial effect of weight loss on diabetes control, but anecdotal clinical experience suggests that it may be long lasting in some patients. The American Diabetes Association recommends attempts at weight loss as essential to the care of obese diabetic patients.

Hyperlipidemia

The association between obesity and hyperlipidemia is not as easily demonstrated as the relationship of obesity to hypertension and diabetes. Still, epidemiologic studies have consistently shown that, in comparison to lean subjects, obese individuals have small to moderate elevations in fasting triglyceride levels, small increases in levels of total and low-density lipoprotein (LDL) cholesterol, and decreased levels of high-density lipoprotein (HDL) cholesterol. These lipid changes are associated with increased rates of cardiovascular morbidity and mortality. The pathophysiology of these lipid changes is not certain but may be related to the effects of hyperinsulinemia on hepatic lipid metabolism. Obesity-related hyperlipidemia may also be the result of increased release of free fatty acids from obese fat cells.

Weight loss through dietary restriction or exercise will tend to lower triglyceride and total and LDL-cholesterol levels to a small degree. Effects on HDL-cholesterol vary, with some studies showing improvements and others demonstrating equivocal results.

CAN WEIGHT REDUCTION DECREASE MORTALITY RATES FOR CARDIOVASCULAR DISEASE?

In contrast to the beneficial effect of weight reduction on individual cardiovascular disease risk factors (i.e., hypertension, diabetes, and hyperlipidemia), no clinical trials have demonstrated that intentional weight loss can actually decrease mortality rates. In evaluating the effect of weight reduction on mortality rates, it is important to distinguish intentional from unintentional weight loss. Data from the Framingham study showed that individuals who lost weight during the observation period of the study had decreased mortality rates. However, the reasons for weight loss in these study subjects are not clear, because data were not collected to determine whether weight loss was intentional or unintentional, or why it occurred. The decrease in mortality rate seen in Framingham subjects certainly suggests that weight loss is beneficial, and this conclusion is strengthened by data discussed above showing improvements in cardiac risk factors with weight loss. However, there are no long-term trials with weight reduction analogous to those with antihypertensive medications to show that weight reduction decreases cardiovascular disease mortality.

Thus, while weight reduction can decrease the risk of cardiovascular disease by improving blood pressure, diabetic control, and lipid profiles, this does not prove that weight loss due to any selected medical intervention will lead to decreased mortality rates. In fact, there are known and perhaps unrecognized deleterious effects of purposeful medical weight-loss programs, such as those that use severe caloric restriction, drugs, or surgery. In addition, limited data have suggested that weight loss and regain (often called yo-yo dieting) can increase mortality rates.

Cholelithiasis

Cholelithiasis and resulting complications, such as biliary colic and cholecystitis, are common among obese individuals. Epidemiologic studies have shown two to four times the incidence of symptomatic gallstone disease among obese compared to lean women. In men, gallbladder disease is much less common, but obesity still increases its incidence. Obese individuals have increased hepatic secretion of cholesterol and supersaturated bile, leading to an increased rate of cholesterol gallstones.

Weight loss has a complex effect on gallbladder disease rates. Many studies have shown that weight reduction can actually increase the incidence of gallstones, presumably through biochemical changes in bile that occur in catabolic states. This risk appears to be much greater if weight loss is rapid or profound, such as occurs on very low-calorie diets or following gastric surgery. Less extreme weight reduction programs, which result in weight loss at a rate of less than 1.5 kg/week, are associated with a lowered risk of inducing gallstone disease.

Pulmonary Problems

Obesity is associated with a variety of pulmonary syndromes. These syndromes include obesity-related hypoventilation, sleep apnea, and measurable lung-function abnormalities, such as decreased expiratory reserve volume, total lung volume, and maximum voluntary ventilation rate.

Obesity-related hypoventilation is an uncommon but clinically important condition. Also known as pickwickian syndrome (named for a character in a Charles Dickens novel), it tends to occur in patients who are severely obese. Obesity-related impairment of chest wall and airway function leads to hypoventilation, which results in hypercapnia and hypoxemia. Patients then become somnolent, ventilate even less vigorously, and become further hypoxemic and hypercapnic. Persons with the pickwickian syndrome may subsequently develop right ventricular failure (cor pulmonale) and/or left-sided congestive heart failure. Weight loss at an early stage in the condition may prevent serious clinical deterioration and may be of some benefit even after severe symptoms are manifest.

There also appears to be a relationship between obesity and obstructive sleep apnea. The relationship is complex, however, since many individuals with sleep apnea are not obese. Nonetheless, in the presence of typical symptoms of sleep apnea (e.g., snoring and daytime sleepiness), obesity should raise the clinician's suspicion that obstructive sleep apnea may be present. A formal sleep study with polysomnography is recommended for diagnosis of this condition.

Osteoarthritis

Osteoarthritis of the lower extremities is associated with obesity. The basis for the relationship is hypothesized to be the increased mechanical load on the weight-bearing joints of the hips, knees, and ankles caused by excessive weight, leading to cartilage deterioration and resultant osteoarthritis. Based on this reasoning, clinicians frequently recommend weight loss to improve symptoms of osteoarthritis, but there is very little evidence that this actually works. On the other hand, since there is evidence that regular exercise can decrease symptoms of osteoarthritis in the knees, it would make good sense to include exercise in any weight-reduction regimen that might be prescribed for obese patients with osteoarthritis.

Cancer

Although data are relatively sparse, several studies have shown an increased prevalence of certain types of cancer in obese persons. In a large study performed by the American Cancer Society during the 1960s, obese men were found to have higher mortality rates from cancer of the colon and prostate, and obese women had increased mortality rates from cancer of the endometrium, breast, gallbladder, cervix, and ovary. Obese persons have a mortality rate from cancer that is 1.3 to 5.4 higher than that for nonobese persons, depending on the site of cancer and the degree of obesity.

The mechanism responsible for the increased frequency of endometrial cancer is probably increased circulating estrogen in obese women due to conversion of adrenal androgens to estrogens in adipose tissue. The mechanism responsible for the increased risk of breast cancer is unclear, but the risk may be more closely associated with central (abdominal) obesity than with gluteal or hip obesity. The mechanism for the association of obesity with other forms of cancer is not yet known, and there has been no evidence of an improvement in cancer risk following weight loss.

Pregnancy

Obesity increases the risk of adverse pregnancy outcomes, mostly complications during delivery related to fetal macrosomia. A very large weight gain during pregnancy appears to increase the risk of adverse outcomes. Recent studies have also suggested an increase in the risk of neural tube defects in infants born to obese women, irrespective of their folic acid status. Despite the risks of obesity during pregnancy, however, most authorities recommend against weight loss during pregnancy, even in markedly obese women, for fear of compromising fetal nutrition.

Social Stigma

Numerous studies have demonstrated that obese individuals suffer from discrimination in school and the workplace. The social bias against obesity appears to begin early in childhood, with schoolchildren showing greater attraction to photographs of persons with severe disabilities than to those of obese individuals. Studies consistently show that obese persons are less likely than nonobese individuals to be successful in college admission and job application processes.

Principal Diagnoses

Common Idiopathic Obesity

Common obesity, as seen in the vast majority of overweight individuals, probably consists of several syndromes or subtypes, each with a different cause and pathogenesis. In the future, it may be possible to separate obese patients into these subtypes and initiate treatments appropriate to the type of obesity identified. In current clinical practice, however, most patients with obesity are grouped together and receive similar treatments based on the common feature of increased adipose tissue mass.

Still, even with today's approach to obesity, we can identify variability among overweight individuals. Some of this variability is important in determining health risk and response to treatment. For example, as mentioned above, obese individuals vary in the way adipose tissue is distributed in the body. Some individuals accumulate relatively more adipose tissue in the hips and gluteal region, while others accumulate it in the abdomen, the latter being associated with increased risk of cardiovascular disease and probably certain cancers. Waist-to-hips ratio and simple waist circumference are common measures used to identify these two types of obesity, but they are probably crude approximations of complex variations in intraabdominal and subcutaneous fat deposition.

Another example of variation in obesity is varying age of onset. Obesity in infants and children under the age of 3 years frequently resolves before adulthood, especially if the child's parents are not overweight. Adolescence, on the other

hand, is a high-risk time for development of obesity, and obesity that begins in adolescence often persists into adulthood. Adolescent-onset obesity can be severe and is associated with more adipose tissue hyperplasia (i.e., an increase in the number of fat cells). Such adolescent-onset obesity is often more resistant to treatment. In contrast, adult-onset and more mild obesity typically exhibit simple adipose cell hypertrophy, instead of hyperplasia. These differences have potential therapeutic implications, because there is some evidence that short-term weight loss is accomplished through decreased adipose cell size and that additional adipose cells, once established, are unlikely to disappear.

ETIOLOGY OF COMMON IDIOPATHIC OBESITY

There has been much research and debate about the causes of obesity, but most authorities agree that the first law of thermodynamics (conservation of energy) applies to development of obesity in biologic systems. According to the first law of thermodynamics, energy consumed (food or calorie intake) equals energy expended (metabolic rate plus activity) plus energy stored (body fat). In a stable system, therefore, weight loss can be achieved only by decreased energy consumption, increased energy expenditure, or both. Conversely, to produce obesity, energy intake must exceed energy expenditure. Maintenance of obesity, once established, requires only a balance between energy intake and expenditure.

Findings from studies of obese populations support the general notion that the first law of thermodynamics applies to the pathogenesis of obesity. Obese people generally consume more calories than lean people of comparable height. Furthermore, studies indicate lower levels of physical activity in obese people than in lean control subjects. In fact, there are even data demonstrating that obese individuals spend more time watching television than do nonobese people.

These concepts appear to make the genesis and treatment of obesity quite simple, but the situation is more complex than it appears. Simple measurements of calorie intake and expenditure carry a large margin of error and do not fully explain the development of obesity in most individuals. Obese people also tend to have increased, not decreased, resting metabolic rates. Obese individuals expend more calories than do lighter persons during comparable exercise.

Part of the problem in understanding the cause of obesity may stem from considering it as a single pathophysiologic condition rather than a group of various syndromes with the common endpoint of obesity. Once methods become available to identify various obesity syndromes, it is likely that their causes will become clear.

At this point, however, several additional factors have been proposed to explain or contribute to the development of obesity. These factors include genetics, diet and exercise, psychological factors, and endocrinologic systems.

GENETICS   Family and twin studies have shown important genetic as well as environmental influences on body weight. There are genetic models of obesity in experimental laboratory animals, and genetic syndromes of human obesity also exist (e.g., Prader-Willi syndrome). The applicability of these genetic syndromes to the common obesity seen in primary care practice is unclear because these syndromes involve specific chromosomal aberrations and patterns of inheritance, while the mode of inheritance in common human obesity appears to be polygenic. Undefined genetic factors are estimated to explain at least 25 percent of body fat variability. Genetic factors are also important in determining the locations of body fat distribution.

DIET AND EXERCISE   Changes in diet and exercise have been suggested as explanations for the increased prevalence of obesity in recent decades. One commonly espoused theory is that high-fat diets have contributed to the increased prevalence of obesity in Western populations during the latter half of the twentieth century because of the marked increase in dietary fat consumption

during this period. Physical inactivity has also been proposed as an etiologic factor and may be an important cause of the increased prevalence of obesity in the general population.

PSYCHOLOGICAL FACTORS   There is a greater prevalence of psychopathology in obese binge eaters than in non-binge eaters who are obese. However, obesity has not been associated with any specific psychological disorder, and obese individuals as a group have not been shown to have a higher prevalence of psychopathology than do nonobese populations.

ENDOCRINE FACTORS: THE SET-POINT THEORY   While the "set-point" theory remains a theory, control of body fat stores appears to be regulated in much the same manner as a thermostatic system with a set point. The set-point theory proposes that signals from adipose tissue trigger homeostatic mechanisms that increase or decrease energy intake and expenditure so as to maintain a constant adipose tissue mass.

This theory involves a peptide hormone called leptin. Leptin is produced by adipose tissue and is thought to signal the hypothalamus about the status of adipose tissue stores. If fat stores rise above a certain set point, through food intake or other processes, leptin secretion by adipose tissue increases. The hypothalamus responds to the increased leptin levels by signaling the cerebral cortex to decrease food-seeking behavior (appetite) and the sympathetic nervous system to increase the metabolic rate. This leptin-induced physiologic response continues until the set-point fat-storage level is reached.

The set-point theory of obesity suggests that this regulatory system is somehow altered and a new, higher set point is established. Weight loss becomes difficult because if adipose tissue mass falls below the higher set point, the leptin response abates, activating physiologic processes that resist weight loss. The resulting desire to eat will be strong, perhaps as strong as the urge to drink when thirsty or seek warmth when cold. It is too soon to tell how research on leptin and the set-point theory will apply to clinical care of human beings. In addition, there may be other mechanisms in the genesis of obesity that have yet to be determined.

Other Clinical Syndromes

Most patients presenting to primary care physicians have common idiopathic obesity, as described above. However, in evaluating obese patients, other obesity syndromes, some common and some rare, must always be considered.

HYPOTHYROIDISM

Hypothyroidism is commonly associated with moderate weight gain. The low metabolic rate seen with hypothyroidism is probably responsible for the weight gain, and thyroid hormone replacement typically results in modest weight loss. Severe obesity, however, is not usually caused by hypothyroidism alone.

CORTICOSTEROID EXCESS

Excess corticosteroid production results in Cushing's syndrome, a constellation of abnormalities that includes obesity, hypertension, central fat distribution, and other findings. Cushing's syndrome can be caused by excess endogenous production of adrenal steroid hormones or by exogenous administration of steroid hormones as treatment for medical conditions. Corticotropin-releasing factor appears to play a role in the control of food intake and body weight at the hypothalamic level, and this hormone may be involved in the pathogenesis of obesity in Cushing's syndrome.

GENETIC ABNORMALITIES

Dysmorphic genetic syndromes have been described in which obesity occurs along with other physiologic and anatomic abnormalities. The most common of these is Prader-Willi syndrome, caused by an abnormality in chromosome 15. The syndrome includes obesity plus short stature, hypogonadism, mental retardation, small hands and feet, hypotonia, and several craniofacial abnormalities. Children with this syndrome tend to have such voracious appetites that families may resort to locking the refrigerator. Since Prader-Willi syndrome occurs in about 1 of every 15,000 children, it is occasionally encountered by primary care clinicians. Other genetic syndromes that involve obesity are uncommon and rarely seen in primary care practice.

HYPOTHALAMIC ABNORMALITIES

In laboratory animals, hypothalamic lesions can cause abnormalities in body weight, either obesity or excessive leanness. Case reports of sudden weight gain and obesity after traumatic or surgical lesions of the hypothalamic area suggest that hypothalamic mechanisms may be responsible for some cases of human obesity. Hypothalamic lesions are, of course, rare and almost never encountered in primary care practice.

Typical Presentation

As discussed earlier, studies indicate that more than half of the patients seen in primary care practice are overweight. Because obesity is commonly associated with such chronic medical conditions as hypertension, diabetes, and hyperlipidemia, many patients in primary care practice seek care for these conditions, and obesity is seen as a concomitant (though perhaps causative) problem. Despite the high prevalence of obesity in primary care practice, it is not clear that primary care clinicians acknowledge and treat it with sufficient frequency. Obesity is included as a diagnosis in the medical record of fewer than half of obese patients, and only 30 percent of obese patients' medical records contain evidence that patients received counseling about the need to lose weight during the past year. When obesity is addressed in primary care practice, there are no published data to indicate how often the problem is addressed on the initiative of the patients versus the initiative of the clinician. There are also no data to compare the frequency with which obesity and weight loss are addressed in primary care offices, specialty offices, or commercial weight reduction programs.

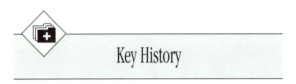

Key History

The diagnosis of obesity is made with physical examination measurements of weight and height. The history is used to help detect secondary causes of obesity (i.e., other than common idiopathic obesity). It also used to assess the patient's need and motivation to lose weight, and to help identify the best method of achieving weight loss in the patient.

Detecting Secondary Causes of Obesity

The history should include questions to screen for symptoms of hypothyroidism (fatigue, dry skin, cold intolerance, voice change, and constipation), Cushing's syndrome (corticosteroid use, menstrual disorder, and muscular weakness), hypothalamic disorders (brain injury or surgery), and genetic disorders (mental retardation). If the history elicits symptoms suggestive of any of these conditions, appropriate diagnostic tests should be performed.

Need for Weight Loss

To evaluate the medical need for weight loss, the clinician should ask about the presence of obesity-related complications such as diabetes, hypertension, hyperlipidemia, gallbladder disease, sleep apnea (snoring, morning headaches, and daytime sleepiness), or osteoarthritis. If present, these complications impart greater urgency to the need for weight reduction.

Motivation

Before counseling a patient about weight loss methods, clinicians should assess the patient's willingness to try losing weight, the effect of obesity on the patient's quality of life, and any life stresses that might impede weight loss efforts. It is generally believed that the chance of successful weight loss is increased by addressing these issues and targeting weight reduction efforts at appropriately motivated patients. However, there is little research evidence to support this point of view.

Weight-Loss Method Selection

At any one time, 25 percent of men and 45 percent of women are trying to lose weight, and $33 billion is spent on weight control products and services in the United States. Thus, most obese patients seen by primary care clinicians will have had some experience with attempts at weight loss. To help in selection of an appropriate weight-loss method, the history should determine methods used for prior weight loss efforts and their results. The history should also determine the role of family members in meal preparation because, when the family meal preparer makes meals that support the patient's weight loss efforts, the chances of successful weight reduction may be increased. The history should also target contraindications to weight reduction (e.g., pregnancy or lactation) or cautions in the use of weight-loss medications (e.g., the presence of cardiac arrhythmias, hepatic or renal failure, or use of serotonergic medications or monoamine oxidase inhibitors for depression).

Physical Examination

The physical examination is targeted at diagnosing obesity, determining the need for weight reduction, and identifying secondary causes of obesity.

Diagnosing Obesity

Simple measurements of height and weight permit calculation of the BMI for diagnosis of obesity. As described above, values over 27 kg/m² indicate the presence of obesity. Values over 30 kg/m² indicate a substantially increased risk of medical complications and death from obesity-related conditions.

Findings Suggesting the Need for Weight Reduction

In general, all patients with a BMI exceeding 27 kg/m² should be encouraged to lose weight. Because of their greatly increased risk of adverse outcomes, those with BMI over 30 kg/m² should be strongly urged to lose weight.

Because of evidence suggesting that abdominal obesity carries particular risk to overweight patients, waist circumference has recently been advocated as a parameter to use in determining the need for weight loss. A recent study suggested that patients are at higher risk for obesity-related complications if their waist circumference exceeds 40 in for males and females under age 40 years or 35 in for males and females over age 40 years. These values can be used to identify "high-risk abdominal obesity" until further norms are available.

A finding of high blood pressure in patients with a BMI over 27 kg/m² definitely warrants an attempt at weight reduction. It is important to keep in mind that, when examining a patient

with obesity, a falsely elevated blood pressure can be obtained if a blood pressure cuff is used that is too small for the patients' arm. The inflation bladder of the blood pressure cuff should encircle at least two-thirds of the arm. If it does not, a larger size (such as a "thigh" cuff) should be used. Using too large a cuff can result in a small artifactual decrease in measured blood pressure, but the magnitude of error when using an overly large cuff is small relative to the error caused by using an inappropriately small cuff.

Other physical examination abnormalities that suggest the need for weight loss are joint findings indicative of osteoarthritis. Finally, patients with findings of cholelithiasis would benefit from weight reduction.

Findings Suggesting Secondary Causes of Obesity

The physical examination of obese patients in primary care should focus on detection of three specific syndromes or disorders. The first is hypothyroidism, with its typical findings of bradycardia, hypothermia, myxedema, and delayed deep tendon reflexes. The second is Cushing's syndrome, with abnormalities including facial plethora, hirsuitism, abdominal striae, edema, and central obesity. The third is findings that might be associated with a genetic syndrome, including short stature or any physical anomaly.

Ancillary Tests

Several blood tests should be ordered for evaluation of obese patients to detect the presence of obesity-related medical problems. These tests include determination of fasting serum glucose and fasting lipids levels to rule out diabetes mellitus, hypercholesterolemia, and hypertriglyceridemia. Since these tests are used to define diabetes and hyperlipidemia, they would have virtually perfect sensitivity and specificity if obtained in the fasting state. If any of these tests results are abnormal, the need for weight reduction becomes more substantial.

Certain additional testing is appropriate if secondary causes of obesity are suspected. In particular, thyroid function tests are useful if hypothyroidism is suspected. Determination of cortisol levels or a dexamethasone suppression test should be performed if there are findings of Cushing's syndrome. Chromosome analysis is in order if there are symptoms or signs suggesting Prader-Willi syndrome.

Finally, patients being considered for a very low-calorie diet or anorectic medication should have additional laboratory testing. In this situation, the clinician should obtain a complete blood count and a chemistry panel including analysis of electrolytes, renal function, and liver enzymes.

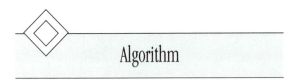

Algorithm

The algorithm summarizes the evaluation of obese patients, and provides possible treatment approaches, which are described in the following section (Fig. 2-3). The BMI is the initial decision point in the algorithm, with obesity defined as a BMI higher than 30 kg/m^2. As discussed earlier, the choice of a BMI cutoff point is somewhat arbitrary, and several authorities consider a BMI higher than 27 kg/m^2 the value at which treatment should be instituted. The algorithm then indicates that patient history, physical examination, and laboratory test results should be used to include or exclude any of the secondary or rare obesity syndromes. Then, once it is established that an obese patient is ready to attempt weight loss, further examination and laboratory results can determine the level of obesity-related risk and appropriate vigor with which treatment should be pursued.

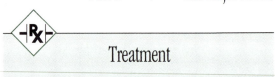

Treatment

Self-Treatment

There are no published data that compare the results of patient-initiated weight loss through self-imposed dieting (with or without the advice of a clinician) with results from any of the various treatments or programs discussed below. Obese patients are constantly bombarded with advice from the popular press about diets and the importance of weight reduction, and all clinicians are aware of individuals who have successfully lost significant weight on their own and kept it off for long periods of time. Such experiences make it imperative that physicians explain the risks of obesity and benefits of weight loss to all of their obese patients. When such simple advice fails to result in weight loss, as is the usual experience, one or more of the treatments discussed below can be considered. Unfortunately, there are no data to aid physicians in selecting the best treatment approach for a particular patient or group of patients. Given the current state of knowledge, treatment approaches must be selected based on the patient's past experiences, preferences, and motivation levels.

General Treatment Principles

There are several approaches to the treatment of obesity, all of which either decrease caloric intake, increase energy expended, or both. A daily caloric deficit of a given number of calories will result in similar fat loss whether it is achieved through decreased food intake or increased activity. A low-carbohydrate, high-fat, calorie-restricted diet will cause an initial diuresis with apparent rapid weight reduction from loss of body fluid, but the amount of fat lost is similar to the loss with a high-carbohydrate diet with the same number of calories. Similarly, treatments such as behavior modification, special diets,

Figure 2-3

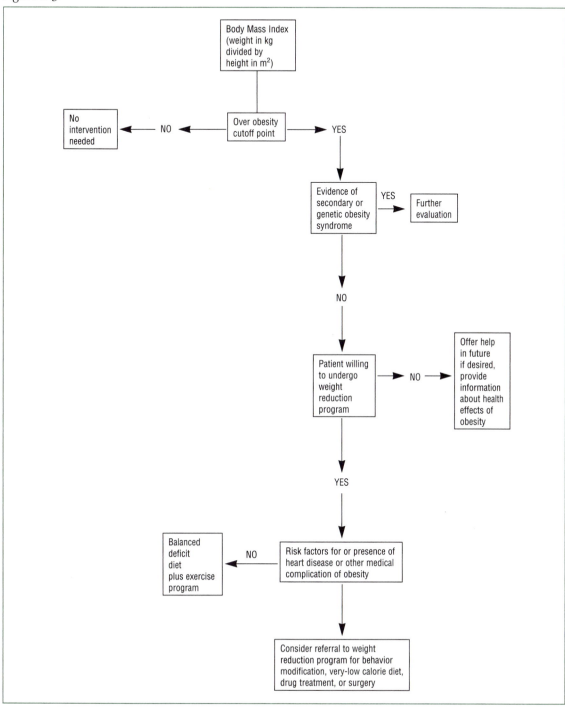

Algorithm for obesity.

medications, and gastric surgery are aimed at decreasing daily caloric intake or increasing activity and exercise. However, despite claims in countless popular publications, there are no quick or magical approaches to weight loss.

Dietary treatment, exercise, and behavior modification are complementary modalities. Reputable weight loss programs should contain all three, as well as a long-term group process to help maintain weight loss. It is clear that these interventions are effective in many patients, but only as long as they are continued. This has led most authorities in the field to view obesity as a chronic disease that should be treated much the same as hypertension or diabetes mellitus, both of which "relapse" when active treatment is discontinued. Running a comprehensive weight loss program is out of the scope of practice for most primary care clinicians. However, because of their long-term relationships with patients, primary care clinicians can play an important role in evaluating and guiding patients into treatment programs, monitoring and reinforcing their progress, and encouraging continued treatment to prevent or deal with relapse.

Finally, clinicians should consider the overall goal of treatment. Achievement of ideal body weight or a BMI of 25 kg/m^2 is certainly desirable, and many clinicians and patients will seek this degree of weight reduction. However, such a goal is elusive for many, if not most, obese patients. Beneficial health effects occur even with modest weight loss in the range of 10 percent of initial weight. Thus, for many patients it is often appropriate to set a weight-loss goal that is more moderate, realistic, and achievable than attainment of ideal body weight.

Diet

BALANCED DEFICIT DIETS

The variety of dietary approaches in the medical literature and the popular press is vast. The most commonly recommended weight loss diet is a balanced-deficit diet, which is composed of whole foods from the major food groups and is designed to be about 500 kcal below the patient's usual intake. As a general rule, a 500-kcal/day reduction will lead to a weight loss of half to 1 lb/week.

Such diets typically contain about 15 percent of calories as protein, 30 percent as fat, and 55 percent as carbohydrate, and comply with dietary recommendations of the American Diabetes and Heart Associations, the American Cancer Society, and the food pyramid promoted by the Food and Drug Administration. Unless the total dietary intake is below 1000 kcal/day, vitamin and mineral supplements are not necessarily required with a balanced-deficit diet.

Patients can learn about balanced-deficit diets from dietitians, primary care clinicians, reading materials from the abovementioned associations and societies, and the popular press. Information is also available from commercial programs such as Weight Watchers, and diets meeting these guidelines can be purchased as prepared foods from programs such as Jenny Craig or Nutri-systems.

VERY LOW-CALORIE DIETS

The very low-calorie diet (VLCD) represents a more aggressive approach to caloric restriction. These diets are usually physician-monitored as part of a comprehensive medical weight-loss program. The nutritional and caloric content of a VLCD can be obtained as whole food or from a powdered formula that is reconstituted to make a meal-replacement beverage. A VLCD is typically 800 kcal/day or less, contains about 1 g protein per kilogram of body weight, and is supplemented with vitamins and minerals. Weight loss in the early phase of this type of diet is usually rapid, on the order of 1 to 2 lb/week.

Supervision of such diets by a physician is recommended because of the possible side effects, including dehydration and postural hypotension, hypokalemia, gallbladder disease, constipation, and hypothyroid-type symptoms. An early version of VLCD was associated with sudden cardiac death after very large weight losses, but modern versions of the diet are supplemented heavily with vitamins and minerals and have not appeared to cause this problem. However, monitoring by electrocardiogram (ECG) for prolonged QT interval, which was associated with the sudden deaths in the early VLCDs, is typically recommended. A VLCD is contraindicated in a number of situations, including severe systemic infections, unstable angina, recent myocardial infarction, malignant dysrhythmias, recent stroke or transient ischemic attack, renal or hepatic failure, severe psychiatric disturbances, and eating disorders.

The VLCD is commonly used for rapid weight loss over a number of months and followed with a balanced calorie-deficit diet for long-term maintenance. However, relapse with regain of lost weight has been a significant problem with VLCD programs.

Exercise

Another common approach to weight loss is exercise. Both aerobic and weight-training exercise appear to promote weight loss, as would be predicted by the first law of thermodynamics. Studies of obese subjects suggest that at least one-half to 1 h of brisk walking 7 d/week is needed before weight loss occurs. However, the amount of weight lost by obese patients with exercise alone is minimal. In fact, when exercise is combined with caloric restriction, the exercise does not appear to add much to the rate of weight loss compared to caloric restriction alone. Nonetheless, studies suggest that regular exercise may still be helpful in a weight loss regimen because it increases the likelihood of maintaining weight loss attained through dietary restriction.

Impediments to exercise in obese patients are significant and include lack of conditioning, discomfort in limbs and joints during weight bearing, lack of opportunity to exercise, and social embarrassment about public exercise with an obese physique. Walking, stationary bicycling, pool aerobics, and weight training appear to be the best form of exercises for obese individuals. Primary care clinicians can provide significant assistance to obese patients by recommending ways to overcome impediments to exercise and by encouraging initiation of and adherence to an exercise plan.

Behavior Modification

The third common element of obesity treatment is behavior modification. Conceptually, caloric restriction and exercise are simple and effective weight loss agents. However, because of the strong biologic resistance to weight change and social, cultural, and familial pressures to maintain established behavior patterns, it is often difficult for obese patients to achieve or maintain weight loss.

Behavior modification refers to a set of skills typically taught by a psychologist and a dietician over 2 to 3 months in a group setting. These skills range from methods of reducing inappropriate eating behaviors, such as snacking while watching television, to cognitive methods of avoiding food consumption as a response to stress. Research has demonstrated that behavior modification programs can result in significant, although moderate, weight loss. When combined with a VLCD, the results are better than with either method used alone. Unfortunately, follow-up studies have shown that nearly all of the lost weight is usually regained after 2 to 5 years. Recent programs have emphasized the importance of continued participation in group behavior modification therapies to increase the chance that attained weight loss is maintained.

Drug Treatment

Pharmacologic agents for weight loss, known as anorectics, have been available for years. Many anorectics have been marketed in the past several decades, but after initial enthusiasm for each drug category, they have fallen into disfavor.

AMPHETAMINES

The first anorectics to see widespread clinical use were amphetamines. These drugs were effective but quickly fell into disfavor because of problems with addiction and abuse as well as side effects such as insomnia, nervousness, euphoria, hypertension, and tachycardia. A number of amphetamine derivatives have since been developed, but they all have similar side effect profiles. Because of concerns generated by amphetamines, the Food and Drug Administration has approved amphetamine anorectics only for short-term use, and some state medical practice laws prohibit use of amphetamines for weight-reduction therapy. Since weight regain upon discontinuation of any of the anorectics is the rule, it makes little sense to use them as short-term treatments for obesity.

SEROTONIN-AUGMENTING AGENTS

In the 1990s, several new anorectics were developed that differed from amphetamine analogues by acting principally on serotonin receptors, rather than catecholamine receptors. These drugs included fenfluramine and dexfenfluramine. They achieved great popularity when it was shown that, in combination with phentermine (an amphetamine derivative), these serotonergic medications were effective in inducing substantial weight loss. Subsequently, however, pulmonary hypertension and serious cardiac valve abnormalities were reported in young women taking these medications for short periods of time. As a result, both fenfluramine and dexfenfluramine were removed from the commercial market.

SEROTONIN AND NOREPINEPHRINE REUPTAKE INHIBITORS

Sibutramine is the first of a new class of medications that inhibit uptake of serotonin and norepinephrine (and, to a lesser degree, dopamine). Sibutramine was approved by the Food and Drug Administration in 1998 for treatment of obesity, defined as a BMI higher than 30 kg/m^2 or higher than 27 kg/m^2 in the presence of cardiovascular risk factors such as hypertension, diabetes, or hyperlipidemia. This approval occurred despite contrary recommendations by a Food and Drug Administration advisory committee because of the fact that, in clinical trials, some patients developed elevated blood pressure. While effective in short-term clinical trials, long-term experience with sibutramine is limited.

FUTURE ROLE OF ANORECTICS

The experience with amphetamines and serotonin reuptake inhibitors has generated controversy about whether medications are ever appropriate for treating obesity. Some argue that the serious health hazards of obesity outweigh the risks of drug complications. However, the life-threatening nature of some side effects and the concern that they may develop without warning in otherwise healthy individuals leads most experts to avoid use of anorectic drugs.

The future role of anorectic medications in the treatment of obesity is unclear. Nonetheless, drug development continues, with sibutramine being only the first of many medications that will be available over the next decade. Table 2-2 lists antiobesity drugs that are currently under development.

Surgery

Past surgical treatments for obesity included jaw wiring to decrease caloric intake and jejunoileal bypass to induce malabsorption and decrease calorie assimilation by the body. Both of these procedures have been abandoned because of unacceptable side effects.

The only surgical approach currently used with any frequency is gastric partitioning, a procedure that attempts to decrease food intake by increasing satiety through decreased stomach size. The two most common gastric partitioning

Table 2-2

Obesity Drugs Under Development

DRUG	MECHANISM OF ACTION
APPROVED DRUGS BEING TESTED FOR OBESITY TREATMENT	
Bromocriptine	Enhances dopamine release, thereby affecting hypothalamic and neostriatal receptors that regulate appetite
Naltrexone	Opiate receptor antagonist
NEW OBESITY DRUGS UNDERGOING CLINICAL TRIALS OR IN DEVELOPMENT	
Orlistat	Interferes with pancreatic lipase causing malabsorption of up to 30 percent of ingested fat
Insulinotropin (GLP-1)	Synthetic glucagonlike peptide-1; slows gastric emptying and elevates insulin levels
Leptin	Regulates appetite and metabolism through feedback based on quantity of body fat
Melanocortin (HP-228)	Binds to melanocortin receptors; suppresses appetite, decreases glucose and insulin
Neuropeptide Y inhibitor (NGD 95-1)	Blocks neuropeptide Y, an appetite stimulant; increases fat catabolism
BTA-243	Binds to the beta$_3$-adrenergic receptor on fat cells, increasing fat catabolism
Batabindide (CCK-8)	Blocks enzyme that restores appetite by breaking down cholecystokinin
Cholecystokinin promoters	Increases availability of receptors that reduce appetite when stimulated by cholecystokinin
Corticotropin-releasing factor	Stimulates stress receptors in the brain to control appetite and regulate metabolism
Uncoupling protein 2	Heat-generating protein that raises metabolism and burns white adipose tissue

SOURCE: Information available from http://www.obesity-news.com.

procedures are (1) horizontal stomach transection with Roux-en-Y gastrojejunostomy and (2) vertical banded gastroplasty (Fig. 2-4). These surgical procedures are generally reserved for patients with severe obesity who have failed less invasive treatments. They are best performed in centers with multidisciplinary teams including psychological and dietary consultants and surgeons experienced with the techniques.

Since the main effect of these surgical procedures is to facilitate decreased food intake, the selection and motivation of patients are impor-

tant. Patients must be motivated to participate in programs to alter their eating behaviors because it is possible to continue consuming a high-calorie diet after gastric partitioning by drinking calorie-dense liquids. However, with appropriate selection of patients, results are often impressive, with as many as 80 percent of patients maintaining losses of 50 percent of excess weight for 10 years.

Advocates of surgical approaches to obesity frequently point out that these procedures are the only treatments with proven long-term effi-

Figure 2-4

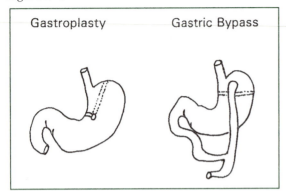

Gastroplasty   Gastric Bypass

Gastric surgical procedures for treatment of obesity. The two most common surgical treatments for obesity are the vertical banded gastroplasty *(left)* and the gastric bypass with Roux-en-Y gastrojejunostomy *(right)*. In the vertical banded gastroplasty, a double row of surgical staples *(dotted lines)* partitions the stomach vertically, effectively decreasing stomach size and creating a pouch that food enters and exits. In the gastric bypass, the stomach is also partitioned, and it is drained though a Roux-en-Y gastrojejunostomy.

cacy, including improved control of diabetes and hypertension as well as weight loss. Nonetheless, complications and side effects of gastric partitioning procedures are significant and include perioperative death (1 percent); surgical morbidity (10 percent), including leakage at the anastomosis, stomal obstruction, and malignant ulceration; and long-term nutritional problems such as persistent vomiting, protein malnutrition, and vitamin and mineral deficiencies. Primary care clinicians contemplating referral of patients for obesity surgery should make referrals to centers experienced in the performance of these procedures.

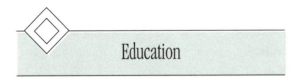

Education

It should be clear from the foregoing discussions that education of the patient is a fundamental part of any obesity treatment. The health risks inherent in obesity are substantial, and clinicians should educate patients about them just as they do about the risks of hypertension or hyperlipidemia. It is also important to be realistic about the difficulty of weight loss. No matter what treatment approach is used, successful weight loss and maintenance require considerable effort. Poorly timed interventions in inadequately motivated patients can do harm by lowering self-esteem or causing depression while producing no beneficial weight loss.

Many patients require substantial amounts of education before they will make the life-style changes needed for successful weight loss. Providing extensive educational support can be difficult for busy primary care clinicians. Therefore, in many cases the best approach may be to refer patients to dietitians or weight loss programs.

Should primary care clinicians wish to provide the counseling themselves, a number of weight-reduction education techniques can be employed. However, since there are no published data evaluating the effectiveness of these methods, they must be used empirically. One example is a guide for education of patients by Moore and Nagle entitled *Physicians' Guide to Outpatient Nutrition*. It can be obtained from the American Academy of Family Physicians (phone 800-274-2237, order no. 939). Other techniques include diet diaries, diet prescriptions, and exercise prescriptions.

Diet Diary

A diet diary is a useful educational tool for determining the quality of a patient's diet, modifying eating patterns, and monitoring progress with weight reduction. The patient is asked to record everything eaten and drunk each day, usually for between 3 to 7 days. When reviewing the diet diary, it is often easy to identify poor eating habits, such as snacking, frequent meals in restaurants (especially "fast-food" restaurants), frequent consumption of high-caloric foods, or potential nutritional problems from diets that exclude certain food groups, such as fresh vegetables. A food diary can also aid in adherence to a prescribed diet. Used on a continuous or intermittent schedule, the food diary can function as a feedback tool to make patients aware of their dietary intake. Knowing that the clinician will review the diary may also help patients adhere to their diets.

Diet Prescription

A diet prescription involves giving patients specific written dietary instructions. It has been common practice to hand out printed diet sheets containing instructions for diets of various calorie levels. While there are no published data to evaluate the effectiveness of using these pre-printed diet handouts, there is general consensus that this practice is not useful. Rather, more useful diet prescriptions involve giving patients a suggested number of servings from each of the food groups with accompanying information about serving sizes in each group. This allows patients to choose from a variety of foods according to personal preference. Within each group, foods can be ranked according to caloric density. Compliance with the diet prescription can be monitored with a diet diary.

Exercise Prescription

After questioning about preferences and impediments to exercise, specific suggestions can be provided about gradually increasing exercise up to a certain goal level. Many suggestions for exercise goals have been published, but a typical regimen involves at least one half h of exercise per day for five or more, and preferably all, days per week. Walking appears to be the most desirable exercise for obese patients. Other options include stationary bicycles, weight training, and water aerobics, as well as the whole range of sports and physical activities. The key appears to be finding an activity that patients enjoy enough to maintain on a consistent, regular basis.

Frequent Follow-Up

While there are no data to evaluate the effects of various frequencies of follow-up on weight-loss success, it has been a common observation in obesity programs that the amount of participation in the program correlates with weight-loss results. One suggestion has been that monthly follow-up checks be performed by an interested office staff member who can give reinforcement for successful weight loss and encouragement and advice for continued adherence to diet, exercise, and behavior modification interventions.

Family Approach

So many of the dietary and physical activity issues in weight control are central to family life that involvement of one or more family members in weight-loss treatment is crucial. Several studies have shown that programs involving parents or spouses were more effective than those that did not. When a family member purchases and prepares food for a patient, that person must be involved in dietary education. Even when this is not the case, a supportive family environment appears to increase adherence to reduced calorie diets and exercise regimens.

Doherty and Harkaway have proposed that obesity can serve several important inclusion functions in families. In families with a high prevalence of obesity, especially across generations, attainment and maintenance of obesity can be a way of showing loyalty to the family. When one parent is obese and the other thin, obesity in a child can help to form a coalition with the obese parent. Obesity can also delay entry into the adult world for obese children who turn to the family for emotional support when ostracized from peer social groups.

The Doherty and Harkaway model also suggests that weight can play a role in relationship control. For example, an obese partner might agree to accept the lean partner's help in weight loss efforts, but over time this "help" may begin to feel coercive, leading to rebellion and failure of weight-loss efforts. The obese partner "wins" the control struggle by remaining overweight. Similarly, a child's obesity can provide the child with control over one or both parents on the family battleground over food.

Obesity can also affect family interactions because of the close ties between sexuality and body weight and body image. Individuals can use changes in body weight to manage sexual closeness and distance. Some obese couples feel that there is a protective value of obesity for marriage stability, since weight loss by one or both partners would increase worry about extramarital affairs.

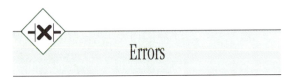

Errors

Studies and commentaries in the literature suggest that clinicians commonly make three errors in evaluating and treating obese patients. The first is ignoring the problem altogether. A study in family medicine clinics suggested that physicians failed to address obesity as often as 70 percent of the time. A second common error is to let personal biases against obese people affect the clinician-patient relationship. Robinson and coworkers have reviewed the literature and found that clinicians express the same negative attitudes about obese people as society in general. They recommend that clinicians make a conscious effort to treat their obese patients with understanding and respect. The third common

error is to suggest or agree with unrealistic weight-loss goals. As discussed earlier, it is unlikely for obese patients to achieve ideal body weight regardless of the treatment method, and loss of as little as a 10 percent of excess body weight can lead to significant improvements in health. Insistence on, or even support of, a goal to reach "ideal weight" could predispose to relapse when the goal is not attained.

In addition, although there is no documentation in the literature, a probable common error in treating obese patients is failing to follow up on treatment recommendations made at prior office visits. There is general agreement that clinicians have significant influence on the health behaviors of patients, and continued attention to patients' efforts at weight reduction will reinforce the importance of the problem.

Another potential problem is failure to obtain informed consent about treatment. This is particularly important when using medications for obesity treatment, but it is also applicable to surgical treatments and enrollment in comprehensive weight-reduction programs.

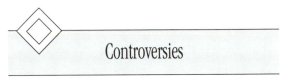

Controversies

Cause

Controversy has existed for years about the cause of obesity. While scientists have recently pointed to the roles of genetics and hypothalamic control of food intake as important factors, there is still a strong feeling among laypersons and professionals alike that obesity is nothing but a manifestation of sloth or lack of personal will power. It appears that opinions are changing to reflect scientific evidence of a genetic and metabolic basis for obesity, but practicing clinicians are only recently becoming aware of this evidence.

Effectiveness of Treatment

There has been considerable controversy in the literature about the effectiveness of obesity treatment. Most authors have suggested that the long-term results of all methods except surgery are universally poor. Others have countered that obesity treatment is held to too high a standard. They argue that obesity treatment is considered a failure if weight is regained after a treatment program but that treatment of diabetes or hypertension is not considered a failure if blood sugar or blood pressure rise after discontinuing medication. These concepts have led to recommendations to refocus the goal of obesity treatment from short-term weight loss to long-term "weight management."

Drug Therapy

Another controversy in obesity management has been over the use of pharmaceutical agents. Concerted efforts were made to discourage their use after earlier negative experiences with amphetamines and other combination treatments, including thyroid hormone. The recent debacle with fenfluramine, phentermine, and dexfenluramine have led many to reevaluate the role of drug treatment, but controversy remains because of the serious adverse health effects of untreated obesity.

Weight Cycling

Epidemiologic studies have suggested that repeated cycles of weight loss and regain (often called "weight cycling" or "yo-yo dieting") may lead to adverse health consequences, such as increased rates of hypertension and coronary disease. If weight cycling does have adverse effects, then any treatment that does not produce sustained weight loss could be harmful upon relapse. Unfortunately, research up to this point has not been sufficient to answer this important clinical question, but a consensus of opinion has been that obesity treatment should not be avoided because of worries over potential risks of weight cycling.

Emerging Concepts

The most likely advances from current research on obesity will be in understanding genetics and brain regulation of appetite and body fat stores, and in development of new pharmaceutical agents for treatment (Table 2-2). In addition, it will be increasingly recognized that the clinical syndrome of human obesity is likely to be polygenic and complex, and molecular biology research may reveal specific genetic defects in subsets of the obese population.

Of the many drugs under development, research on leptin, the chemical messenger from adipose tissue that conveys information about the status of body fat stores to the central nervous system, is progressing rapidly. Mouse models with either deficiencies of or resistance to leptin have been described. Mice that are deficient in leptin become obese, leading to the theory that leptin can be used to promote weight loss. The gene for leptin has been cloned, and leptin is currently undergoing trials in humans as a treatment agent for obesity.

A number of other important peptides, such as neuropeptide Y and corticotropin-releasing factor, are also being studied for their roles in the regulation of appetite and body fat. Still other agents are in the preclinical research phase (Table 2-2). While past pharmaceutical treatments for obesity have generally been disappointing, many of these new agents offer novel mechanisms for stimulating metabolism or decreasing appetite, and may have fewer side effects than current or past anorectics. With further characterization of appetite- and body fat-regulating peptides and receptors, production of more focused pharmaceutical agents should be relatively straightforward.

Bibliography

American Dietetic Association: Position of the American Dietetic Association: Weight management. *J Am Diet Assoc* 97:71, 1997.

Andersen RE, Crespo CJ, Bartlett SJ, et al: Relationship of physical activity and television watching with body weight and level of fatness among children: Results from the Third National Health and Nutrition and Examination Survey. *JAMA* 279:938, l998.

Benotti PN, Bistrian B, Benotti JR, et al: Heart disease and hypertension in severe obesity: The benefits of weight reduction. *Am J Clin Nutr* 55:586S, 1992.

Bray GA, Gray DS: Obesity: I. Pathogenesis. *West J Med* 149:429, 1988.

Brownell KD, Wadden TA: Etiology and treatment of obesity: Understanding a serious, prevalent, and refractory disorder. *J Consult Clin Psychol* 60:505, 1992.

Caro JF, Sinha MK, Kolaczynski JW, et al: Leptin: The tale of an obesity gene. *Diabetes* 45:1455, 1996.

Foreyt JP, Goodrick GK: Evidence for success of behavior modification in weight loss and control. *Ann Intern Med* 119:698, 1993.

Goldenberg RL, Tamura T: Prepregnancy weight and pregnancy outcome. *JAMA* 275:1127, 1996.

Goldstein DJ: Beneficial health effects of modest weight loss. *Int J Obes* 16:397, 1992.

Gray DS: Diagnosis and prevalence of obesity. *Med Clin North Am* 73:1, 1989.

Kannel WB, Gordon T, Castelli WP: Obesity, lipids, and glucose intolerance: The Framingham Study. *Am J Clin Nutr* 32:1238, 1979.

Kirschenbaum DS, Fitzgibbon ML: Controversy about the treatment of obesity: Criticisms or challenges? *Behav Ther* 26:43, 1995.

Kuczmarski RJ, Flegal KM, Campbell SM, et al: Increasing prevalence of overweight among U.S. adults. *JAMA* 272:205, 1994.

Lemieux S, Prud'homme D, Bouchard C, et al: A single threshold value of waist girth identifies normal-weight and overweight subjects with excess visceral adipose tissue. *Am J Clin Nutr* 64:685, 1996.

Lew EA, Garfinkel L: Variations in mortality by weight among 750,000 men and women. *J Chron Dis* 32:563, 1979.

Loube DI, Loube AA, Mitler MM: Weight loss for obstructive sleep apnea: The optimal therapy for obese patients. *J Am Diet Assoc* 94:1291, 1994.

McDaniel SH, Hepworth J, Doherty WJ: *Medical family therapy.* New York, Basic Books, 1992, pp 112–121.

National Task Force on the Prevention and Treatment of Obesity: Very low-calorie diets. *JAMA* 270:967, 1993.

National Task Force on the Prevention and Treatment of Obesity: Weight cycling. *JAMA* 272:1196, 1994.

National Task Force on the Prevention and Treatment of Obesity: Long-term pharmacotherapy in the management of obesity. *JAMA* 276:1907, 1996.

NIH Technology Assessment Conference Panel: Methods for voluntary weight loss and control. *Ann Intern Med* 116:942, 1992.

Olefsky JM, Kolterman OG, Scarlett JA: Insulin action and resistance in obesity and noninsulin-dependent type II diabetes mellitus. *Am J Physiol* 243:E15, 1982.

Pi-Sunyer FX: Medical hazards of obesity. *Ann Intern Med* 119:655, 1993.

Robinson BE, Gjerdingen DK, Houge DR: Obesity: A move from traditional to more patient-oriented management. *J Am Board Fam Pract* 8:99, 1995.

Rosenbaum M, Leibel RL, Hirsch J: Obesity. *New Engl J Med* 337:396, 1997.

Schwartz MW, Seeley RJ: The new biology of body weight regulation. *J Am Diet Assoc* 97:54, 1997.

Stampfer MJ, Maclure KM, Colditz GA, et al: Risk of symptomatic gallstones in women with severe obesity. *Am J Clin Nutr* 55:652, 1992.

Steven J, Jianwen C, Pamuk ER, et al: The effect of age on the association between body-mass index and mortality. *New Engl J Med* 338:1, l998.

Weinsier RL, Wilson LJ, Lee J: Medically safe rate of weight loss for the treatment of obesity: A guideline based on risk of gallstone formation. *Am J Med* 98:115, 1995.

Whitaker RC, Wright JA, Pepe MS, et al: Predicting obesity in young adulthood from childhood and parental obesity. *New Engl J Med* 337:869, 1997.

Stephen A. Brunton
Louis Kuritzky

Chapter 3

Hypertension

Errors	Controversies
Inappropriately Switching Medications	Target Blood Pressure
Inappropriately Assuming a Class of	Ambulatory Blood Pressure Monitoring
Medications Will Be Ineffective	The Role of Echocardiography
Failure to "Step Down" Therapy	**Emerging Concepts**
Inappropriately Blaming Patients	

How Common Is Hypertension?

Hypertension is the most common chronic condition seen by primary care clinicians. It is the "bread and butter" of office practice, resulting in approximately 90 million office visits per year in the United States. The population's awareness of hypertension has increased over the last two decades, and there has been a progressive decline in blood pressure-related morbidity and mortality rates during that time (Fig. 3-1). However, new data suggest that during the late 1990s, the public's awareness of hypertension may have decreased, and the decline in blood pressure-related mortality rates has leveled off. It is now estimated that about 50 million Americans have elevated blood pressure, of whom up to 75 percent have not achieved satisfactory blood pressure control.

The nomenclature and definition of hypertension pose problems for both patients and clinicians. For patients, the nomenclature implies a condition in which patients are either "hyper" or "tense," creating misunderstandings about the cause and symptoms of high blood pressure. It is not surprising, therefore, that patients have manifested various negative feelings and behaviors after being diagnosed as "hypertensive," including lowered self-esteem, increased sickness behavior, and increased absenteeism from work, all of which have a deleterious effect on their quality of life.

For clinicians, difficulty is created by the common definition of hypertension, which is a persistent elevation of blood pressure to above 140 mmHg systolic and 90 mmHg diastolic. This definition does not recognize that elevation of only the systolic or only the diastolic blood pressure is associated with increased rates of cardiovascular disease, renal disease, and mortality. Nor does it recognize that there is actually a continuum of risk associated with blood pressures, rather than a specific point at which risk begins. Indeed, epidemiologic studies show that morbidity and mortality rates rise progressively as both (or either) systolic and diastolic blood pressures increase. The progressive increase in morbidity and mortality rates occurs even within what is considered the high-normal range for blood pressures (i.e., diastolic pressures from 80 to 90 mmHg and systolic pressure from 120 to 140 mmHg) as well as at higher blood pressure levels.

The recognition that both systolic and diastolic blood pressures are independent variables for hypertension-related sequelae, as well as recognition of the risk associated with so-called "high-normal" or "borderline" hypertension, has given rise to a new classification for hypertension in adults (Table 3-1). The stages of hypertension shown in Table 3-1 represent progressively increased risk for nonfatal and fatal cardiovascular and renal disease.

Figure 3-1

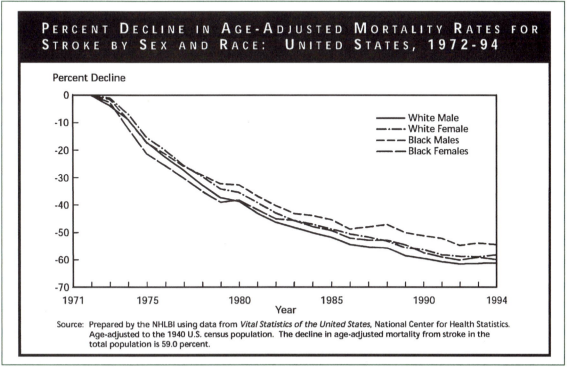

PERCENT DECLINE IN AGE-ADJUSTED MORTALITY RATES FOR STROKE BY SEX AND RACE: UNITED STATES, 1972-94

Source: Prepared by the NHLBI using data from *Vital Statistics of the United States*, National Center for Health Statistics. Age-adjusted to the 1940 U.S. census population. The decline in age-adjusted mortality from stroke in the total population is 59.0 percent.

The death rate from hypertension-related complications has been declining. Data from the U.S. National Center for Health Statistics indicate that since the 1970s there has been a progressive decline in death from stroke. A similar decrease has occurred in death from coronary artery disease. *(From Sheps et al, 1997.)*

Table 3-1

Classification of Blood Pressure in Adults

CATEGORY	SYSTOLIC, mmHg		DIASTOLIC, mmHg
Optimal	<120	and	<80
Normal	<130	and	<85
High-normal	130–139	or	85–89
Hypertension			
Stage 1	140–159	or	90–99
Stage 2	160–179	or	100–109
Stage 3	≥180	or	≥110

NOTE: Blood pressure levels are the average of two or more readings taken at each of two or more visits following an initial screening blood pressure for persons who are not taking antihypertensive medications and are not acutely ill.

SOURCE: Adapted and modified from Sheps et al, 1997.

Epidemiology

The prevalence of hypertension varies among nations, with higher rates in industrialized nations than in nonindustrialized nations. This is thought to occur, at least in part, because of the higher rates of obesity and salt consumption in industrialized countries. In addition, the measured prevalence of hypertension may be higher in countries with well-organized health care systems that are better able to detect hypertension.

In the United States, hypertension occurs more frequently in men and the elderly. The incidence of hypertension increases by approximately 10 percent for each decade over the age of 18 years, such that approximately 60 percent of adults aged 65 to 75 have elevated blood pressure. Stage 1 high blood pressure (formerly known as mild hypertension) is the most common form, and it is responsible for most hypertension-associated morbidity and mortality.

The prevalence of hypertension also differs among racial groups. Of most importance, African Americans are more likely to develop hypertension. Furthermore, when hypertension develops in African Americans, it tends to appear earlier in life, is more severe, and is associated with a greater rate of cardiovascular and renal complications than in other racial groups.

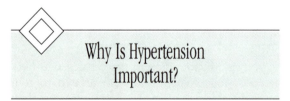

Why Is Hypertension Important?

Hypertension results in numerous pathophysiologic changes in the circulatory system. The most important of these are (1) structural alterations in arteries and arterioles that contribute to atherosclerosis and (2) hypertrophy of the myocardium. These cardiovascular changes are responsible for a variety of end-organ complications.

Hypertension-related end-organ complications most commonly involve the heart, brain, and kidneys. Some patients also develop hypertensive eye disease. Without treatment, approximately 70 percent of hypertensive patients will die of coronary artery disease or heart failure, 15 percent of cerebrovascular disease, and 10 percent of renal failure. Fortunately, as a result of blood pressure education and control efforts over the last two decades, mortality rates from coronary heart disease and stroke have decreased by 50 and 57 percent, respectively.

Hypertensive Heart Disease

Heart disease is the principal cause of death in persons with hypertension. The major cardiac manifestations of hypertension are atherosclerotic coronary artery disease and congestive heart failure. In many patients, atherogenic risk factors such as hyperlipidemia, smoking, and hyperinsulinemia are also present, and they further contribute to the prevalence and severity of cardiovascular complications. However, uncontrolled hypertension represents a stronger risk for heart disease than do these other factors.

CORONARY ARTERY DISEASE

About 11 million people in the United States have coronary artery disease, and 1.5 million of them have myocardial infarctions each year, from which the death rate is about 30 percent. Hypertension is a major contributor to coronary artery disease and myocardial infarction.

In hypertension, changes in arterial and arteriolar structure contribute to development of atherosclerotic plaques, with arterial narrowing throughout the systemic circulation, including the coronary arteries. Most myocardial infarctions occur when a coronary artery plaque becomes unstable and fissures, leading to platelet aggregation and thrombus formation with occlusion of the involved coronary artery.

In addition to contributing to coronary artery atherosclerosis, elevated systemic arterial pressure increases the work load on the heart, thereby increasing myocardial oxygen requirements. The combination of increased oxygen demand and a limited coronary circulation that is unable to meet these oxygen requirements predisposes hypertensive patients to myocardial ischemia, clinically manifested as angina and/or myocardial infarction. Inability of the coronary circulation to meet oxygen requirements typically occurs when the cross-sectional diameter of a coronary artery is reduced to about 75 percent of normal.

Coronary ischemia also predisposes to cardiac rhythm disturbances, including lethal arrhythmias (usually ventricular tachycardia or fibrillation), which cause sudden death. Sudden death may occur without premonitory symptoms and thus be the first manifestation of coronary artery disease.

CONGESTIVE HEART FAILURE

Congestive heart failure is the major cause of hospitalization in the United States. Each year in the United States, about 400,000 persons develop and 40,000 die from congestive heart failure. While the rates of many cardiovascular conditions (e.g., myocardial infarction) have been decreasing in the United States, the incidence and prevalence of congestive heart failure is increasing. In the majority of cases, heart failure is caused either by chronic hypertension or by coronary artery disease (to which hypertension is a major contributor).

In persons with hypertension, the left ventricular muscle undergoes compensatory thickening in response to increased systemic vascular pressure. In fact, echocardiographic studies suggest that as many as 50 percent of hypertensive patients have some degree of left ventricular hypertrophy (LVH). This initial ventricular enlargement is often viewed as an adaptive response to increased systemic vascular resistance, but LVH is a significant risk factor for ventricu-

lar arrhythmias and sudden death, as well as for myocardial ischemia, because of the increased oxygen requirements of hypertrophied cardiac muscle.

With sustained hypertension, the ventricular chamber becomes dilated, ventricular function deteriorates, and clinical congestive heart failure develops. Heart failure is often the result of impaired systolic function, especially when coronary ischemia or infarction further diminishes ventricular contractile function. However, diastolic dysfunction can also occur when chronic hypertrophy impairs the ability of the ventricle to relax during diastole. Control of hypertension can prevent development of heart failure from both systolic and diastolic dysfunction.

Cerebrovascular Disease

Improved awareness and treatment of hypertension has led to a decrease in death from stroke over the last 25 years. Nonetheless, over 400,000 persons in the United States suffer a stroke each year. About half of these individuals die, and many survivors have chronic neurologic disabilities. About 85 to 90 percent of strokes are caused by ischemia, due either to intracerebral atherosclerotic disease or embolism from the cerebrovascular circulation or from the heart. The remaining 10 to 15 percent of strokes are the result of intracerebral hemorrhage. For all of these pathogenic mechanisms, hypertension is a major risk factor. Elderly individuals with isolated systolic hypertension are at two to four times greater risk of stroke than their normotensive peers.

Severe uncontrolled hypertension can also cause an acute syndrome of hypertensive encephalopathy. The clinical syndrome includes extreme elevation of blood pressure, impaired consciousness, and papilledema; seizures and death may occur. The precise pathophysiologic mechanisms are uncertain, but disordered cerebral circulatory function is probably involved.

Renal Disease

Each year, approximately 140,000 Americans develop hypertension-related impairment of renal function, and 5300 develop hypertension-related end-stage renal disease; recent evidence indicates that the incidence of hypertension-related renal impairment is increasing. The most common pathophysiologic mechanisms in hypertensive renal disease are atherosclerosis of the large arteries of the kidney and thickening with deposition of lipoproteinaceous material in the walls of the efferent arterioles (arteriolar nephrosclerosis). In some patients, the process progresses to "malignant" arteriolar nephrosclerosis, with necrosis of arterioles. This malignant form of hypertensive renal disease can progress rapidly to end-stage renal failure and is more common in persons of African descent. By controlling blood pressure, renal function can be preserved and progression of renal failure slowed.

Eye Disease

Persons with hypertension can develop vascular changes in the retina of the eye [Fig. 3-2 (Plate 1)]. Milder changes of hypertensive retinopathy include narrowing and focal spasm of arterioles. With more advanced retinopathy, obliteration of arterioles may occur, along with retinal hemorrhages and exudates. These retinal lesions may produce scotomata or even blindness if they involve the macular area of the retina.

Hypertension is also a risk factor for occlusion of the central retinal vein or one of its branches [Fig. 3-3 (Plate 2)]. This is a serious condition that may sometimes resolve spontaneously but that can also progress to overt retinal hemorrhage and visual loss.

Figure 3-2 (Plate 1)

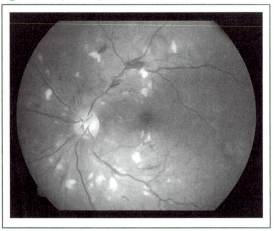

In hypertensive retinopathy, the retina may develop flame, or splinter, hemorrhages (seen in the upper part of the photo) and cotton wool spots (light-colored areas), which represent infarction of the nerve fiber layer of the retina. *(Reproduced with permission from AS Fauci et al, eds: Harrison's Principles of Internal Medicine. New York, McGraw-Hill, 1998.)*

Figure 3-3 (Plate 2)

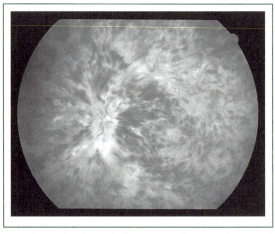

Central retinal vein occlusion can produce massive retinal hemorrhage, retinal ischemia, and visual loss. Its typical appearance, shown in this fundus photograph, is of "blood and thunder." *(Reproduced with permission from AS Fauci et al, eds, Harrison's Principles of Internal Medicine. New York, McGraw-Hill, 1998.)*

Principal Diagnoses

Hypertension is typically classified as either primary or secondary. Secondary hypertension is hypertension for which a specific underlying (and sometimes reversible) cause can be identified. Primary hypertension, also referred to as "essential" hypertension, is blood pressure elevation for which an underlying cause cannot be determined. In evaluating patients in primary care practice, the principal diagnosis to consider is essential hypertension. However, clinicians should always consider the possibility that a secondary cause is responsible for blood pressure elevation.

Essential Hypertension

The vast majority (over 95 percent) of hypertensive patients seen in primary care practice have "essential," or primary, hypertension. There has been a plethora of hypotheses regarding the pathogenesis of essential hypertension, including theories regarding genetics, diet, socioeconomics, and the renin-angiotensin system. However, no unifying theory has been generated. In any given individual, hypertension probably represents a complex interaction between these factors, which converge in a final common pathway that ultimately results in increased peripheral resistance, manifested clinically as hypertension.

GENETICS

It is likely that many individuals have a genetic predisposition to develop hypertension, but the mode of inheritance is complex and has not been delineated. Persons of African descent have higher rates and greater severity of hypertension, presumably due to genetic factors. It is likely that, when a genetically predisposed individual is exposed to "triggering" environmental influences, hypertension develops. Environmental influences may include diet and socioeconomic factors.

DIET

A number of dietary factors have been linked to the genesis of hypertension. The most well studied of these are obesity and dietary intake of sodium, potassium, and calcium.

OBESITY   As described in Chap. 2, "Obesity," excess body weight is associated with hypertension. The mechanism for this relationship probably involves obesity-related hyperinsulinemia and its effects on renal sodium retention.

SODIUM   The link between sodium intake and hypertension is demonstrated by comparing diets in nonindustrialized societies with diets in industrialized nations. In nonindustrialized societies with low-sodium diets, hypertension is uncommon, and adult blood pressures are considerably lower than "normal" blood pressures in industrialized nations with higher sodium intakes. However, sodium intake is not involved in all cases of hypertension. In fact, sensitivity to sodium is thought to be involved in only about half of cases of essential hypertension.

POTASSIUM   Evidence suggests that high dietary potassium intake lowers the risk of hypertension and inadequate dietary potassium intake increases blood pressure. However, dietary potassium is not thought to be a key factor in the cause of most patients' hypertension.

CALCIUM   Calcium intake has also been linked to hypertension. Epidemiologic studies have shown that populations living in areas with "hard" water (i.e., water with higher mineral content, including calcium) tend to have lower rates of hypertension than populations in "soft"-water areas. Conversely, populations with low-calcium diets tend to have higher blood pressures. The significance of these findings for prevention and treatment of essential hypertension is unclear, however, and there is insufficient evidence to support recommending calcium supplementation to prevent hypertension.

SOCIOECONOMICS

Hypertension is more frequent among those living in large families and/or crowded living conditions. It is also more common in "white collar" workers with high-stress occupations. The physiologic basis for these relationships is unclear.

RENIN-ANGIOTENSIN SYSTEM

Renin, an enzyme secreted by juxtaglomerular cells of the kidney in response to low circulatory blood volume or decreased renal blood flow, is probably involved in the pathogenesis of essential hypertension. When released into the circulation, the enzymatic activity of renin results in production of the vasoconstricting substance angiotensin II. Several studies have shown that some patients with hypertension have low plasma renin activity, others have normal renin levels, and still others have high renin activity. However, despite numerous attempts to translate these abnormalities into meaningful diagnostic and therapeutic categories, the significance and practical application of these findings remain unclear. Nonetheless, suspicion remains that the renin-angiotensin system plays a role in many cases of essential hypertension.

Secondary Hypertension

A variety of identifiable conditions can cause "secondary" hypertension. Chronic alcohol ingestion may be the most common, followed by renal disease. Other secondary causes are uncommon in primary care practice and some, such as pheochromocytoma, Cushing's syndrome, and coarctation of the aorta, may never be encountered in the practice career of a primary care clinician. Still others, such as sleep apnea or medication-induced hypertension, may be relatively common, although the incidence is unknown. However, because all of these conditions have important therapeutic and/or prognostic implications, they each should be considered as possible diagnoses when evaluating patients with hypertension.

ALCOHOL INGESTION

Alcohol ingestion is a frequently unrecognized cause of hypertension. In contrast to the ability of alcohol to lower cardiovascular disease risk when consumed in small quantities, larger quantities of alcohol are associated with development of hypertension. There is a direct linear relationship between alcohol use and blood pressure that begins with daily alcohol ingestion in excess of two drinks (with a drink defined as a 12-oz glass of beer, a 5-oz glass of wine, or a 1-oz shot of hard liquor). Considering the widespread use and abuse of this substance, some experts believe that as much as 10 percent of supposed essential hypertension in men may be related to alcohol, but most cases are unrecognized. In addition to causing hypertension, chronic alcohol ingestion also may explain some patients' apparent refractoriness to treatment of hypertension.

The mechanism for the association between alcohol ingestion and hypertension is unclear. Alcohol may exert its hypertensive effect by stimulating the sympathetic nervous system, increasing insulin resistance, increasing cortisol secretion, and/or inducing cellular changes that affect calcium and sodium transport.

RENAL DISEASE

Patients with primary renal diseases develop hypertension. Renal disease is probably responsible for between 2 and 5 percent of all cases of hypertension. Several forms of renal disease can cause hypertension; they fall into two major categories.

One important category is renovascular disease, in which renal hypoperfusion develops because of atherosclerotic renal artery stenosis, fibromuscular dysplasia of the renal artery, or inflammatory disease involving the renal arteries. Decreased perfusion of the kidney leads to release of renin and subsequent angiotensin II-induced vasoconstriction. Surgical or angioplastic repair of stenotic renal artery lesions can result in significant reduction in blood pressure.

The other major category of hypertension-inducing renal problems is parenchymal disease, such as acute or chronic glomerulonephritis, diabetic nephropathy, or polycystic kidney disease. While these processes are not generally reversible, control of blood pressure is important to prevent development of a vicious cycle whereby hypertension worsens renal disease, resulting in further blood pressure elevation and continued deterioration of renal function.

ENDOCRINE DISORDERS

The most common endocrine disorders that can cause hypertension are hyperthyroidism, pheochromocytoma, primary hyperaldosteronism, and Cushing's syndrome.

HYPERTHYROIDISM Hyperthyroidism is relatively common and is often associated with tachycardia and hypertension. Because it is easily treatable, hyperthyroidism should be considered as a cause of hypertension in all patients with elevated blood pressure.

PHEOCHROMOCYTOMA Pheochromocytoma occurs in less than 1 of every 10,000 persons with hypertension. Pheochromocytomas are chromaffin-cell tumors that synthesize, store, and secrete catecholamines (the name "*pheochromocytoma*" refers to the affinity of the tumor cells for chromium-containing histologic stains). Pheochromocytoma occurs predominantly in the adrenal medulla. However, in 15 percent of adults and 30 percent of children with pheochromocytoma, the tumor develops in extraadrenal chromaffin tissue.

The classic presentation of pheochromocytoma consists of severe, symptomatic hypertensive episodes that may include palpitations, tachycardia, headache, sweating, agitation, pallor, and/or tremulousness. The timing and severity of the symptoms, however, are related to the pattern of catecholamine secretion. With paroxysmal secretion, the classic symptom complex may occur. However, in more than half of patients with pheochromocytoma, catecholamine secretion is continuous, resulting in chronic, sustained, and sometimes marked, hypertension.

PRIMARY HYPERALDOSTERONISM Usually seen in patients between the ages of 30 and 50, primary hyperaldosteronism accounts for approximately 1 in 200 cases of hypertension. It results from secretion of excessive amounts of aldosterone produced by either a solitary adrenal adenoma or by bilateral hyperplasia or adenomas of the adrenal cortex. Surgical removal of the lesions can reduce blood pressure substantially.

The typical clinical presentation of primary hyperaldosteronism is hypertension with unexplained hypokalemia. The hypertension is caused by aldosterone-induced vasoconstriction and sodium retention. Hypokalemia results from aldosterone-induced hyperkaluria.

CUSHING'S SYNDROME Cushing's syndrome is the result of excessive glucocorticoid (cortisol) secretion from adrenal tumors or hyperplasia, ectopic tumors that produce adrenocorticotropic hormone (ACTH), or ACTH hypersecretion from the pituitary gland (Cushing's disease). Besides hypertension, which is present in about 80 percent of cases, the typical syndrome includes features such as truncal obesity, hirsutism, purple cutaneous striae, bruising, edema, menstrual irregularities, and emotional changes (ranging from depression to overt psychosis).

The commonly cited explanation for hypertension in Cushing's syndrome is the sodium-retaining property of cortisol. However, other adrenal mineralocorticoids and renin activity may also contribute to the sodium retention and increased peripheral vascular resistance that occur in Cushing's syndrome.

COARCTATION OF THE AORTA

Coarctation is a congenital narrowing of the aorta that most commonly occurs just distal to the origin of the left subclavian artery. Presentation is typically in infancy or childhood, but with less severe narrowing the condition may not be recognized until later in life. Coarctation of the aorta should be suspected when hypertension is present in the upper extremities in association with weak femoral pulses. The mechanism of hypertension is probably renal hypoperfusion distal to the aortic constriction, causing activation of the renin-angiotensin system.

SLEEP APNEA

Obstructive sleep apnea is characterized by intermittent soft tissue airway obstruction during sleep, generally in the pharynx or hypopharynx. While its true prevalence is unknown, obstructive sleep apnea is thought to' occur in about one-fifth of community-dwelling geriatric-aged individuals. Thus, sleep apnea is probably a more common cause of hypertension than realized, perhaps accounting for 1 percent or more of hypertension cases.

The relationship between sleep apnea and hypertension may partly be explained by the obesity that frequently accompanies sleep apnea, since obesity is associated with both sleep apnea and hypertension. The hypertension of sleep apnea may also be related to the catecholamine release and increased systemic vascular resistance that occur in response to apnea-related hypoxemia and hypercapnia. In addition to hypertension, obstructive sleep apnea has also been associated with a number of other cardiovascular problems, including coronary artery disease, stroke, left ventricular hypertrophy, and dilated cardiomyopathy.

The syndrome of obstructive sleep apnea is characterized by loud snoring, typically in overweight, middle-aged men, which may be followed by periods of apnea that are terminated by gasping or snorting. This disruptive sleep results in daytime somnolence and morning headaches. A polysomnographic sleep study is usually required for definitive diagnosis.

MEDICATIONS

A number of medications can cause hypertension, and medication-induced hypertension should always be considered. Several common nonprescription medications have been linked to hypertension when ingested on a chronic basis. These medications include nonsteroidal anti-inflammatory drugs, sodium-containing antacids, decongestants (e.g., pseudoephedrine), and various drugs used for treatment of obesity, including sibutramine and appetite suppressants such as phenylpropanolamine. Hypertension is also caused by several prescription medications, including cyclosporin, steroids, erythropoetin, monoamine oxidase inhibitors, and bromocriptine. Finally, illicit drugs, such as cocaine and amphetamines, can cause hypertension; these drugs should be considered, especially with severe hypertension or when complications such as stroke or myocardial infarction occur early in the course of hypertension. Use of any of these prescription or nonprescription drugs can also explain a poor response to treatment of hypertension.

Typical Presentation

Hypertension is usually asymptomatic and is typically discovered incidentally during a routine office visit or during investigation of symptoms associated with some other problem, including hypertension-related end-organ damage. Usually, it is a primary care clinician who detects and evaluates hypertension. Occasionally, however, patients may be referred to a specialist, such as a cardiologist, when elevated blood pressures are detected through mass screenings or when surgical or other limited specialists detect hypertension and refer patients to cardiologists. Evaluation and management, however, are essentially the same regardless of the specialty of the clinician seeing the patient.

Another presentation of hypertension is that of patients complaining of apparent "pressure-related" symptoms, such as headache, dizziness, or lightheadedness. These individuals may have hypertension. However, such symptoms are commonly independent of hypertension, or, if elevated blood pressure is found, it may be a temporary manifestation of pain or anxiety associated with a patient's symptoms.

A third common presentation is that of hypertension that has been treated in the past but that is currently untreated. Many patients assume that they are aware of when their pressure is high, believing that feelings of anxiety or tension signal a rise in blood pressure. This erroneous perception leads some patients to believe their hypertension has resolved when there are no reinforcing symptoms, and they discontinue their medication. Then, at a future date, hypertension is detected again by a subsequent clinician. Finally, some patients who know they have hypertension may avoid standard medical care altogether and instead attempt self-treatment with relaxation to be less "hypertense."

Key History

The primary focus of the history is to (1) evaluate cardiovascular risk and need for treatment, (2) identify modifiable life-style factors, (3) elucidate symptoms suggesting secondary hypertension, and (4) screen for future noncompliance. Topics that should be covered in the history are listed in Table 3-2. Clinicians should also inquire as to the patient's understanding of blood pressure complications and treatment side effects. This conversation will provide an opportunity to clarify misunderstandings, as well as deal proactively with potential compliance problems.

In addition to the questions listed in Table 3-2, it is appropriate to ask men about sexual function, since impotence is often attributed to the use of antihypertensive medications. While antihypertensive medications can cause impotence, it may also occur in up to one-third of untreated hypertensive men as a result of psychosocial problems or penile vascular insufficiency.

Headaches are also a common concern, but they usually only occur in patients with severe hypertension. Distinguishing characteristics of hypertension-related headaches include presence upon awakening and location in the occipital area. Early-morning headaches also occur with sleep apnea.

Finally, the history should be used to identify situations that might contraindicate use of certain pharmacologic therapies. For example, patients with asthma or tightly controlled insulin-dependent diabetes are usually poor candidates for treatment with beta blockers. Patients with gout may not be good candidates for diuretic therapy, since diuretics raise uric acid levels. Other drugs that interact with antihypertensive medications are listed in Table 3-3.

Physical Examination

The most important aspect of the examination is to establish whether hypertension does indeed exist. Additional objectives of the examination are to detect evidence of secondary hypertension and identify signs of end-organ damage.

Measuring Blood Pressure

A critical, but often overlooked, aspect of the examination is the method by which blood pressure is measured. Patients often have rushed to or are late for an appointment, leading to short-term anxiety that may result in elevated blood pressure readings if sufficient time (usually at

Table 3-2

Topics for Questions in the History of Patients with Hypertension

ASSESSING CARDIOVASCULAR RISK
Family history of high blood pressure, premature coronary heart disease, stroke, diabetes mellitus, or dyslipidemia History or symptoms of cardiovascular, cerebrovascular, or renal disease; diabetes; or dyslipidemia Duration and level of hypertension
IDENTIFYING MODIFIABLE LIFE-STYLE FACTORS
Need for weight loss or smoking cessation Leisure-time physical activities Intake of sodium, alcohol, cholesterol, and saturated fats
IDENTIFYING CLUES TO SECONDARY HYPERTENSION
Muscle weakness, kidney problems, episodes of tachycardia, sweating, or tremor Alcohol use Use of prescribed and/or nonprescription medications
IDENTIFYING RISKS FOR NONCOMPLIANCE
Results and side effects of previous antihypertensive therapy Psychosocial and environmental factors (e.g., unstable family situation, employment status, or working conditions; poverty; and illiteracy or low educational level)

SOURCE: Adapted and modified from Sheps et al, 1997.

Table 3-3

Medications That May Interact with Antihypertensive Medications

MEDICATION	INTERACTION
Antacids	Decrease effect of ACE inhibitors
Antidepressants	Decrease effect of clonidine and other central alpha$_2$ agonists
Cyclosporin	Cyclosporin levels raised by some calcium channel blockers
Hepatic enzyme antagonists (e.g., cimetidine)	Increase effect of beta blockers and calcium antagonists
Hepatic enzyme inducers (e.g., rifampin, phenobarbital)	Decrease effect of calcium antagonists
Lithium	Lithium levels raised by diuretics, ACE inhibitors
NSAIDs	Decrease effect of diuretics, beta blockers, ACE inhibitors
Steroids	Decrease effect of diuretics

ABBREVIATIONS: ACE, angiotensin-converting enzyme;
NSAIDs, nonsteroidal anti-inflammatory drugs.
SOURCE: Adapted and modified from Sheps et al, 1997.

least 5 min) is not provided for relaxation. Other factors, such as smoking a cigarette or drinking coffee within 30 min of measurement, can also temporarily elevate blood pressure.

To ensure standardization of results, the following technique should be used to measure blood pressure. First, patients should rest for at least 5 min and then be seated with their arm bared and supported at heart level. Second, it is essential to use an appropriate-size cuff. The bladder of the cuff should nearly (at least 80 percent) or completely encircle the patient's arm. Blood pressure is then measured with a mercury sphygmomanometer, a recently calibrated aneroid manometer, or a calibrated electronic device. Both systolic and diastolic pressures should be recorded, using disappearance of sound (Korotkoff phase V) for the diastolic reading.

Two or more readings separated by at least 2 min should be averaged, and if the first two readings differ by more than 5 mmHg, additional readings should be obtained. If blood pressure is increased, elevated pressure should be verified in the contralateral arm. If values are different in each arm, the higher value should be used.

After detecting an elevated blood pressure, it should be confirmed on at least two subsequent visits at a follow-up interval determined by the initial reading (Table 3-4). If blood pressure is 180 mmHg systolic and/or 110 mmHg diastolic or greater, management should be begin within

1 week. Treatment should begin immediately if patients have symptoms of acute cardiac, renal, or central nervous system dysfunction.

Detecting Causes of Secondary Hypertension

The patient's body habitus should be noted, as truncal obesity and purple striae may indicate the presence of Cushing's syndrome. Signs of hyperthyroidism, such as tremor, exophthalmos, and thyroid enlargement, should also be sought.

Examination of the abdomen may reveal renal artery or aortic bruits, or enlarged kidneys, suggesting the possibility of renovascular hypertension or polycystic kidneys, respectively. Absent or reduced femoral pulses indicate the possibility of aortic coarctation.

Detecting End-Organ Damage

Ophthalmoscopic examination of the retina should be performed to detect signs of hypertensive retinopathy. In the earliest stage (stage 1) of hypertensive retinopathy, narrowing of arterioles is seen. In stage 2 retinopathy, "nicking" of retinal veins occurs where they are crossed by rigid arterioles. Stage 3 hypertensive retinopathy [Fig. 3-2 (Plate 1)] is manifested as hemorrhages

Table 3-4

Recommended Follow-Up Interval Based on Initial Blood Pressure

INITIAL BLOOD PRESSURE, MMHG		FOLLOW-UP INTERVAL
SYSTOLIC	DIASTOLIC	
<130	<85	Recheck in 2 years
130–139	85–89	Recheck in 1 year
140–159	90–99	Confirm within 2 months
160–179	100–109	Evaluate within 1 month
≥180	≥110	Evaluate within 1 week or immediately, depending on clinical situation

NOTE: If systolic and diastolic pressures are in different categories, follow-up should be based on the pressure warranting the shorter follow-up interval.
SOURCE: Adapted and modified from Sheps et al, 1997.

and exudates. Papilledema occurs in stage 4 retinopathy.

Neck examination should include auscultation of the carotid arteries to detect bruits, suggestive of carotid artery stenosis. The heart should be examined for evidence of left ventricular enlargement (manifested as a precordial heave and displaced point of maximal impulse) or aortic regurgitation (which causes systolic hypertension). The lungs should be examined to check for the presence of rales, suggestive of congestive heart failure.

Vascular examination may detect a pulsatile mass in the abdomen, suggesting abdominal aortic aneurysm. It may also reveal peripheral vascular disease, as evidenced by bruits or reduced pulses in the lower extremities.

Ancillary Tests

A variety of laboratory tests have been recommended for evaluating patients with hypertension. As with the history and physical examination, the purpose of ancillary tests is to assess other risks for cardiovascular disease, detect evidence of secondary hypertension, and identify the presence of end-organ damage. In addition, home and ambulatory blood pressure monitoring can be used when the presence or control of hypertension is in doubt.

Tests for Other Cardiovascular Risk Factors

Blood testing should be performed to measure fasting glucose or glycosylated hemoglobin levels for detection of diabetes, and fasting lipid levels to detect hyperlipidemia. Lipid profiles should usually include total cholesterol, high-density cholesterol, and triglyceride. Measurement of low-density lipoproteins should be performed if the total cholesterol level is high.

Tests to Detect Secondary Hypertension

Serum electrolytes and creatinine levels are measured, and urinalysis is performed, to detect clues to causes of secondary hypertension, such as hyperaldosteronism and renal disease. Thyroid function tests are appropriate if hyperthyroidism is suspected. Appropriate endocrine tests are needed if there is suspicion of any of the syndromes discussed above.

Tests for End-Organ Damage

A 12-lead electrocardiography (ECG) is often performed in patients with hypertension to detect evidence of LVH. Unfortunately, ECG is an insensitive tool for detecting LVH, since it identifies LVH in only 5 to 10 percent of persons with hypertension. Based on echocardiographic studies, however, some degree of LVH is present in up to half of hypertensives. This has led some experts to recommend echocardiographic screening of patients with hypertension to detect LVH. Limited M-mode scanning, directed specifically at LVH detection, is the most widely used approach. The clinical relevance of occult LVH detected by ultrasound, however, is unclear.

Renal end-organ damage can be detected by the presence of proteinuria or diminished glomerular function; urinalysis and measurement of serum creatinine levels are the standard tests. Measurements of creatinine clearance and urinary protein excretion may be useful in some patients.

Tests to Confirm the Presence or Control of Hypertension

Blood pressure measurements performed outside a clinician's office may provide more accurate assessments of blood pressure control than in-office measurements. These out-of-office measurements are performed at home by the patient using a personal sphygmomanometer or with a continuous ambulatory blood pressure monitor.

PERSONAL BLOOD PRESSURE MONITORS

While mercury sphygmomanometers are the most accurate, they are expensive and often difficult for patients to use. A variety of home devices, which use aneroid or electronic mechanisms, are available for measuring blood pressure, and they are reasonably accurate compared to mercury devices. Finger blood pressure monitors, however, are not sufficiently accurate to provide reliable measurements of blood pressure.

CONTINUOUS AMBULATORY BLOOD PRESSURE MONITORS

Ambulatory blood pressure monitors are electronic devices that are programmed to take blood pressure readings throughout the day and night, typically every 15 to 30 min. Results are stored in the device and then downloaded and analyzed on a computer.

While not part of the routine evaluation of hypertension, ambulatory blood pressure monitoring provides an opportunity to evaluate blood pressure in a more natural setting than a clinician's office. There is strong evidence that target-organ damage may correlate better with ambulatory blood pressure measurements than with measurements obtained during isolated office visits. However, there has been no formal evaluation of managing blood pressure solely with ambulatory blood pressure measurements, and the cost of using these devices for routine treatment would be high.

Currently, there are several situations in which continuous ambulatory blood pressure monitoring devices are considered useful. The most frequent is when a clinician suspects "office," or "white coat," hypertension, a situation in which blood pressure is repeatedly elevated in the office setting but repeatedly normal out of the office. In some studies, fully one-third of persons thought to be hypertensive based on office blood pressure measurements are not really hypertensive. Rather, they were falsely designated as hypertensive based on an office measurement. Other uses of continuous monitoring devices include the evaluation of patients who respond poorly to treatment, measuring night-time blood pressure, detecting episodic hypertension (e.g., in pheochromocytoma), and identifying hypotensive symptoms associated with antihypertensive medications or autonomic dysfunction.

Algorithm

The algorithm (Fig. 3-4) outlines the basic diagnostic and management approach to hypertension. After confirming the diagnosis of hypertension and excluding secondary causes, treatment is instituted. Appropriate initial treatment almost always includes lifestyle modifications, as outlined below. Medications are used if lifestyle modifications fail to control blood pressure or, depending on the severity of hypertension, as part of the initial treatment regimen.

Treatment

The goal of hypertension treatment is to prevent end-organ complications by lowering blood pressure through lifestyle modifications and pharmacotherapy. The traditional target for treatment is to lower blood pressure to below 140 mmHg systolic and below 90 mmHg diastolic. However, the sixth report from the Joint National Committee (JNC-VI) on the Prevention, Detection, Evaluation and Treatment of High Blood Pressure, issued in late 1997, suggests that 130/80 mmHg may be a more appropriate goal if it can be achieved without treatment side effects. This lower level is particularly appropriate for persons over 60 years of age and for those with cardiovascular risk factors, such as smoking, hy-

Figure 3-4

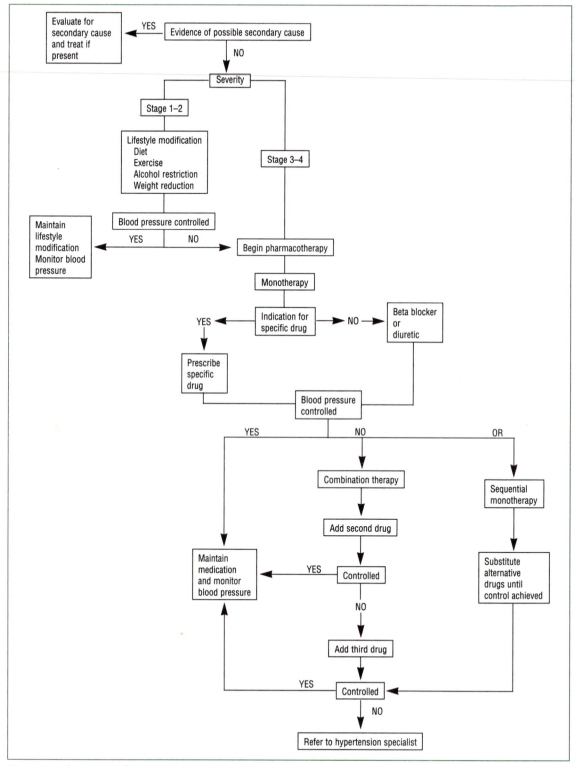

Diagnosis and treatment of hypertension.

perlipidemia, diabetes, or a family history of premature cardiovascular disease. Patients with renal insufficiency and proteinuria (more than 1 g/d) should have a goal blood pressure of 125/75 mmHg.

Lifestyle Modifications

Lifestyle modification is an appropriate initial step in all stages of hypertension, although most patients will also require pharmacotherapy for optimal blood pressure control. Even though stages 3 and 4 hypertension will almost always necessitate pharmacotherapy, appropriate lifestyle modification will enhance the effect of such therapy and probably further reduce the risk of cardiovascular disease. Lifestyle modifications include changes in diet and exercise patterns, and smoking cessation for those who smoke. Studies of relaxation interventions, such as biofeedback and meditation, have had equivocal results, and these interventions are not recommended as standard treatments.

DIET

Dietary change is difficult for most patients. Hence, they must be informed of the rationale for and anticipated benefits of diet modification to help motivate the personal investment of energy required to successfully alter dietary habits. For most clinicians and patients, dietary modification will require consultation with a nutrition expert, since simply providing patients with diet information handouts or basic diet instructions is generally insufficient to evoke major dietary change. Clinicians can reinforce successful diet modifications with positive comments and by pointing out favorable changes in blood pressure, lipid levels, glucose levels, and weight when they occur.

SODIUM Individuals vary widely in their response to sodium intake, but it is generally recommended that all persons with hypertension aim to keep daily sodium intake below 2.4 g

(6 g of salt). Many individuals can achieve even lower intakes of sodium, which may be worthwhile if their hypertension is salt-sensitive. Reduction in consumption of processed foods and overtly salty foods, the principal sources of sodium in most American diets, is the most effective first step in reducing salt intake. On average, dietary sodium restriction will lower systolic blood pressure by about 6 mmHg and diastolic pressure by about 2 mmHg.

POTASSIUM AND CALCIUM Addition of potassium to the diet, ideally via fruits and vegetables, may improve blood pressure control. Patients on low-sodium diets may elect to use a potassium-chloride salt substitute as long as they have normal renal function and are not taking potassium-sparing diuretics. Because some data indicate that higher dietary intakes of calcium are associated with lower blood pressure, adequacy of calcium intake should be assured.

WEIGHT REDUCTION Research indicates that as many as 60 percent of overweight patients with mild hypertension may be able to control blood pressure with weight reduction alone. If antihypertensive medications are necessary, weight loss will enhance the effect of the medications. While achievement of ideal body weight is an unrealistic goal for most overweight patients, loss of even 10 to 15 percent of body weight is associated with substantial changes in blood pressure. In fact, a 20-lb weight loss has been associated with a reduction in blood pressure of as much as 26 mmHg systolic and 20 mmHg diastolic. Additional information about weight loss is provided in Chap. 2.

EXERCISE

Regular exercise is associated with lower blood pressure and also with weight reduction, improved glucose levels and insulin resistance, and better sleep. In contrast to dietary counseling, for which a nutritional expert is generally required, clinicians can often prescribe an exercise program themselves.

To be successful, an exercise plan must fit a patient's lifestyle. However, since a substantial majority of hypertensive patients do not exercise, an exercise program will represent a major life-style change for them. Thus, to facilitate this change, patients should be offered specific programs they can realistically follow. Clinicians should inquire about activities that patients enjoy and to which they have access. Exercise programs may begin with as little as 3 to 4 min of brisk walking daily and progress from there. The goal, however, is to have at least moderate aerobic physical activity (e.g., brisk walking or more strenuous activity) for 30 to 45 min on most or all days of the week. Men over 40, women over 50 (or younger if they are postmenopausal), or anyone with multiple risk factors for coronary artery disease should be evaluated for coronary artery disease before initiating a vigorous exercise program. Typically, this evaluation involves an exercise treadmill test.

SMOKING CESSATION

Because cigarette smoking raises blood pressure and is a strong risk factor for cardiovascular disease, it is essential that patients with hypertension be counseled not to smoke. The recommended approach to smoking cessation is described in Chap. 1.

Pharmacotherapy

Despite institution of lifestyle modifications, most patients with hypertension eventually require pharmacotherapy. Thus, clinicians must be familiar with the approach to pharmacotherapy, and the advantages and disadvantages of the various classes of antihypertensive medication.

The general approach to drug therapy is to begin treatment and attempt to achieve blood pressure control with one medication (monotherapy). If unacceptable side effects occur with this initial medication, the clinician should substitute a drug from another class. There are suf-

ficient alternative medications so that satisfactory blood pressure control can be achieved in nearly all patients without unacceptable side effects.

If the initial medication is tolerated without adverse effects but blood pressure is not controlled at the target level (140/90 mmHg for most patients), the clinician must consider using an alternative medication. This is a common scenario, because no single agent used for stages 1 and 2 hypertension is routinely effective as monotherapy for more than 50 to 60 percent of patients. There are two possible approaches when control is not achieved with the initial medication. One approach is to add a second drug from a different class. In general, the second drug should be a diuretic if the first drug was not. The other approach is "sequential monotherapy," which is the substitution of a drug from a different class in an attempt to achieve control with a single medication. Either approach is acceptable, but many clinicians prefer sequential monotherapy because, if successful, monotherapy yields the highest compliance and satisfaction from patients. However, if a patient's preference, economics, or other factors (e.g., concomitant medical illnesses) so dictate, combination therapy may be the treatment of choice.

SELECTING INITIAL THERAPY

Major consensus groups, such as the JNC-VI, have concluded that, all things being equal, beta blockers or diuretics should be the initial therapy for uncomplicated hypertension. This conclusion is based on the low cost of and long experience with these drugs, and the fact that meta-analyses of randomized, placebo-controlled trials have shown that beta blockers and diuretics lower morbidity and mortality rates from hypertension (up to a 14-percent reduction in cardiac morbidity and mortality rates and a 40-percent reduction in stroke).

However, the recommendation to use beta blockers and diuretics is by no means universally accepted. In fact, a recent study of antihypertensive-drug sales involving 35,000 retail pharmacies in the United States showed that most clinicians do not follow this recommendation. Instead, the antihypertensive medications most often prescribed in the United States are calcium channel blockers and angiotensin-converting enzyme (ACE) inhibitors. Medications from these two classes represent over 70 percent of antihypertensive prescriptions in the United States. In contrast, beta blockers and diuretics together account for only 19 percent of antihypertensive prescriptions, with other medications making up the remainder.

Most clinicians base selection of an antihypertensive agents on factors such as (1) effect on cardiac risk factors or medical conditions other than blood pressure, (2) side effect profile (including preservation of exercise and sexual function), and (3) interactions with other drugs. The low side-effect profile of ACE inhibitors has made them particularly popular with clinicians and patients. Calcium channel blockers have also been popular because they have few day-to-day side effects. However, their popularity has diminished because of concerns that these drugs (especially the immediate-release and short-acting calcium blockers) might increase the risk of myocardial ischemia and infarction. Alpha-adrenergic blockers will probably increase in popularity because they favorably affect lipid profiles in patients with hyperlipidemia.

Nonetheless, the JNC-VI report advises that beta blockers or diuretics should be the first-line treatment for uncomplicated essential hypertension that is not accompanied by other illness or risk factors. However, JNC-VI acknowledges that in a variety of special situations, other medications may be more appropriate choices for first-line treatment (Table 3-5).

Table 3-5

Selection of Medications for First-Line Treatment of Essential Hypertension

MEDICATION CLASS	INDICATIONS
Diuretics	Uncomplicated essential hypertension
	Isolated systolic hypertension in older patients
	Osteoporosis
Beta blockers	Uncomplicated essential hypertension
	Myocardial infarction
	Angina
	Atrial tachycardia and fibrillation
	Essential tremor
	Hyperthyroidism
	Migraine
ACE inhibitors	Diabetes with proteinuria or microalbuminuria
	Congestive heart failure
	Renal insufficiency
Alpha-adrenergic blockers	Hyperlipidemia
	Prostatic hypertrophy
Calcium channel blockers (long-acting, nondihydropyridine)	Isolated systolic hypertension in older patients
	Angina
	Atrial tachycardia or fibrillation
	Migraine
	Asthma

SOURCE: Adapted and modified from Sheps et al, 1997.

SPECIFIC ANTIHYPERTENSIVE MEDICATIONS

The principal medications used for antihypertensive treatment are diuretics, beta blockers, ACE inhibitors, angiotensin II-receptor blockers, alpha blockers, and calcium antagonists.

DIURETICS When diuretics are used for first-line therapy, thiazides are generally the agents of choice because of their low cost and overall tolerability. Because thiazides decrease urinary calcium excretion, they are often a good choice for patients with osteoporosis. Thiazides are also recommended for isolated systolic hypertension in older patients.

Symptomatic side effects of thiazides are limited, but some of their metabolic effects are of concern. In particular, hypokalemia (responsible on rare occasions for cardiac rhythm disturbances) occurs in a substantial percentage of patients. It is recommended, therefore, that electrolytes be checked 1 month after initiation of diuretic therapy and every 6 to 12 months thereafter. Potassium levels should be checked more often if symptoms of hypokalemia (e.g., muscle cramps or palpitations) occur.

Thiazide diuretics can also cause hyperglycemia and elevate blood lipids and therefore may not be suitable for patients with diabetes or hyperlipidemia. However, very low-dose diuretic therapy (e.g., 6.25 mg/d of hydrochlorothiazide) can be used in patients with diabetes or hyperlipidemia because at this dose thiazides have no metabolic effects and can augment blood pressure control achieved with other antihypertensive agents. Thiazides also cause hyperuricemia and therefore are not appropriate for patients with gout. Thiazide-induced hyperuricemia in the absence of gout, however, is not a contraindication to continued diuretic therapy.

Other diuretics, such as spironolactone, are also inexpensive and equally effective as thiazides in stages 1 and 2 hypertension. Because it is well tolerated at doses up to 50 mg/d and it is potassium and magnesium sparing, some experts regard spironolactone as a reasonable alternative to thiazide therapy. However, caution must be observed when using spironolactone because this medication can cause potassium retention and hyperkalemia. Hyperkalemia may occur when spironolactone is used alone but is more likely when spironolactone is used in combination with ACE inhibitors, potassium supplementation, or other potassium-sparing diuretics, or in renal failure. Spironolactone may also be inadvisable for patients with diabetes because such patients often manifest hyporeninemic hypoaldosteronism and therefore have a higher risk of hyperkalemia.

Other diuretics include loop diuretics and indapamide. Short-acting loop diuretics such as furosemide are not useful for hypertension management because they are active for only a few hours, and excessive symptomatic diuresis is a bothersome side effect. Indapamide, a diuretic that may also have calcium channel blocking actions, appears to have a beneficial effect on hypertension-related end-organ problems, such as microalbuminuria and LVH. Indapamide is also less likely than thiazides to cause hypokalemia, and it is magnesium sparing. However, the ideal role for indapamide in treating hypertension is unclear.

BETA BLOCKERS Beta blockers are the other agents recommended by JNC-VI as first-line therapy, and they are the antihypertensives of choice in a variety of special situations (Table 3-5). Because once-daily therapy enhances compliance, long-acting agents like atenolol are often preferable. However, short-acting beta blockers (e.g., propranolol) are considerably less expensive and equally effective for controlling blood pressure. Because beta blockers can worsen depression, asthma, congestive heart failure, second- or third-degree heart block, and hyperlipidemia, beta blocker therapy is often unsuitable for persons with these conditions. Beta blockers also interfere with the physiologic response to hypoglycemia, making them undesirable for diabetic patients who are on tightly controlled insulin therapy.

Finally, recent analyses suggest that beta blockers may lack effectiveness in preventing cardiovascular and cerebrovascular complications in elderly patients with hypertension. Thus, beta blockers may not be a desirable first-line antihypertensive in geriatric patients.

ACE INHIBITORS   ACE inhibitors block the action of the enzyme that converts angiotensin I to the vasoconstrictor angiotensin II. Although ACE inhibitors were not recommended as the preferred initial therapy by the JNC-VI consensus report, many experts consider them first-line therapy. Not only do these agents control blood pressure with high levels of patient acceptance and low rates of side effects, but they also have favorable effects on LVH and insulin resistance. Furthermore, they do not increase cardiac risk factors and can be combined with diuretic therapy in most patients.

There is no one best ACE inhibitor, since all medications in this class have similar actions, contraindications, and side effects. The most common side effect is cough, which occurs because ACE also catalyzes the breakdown of the inflammatory mediators, such as bradykinin and substance P. Increased bradykinin and substance P levels cause bronchial cough. In some patients, elevated bradykinin levels result in ACE-induced angioedema, which is a contraindication to using any other ACE inhibitor.

As noted in Table 3-5, ACE inhibitors are preferred first-line medications for patients with diabetes who have proteinuria or microalbuminuria, in whom they reduce the frequency and rate of development of end-stage renal disease. ACE inhibitors may be combined with all other classes of antihypertensive agents, but caution must be exercised when they are combined with potassium-sparing agents because ACE inhibition can induce hyperkalemia.

ANGIOTENSIN-RECEPTOR BLOCKERS   In contrast to ACE inhibitors, which block production of an-

giotensin II, angiotensin-receptor blockers block the receptor on which angiotensin II acts. Angiotensin II-receptor blockers include medications such as losartan, valsartan, irbesartan, candesartan, and eprosartan.

Trials to date in patients with heart failure and hypertension indicate that angiotensin-receptor blockers are generally as effective and well tolerated as ACE inhibitors, and, because they do not interfere with bradykinin metabolism, they are not associated with cough. This makes angiotensin receptor blockers an excellent choice for patients in whom ACE inhibition is desired but who are intolerant of ACE inhibitors because of cough. Rare cases of angioedema have been reported with angiotensin-receptor blockers, but they are thought to be idiosyncratic and unrelated to drug action. For unexplained reasons, these drugs are not associated with hyperkalemia.

ALPHA-RECEPTOR BLOCKERS   Some experts consider alpha blockers an appropriate choice as first-line therapy because, in addition to lowering blood pressure, they decrease insulin resistance, improve LVH, and increase high-density lipoprotein cholesterol. Because alpha blockers induce relaxation of the urethral sphincter, they are often considered first-line therapy for patients who also require treatment for benign prostatic hypertrophy. However, alpha blockers can cause orthostatic hypotension in some patients, making some clinicians reluctant to prescribe these medications in full doses, and this reluctance leads to treatment failure.

CALCIUM CHANNEL BLOCKERS   Calcium channel blockers are reasonable first-line choices for hypertension, and they are particularly effective in older patients with isolated systolic hypertension. In addition, calcium channel blockers have beneficial effects for asthma, migraine, and urge urinary incontinence, making them a good choice for patients who also have these conditions.

However, as mentioned earlier, there have been several reports of the association of calcium channel blockers with unfavorable cardiac outcomes. These studies were all retrospective case-control studies, limiting the certainty of findings; and they only involved short-acting agents. Recent publications stress that long-acting calcium channel blockers have not been associated with adverse cardiac outcomes, and the studies on short-acting agents are not applicable to long-acting agents. Thus, if calcium channel blockers are prescribed, only the long-acting preparations should be used.

Another concern has been that the dihydropyridine calcium channel blockers (e.g., felodipine, nicardipine, nifedipine, amlodipine, and isradipine) are associated with edema precipitated, not by total-body water accumulation, but rather by a local vasoactive phenomenon related to arteriolar dilation and reflex venoconstriction. For this reason, nondihydropyridine agents (e.g., diltiazem and verapamil) are often preferred if calcium channel blockers are used. However, some nondihydropyridines have been associated with bradycardia and cardiac conduction abnormalities. In addition, verapamil can cause constipation, especially in older patients.

Finally, recent investigations suggest that hypertensive patients treated with either dihydropyridine or nondihydropyridine calcium channel blockers may be more likely to develop central nervous system white-matter lesions and evidence of mild cognitive impairment than patients treated with other antihypertensive agents. Though these findings are preliminary and their clinical significance is uncertain, they have raised further concerns about the benefits and risks of calcium channel blocking drugs.

CENTRAL ALPHA AGONISTS   Central alpha agonists (guanfacine, guanabenz, and clonidine) are rarely chosen as first-line agents because a high percentage of patients experience side effects such as drowsiness, fatigue, or dry mouth. Furthermore, rebound hypertension can occur upon abrupt discontinuation of therapy after prolonged use. One exception is clonidine administered by transdermal patch. Transdermal clonidine therapy has rarely, if ever, been associated with rebound hypertension. This is probably due to the fact that the skin reservoir of drug produces a physiologic tapering system. Because clonidine patches are applied once per week, they may enhance compliance with therapy. However, dermatologic intolerance of the patch is common, occurring in up to 15 to 18 percent of Caucasian women and 8 to 10 percent of darker-skinned individuals.

One central alpha agonist, methyldopa, has special applicability for treating hypertension that develops during pregnancy. Methyldopa is effective for pregnancy-induced hypertension, and long experience with the drug has shown it to be safe during pregnancy.

OTHER MEDICATIONS   A variety of other medications are available for the treatment of hypertension but are rarely used. Notable among these drugs are hydralazine and reserpine. Hydralazine, because of its vasodilating (afterload reducing) properties, may have a role in selected patients with congestive heart failure who are intolerant of other standard treatments. However, hydralazine is associated with fluid retention and a lupus-like syndrome and must be administered four times daily. Reserpine, formerly a first-line medication, has been all but discarded from the therapeutic armamentarium due to its association with depression, including suicide. Nonetheless, in patients without underlying depression, reserpine may represent a reasonable choice when other standard medications have failed to control blood pressure.

MULTIDRUG TREATMENT

When patients do not respond adequately to monotherapy, a second drug may be added to the therapeutic regimen. Diuretics are commonly selected as the second drug (unless they were used as the initial therapy), but, in the absence of specific contraindications, most antihypertensive agents can be used with any of the others.

In addition, there are a variety of commercially available preparations that combine two medications into a single pill (Table 3-6). Most of these preparations combine a diuretic with another agent. Combination drugs offer ease of administration and therefore probably improve compliance. However, some combination drugs are more expensive than the constituent drugs used separately.

Several issues related to combination therapy with calcium channel blockers deserve special comments. First, combining diuretics with calcium channel blockers has little, if any, synergistic effect and is not usually recommended. Second, combining calcium channel blockers with beta blockers may adversely affect cardiac conduction and systolic pump function and, in general, should be avoided. Third, there have been a few reports of successfully combining different classes of calcium channel blockers (i.e., dihydropyridines plus nondihydropyridines), but the benefits of such combinations are unclear. Finally, preparations that combine an ACE inhibitor with dihydropyridine calcium channel blockers are commercially available and cause considerably less edema than dihydropyridines alone.

Table 3-6

Commercially Available Antihypertensive Drug Combinations

Combinations with diuretics
Beta blocker + thiazide diuretic
ACE inhibitor + thiazide diuretic
Angiotensin II-receptor antagonist + thiazide diuretic
Alpha blocker + diuretic
Diuretic-diuretic combinations
Potassium-sparing diuretic + thiazide diuretic
Other combinations
Calcium channel blocker + ACE inhibitor

SOURCE: Adapted and modified from Sheps et al, 1997.

EVALUATING TREATMENT FAILURE

When patients fail to respond to treatment, clinicians should try to determine why this has occurred. Common reasons include noncompliance with therapy and use of hypertension-inducing substances (e.g., alcohol, cocaine, or nonsteroidal anti-inflammatory drugs). Patients who require more than three drugs to control their hypertension are considered refractory to therapy. Such individuals merit reconsideration of secondary causes of hypertension and, generally, consultation with a specialist.

DISCONTINUING TREATMENT

After a period of successful blood pressure control (usually 1 year or more), clinicians should consider "step-down" therapy—attempting to reduce or eliminate hypertensive medications. Many patients can be controlled with fewer medications or a lower dose of the same medication, particularly if they have successfully implemented lifestyle modifications while on medication. Such individuals should be closely monitored, however, because blood pressure may subsequently rise after medications have been lowered or discontinued.

The literature indicates that approximately 15 percent of persons with stages 1 and 2 hypertension can have their medication discontinued and will remain normotensive without treatment for prolonged periods of time. Some of these patients probably never had hypertension and were falsely diagnosed because of the "white coat" phenomenon, improper blood pressure measurement techniques, or other factors. In others, however, it is thought that hypertension was truly present but that medication therapy somehow "reset" the homeostatic mechanisms responsible for blood pressure control such that medication is no longer needed to maintain normotension. All patients who have been successfully withdrawn from antihypertensive medications should be monitored for return of hypertension.

Education

Education of patients with hypertension should focus on lifestyle modifications and compliance with medication regimens. Lifestyle modifications were discussed above, but clinicians should repeatedly acknowledge and reinforce patients' success with weight loss, smoking cessation, dietary lipid and sodium reduction, and exercise regimens.

Counseling regarding compliance is also essential, because hypertension generally has no symptoms, and treatment does not cause the symptom relief that promotes compliance with other chronic medical treatments. Because of extensive media publicity, most Americans are familiar with the concept that high blood pressure is dangerous, and clinicians should reinforce this awareness with information about the end-organ consequences of uncontrolled hypertension. If convinced that close adherence to a therapeutic regimen will reduce the likelihood of such consequences, patients can become motivated to comply with therapy.

For some patients, monitoring blood pressure at home and preparing a diary of readings can enhance compliance. In addition, blood pressure diaries may provide clinicians with a more accurate picture of blood pressure control than can be obtained only with office blood pressure measurements.

Family Approach

Upon receiving a diagnosis of hypertension, patients and their families may experience a number of emotional and/or behavioral changes. For example, spouses may fear loss of their partner to premature death. Antihypertensive medica-

tions may affect mood, sleep, or overall energy level. Medications may also impair sexual function, leading to stress between patients and their sex partners. Finally, adopting new habits of diet and exercise may alter family behavior patterns and tax an already stressful family schedule or living situation.

The best tools to combat these consequences are anticipation, guidance, and written (or audiovisual) educational information. Enlisting the participation of spouses or caregivers in the care of hypertension can be beneficial on numerous levels. For instance, a food-preparing spouse who recognizes the rationale for dietary changes may be more motivated to adopt those changes in food preparation. A caregiver who knows a patient's daily activities may be able to choose the optimal time for medication administration, resulting in the fewest omissions of medication. Candid discussions of the potential for medication side effects and medication costs will probably open the door for early reporting and resolution of problems.

Sometimes, family members can become overprotective, insisting that hypertensive patients not participate in healthful energetic activity for fear of increasing blood pressure or causing sudden death. Patients and their families should be encouraged that, with few exceptions, hypertension should not close the door to full participation in normal activities.

Errors

Several errors are commonplace in the clinical management of hypertension. For the most part, these errors are preventable.

Inappropriately Switching Medication

Some clinicians institute therapy with one medication and, when the target blood pressure is not achieved, switch the patient to another medication without having first increased the initial medication to its maximum recommended dose (or until side effects develop). This inappropriate discontinuation of medications without a therapeutic trial at appropriate doses leads to patients being labeled as resistant to medications when, in fact, they are not.

A related error is failure to continue a medication long enough to determine if it is effective. Although most antihypertensive agents manifest their effects within a few hours or days, some require longer intervals. For example, the diuretic indapamide may not manifest a full therapeutic effect for up to 6 weeks. It would be inappropriate to conclude that this drug is ineffective after treatment for shorter intervals of time.

For more than 95 percent of patients with hypertension, the urgency to control blood pressure is not so great that medications cannot be given a full therapeutic trial (of both appropriate dose and duration) before concluding that a medication is ineffective. The need for a full therapeutic trial and the avoidance of premature discontinuation of a medication are particularly important if a certain class of agents is likely to be of particular benefit for a given patient.

Inappropriately Assuming a Class of Medications Will Be Ineffective

Numerous investigations have demonstrated varying levels of responsiveness to different classes of agents by persons of different ages and ethnic backgrounds. For example, research has shown that older patients, as a group, are less responsive to ACE inhibitors than other patients. However, "less effective" does not mean "ineffective." It is not appropriate to eliminate an entire class of medications from consideration for a particular patient based on literature that reports it as "less effective" for that patient's demographic group. For individual patients in specific circumstances, the "less effective" medication may be the drug of choice.

Failure to "Step Down" Therapy

It is not uncommon to find hypertensive persons who have been treated with progressively newer antihypertensive agents for as long as 30 to 40 years with no attempt ever having been made to discontinue therapy. There are a variety of reasons to "step down" therapy by attempting to wean and discontinue antihypertensive medications. First, as noted earlier, the diagnosis of hypertension may have been erroneous. Second, factors contributing to hypertension at the time of initial diagnosis may no longer be present. For example, heavy drinkers may have decreased alcohol intake, cocaine users may have discontinued use, cigarette smokers may have stopped smoking, and overweight patients may have lost weight. Similarly, patients may have adopted exercise routines, or they may no longer be taking drugs that contributed to hypertension (e.g., nonsteroidal anti-inflammatory drugs). Thus, most patients with well-controlled hypertension should periodically be given a trial at reduction or cessation of therapy.

Inappropriately Blaming Patients

Clinicians sometimes explicitly or implicitly suggest that hypertension is the patients' fault, because of cigarette smoking, diet, lack of exercise, and so on. Furthermore, many patients may not achieve blood pressure control with lifestyle modifications, and clinicians may give these patients a stated or implied message that they have "failed." The reality, however, is that lifestyle interventions do not always result in blood pressure control, even if patients conscientiously adhere to recommended regimens. Few hypertensive patients will be able to control blood pressure with a low-sodium diet, and substantial weight loss may be difficult or unachievable even for highly motivated patients. Using the concepts of "responders" and "nonresponders" when discussing lifestyle interventions with patients can lessen the chance that nonresponders will feel guilty.

Controversies

Target Blood Pressure

Although achieving a blood pressure of 140/90 mmHg has traditionally been the goal of therapy, considerable epidemiologic evidence suggests that lower blood pressures may be preferable. On the other hand, some investigators have reported a "J" phenomenon, in which individuals with both the lowest and the highest blood pressures have the highest rates of morbidity and mortality, while an intermediate blood pressure level is associated with the best outcomes (Fig. 3-5). This issue has become even more controversial with the recent publication of results from the Hypertension Optimal Treatment (HOT) study. HOT involved 18,790 subjects randomized to different target blood pressures. The lowest incidence of major cardiovascular events and death occurred with diastolic blood pressures of 82.6 and 86.5 mmHg, respectively.

Figure 3-5

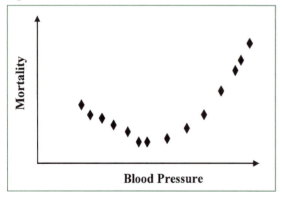

The "J"-shaped curve relates mortality rates to blood pressure. The highest levels of blood pressure are associated with a higher mortality rate. With decreasing blood pressure, the mortality rate from cardiovascular complications decreases, but only to a point of optimal blood pressure control. Below that optimal level, which has not been clearly defined, the mortality rate progressively increases.

Ambulatory Blood Pressure Monitoring

The role of continuous ambulatory blood pressure monitoring (and, for that matter, home self-monitoring with a personal sphygmomanometer) remains controversial. Although continuous ambulatory blood pressure levels are more closely correlated with end-organ damage than are office blood pressure measurements, all major clinical trials of antihypertensive medications have been based on office blood pressure measurements. Patients with elevated office blood pressures, as a group, are at higher risk of adverse outcomes, and this risk is reduced by antihypertensive therapy. Whether ambulatory monitoring can define who in that risk group would most benefit from therapy is unknown.

The Role of Echocardiography

Left ventricular hypertrophy is the most potent known risk factor for increased rates of cardiovascular morbidity and mortality. Some experts, therefore, advocate routine echocardiography in the evaluation of hypertension to identify patients with LVH so that antihypertensive medications can be selected based on their ability to reverse or prevent progression of LVH. However, there currently is insufficient information to permit ranking of pharmacologic agents by their ability to reverse LVH. For example, ACE inhibitors are generally considered most potent in this regard, but there is some suggestion that central alpha agonists (e.g., clonidine) may be even more effective, and data comparing these two drug classes for their ability to reverse LVH are unavailable. In addition, diuretic-based regimens, with and without simultaneous use of beta blockers, decrease left ventricular size in patients with isolated systolic hypertension, but these agents have not been compared to ACE inhibitors and alpha agonists. Finally, while the presence of LVH is a risk factor for increased rates of morbidity and mortality and drug therapy appears to reverse LVH, there is no definite evidence that reversing LVH through antihypertensive therapy will decrease morbidity and mortality rates. More research is needed to clarify the role of echocardiography in routine evaluation and management of hypertension.

Emerging Concepts

Blood pressure control alone does not completely prevent adverse cardiovascular outcomes. For example, even when blood pressure is well controlled, the risk of stroke and heart disease is not reduced to that of the general population. This suggests the possibility that some other factor or factors may be at least partly responsible for both hypertension and its associated cardiovascular outcomes.

Perhaps the most intriguing direction of current research focuses on the possibility that dysfunction of vascular endothelium, the single-cell layer lining the vascular system, is a factor. Endothelial dysfunction in patients with hypertension involves (1) hypersensitivity of vascular structures to vasoconstricting catecholamines, even at normal catecholamine levels; (2) subnormal vasodilatory capacity (due to low levels of nitric oxide, the principal vasodilating substance in endothelium); (3) free-radical oxidation of the endothelium, resulting in destruction of nitric oxide; and (4) imbalance in the coagulation-thrombolysis system that favors coagulation. Research indicates that these endothelial abnormalities occur early, antedating development of hypertension, raising the possibility that endothelial dysfunction could be responsible for both hypertension and cardiovascular complications.

Endothelial dysfunction can be lessened by control of dyslipidemia, glucose control, and smoking cessation. It is not clear, however, that blood pressure control itself is capable of reducing endothelial dysfunction. Thus, there would be great conceptual appeal to antihypertensive agents that focus on endothelial cell dysfunction by increasing production of nitric oxide or limiting oxidative destruction of nitric oxide by free radicals.

In fact, a few currently available drugs have some of these properties. For example, ACE inhibitors increase production of nitric oxide, indapamide is a scavenger of free radicals, and nitroglycerin is metabolized to nitric oxide. In addition, 3-hydroxy-3-methylglutaryl coenzyme-A reductase inhibitors ("statin" drugs for hyperlipidemia), beta carotene, and vitamins C and E are currently being used in research settings for their antioxidant properties to prevent or limit endothelial damage in patients with established atherosclerotic cardiovascular disease.

Thus, it is likely that, in the coming years, the consequences of hypertension will be viewed as a result of endothelial disease, rather than of hypertension itself, and agents will be developed that are specifically designed to enhance nitric oxide production and protect arterial endothelium.

Bibliography

Awan NA, Mason DT: Direct selective blockade of the vascular angiotensin II receptors in therapy for hypertension and severe congestive heart failure. *Am Heart J.* 131:177, l996.

Borhani N, Mercuri M, Borhari P, et al: Final outcome results of the multi-center isradipine diuretic atherosclerosis study. *JAMA* 276:785, l996.

Burt VL, Whelton P, Roccella EJ, et al: Prevalence of hypertension in the U.S. adult population: Results from the third National Health and Nutrition Examination Survey, 1988–1991. *Hypertension* 25:305, 1995.

Cappuccio FP, Elliot P, Allender PS, et al: Epidemiologic association between dietary calcium intake and blood pressure: A meta-analysis of published data. *Am J Epidemiol* 142:935, 1995.

Chobanian A: Changing patterns in the treatment of hypertension. *Prim Cardiol* special edition 2:6, l986.)

Curb JD, Pressel SL, Cutler JA, et al: Effect of diuretic-based antihypertensive treatment on cardiovascular disease risk in older diabetic patients with isolated systolic hypertension. *JAMA* 276:1886, 1996.

Cutler JA: Calcium-channel blockers for hypertension: Uncertainty continues. *New Engl J Med* 338:679, 1998.

Devereux RB: Do antihypertensive drugs differ in their ability to regress left ventricular hypertrophy? *Circulation* 95:1983, 1997.

Elliott W: Glucose and cholesterol elevations from diuretic therapy: Intention to treat vs actual on-therapy experience. *Am J Hypertension* 6(suppl): 9A, l993.

Furberg CD, Psaty BM, Meyer JV: Nifedipine: Dose-related increase in mortality in patients with coronary heart disease. *Circulation* 92:1326, 1995.

Garg R, Yusuf S: Overview of randomized trials for angiotensin-converting enzyme inhibitors on mortality and morbidity in patients with heart failure. Collaboration group on ACE inhibitor trials. *JAMA* 273:1450, 1995.

Gavras H, Gavras I: Modern approaches to initiating antihypertensive therapy. *Cardiol Clin* 13:593, l995.

Hansson L, Zanchetti A, Carruthers SG, et al: Effects of intensive blood-pressure lowering and low-dose aspirin in patients with hypertension: Principal results of the Hypertension Optimal Treatment (HOT) randomised trial. *Lancet* 351:1748, 1998.

Heckbert SR, Longstreth WT, Psaty BM, et al: The association of antihypertensive agents with MRI white matter findings and with modified mini-mental state examination in older adults. *J Am Geriatr Soc* 45:1423, l997.

Insua J, Sacks H, Lau T, et al: Drug treatment of hypertension in the elderly: A meta-analysis. *Ann Intern Med* 121:355, l994.

Kannel W: Blood pressure as a cardiovascular risk factor. *JAMA* 275:1571, 1996.

Kannel WB: Framingham study insights into hypertensive risk of cardiovascular disease. *Hypertens Res* 18:181, 1995.

Kaplan NM: *Clinical Hypertension*. Baltimore, Williams & Wilkins, 1994.

Kaplan NM, Gifford RW: Choice of initial therapy for hypertension. *JAMA* 275:1577, 1996.

Lewis EJ, Hunsicker LG, Bain RP, Rohde RD: The effect of angiotensin-converting enzyme inhibition on diabetic nephropathy. *New Engl J Med*. 329: 1456, 1993.

Messerli FH, Grossman E, Goldbourt J: Are beta-blockers efficacious as first-line therapy for hypertension in the elderly? A systemic review. *JAMA* 279:1903, 1998.

Middgley JP, Matthew AG, Greenwood GMT, et al: Effect of reduced dietary sodium on blood pressure: A meta-analysis of randomized controlled trials. *JAMA* 275:1590, 1996.

Neutel JM, Smith DHG, Graettinger WF, et al: Heredity and hypertension: Impact on metabolic characteristics. *Am Heart J* 124:435, 1992.

Ofilli EO, Cohen JD, St Vrain JA, et al: Effect of treatment of isolated systolic hypertension in left ventricular mass. *JAMA* 279:778, 1998.

Price DW: The hypertensive patient in family practice. *J Am Board Fam Pract* 7:403, 1994.

Psaty BM, Heckbert SR, Koepsell TD, et al: The risk of myocardial infarction associated with antihypertensive drug therapies. *JAMA* 274:620, 1995.

Psaty BM, Smith NL, Siscovick DS, et al: Health outcomes associated with antihypertensive therapies used as first-line agents: A systematic review and meta-analysis. *JAMA* 227:739, 1997.

SHEP Cooperative Research Group: Prevention of stroke by antihypertensive drug treatment in older persons with isolated systolic hypertension: Final results of the Systolic Hypertension in the Elderly Program (SHEP). *JAMA* 265:3255, 1991.

Sheps SG et al: *The Sixth Report of the Joint National Committee on Prevention, Detection, Evaluation, and Treatment of High Blood Pressure*, NIH publication no 98-4080. Bethesda, National Institutes of Health, National Heart, Lung, and Blood Institute, 1997.

Siegel S, Lopez J: Trends in antihypertensive drug use in the United States: Do the JNC-V recommendations affect prescribing. *JAMA* 278:1745, 1997.

Staessen J, Fagard R, Thijs L, et al: Randomised double-blind comparison of placebo and active treatment for older patients with isolated systolic hypertension. *Lancet* 350:757, 1977.

Whelton PK, Appel LJ, Espeland MA: Sodium reduction and weight loss in the treatment of hypertension in older persons: A randomized controlled trial of nonpharmacologic interventions in the elderly (TONE). *JAMA* 279:839, 1998.

Judith Gore Gearhart

Chapter 4

Diabetes Mellitus, Type 2

How Common Is Type 2 Diabetes?

Approximately 16 million people in the United States (6 percent of the population) have diabetes mellitus. Of these, 90 to 95 percent have type 2 disease, which has also been referred to as adult-onset diabetes, non-insulin-dependent diabetes mellitus (NIDDM), and non-ketosis-prone diabetes. Nearly all of the remaining 5 to 10 percent of patients with diabetes have type 1 disease, also referred to as juvenile-onset diabetes, insulin-dependent diabetes mellitus (IDDM), or ketosis-prone diabetes. The classification of diabetes is outlined in Table 4-1. This chapter focuses on type 2 diabetes, which is one of the most common problems seen in primary care practice.

Type 2 diabetes is the second most common reason for outpatient visits to clinicians in the

Table 4-1

Classification of Diabetes and Abnormal Glucose Metabolism

CLASSIFICATION	DISTINGUISHING CHARACTERISTICS
Diabetes mellitus	
Type 1 (also known as insulin-dependent, IDDM, ketosis prone, or juvenile onset)	Onset at any age, but more commonly in childhood or adolescence
	Onset usually abrupt
	Usually not obese
	Insulinopenia before age 30
	Dependent on insulin to prevent ketosis
	One form characterized by beta-cell destruction; other forms idiopathic
Type 2 (also known as non-insulin-dependent, NIDDM, adult onset, or ketosis resistant)	Onset usually after age 30
	Typically obese at diagnosis
	Ketosis-prone during stress
	Tissues are insulin resistant
	May need insulin to control hyperglycemia
Secondary diabetes	See Table 4-4
Malnutrition-related diabetes	Young (age 10–40 years)
	Symptomatic
	Not prone to ketosis but require insulin
Impaired glucose metabolism	Plasma blood sugar higher than normal, but not diagnostic for diabetes mellitus; is a risk factor for subsequent overt diabetes and its complications
Gestational diabetes	Onset of glucose intolerance during pregnancy

SOURCE: Adapted with permission from American Diabetes Association: *Medical Management of Insulin-Dependent (Type 1) Diabetes*, 2d ed. Alexandria, VA, American Diabetes Association, 1994.

United States, and primary care clinicians provide care for almost 95 percent of adults who have type 2 diabetes. It is the fourth leading reason for visits to family physicians and the third most common reason for visits to internists. For geriatric-aged individuals, diabetes is involved in nearly one of every ten visits to primary care clinicians.

Each year in the United States, between 400,000 and 600,000 new individuals are diagnosed as having diabetes mellitus. About half of these new cases occur in persons over 55, and nearly all of them are type 2. The incidence and prevalence of diabetes is slightly higher in women than in men. It also increases with age, such that about one in every nine Americans between ages 65 and 74 has diabetes.

Epidemiology

The prevalence of diabetes varies by ethnic group. Type 2 diabetes is least common in non-Hispanic whites, more common in African Americans, and even more common in persons of Hispanic descent. Prevalence is highest in the Pima Indians of central Arizona (reaching 50 percent in Pimas aged 30 to 64). Diabetes is also common in other Native American groups.

Type 2 diabetes has a genetic basis, since it is more common in relatives of patients with diabetes. The genetic mechanism, however, has not been completely identified.

Overall, the prevalence of diabetes in the United States has increased during the past 35 years. This increase is partially due to aging of the United States population and the higher rate of diabetes in older individuals. The higher prevalence may also be due to reduction in diabetes-associated mortality rates, especially those for cardiovascular disease, permitting more individuals with diabetes to live longer, thereby increasing the total population of diabetics. Increased prevalence of obesity and decreased rates of physical inactivity, both of which are risk factors for diabetes, have also occurred in recent decades and have probably contributed to the rising prevalence of diabetes. An additional factor in the increased prevalence may be detection bias, in that new tests for detection of diabetes have increased sensitivity, and these tests have been used to detect diabetes in an increasing proportion of the population. Other risk factors for diabetes are listed in Table 4-2.

UNDIAGNOSED DIABETES

Finally, the prevalence of undiagnosed type 2 diabetes is estimated to be twice that of diagnosed cases. This has important clinical consequences because, by the time type 2 diabetes is diagnosed, a significant number of patients have already developed complications. Thus, better and earlier detection of diabetes could permit more timely treatment and prevention of complications. For this reason, the U.S. Public Health Service Preventive Services Task Force and others indicate that screening for diabetes may be appropriate for persons at high risk (Table 4-2). However, routine diabetes screening of all adults is not recommended.

Table 4-2

Risk Factors for Diabetes Mellitus

TYPE	RISK FACTORS
Diabetes mellitus type 1	Genetic susceptibility (specific HLA types)
Viral insulitis	
Autoimmune (islet cell antibody) phenomena	
Diabetes mellitus type 2	Family history of diabetes
Obesity (>20% over ideal body weight)	
Ethnic background	
African American	
Hispanic American	
Native American	
Asian American	
Pacific Islander	
Age over 45 years	
Previous impaired glucose tolerance	
Hypertension	
HDL-cholesterol <35 mg/dL	
Triglyceride >250 mg/dL	
Physical inactivity	
History of gestational diabetes	
Previous delivery of infant >4000 gm	

Pathophysiology

Type 2 diabetes is defined by the presence of endogenous insulin secretion sufficient to prevent ketoacidosis but inadequate to meet the body's requirements for insulin due to tissue insensitivity to insulin. The primary defect is a tissue insulin receptor disorder resulting in resistance to insulin action. Compensatory hyperplasia of pancreatic beta cells and increased insulin production occur and account for fasting hyperinsulinism and an exaggerated insulin response to glucose ingestion. Prolonged exposure over time to fasting hyperglycemia causes beta cell desensitization and failure of insulin secretion by the beta cells.

The pathophysiology of type 2 diabetes contrasts with that of type 1 diabetes, in which there are an absence of endogenous insulin production, beta-cell failure in response to insulinogenic stimuli, and elevated glucagon levels. Autoimmune mechanisms appear to be involved in type 1 diabetes, but not in type 2 disease.

It is interesting to note that the relative prevalence of type 1 and type 2 diabetes differs in various parts of the world. Whereas 5 to 10 percent of diabetes in the United States is type 1, the corresponding figure in Japan is only 1 percent, while it is 50 percent in Norway. The reasons for these differences are unclear.

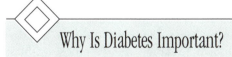

Why Is Diabetes Important?

Type 2 diabetes mellitus is one of the most important health problems in the United States. Its importance, however, lies less with its prevalence than with its complications. Persons with diabetes develop problems in a variety of organs and systems, including the heart, vascular system, kidneys, nervous system, and eyes. One or more of these "end-organ" complications, discussed below, causes premature death and disability in the majority of persons with diabetes.

The results of these complications are of considerable importance to the U.S. health care economy. Caring for diabetes and its complications in the United States costs more than $90 billion per year. Nearly half of this amount is spent on hospital care, with $10 billion of the hospital cost related to chronic complications of diabetes. The annual average direct cost per patient exceeds $11,000, and lost workdays because of premature disability or death account for further indirect costs. Cost-effectiveness research makes it clear that prevention of complications is important in reducing the costs of diabetes care.

Acute Complications of Diabetes

Acute complications of diabetes mainly pertain to disorders of metabolic homeostasis. In type 2 diabetes, the most common serious acute complication is a hyperosmolar nonketotic state. On rare occasions, diabetic ketoacidosis can occur.

HYPEROSMOLAR NONKETOTIC STATE

Hyperosmolar nonketotic state occurs predominantly in older patients with type 2 diabetes. It typically develops in response to extreme stress, such as during or following myocardial infarction, stroke, or infection. The condition is characterized by marked hyperglycemia and massive glycosuric osmotic diuresis, which, in turn, leads to severe dehydration. Mental status changes, including coma, are not uncommon. Because these patients usually have sufficient circulating insulin, ketoacidosis does not occur. Management in the hospital involves replacement of fluids, correction of hyperglycemia with insulin, and identification of any precipitating illness.

DIABETIC KETOACIDOSIS

Ketoacidosis results from severe insulin deficiency, and, therefore, it most commonly occurs in type 1 diabetes. It can, however, occur in type 2 disease in situations of extreme physiologic stress. The inability of the body's tissues to take up and metabolize glucose results in hyperglycemia, hypovolemia from glycosuric diuresis, and acidosis with ketosis. Diabetic ketoacidosis is a life-threatening condition that requires in-hospital management, often in an intensive care setting. Treatment involves intravenous administration of insulin, replacement and management of fluids and electrolytes, and identification of conditions that may have precipitated development of ketoacidosis.

Chronic Complications of Diabetes

Patients with diabetes develop two main categories of complications: macrovascular complications (involving the coronary, cerebrovascular, and peripheral vascular circulations) and microvascular complications (retinopathy, nephropathy, and neuropathy). Diabetic foot disease results from a combination of both macrovascular and microvascular abnormalities.

Studies show a strong relationship between hyperglycemia and the incidence and progression of microvascular and macrovascular complications. New research indicates that biochemical abnormalities, including hyperinsulinemia, and endothelial abnormalities, including nitric oxide production, are probably involved in the pathogenesis of these vascular complications.

MACROVASCULAR DISEASE

The prevalence of angina, stroke, and myocardial infarction in diabetics is two to three times that of the general population, and the risk of death due to cardiovascular disease is approximately three times higher, regardless of age, ethnic group, cholesterol level, systolic blood pressure, or tobacco use. Diabetic patients not only have an increased incidence of coronary artery disease, but they also have more extensive coronary disease in multiple vessels. Thus, they are at higher risk for complications of myocardial infarction, including congestive heart failure, recurrent infarction, arrhythmias, and cardiogenic shock.

These poor outcomes are attributable to several factors. First, as already noted, persons with diabetes have more extensive atherosclerotic disease and a higher prevalence of prior infarction than do nondiabetics. Second, diabetic patients have a blunted sensation of ischemic pain due to autonomic denervation of the heart. As a result, they may not experience chest symptoms with an infarction, and so the time between onset of infarction and presentation for health care may be prolonged. This is unfortunate because the benefits of therapeutic interventions such as thrombolytic agents are greater in diabetic patients, but thrombolytics must be given early to have maximum effect. Thus, in-hospital death from acute infarction is twice as likely in diabetic patients as in nondiabetic patients and twice as likely in diabetic women as in diabetic men. In fact, diabetes negates the cardioprotective effect of female gender, and the incidence of congestive heart failure after myocardial infarction is 10 times greater in women with diabetes than in those without diabetes. Outcomes are also poor in diabetic men, with a sixfold increase in congestive heart failure for men with diabetes compared with those without diabetes.

Several factors contribute to the cardiovascular disease process in diabetes. These include hyperinsulinemia, hypertension, hyperlipidemia, and coagulation abnormalities.

HYPERINSULINEMIA Type 2 diabetes is characterized by insensitivity or resistance of tissue insulin receptors to the action of insulin. This insulin resistance is frequently associated with obesity.

Early in the course of type 2 diabetes, when pancreatic insulin production still occurs, feedback mechanisms react to tissue insulin insensitivity with an increase in pancreatic insulin secretion, resulting in higher-than-normal blood insulin levels (i.e., hyperinsulinemia). Later in the course of type 2 diabetes, pancreatic insulin production falls, but insulin resistance persists. Thus, if insulin therapy is used for treatment of type 2 diabetes, it is not uncommon to need large doses (100 U/d or more), which maintains the state of hyperinsulinemia.

Hyperinsulinemia, whether from endogenous or exogenous insulin, has a variety of adverse effects. These include hypertension, lipid and coagulation abnormalities, and stimulation of tissue growth factor receptors, leading to endothelial proliferation and atherosclerosis. These and other hyperinsulinemia-related abnormalities combine in a clinical syndrome, often known as "syndrome X," that markedly increases the risk of macrovascular complications.

Hypertension   Hypertension is closely associated with, and involved in the development and progression of, diabetic complications. The pathogenesis of hypertension in diabetes is uncertain, but several mechanisms are probably involved. One mechanism is an increase in total body sodium. Typically, the increase is about 10 percent, and it results in intravascular volume expansion, leading to hypertension. Sodium retention is probably caused by hyperglycemia and hyperinsulinemia, both of which act on the renal tubules to inhibit sodium excretion. In addition, decreased renal blood flow through artherosclerotic or glomerulonephritic renal vessels causes increased activity of the renin-angiotensin-aldosterone system, which in turn further exacerbates sodium retention. Finally, other factors may be involved, including an insulin-mediated increase in vasomotor tone, glomerular hyperfiltration, and the action of norepinephrine and/or endothelin.

Lipid Abnormalities   High blood insulin levels decrease production of high-density lipoproteins (HDL) and augment production of very-low-density lipoprotein, which increases the level of serum triglyceride. High total cholesterol and low-density lipoprotein (LDL) levels also occur. The lipid abnormalities are so characteristic that an incidental finding of fasting hypertriglyceridemia and/or low HDL levels on routine blood testing should raise suspicion of hyperinsulinemia.

This so-called hyperinsulinemia-associated dyslipidemia of diabetes may be worsened by some antihypertensive drugs. The choice of antihypertensive medications for patients with diabetes should therefore include consideration of agents that decrease insulin resistance or at least do not worsen it (Table 4-3). Alpha-adrenergic blocking agents, in particular, lower blood pressure while lessening insulin resistance and improving lipid profiles.

The mechanism by which these lipid abnormalities contribute to macrovascular disease includes oxidation of the lipoproteins. Oxidation, especially of LDL, results in a product that is cytotoxic to vascular endothelial cells and smooth muscle cells, contributing to atherogenesis. This effect can be suppressed to some extent by antioxidant therapy.

Coagulation Abnormalities   Diabetic patients' platelets release higher levels of thrombogenic chemicals, such as thromboglobulin and platelet factor 4, and have an increased tendency to aggregate in response to platelet stimulants. The biochemical basis for these alterations in platelet function is unknown, but it is probably linked to hyperinsulinism and insulin resistance. The most important result of these coagulation abnormalities is a predisposition to coronary thrombosis.

Syndrome X   The constellation of abnormalities associated with insulin resistance and hyperinsulinemia—diabetes mellitus, hypertension, hypertriglyceridemia, and coagulation abnormalities—along with the obesity that frequently

Table 4-3

Antihypertensive Drugs in Diabetes

Effects	Thiazides	Beta Blockers	Alpha Blockers	ACE Inhibitors	ACE Receptor Antagonists	Calcium Antagonists
Glycemic control						
Glucose	↑	↑	0	0 or ↓	0	0 or ↑
Insulin	↑	↑	↓	0	0	0
Insulin resistance	↑	0 or ↑	0 or ↓	0	0	0
Lipids						
HDL	↓	↓	0 or ↑	0	0	0
LDL	↑	↓ or ↑	↓	0	0	0
Triglyceride	↑	0 or ↑	↓	0	0	0
Obesity	0		0			0
Complications						
Nephropathy						
Potassium	↓	0	0	0 or ↑	0	0
Renal impairment	0	0	↓	?↓	?	0
Proteinuria	0 or ↓	0 or ↓		↓	?↓	?↓
					(dihydropyridines ↑)	
Neuropathy						
Impotence	↑	↑	0 or ↑	0	0	0 or ↑
Orthostatic						
Hypotension	↑	↑	↑	0	0	0
Cardiovascular disease						
Peripheral vascular disease	?	↑	0	0	?	0
Renal artery stenosis	0	0	0	↑	?	0
Coronary heart disease	?	↓	0	?↓	?	?

NOTE: ↑, level or effect is increased; ↓, level or effect is decreased; 0, level or effect is unchanged; ?, level or effect is uncertain.

accompanies hyperinsulinemia, is often considered a discrete clinical syndrome. The syndrome has been given the names "syndrome X," insulin resistance syndrome, and "CHAOS" (an acronym for coronary artery disease, hypertension, atherosclerosis, obesity, and stroke). Increased sympathetic nervous system activity is also frequently present.

The precise mechanisms by which this syndrome causes vascular disease are unknown, and, indeed, it is not certain whether a syndrome actually exists. The main point of conceptualizing such a syndrome, however, is to emphasize that the goal of treating diabetes is not just to correct elevated glucose values. It is also to treat the multiple metabolic disturbances that occur in diabetes, especially insulin resistance and hyperinsulinemia, because hyperinsulinemia itself is linked to multiple abnormalities that cause cardiovascular disease. Insulin resistance is reversible with improvement in diet, glucose control, weight reduction, and exercise. Smoking may also worsen insulin resistance and therefore should be avoided. A variety of drugs, including low-dose insulin, troglitazone, and metformin, all improve insulin sensitivity of peripheral tissues.

MICROVASCULAR DISEASE

The three principal microvascular complications of type 2 diabetes are nephropathy, eye disease, and neuropathy.

NEPHROPATHY Diabetic nephropathy is the leading cause of end-stage renal disease in the United States and in Europe. Nearly half of all new cases of end-stage renal disease (ESRD) are caused by diabetic nephropathy, and the risk of developing renal disease in diabetes is 17 times that in the general population. Older African Americans are at particularly high risk, with a seven-times greater likelihood of developing diabetes-related renal failure than Caucasians.

Pathogenesis Mogensen proposed a five-stage sequence for the development of diabetic renal

disease. The first stage is glomerular hyperfiltration and renal enlargement. This probably occurs because hyperinsulinemia causes glomerular efferent arterioles to constrict to a greater extent than afferent arterioles, leading to increased glomerular capillary hydraulic pressure and, as a result, increased glomerular filtration.

The second stage is the onset of glomerular basement membrane thickening and mesangial expansion, both resulting from the increased glomerular hydraulic pressure. This second stage often has no symptoms but may be evidenced by exercise-induced microalbuminuria.

The third stage is the presence of relatively constant microalbuminuria, defined as a daily urinary albumin excretion rate of 20 to 200 μg/min. Development of microalbuminuria predicts renal function deterioration and poor outcome. Only 3 to 8 percent of all type 2 diabetics will develop ESRD, but ESRD ultimately occurs in 20 to 50 percent of those who develop microalbuminuria.

In the fourth stage, overt nephropathy develops with gross albuminuria, defined by proteinuria greater than 0.5 g/d. This proteinuric stage of diabetic nephropathy is often accompanied by hypertension and retinopathy. It will generally progress to ESRD, and suboptimal treatment results in more rapid progression, in as little as 2 to 3 years after the appearance of proteinuria.

The fifth and final stage is ESRD. This is a fatal condition unless transplantation or dialysis is undertaken. Concomitant medical problems, such as hypertension, urinary infections, and renovascular disease, may increase the likelihood that ESRD will develop.

Epidemiology In type I diabetes, 70 to 80 percent of patients with microalbuminuria will develop nephropathy within 10 years. However, less is known about the timing of renal involvement in type 2 diabetes because of imprecision in dating the onset of type 2 disease. Between 20 and 37 percent of patients with type 2 diabetes have microalbuminuria at the time diabetes is first diagnosed, probably reflecting a long period of unrecognized disease.

EYE DISEASE   Diabetes (both type 1 and type 2) is the leading cause of blindness in working-age Americans, involving 8000 new individuals per year. The risk of developing retinopathy with diabetes is 25 times that in the general population. Thirty-seven percent of patients with type 2 diabetes have retinopathy at the time diabetes is diagnosed.

Diabetic Retinopathy   The development of retinopathy is broadly categorized into three stages: (1) nonproliferative, (2) proliferative, and (3) quiescent.

The first stage, nonproliferative retinopathy, initially involves cellular and hemodynamic al-

terations in the retinal vasculature. With progression in the nonproliferative stage, classic ophthalmoscopic findings develop, including dot and blot retinal hemorrhages, "cotton-wool" spots (nerve fiber layer infarctions with stasis of axoplasmic flow), venous loops, venous caliber changes (venous tortuosity and beading), and retinal capillary dropout [Fig. 4-1 (Plate 3)]. The prevalence of nonproliferative retinopathy approaches 100 percent after 15 years of disease. Retinal ischemia and resultant vasoproliferation ensue, leading to the second and more advanced stage: proliferative retinopathy.

In proliferative retinopathy, proliferating vessels (neovascularization) and glial tissue cause traction on the retina and may cause vitreous hemorrhage, retinal detachment, and/or edema that interferes with retinal function [Fig. 4-2*A* (Plate 4), p. 89, and Fig. 4-2*B* (Plate 5), p. 90].

Figure 4-1 (Plate 3)

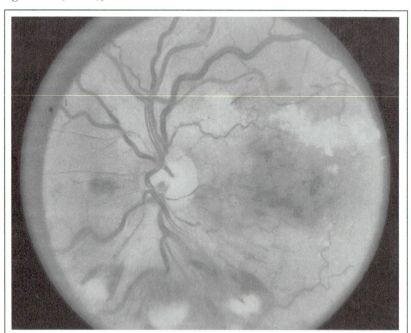

Nonproliferative diabetic retinopathy. The optic fundus photograph shows nonproliferative diabetic retinopathy with hemorrhages (red areas) and "cotton-wool" spots (pale areas). (*Courtesy of Dr. Ching-Jygh Chen, University of Mississippi School of Medicine.*)

Figure 4-2 (Plate 4)

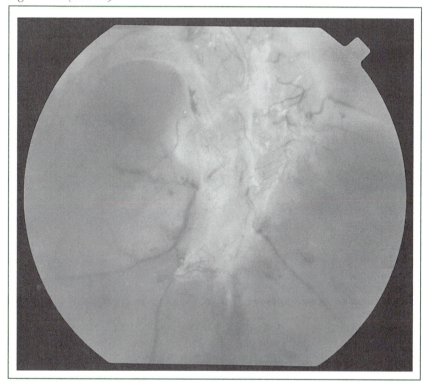

A

A. Proliferative diabetic retinopathy. Neovascularization from the disc extends to surrounding retina. Localized tractional retinal detachment is also seen (pale areas).

The final stage is quiescent retinopathy, which occurs spontaneously over time or after laser photocoagulation. Laser therapy accelerates the progression to quiescence and reduces the retinal vascular leakage that causes macular edema. Laser therapy effectively reduces the risk of visual loss in selected patients.

Nonretinal Eye Disease In addition to retinal visual loss from vitreous hemorrhage, traction retinal detachment, and macular edema, patients with diabetes also develop nonretinal eye disease. The nonretinal causes of visual loss include fibrovascular proliferation across the visual axis, neovascular glaucoma, and cataracts.

NEUROPATHY Metabolic abnormalities and ischemia or infarction of peripheral, cranial, and/or autonomic nerves result in diabetic neuropathy.

Peripheral Neuropathy The most common diabetic neuropathy is distal symmetric sensorimotor neuropathy, clinically evidenced as "glove-and-stocking" sensory loss. Other neuropathies include cranial mononeuropathy, isolated peripheral neuropathy (e.g., superficial cutaneous femoral neuropathy), proximal motor neuropathy, and autonomic neuropathy. Autonomic neuropathy includes such cardiovascular effects as tachycardia, exercise intolerance, and orthostatic hypotension. The latter is likely to be worsened by

Figure 4-2 (Plate 5)

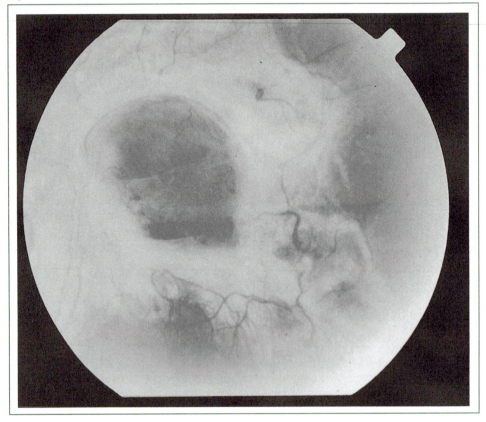

B

B. Advanced proliferative diabetic retinopathy. In more advanced disease, fibrovascular proliferation and preretinal hemorrhages occur. Progressive traction on the retina leads to extensive areas of detachment (pale areas). (*Courtesy of Dr. Ching-Jygh Chen, University of Mississippi School of Medicine.*)

diuretics, beta blockers, and short-acting, but not long-acting, alpha blockers.

Gastrointestinal Neuropathy   Gastrointestinal autonomic neuropathy deserves special mention because of its frequency and morbidity. The precise prevalence of gastrointestinal neuropathy among diabetics is unknown but is reported in some studies to be as high as 75 percent. Gastrointestinal dysfunction may result from vagus nerve dysfunction, sympathetic nerve damage, and alterations in glucose counterregulatory hormones that affect gastrointestinal motility. Symptoms include dysphagia, nausea and vomiting, diarrhea, constipation, and abdominal pain. Abnormal mucosal sensation secondary to pudendal nerve dysfunction may result in constipation and anorectal incontinence. There is an increased prevalence of altered gallbladder contractility and gallstones. Mesenteric ischemia due to vascular disease can also occur.

In terms of activities of daily living and lifestyle, diabetic diarrhea and gastroparesis are particularly debilitating manifestations of gastrointestinal autonomic neuropathy. Reversal of metabolic derangements and medical therapy for motility disorders are only partially successful in alleviating symptoms. Therefore, evaluation should also exclude other reversible causes of enteropathy. Interventions for diarrhea include pancreatic enzymes, biofeedback, loperamide, clonidine, verapamil, and somatostatin. Medications to control gastroparesis include metoclopramide, domeperidone, cisapride, and erythromycin.

Genitourinary Neuropathy Genitourinary neuropathy includes neurogenic bladder and sexual dysfunction. Impotence may be a presenting symptom of diabetes. Impotence may be worsened by antihypertensive medication, except alpha blockers.

FOOT DISEASE

The pathogenesis of diabetic foot disease was once thought to be vasculo-occlusive, but it is now known that many factors contribute to this condition. First, the circulation is abnormal, with defective vascular capillary basement membranes that allow leakage of albumin into the perivascular tissues of the foot. Second, motor neuropathy may result in the development of claw toes and other deformities, with prominent pressure points over the metatarsal heads and elsewhere leading to skin ulceration. Third, sensory neuropathy leads to faulty perception of pressure or trauma, leading to unperceived injuries. Finally, autonomic neuropathy causes loss of sweat and oil gland activity, resulting in fissured dry skin. Cracks and fissures predispose to infection.

The combined effects of ischemia, neuropathy, and infection markedly increase the risk of catastrophic foot complications. The risk for gangrene in patients with diabetes is 50 times that of the general population, and diabetic gangrene is a major reason for lower-extremity amputation

in the United States. Prevention and surveillance for foot injuries and infections are critical to management.

Principal Diagnoses

The principal diagnosis to consider in adult patients who present to primary care clinicians with hyperglycemia or other symptoms and signs of diabetes is type 2 diabetes. Type 1 diabetes, however, is also seen in primary care practice and should always be considered as a possible diagnosis, particularly in children, adolescents, and young adults. In fact, some individuals with type 1 diabetes will initially have sufficient beta-cell function to produce insulin and avoid ketosis, thus appearing to have type 2 diabetes. As their beta-cell function decreases with age, they will become dependent on insulin, and the diagnosis of type 1 diabetes will become evident.

In addition, clinicians should consider a number of uncommon causes of hyperglycemia in patients suspected of having diabetes. These conditions are listed in Table 4-4.

Typical Presentation

While specific data are lacking, perhaps the most common presentation of diabetes in primary care practice is an incidental finding of hyperglycemia on a blood test—often a blood test that was not drawn with the specific intent of diagnosing diabetes. In primary care practice, patients also often present with symptoms they believe are due to diabetes, not infrequently because the symptoms bear a resem-

Table 4-4

Secondary and Other Causes of Hyperglycemia

Pancreatic disease	Pancreatectomy, hemochromatosis, viral infection, cystic fibrosis, chronic pancreatitis, tumors, trauma
Other endocrine diseases	Cushing's syndrome, acromegaly, thyrotoxicosis, pheochromocytoma, primary hyperaldosteronism, glucagonoma, somatostatinoma
Drugs	Steroids, high doses of thiazides, propranolol, phenytoin, diazoxide, oral contraceptives, alloxan, streptozotocin, nicotinic acid, catecholamines, pentamidine, possibly protease inhibitors
Other diseases	Chronic renal failure, chronic liver disease, hemochromatosis, cirrhosis, infection, truncal obesity
Insulin receptor abnormalities	Acanthosis nigricans (insulin receptor antibodies), leprechaunism
Genetic syndromes	Lipodystrophic syndromes, muscular dystrophies, Huntington's chorea

Table 4-5

Frequency of Typical Presenting Symptoms of Diabetes

SYMPTOM	TYPE 1 DIABETES	TYPE 2 DIABETES
Abrupt onset	++	−
Polyuria, polydypsia	++	+
Weakness/fatigue	++	+
Polyphagia with weight loss	++	±
Vomiting	++	−
Recurrent blurred vision	++	++
Vulvovaginitis/pruritis or balanitis	+	++
Cardiovascular complications	−	++
Peripheral neuropathy	+	++
Impotence	−	+
Nocturnal enuresis	++	+
Altered sensorium	++	−
Clinical dehydration	++	−
Absence of symptoms	−	++

NOTE: ++, very common; +, somewhat common; −, quite uncommon.

blance to those of a family member or friend who has had diabetes. These symptoms are outlined on Table 4-5, where they are contrasted with symptoms of type 1 diabetes. It is important to note that type 2 diabetes presents with the classic symptoms of polydypsia, polyuria, and polyphagia with weight loss less often than does type 1.

The presentation of type 2 diabetes can be different in primary care practice than in the practice of subspecialists. Patients may present to either kind of clinician with a known diagnosis of diabetes, in which case the diagnosis is already established and the patient may already be under treatment. Ongoing care for diabetes is most often provided by primary care clinicians, whereas visits to subspecialists are frequently for treatment of complications such as retinopathy, nephropathy, foot infections, and others. Visits to diabetologists and endocrinologists comprise less than 5 percent of all visits to physicians for diabetes.

Key History

While the diagnosis of type 2 diabetes is made with blood testing, the history should focus on questions that clarify the urgency and type of treatment that is required. The American Diabetes Association (ADA) has published standards of care for management of diabetes, which recommend that the medical history of persons with diabetes include the elements shown in Table 4-6. The intent of the history is to identify

Table 4-6

Recommended Elements of the Medical History in Patients with Diabetes Mellitus

Symptoms, results of laboratory tests and special examinations related to the diagnosis of diabetes, prior glycated hemoglobin records

Eating patterns, nutritional status, and weight history; growth and development in children and adolescents

Details of previous treatment programs, including nutrition and diabetes self-management training

Current treatment of diabetes, including medications, meal plan, and results of glucose monitoring and patient's use of the data

Exercise history

Frequency, severity, and cause of acute complications, such as ketoacidosis and hypoglycemia

Prior or current infections, particularly skin, foot, dental, and genitourinary

Symptoms and treatment of chronic complications associated with diabetes (eye, kidney, nerve, genitourinary, sexual, bladder, and gastrointestinal function, heart, peripheral vascular, foot, and cerebrovascular)

Other medications that may affect blood glucose levels

Risk factors for atherosclerosis (smoking, hypertension, obesity, dyslipidemia, and family history)

History and treatment of other conditions including endocrine and eating disorders

Family history of diabetes and other endocrine disorders

Gestational history (hyperglycemia, delivery of an infant weighing >9 lb, toxemia, stillbirth, polyhydramnios, other complications of pregnancy)

Life-style, cultural, psychosocial, educational, and economic factors that might influence the management of diabetes

Source: Adapted with permission from American Diabetes Association: Standards of medical care for patients with diabetes mellitus (position statement).

complications of diabetes, determine an optimal method of treatment, and exclude causes of hyperglycemia other than diabetes.

History Suggesting Diabetic Complications

The history should include questions to identify early or overt signs of complications for which persons with diabetes are at risk. For example, clinicians should ask about visual changes (suggesting eye disease); chest discomfort, shortness of breath, or swelling (suggesting cardiovascular complications); or loss of sensation in the extremities (suggesting neuropathy).

History Influencing the Type of Treatment

The patient's level of comprehension and comfort with self-care will affect decisions about the complexity of the treatment regimen. Tightly controlled insulin regimens require motivated patients who understand the basic concepts of diabetes treatment. For patients who live alone, especially older or debilitated individuals, tight control of blood sugar may not be appropriate because of the dangers of inducing hypoglycemia. Positive or negative experiences with previous treatments may affect the choice of and compliance with any new treatments prescribed. Finally, insurance coverage may affect choice of treatment. For example, some insurers will not cover home glucose meters, which might influence the clinician to choose a treatment regimen that does not seek tight control of glucose levels.

A clinical presentation consistent with type 1 disease (young age, abrupt onset, marked symptoms, and ketoacidosis) is a contraindication to oral agents. Patients with liver disease should not be treated with metformin or troglitazone, and renal disease is a contraindication to metformin therapy.

History Suggesting Other Causes of Hyperglycemia

The history should explore the possibility of other causes of hyperglycemia, such as steroid use (athletics or bodybuilding), thyroid disease (heat or cold intolerance, weight changes, tremulousness, or fatigue), other endocrinopathies (changes in appearance, skin, or weight), or other conditions listed in Table 4-4.

Physical Examination

The ADA Standards of Care state that a comprehensive physical examination of a patient with diabetes should include the items listed in Table 4-7. Like the medical history, the physical examination is directed at detecting complications of diabetes, identifying factors that might influence the method of treatment, and excluding causes of hyperglycemia other than diabetes.

Examination Findings Suggesting Diabetic Complications

The physical examination should include a careful search for manifestations of end-organ damage. Postural hypotension suggesting autonomic neuropathy may be detected by checking the blood pressure with the patient supine and then standing. Funduscopic examination may reveal retinopathy. Manifestations of cardiovascular disease may include hypertension, a precordial lift, a displaced point of maximal palpable precordial impulse, and/or presence of an S_3 or S_4 on cardiac examination. In assessing the peripheral vascular system, absence of a posterior tibial pulse is the most valuable physical examination indicator of circulatory compromise. Peripheral edema may be a sign of congestive heart failure or nephrop-

Table 4-7

Recommended Elements of the Physical Examination in
Adults with Diabetes Mellitus

Height and weight
Blood pressure determination (with orthostatic
    measurements when indicated by history)
Ophthalmoscopic examination (preferably with
    dilation of pupils)
Oral examination
Thyroid palpation
Cardiac examination
Abdominal examination (including aortic or
    renal artery bruits)
Evaluation of pulses (by palpation and
    auscultation)
Hand/finger examination
Foot examination (callus, nail abnormalities,
    cracks, fissures, ulcers)
Skin examination (insulin-injection sites,
    wounds, infections)
Neurologic examination

Source: Adapted with permission from American Diabetes
Association: Standards of medical care for patients with diabetes mellitus (position statement).

athy. Peripheral neuropathy is often manifest as
"stocking-and-glove" sensory loss. Skin changes,
diminished pulses, and hair loss on the feet suggest peripheral vascular disease.

Examination Findings Influencing
the Type of Treatment

Visual acuity and manual dexterity affect the patient's ability to self-monitor blood sugars and
administer medication. This may influence decisions about type, route, frequency, and timing of
medications and monitoring. Obesity indicates
the need for weight reduction.

The physical examination may also reveal
contraindications to certain methods of treatment. In particular, the presence of pulmonary

rales or edema may signify congestive heart failure or renal impairment and would preclude the
use of metformin. Stigmata of active or chronic
liver disease would contraindicate metformin
and troglitazone.

Examination Findings Suggesting
Other Causes of Hyperglycemia

The clinician should check for physical signs of
unusual or secondary causes of hyperglycemia,
such as findings suggestive of hemochromatosis
(hepatomegaly or altered skin color), pancreatic
disease (jaundice or abdominal pain), exogenous steroids (steroid facies), and endocrine disorders such as Cushing's syndrome, acromegaly,
and pheochromocytoma. Thyroid disease (glan-
dular enlargement or nodules or skin changes)
when untreated can complicate glucose control.
Obesity, hirsutism, and a history of infertility are
suggestive of the polycystic ovary syndrome,
which is accompanied by insulin resistance.

Ancillary Tests

A variety of laboratory tests have been recommended for patients with known or suspected
diabetes. Some of these tests are used for diagnosing diabetes. Others assess its severity or
adequacy of control, or detect and monitor complications. Still other tests are used to exclude
causes of hyperglycemia other than type 2 diabetes. Useful tests are described below and outlined in Table 4-8.

Tests for Diagnosing Diabetes

Fasting Plasma Glucose

The test of choice for diagnosing diabetes is
measurement of the fasting plasma glucose level,

Table 4-8

Tests for Assessment of Diabetes

TESTS	COMMENTS
Self-monitoring of blood glucose	Highly preferable to laboratory monitoring for achieving control; recommended qid for patients with type 1; desirable for type 2 (optimal frequency not known)
	Affected by hematocrit (Hct); high Hct yields false low glucose, low Hct yields false high glucose; avoid generic test strips as results are variable
Fasting blood sugar	Test of choice for diagnosis; normal 70–110 mg/dL; increases with age; glucose ≥ 126 mg/dL diagnostic of diabetes
Glucose tolerance test	Obtain after 8-h overnight fast and 75-g glucose load; diagnosis of diabetes if glucose over ≥200 mg/dL prandial; sensitive but not specific
C peptide	Used to assess insulin secretion; indicates only if beta-cell secretion is present; cannot use to accurately quantitate secretion; can distinguish type 1 (no insulin) from type 2 diabetes. In hypoglycemia, useful for diagnosis of insulinoma or surreptitious injection of insulin
Urine glucose testing	Gives no information on glucose below renal threshold (180 mg/dL); negative urine glucose test results could correspond to a wide range of levels
	Causes of false positive: L-dopa, salicylate, sodium fluoride
	Causes of false negative: hydrogen peroxide, bleach (with glucose oxidase reagent strips)
	Affected by ketones (falsely low urine glucose) and the lower renal glucose threshold in pregnancy
Urine ketones	Should be checked during acute illness, when glucose levels are consistently >300, during pregnancy, or symptoms of ketoacidosis (nausea, vomiting, abdominal pain); up to 50 mg/dL of acetoacetic acid may be present without clinical evidence; does not detect β-hydroxybutyrate
	Causes of false positive: sulfhydryl drugs (e.g., captopril)
	Causes of false negative: prolonged exposure of test strips to air, highly acidic urine, ascorbic acid
	Nondiabetic causes of positive results: fever, dehydration, vomiting, pregnancy, low-carbohydrate diet, cold, strenuous exercise
Microalbuminuria	Standard of care for early detection of complications; by 24-h timed specimen of spot ratio or special sensitive dipsticks

Table 4-8

Tests for Assessment of Diabetes (*Continued*)

TESTS	COMMENTS
Proteinuria	May be increased after exercise
	False positive: Alkaline urine, excessive wetting, quaternary ammonium compounds for cleaning skin, amidoamines in fabric softener
	False negative: Globulinuria (reagent strips more sensitive to albumin)
Serum ketones	Elevated in diabetic ketoacidosis; ketones include (1) acetoacetic acid; also detected on urine reagent strips; forms acetone and beta hydroxybutyrate; (2) β-hydroxybutyric acid; formed reversibly from acetoacetic acid; not detected on urine reagent strips. Other tests not yet widely used.
	Not elevated in hyperosmolar nonketotic state
Glycated hemoglobin (GHb)	Also known as glycohemoglobin, glycated hemoglobin, Hgb A_{1c}, or HbA_1; of all methods, most accurate for diagnosis and follow-up of diabetes; formation directly proportional to glucose levels; most accurately reflects glycemia over previous 120 days; predicts complications of diabetes
	Obtain initially or with change in treatment, then q 3 months until controlled; at least 1–2 times/year if well controlled and stable
	Affected by hemoglobinopathies, chronic ingestion, salicylates, carbamylation products in uremia
	Assay methods and reference levels vary between laboratories not standardized; national program in progress
Glycated serum protein (GSP)	Mostly albumin; shorter half-life (14–20 days) than GHb; reflects preceding 1–2 weeks; total GSP correlates well with glycated serum albumin and with GHb; useful when GHb cannot be measured or not of value (e.g., in patients with hemoglobinopathies) or when short-term evaluation desired (e.g., pregnancy, change in regimen)
	Unlike GHb, not yet correlated with complications; varies with change in serum proteins (illness, liver disease)
	One method is fructosamine assay; debate exists whether fructosamine should be corrected for serum protein or albumin concentration
Serum osmolarity	To identify hyperosmolar hyperglycemic nonketotic coma
Diabetes-associated antibodies	Include islet cell antibodies, insulin associated antibodies, and anti-glutamic acid decarboxylase antibodies present in patients with or destined to have type 1 diabetes; increased titers predict development of diabetes in the future; not routine; may identify high-risk individuals for prevention

defined as a glucose level obtained when there has been no caloric intake for at least 8 h. Values greater than 125 mg/dL (normal is less than 110 mg/dL) indicate the presence of diabetes. Fasting glucose levels increase with age, and slightly elevated values are acceptable in patients over the age of 70.

Alternatively, diabetes can be diagnosed by obtaining a 2-h postprandial glucose level of 200 mg/dL or higher or a random glucose level of 200 mg/dL or more in the presence of diabetes symptoms. Impaired glucose tolerance (but not overt diabetes) is defined as a fasting plasma glucose level of 110 mg/dL or higher but less than 126 mg/dL, or a 2-h postprandial glucose level between 140 mg/dL and 200 mg/dL (normal is less than 140 mg/dL).

GLYCATED HEMOGLOBIN

Measurement of hemoglobin A_{1C}, or glycated hemoglobin, gives the percentage of hemoglobin that has been glycated by circulating blood glucose, with higher glucose levels leading to higher levels of glycated hemoglobin. Because of the long half-life of hemoglobin molecules, glycated hemoglobin levels give an indication of mean glucose levels during the preceding 3 months. Normally, less than approximately 7 percent of hemoglobin is glycated.

Measurement of glycated hemoglobin levels has been advocated by some as a diagnostic test for diabetes. If the glycated hemoglobin level is elevated, especially in the presence of an elevated plasma glucose level, diabetes is likely to be present. However, the test of choice for diabetes, or for diabetes screening in high-risk individuals, is determination of the fasting plasma glucose level.

GLUCOSE TOLERANCE TESTS

The oral or intravenous glucose tolerance test (GTT) is no longer recommended for routine use, including screening for diabetes, because

it lacks age-related normal values. The GTTs may still have a role in pregnancy, however. Although controversial, current recommendations from the Centers for Disease Control and Prevention are that all pregnant women should undergo measurement of plasma glucose between 24 and 28 weeks of gestation and also at the first prenatal visit if they are at high risk for diabetes. A 50-g glucose solution is administered without regard to time of day or last meal, and blood is drawn 1 h later. A 1-h postingestion value of 140 mg/dL or more warrants further testing with a full 3-hour oral glucose tolerance test.

Tests to Document the Adequacy of Diabetes Control

GLYCATED HEMOGLOBIN

Determination of the glycated hemoglobin level is the test of choice to measure the adequacy of diabetes control. Ideally, glycated hemoglobin should be measured when diabetes is initially diagnosed and again at approximately 3-month intervals during treatment to assess the effect of treatment. Random plasma glucose levels can have substantial day-to-day variation and do not give an accurate indication of overall diabetes control.

Tests to Detect Risk Factors for Complications of Diabetes

LIPID LEVELS

Given that abnormalities of blood lipids are strong risk factors for development of cardiovascular complications in patients with diabetes, the National Cholesterol Education Program recommends that lipids be measured in all diabetic patients at the time of diagnosis and again after glucose control has been established. Lipids should be measured in the fasting state and should include total cholesterol, HDL cholesterol, LDL cholesterol, and triglycerides.

MICROALBUMINEMIA

As discussed previously, microalbuminuria is an important early finding that indicates risk of developing overt diabetic nephropathy. Microalbuminuria can be detected with a timed urine specimen (e.g., 24-h collection) or with special dipsticks sensitive to low levels of albumin. Standard urine dipsticks do not detect microalbuminuria.

Testing for microalbuminuria should be performed in all patients with type 2 diabetes at the time of diagnosis. If detected, the presence of persistent microalbuminuria should be confirmed with one or two additional measurements over 3 to 6 months because there is considerable variability in daily albumin excretion. If the initial test is normal, testing for microalbuminuria should be repeated annually.

Tests to Detect Complications of Diabetes

GLUCOSE AND KETONES

Tests for blood glucose and urine ketones should be immediately available in all outpatient primary care settings to permit detection of acute diabetes complications, such as ketoacidosis or a hyperosmolar state. Additional laboratory tests that help assess the severity of these complications include electrolytes and arterial blood gas measurements.

RENAL FUNCTION TESTS

Serum creatinine should be measured at intervals in all adults with diabetes. In the absence of renal disease in a stable patient, measurements can be repeated approximately once per year. Renal function can also be assessed with measurement of creatinine clearance. Referral to a

nephrologist should be considered when creatinine clearance falls to below 70 $(mL/min)/m^2$ or creatinine has risen above 2.0 mg/dL, since such patients are at high risk of developing ESRD.

EYE EXAMINATIONS

Patients with diabetes should undergo formal annual eye examinations with funduscopy and slit-lamp evaluation for early detection of retinopathy and other ocular abnormalities. In general, because of the uncertain time of onset in most cases of type 2 diabetes and because eye disease is often present when diabetes is first detected, these examinations should begin at the time diabetes is diagnosed.

NEUROPHYSIOLOGIC TESTS

Nerve conduction and electromyographic studies are useful for confirming the diagnosis of neuropathy in patients with symptoms or physical findings suggestive of this complication. These tests are not, however, recommended as screening tests if neuropathy is not suspected after the history and physical examination.

TESTS FOR VASCULAR INSUFFICIENCY

When evaluating the peripheral circulation because of a nonhealing ulcer with bone, joint, or tendon involvement, arteriographic studies should be considered. When lower extremity blood pressures are measured with a sphygmomanometer and stethoscope or hand-held Doppler device, the results may be misleading because of noncompressible, calcified arteries that lead to falsely elevated blood pressure readings.

ELECTROCARDIOGRAPHY

Because patients with diabetes often do not experience typical symptoms of angina and myocardial infarction, baseline and interval electrocardiograms are appropriate in older adult diabetic patients for detection of previous asymptomatic infarction.

URINALYSIS

Interval urinalyses should be performed on patients with diabetes to detect infection. The urinalysis should include dipstick testing for glucose, ketones, protein, nitrites, and leukocyte esterase, as well as microscopic examination of the urine sediment. Urine culture is appropriate if urinalysis suggests infection, or if symptoms of infection are present.

Other Tests

INSULIN SECRETION AND AUTOANTIBODY TESTS

Clinicians need not measure levels of C peptide (a precursor protein involved in insulin secretion) to document the presence or absence of insulin secretion unless there is uncertainty about whether a patient has type 1 or type 2 diabetes. Nor is it necessary to test for islet-cell antibodies, which occur in type 1 diabetes. In most clinical settings, the diagnosis of type 1 diabetes will be apparent when it presents with ketoacidosis or ketonuria in the presence of hyperglycemia.

TESTS FOR OTHER CAUSES OF HYPERGLYCEMIA

If diabetes is difficult to control or if diagnoses other than type 1 or type 2 diabetes are suspected, a variety of laboratory tests may help rule out other causes of hyperglycemia. The most commonly used tests are urine drug screens when substance abuse (e.g., steroids) is suspected and an overnight dexamethasone suppression test for Cushing's syndrome. Thyroid function tests are indicated in the presence of history, physical, or laboratory abnormalities that

suggest thyroid disease (e.g., marked hypertriglyceridemia).

Treatment

Self-Treatments

There is little information available on the frequency with which patients use self-treatments and/or alternative therapies for diabetes. Acupuncture has been used with some success to treat diabetic neuropathy. Preliminary studies have suggested that biofeedback, yoga, and guided imagery techniques can lower blood glucose levels by decreasing stress-induced gluconeogenesis. However, large-scale controlled studies of these techniques have not been published.

The ADA stresses that alternative therapies, or "complementary medicine," should only be used to complement traditional diabetes care techniques, not replace them. The ADA Web site (http://www.diabetes.org) lists sources of information on alternative and/or complementary treatments for diabetes.

Inpatient versus Outpatient Management of Newly Diagnosed Diabetes

Outpatient management is often possible, and it is preferable to hospitalization because it is less costly and less emotionally traumatic for patients. The home environment is usually a more reassuring setting for patients and a better site for education about diabetes, a condition for which lifelong self-management in an outpatient (not inpatient) setting will be required. Studies demonstrate significant financial savings for patient and the health care system when newly diagnosed diabetic patients receive outpatient management, with no difference in outcome compared to patients treated in hospitals.

On the other hand, hospitalization is almost always needed in certain acute situations. Patients presenting with significant vomiting, dehydration, altered mental status, hyperosmolar state, or ketoacidosis should be hospitalized. Hospitalization is also frequently required for patients who have such coexisting medical conditions as poorly controlled angina, hypertension, asthma, or chronic obstructive pulmonary disease. Finally, treatment might also be initiated in the hospital for patients with a poor home environment or with psychiatric problems precluding the ability to initiate self-care at home. Table 4-9 lists criteria for admission of patients

Table 4-9

Indications for Hospital Admission for Patients with Diabetes

Arterial pH ≤7.2
Serum bicarbonate ≤15 meq/L
Persistent vomiting
Nonketotic hyperosmolar coma
Changes in sensorium
Infection or significant coexisting medical illness
Life-threatening acute or chronic complications of diabetes
Newly diagnosed diabetes in children and adolescents
Uncontrolled or newly diagnosed diabetes in pregnancy
Institution of insulin pump or other intensive treatment regimen
Poor home environment; unwilling/unable to initiate self-care

NOTE: These are guidelines only; clinical judgment must be used.
SOURCE: Reproduced from Gearhart et al, with permission from the June 1995, vol 51 issue of *American Family Physician*. Copyright by the American Academy of Family Physicians. All rights reserved.

with diabetes. Since the focus of this chapter is on outpatient management of diabetes, inpatient management of hyperosmolar state, ketoacidosis, and other complications of diabetes is not discussed.

Treatment Objectives for Outpatient Management of Type 2 Diabetes

CONTROLLING BLOOD GLUCOSE

A principal objective of diabetes management is to normalize blood glucose levels, an intervention that has proven benefits. It reduces the danger of acute metabolic decompensation. Symptoms and risks of skin infection, blurred vision, polyuria, fatigue, weight loss, polyphagia, vaginitis, or balanitis may be also prevented or improved.

Of perhaps greater importance, however, is the fact that tightly controlling glucose levels can reduce the risk of microvascular complications. The Diabetes Control and Complications Trial (DCCT) clearly indicated such benefits for patients with type 1 diabetes, with reductions of microvascular complications by 50 to 75 percent in patients who achieved normal glycated hemoglobin levels. A smaller randomized trial, similar in design to the DCCT, showed that improved control also decreases microvascular complications in patients with type 2 diabetes.

CONTROLLING CARDIOVASCULAR DISEASE RISK FACTORS

While the DCCT showed that control of glucose levels is related to reduced rates of microvascular disease, glucose control may not prevent or retard the development of macrovascular complications. In both men and women, the rate of macrovascular complications is similar regardless of the level of glucose control. Thus, control of other risk factors, such as hypertension, hyperlipidemia, hyperinsulinemia, and cigarette smoking, is probably the most reasonable approach to preventing macrovascular complications in diabetes.

An example of how control of risk factors can reduce macrovascular complications is seen in the relationship of hyperlipidemia to cardiovascular death rates in diabetes. In the United Kingdom, 80 percent of patients with type 2 diabetes die from coronary artery disease. In Japan, however, only 7 percent die from coronary artery disease, despite similar rates of smoking and hypertension. The difference is attributed to the fact that the Japanese population has lower lipid levels, probably related to differences in diet. This underscores the importance of normalizing lipid levels to improve outcome in diabetes.

AVOIDING HYPOGLYCEMIA

While control of blood glucose is important, tight control carries with it the risk of inducing hypoglycemia. Severe hypoglycemia can cause cardiac and cerebral dysfunction, and in extreme cases can be fatal. Hypoglycemia is poorly tolerated by elderly individuals, and this may lead to a decision to avoid tight control in older patients. Close self-monitoring of glucose levels and appropriate synchronization of diet with drug and insulin treatments helps to prevent hypoglycemia.

Treatment Strategies

Standard therapy for patients with type 2 diabetes begins with controlled diet and exercise, along with weight reduction in overweight patients. The net result of these interventions is to improve insulin resistance. Only a minority of patients will achieve adequate blood glucose control with these measures, however, and medications are frequently needed.

If medications are required, prescription of a single oral medication is usually the first step. If adequate glucose control is not achieved with a single oral agent, several treatment options exist. The most common of these are adding a second oral medication to the first, combining insulin with the single oral agent, and substituting insulin for the oral medication.

Oral Medications

Patients most likely to respond to oral medications are those who develop diabetes after age 40, have had diabetes less than 5 years, and have never received insulin (or, if taking insulin, have been well controlled on less than 20 to 40 U/d). Contraindications to oral agents are ketoacidosis, severe infection, pregnancy, impaired hepatic or renal function, chronic debilitating disease, and allergy to the drugs. Oral agents are inappropriate when there is acute stress, such as trauma or myocardial infarction.

SELECTING AN ORAL AGENT

Until the 1990s, the only class of oral antidiabetic medications in the United States was the sulfonylureas. Since then, several new oral agents have become available, including repaglinide, metformin, troglitazone, and acarbose (Table 4-10). There are no hard and fast rules for predicting the medication or the dose to which patients will have the best response. Titration of medication usually begins with the lowest dose of an oral agent, and the dose is increased as needed to achieve a satisfactory response.

SULFONYLUREAS   Oral sulfonylureas increase the function of tissue insulin receptors and stimulate endogenous insulin secretion by the pancreas through binding to specific membrane receptors and pancreatic beta cells. All sulfonylureas are similarly effective for reducing blood glucose levels, but they differ in duration of action, routes of metabolism and excretion, and side effects (Table 4-10).

Certain sulfonylureas have important side effects. In particular, chlorpropamide, which has

Table 4-10

Characteristics of Oral Drugs for Diabetes

AGENT	DAILY DOSE RANGE MG	DURATION OF ACTION, H	COMMENTS
Sulfonylureas			Increase insulin secretion; all similar in efficacy
First generation			
Tolbutamide (Orinase)	500–3000	6–12	Metabolized by liver to inactive product*; taken 2–3 times per day
Chlorpropamide (Diabinese)	100–500	60	Metabolized by liver (~70%) to less active metabolites and excreted intact (~30%) by kidneys; can cause inappropriate antidiuretic hormone secretion; taken 1 time per day
Tolazamide (Tolinase)	100–1000	12–24	Metabolized by liver to both active and inactive products; excreted by kidney; taken 1–2 times per day
Second Generation			
Glipizide (Glucotrol)	5–50	12–24	Metabolized by liver to inert products*; taken 1–2 times per day
Glipizide extended release	5–20	24	Taken 1 time per day; dose based on total daily dose of regular glipizide
Glyburide (Diabeta)	2.5–20	16–24	Metabolized by liver to mostly inert products; taken 1–2 times per day
Glyburide micronized (Glynase Prestabs)	1.5–12	24	Taken 1 time per day (if dose >6 mg/d, may use twice-a-day dosage)
Third generation			
Glimepiride (Amaryl)	1–6	24	Taken 1 time per day
Meglitinides			
Replaginide (Prandin)	4–16	†	Stimulates insulin release; taken before each meal
Biguanides			
Metformin (Glucophage)	1500–2500	‡	Not metabolized; excreted by kidneys; may be used alone or in combination therapy; decreases gluconeogenesis; taken tid with meals
α-glucosidase inhibitors			
Acarbose (Precose)	75–300	§	Delays and reduces glucose rise after meal; taken tid with meal; metabolized in intestinal tract by bacteria; causes flatulence
Thiazolidinediones			
Troglitazone (Rezulin)	200–400	¶	Promotes tissue utilization of glucose; lowers triglycerides; decreases gluconeogenesis; taken once a day at breakfast or lunch; mainly fecal elimination

* Safer in renal failure than other drugs; plasma elimination half-life is † 1 h   ‡ 5.5 h   § 2 h   ¶ 16–34 h.
SOURCE: Adapted with permission from *Medical Management of Non-Insulin Dependent (Type II) Diabetes.* 3d ed. Alexandria, VA, American Diabetes Association, 1994.

a long half-life (60 h) and undergoes renal excretion, may accumulate in patients with impaired renal function and cause hypoglycemia. Chlorpropamide may also cause inappropriate antidiuretic hormone secretion, which can be dangerous for patients with cardiovascular disease. Because elderly patients are more likely to have congestive heart failure, renal failure, and hypoglycemia due to missed meals, a short-acting agent that is not dependent on renal function for elimination is preferred for this age group. Tolbutamide, glipizide, and glyburide are metabolized by the liver to mostly inactive products, which are excreted in the urine. Therefore, these drugs, particularly glipizide, are safer for patients with renal failure.

MEGLITINIDES Meglitinides are nonsulfonylurea agents that have actions similar to those of the sulfonylureas. They lower blood glucose by stimulating release of insulin from the pancreas, and, as with sulfonylureas, their effect is dependent on having functional beta cells in the pancreas. The prototype drug in this class is repaglinide, a short-acting agent that usually is taken 15 min before each meal. Its short duration of action (half-life 1 h) offers the potential to control glucose levels in persons who are usually diet controlled but who experience transient loss of control during illness or other episodic event. Repaglinide may be used in combination with metformin.

METFORMIN Metformin is a biguanide drug that has two principal mechanisms of action. First, it decreases hepatic gluconeogenesis. Second, it improves insulin resistance by increasing peripheral tissue sensitivity to insulin, thereby decreasing the feedback-mediated increase in insulin levels. The lowering of insulin levels makes metformin unlikely to produce hypoglycemia, and it causes no weight gain. These actions have particular benefit for obese patients, in whom insulin resistance is increased. Thus, many experts consider metformin to be an ideal drug for obese patients with type 2 diabetes.

Metformin can be used as monotherapy, or it can be combined with a sulfonylurea, troglitazone, meglitinide, or insulin. Metformin is contraindicated in patients with liver and renal impairment because of the risk of lactic acidosis in such individuals. Caution is also advised if patients are to undergo radiologic procedures with contrast media, because of the transient renal impairment that may occur after contrast administration. Metformin should be withheld for at least 1 day prior to such radiographic procedures.

TROGLITAZONE Troglitazone acts primarily on insulin receptors to decrease insulin resistance, thereby enhancing insulin action, increasing peripheral glucose uptake in skeletal muscle, and lowering insulin levels. Like metformin, it also decreases gluconeogenesis. Because there is no increase in insulin levels, troglitazone does not cause hypoglycemia.

Troglitazone can be used in combination with insulin, sulfonylureas, or metformin. Furthermore, troglitazone can be used as monotherapy to improve sensitivity to endogenously produced insulin. As monotherapy, it can be the initial treatment, in which case its effectiveness is similar to that of monotherapy with a sulfonylurea. Troglitazone should not, however, be substituted for a sulfonylurea in patients whose diabetes is already well controlled on a sulfonylurea. In those whose diabetes is not well controlled on sulfonylureas, troglitazone can be added as a second medication.

Additional benefits of troglitazone are its lowering of triglycerides levels and blood pressure, and elevation of HDL levels, all probably mediated through reduction of insulin levels. Clinical trials indicate that troglitazone may be effective, even in patients who have impaired glucose tolerance, in preventing progression to the overt diabetic state. It also appears that troglitazone may reduce hirsutism and induce ovulation in polycystic ovary syndrome, an insulin-resistant condition.

Troglitazone's most serious toxicity is hepatic injury, but this effect is uncommon. Postmarketing surveillance as of 1998 revealed 150 cases of liver toxicity and three deaths among 800,000 patients who have taken the drug. The Food and Drug Administration recommends that liver function tests be monitored monthly for the first 6 months of treatment, every other month for the next 6 months, and periodically thereafter. In contrast, the drug has no reported nephrotoxic side effects, and no dose adjustments are necessary for patients with renal disease.

α-GLUCOSIDASE INHIBITORS This category of drug is represented by acarbose. Acarbose inhibits α-glucosidase enzymes in the brush border of the small intestine, thereby slowing cleavage of oligo- and disaccharides into monosaccharides that can be absorbed. This action delays and blunts the blood glucose rise after a meal. It has no effect, however, on fasting hyperglycemia, nor is it useful in achieving weight loss. Acarbose can be used in combination with insulin or any of the oral medications discussed above. A common side effect of acarbose is flatulence, which can be reduced by starting with one-half tablet once per day and gradually increasing to the recommended dose of three times a day. Acarbose must be taken at the beginning of a meal to achieve its effects.

INSULIN Insulin is a standard and effective treatment for diabetes. It should not be used as a "last resort" treatment or as a threat to encourage compliance with diet, exercise, or oral agents. In fact, starting insulin early in the course of diabetes may improve the outcome. This is because high glucose levels cause toxic injury to beta cells, resulting in decreased insulin secretion, increased hyperglycemia, and therefore more beta-cell destruction. Early administration of insulin may help slow this cycle of hyperglycemia, glucotoxicity, and further beta-cell destruction.

In addition, combination therapy with insulin and an oral agent may help achieve glycemic control in some patients with type 2 diabetes that is uncontrolled on diet, exercise, and oral agents. Possible combination regimens include a concomitant oral agent and insulin throughout the day, a daytime oral agent and supper-time insulin, or a daytime oral agent and bedtime insulin. In addition to its use when patients cannot be controlled on diet, exercise, and oral medications, insulin is also indicated during acute injury, stress, infection, surgery, and pregnancy. Furthermore, insulin is a useful treatment in patients who are allergic to sulfonylurea drugs. Because of insulin resistance, large insulin doses may be needed for the patient with type 2 disease. Dose requirements are decreased, however, when insulin is used in combination with metformin or troglitazone.

Intensive Insulin Therapy Modern insulin therapy is relatively intensive and involves an ongoing system of diabetes management consisting of several components. The principal components of intensive regimens are multiple daily injections of insulins with varying durations of action and self-monitoring of blood glucose levels. Other essential components are adjustments in the patient's diet and increasing or decreasing insulin doses to maintain target glucose levels. Representative target glucose values are given in Table 4-11.

The ideal candidate for intensive therapy is a patient who is otherwise healthy and well motivated, and does not yet have signs of diabetic complications. However, intensive therapy is not appropriate for every newly diagnosed diabetic patient. Some patients need time to adjust emotionally to the diagnosis and to learn basic information about diabetes before attempting tight control. Tight control is contraindicated in a patient who cannot recognize hypoglycemic symptoms or has counterregulatory insufficiency, angina pectoris, or other complicating conditions. For some patients who live alone, hypoglycemia presents an unacceptable risk. Finally, the risk-benefit ratio of intensive therapy may be unacceptable in elderly individuals because severe hypoglycemia may have adverse effects on brain function in this age group.

Table 4-11

Glycemic Control Targets for Persons with Diabetes

SUBSTANCE	GOALS	MODIFY TREATMENT IF
Premeal glucose	80–120 mg/dL	<80 mg/dL or >140mg/dL
Bedtime glucose	100–140 mg/dL	<100 mg/dL or >160 mg/dL
Glycated hemoglobin	<7%	>8% (normal 4–6%)

SOURCE: Adapted with permission from American Diabetes Association: Standards of medical care for patients with diabetes mellitus (position statement).

Beginning Insulin Therapy A variety of insulin regimens have been recommended. The ideal regimen for a given patient should be individualized for meal schedule, exercise, and life-style. Several possible insulin regimens are displayed in Fig. 4-3, p. 108, and some of them are discussed below.

Single-Daily Insulin Injections In the past, many patients were treated with a single daily dose of intermediate-acting insulin, but this method rarely results in normalization of glycated hemoglobin levels. Nonetheless, this approach may still be appropriate for selected individuals in whom the dangers of hypoglycemia from attempting tight control are unacceptable or for patients who lack the motivation or understanding necessary to administer more complicated insulin regimens. Most patients are now treated with more intensive insulin regimens.

Twice-Daily Insulin Injections One common regimen used to begin outpatient insulin therapy involves dividing the total daily dose of intermediate-acting human insulin into two injections, with approximately two-thirds given in the morning before breakfast and the remaining one-third given before supper or bedtime. This traditional approach of twice-daily intermediate-acting insulin injections is based on the assumption that caloric intake and insulin needs are greater during daytime hours. In some cases, the total daily insulin dose is known; for example, when insulin was begun in the hospital during

an admission for hyperosmolar state or when patients are already taking insulin. If a patient's daily insulin dose is unknown, therapy can be instituted beginning with 20 to 30 units of intermediate-acting insulin per day.

This regimen of twice-daily intermediate-acting insulin is not likely to achieve tight control of blood glucose levels. However, the regimen can be modified to achieve better control as dictated by glucose levels, by changing the dose of intermediate-acting insulin or by adding short-acting insulin to each of the injections.

For example, after the total daily insulin dose is stabilized, two-thirds of the total daily dose can be injected before breakfast, and one-third is injected before dinner, with each of the two injections containing a mixture of intermediate- and short-acting insulin (Fig. 4-3, *A*). The combination of short-acting and intermediate-acting insulin is available commercially in a premixed solution, or it can be mixed in one syringe by the patient.

The proper dose of each component of the insulin regimen can be determined by monitoring glucose levels throughout the day. In this regimen, the short-acting insulin administered in the morning determines the prelunch glucose level, while the intermediate-acting insulin taken in the morning determines the late-afternoon glucose level. Similarly, the short-acting insulin given before supper determines the prebedtime blood glucose level, while the presupper intermediate-acting insulin controls the glucose level during the night and determines the fasting glucose level.

Three to Four Daily Insulin Injections A more intensive regimen involves three or four injections per day (Fig. 4-3, *C* and *D*). With four injections, regular, short-acting insulin is given: approximately 35 percent of the total daily dose before breakfast, 20 percent before lunch, 30 percent before supper, and 15 percent at bedtime or midnight. A small daily dose of intermediate, or more commonly long-acting, insulin can be given to cover hours in between doses of regular insulin and will be required for between-dose coverage if lispro is used as the short-acting insulin (see below).

This method offers the advantage of flexibility in the timing of meals, because regular insulin is only administered before each meal. If a meal is missed or delayed, the corresponding insulin dose can be omitted or adjusted accordingly. With experience, this method also provides flexibility for dealing with meals that are unexpectedly large or small, since the dose of regular insulin can be adjusted upward or downward as needed.

Incorporating Insulin Lispro With the introduction of lispro insulin, it is likely that new insulin treatment regimens will be developed to achieve even better control of blood glucose levels. Insulin lispro is an analogue of human insulin, originally named "lyspro," because the sequence of amino acids at positions 28 (*lys*ine) and 29 (*pro*line) of the β-insulin chain is reversed. This change results in a drug that is more rapidly absorbed and therefore more rapid acting than regular, short-acting human insulin.

The onset of action of insulin lispro occurs within 15 min of subcutaneous injection. Its peak effect is at 0.5 to 2.5 h, and its duration of action is 3 to 4 h. This time sequence more closely simulates the normal human insulin response to a meal. Because of the timing of its peak activity, it has greater effect on the 1- and 2-h postprandial glucose values than does regular insulin, which has its peak effect about 2 to 4 h after injection. Table 4-12 shows a comparison of insulin lispro and various other types of insulin.

The purpose of multiple injection regimens that include regular insulin is to control postprandial elevations of blood glucose. To achieve this goal with regular insulin, with its 30- to 60-min onset of action and 2- to 4-h peak of action, pa-

Table 4-12

Onset, Peak, and Duration of Action of Different Insulins

INSULIN	ONSET, H	PEAK, H	DURATION THERAPEUTIC, H*	DURATION PHARMACEUTIC, H†
Rapid acting, rapid peaking (Lispro)	0.25	0.5–1.5	3–4	4–6
Short Acting (regular, semilente)	0.5–1	2–4	6–8	5–12
Intermediate acting (NPH, lente, human ultralente)	1–4	8 ± 2	10–16	16–24
Long acting (animal ultralente)	4–6	8	24–36	36 +

*Therapeutic (or effective duration of action): the duration of action of insulin to keep blood glucose levels in normal limits.
†Pharmaceutic (or pharmacokinetic): duration of measurable levels.

Figure 4-3

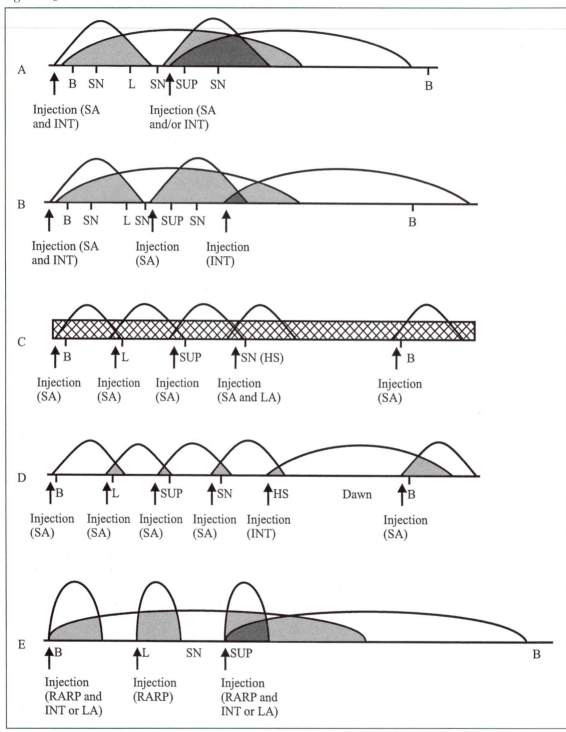

tients should inject regular insulin 30 to 60 min before meals to ensure that peak insulin activity and peak nutrient absorption coincide. Unfortunately, studies show that most patients do not inject their insulin in this fashion, even if recommended by their clinician, and instead administer insulin right before or immediately after meals. Therefore, the peak of regular insulin activity comes too late after injection to coincide with glucose elevation. Hypoglycemia may result about 3 h after the meal. Furthermore, the 4- to 6-h duration of action of regular insulin may increase premeal hunger and weight gain.

Insulin lispro, because of its rapid onset and peak action, can be given immediately prior to a meal (Fig. 4-3, *E*). Thus, it allows for more flexibility of meal times and injections than does regular insulin. However, the shorter duration of action of insulin lispro may result in lack of insulin coverage after 3 to 4 h or premeal if given alone. For patients with type 2 diabetes, insulin lispro may also be used as a short-acting supplement to dietary treatment, oral agents, or intermediate- or long-acting insulin.

Insulin lispro is dosed the same way as other insulins. When initiating short-acting, rapid-peaking insulin lispro in a patient who has been accustomed to older short-, intermediate-, or longer-acting insulins, the patient should be informed of the rapid onset and the need to eat immediately after an injection. It also may be prudent to reduce the usual dose initially until the patient adjusts to the change in regimen. Insulin lispro is compatible with intermediate- and long-acting human insulins and may be mixed with them in the same syringe, provided it is injected immediately. As with regular insulin, lispro should be drawn into the syringe before longer-acting insulins to prevent contamination of the short-acting insulin vial with longer-acting agents. Lispro should not be mixed with animal insulins.

Monitoring and Adjusting Glucose Control

Self-monitoring of blood glucose is essential to optimal glucose control with any treatment regimen. The optimal frequency of monitoring for patients with type 2 diabetes is not known but should be individualized to achieve glucose targets.

Typically, glucose monitoring begins with at least prebreakfast and presupper finger-stick checks. The initial goal for preprandial blood glucose levels is 150 to 200 mg/dL. As the patient becomes more accustomed to the treatment regimen and the concept of tight control, the goal becomes 100 mg/dL. The patient then learns to adjust diet, oral medications, insulin, or activity to correct for a given value.

When tight control with insulin is the objective, values should be checked before each meal

Common multiinjection insulin regimens. The figure illustrates several common insulin-delivery schemes not yet individualized for meal plan, exercise, and life-style. **A.** Standard twice-daily insulin regimen (intermediate- and short-acting, mixed or premixed). **B.** Three-times daily insulin regimen, suggested for patients with early-morning hypoglycemia followed by rebound hyperglycemia, or for patients with early-morning hyperglycemia (dawn phenomenon). **C.** Multidose insulin regimen of four injections per day (short-acting insulin before meals and long-acting animal insulin at bedtime). Continuous subcutaneous infusion (hatched area) would have a similar appearance. **D.** Alternative multidose regimen of five injections (short-acting insulin before meals and intermediate-acting insulin at bedtime). **E.** Three-times daily regimen using lispro and intermediate insulin. NOTE: Shaded areas illustrate overlap between insulin peaks. Human long-acting insulin has a curve only slightly more prolonged than intermediate-acting insulin. Arrows indicate injections. B, = breakfast; HS, bedtime; INT, intermediate-acting insulin; L, lunch; LA, long-acting insulin; RARP, = rapid-acting, rapid-peaking insulin lispro; SA, = short-acting insulin; SN, snack; SUP, supper.
(*Adapted with permission from American Diabetes Association: Medical Management of Insulin-Dependent [Type 1] Diabetes, 2d ed, Alexandria, VA, American Diabetes Association, 1994; and Gearhart et al with permission from the June 1995, vol 51 issue of American Family Physician. Copyright by the American Academy of Family Physicians. All rights reserved.*)

and at bedtime. Once fasting and premeal values improve, postprandial and middle-of-the-night levels can be monitored to tighten control and avoid hypoglycemia. For patients being treated with oral agents, less frequent measurements (once or twice daily at different times during the day) may be sufficient.

For patients who are unable or unwilling to perform finger-stick blood checks in outpatient settings, urine glucose checks can be used. However, urine tests are unequivocally less desirable than blood testing because urine glucose testing gives only a rough estimate of blood glucose values. Urine testing should not be used to fine-tune and adjust insulin dosage to obtain tight control because it does not quantify blood glucose levels below the renal threshold of approximately 180 mg/dL.

Insulin Adjustments Based on Blood Glucose Monitoring

When making adjustments in insulin dosage, one should take into account the type of insulin; the time to onset, peak, and duration of action; and mealtimes and size of meals. Adjustments in dose should be based on a pattern of glucose values observed over 3 or more days, with the goal of achieving blood glucose levels outlined in Table 4-11. Insulin decrements or supplements should attempt to correlate the peak of action of the insulin used with the anticipated glucose peaks.

To make adjustments, it is usually best to adjust one injection or one type of insulin at a time unless all glucose values are greater than 200mg/dL. Adjustments typically begin with the insulin affecting the fasting (prebreakfast) glucose value. This is usually the evening dose of intermediate- or long-acting insulin. Adjustments of 1 to 2 U are made until the fasting glucose level is corrected.

After prebreakfast glucose values are under control, adjustments in the morning dose of intermediate- or long-acting insulin can be made

to correct the predinner glucose levels. Addition of regular insulin before meals should affect both the postprandial and the following premeal glucose values. The premeal insulin lispro dose will affect the postprandial glucose level.

Sliding-scale therapy should be avoided, since it represents an attempt to control hyperglycemia in a retrospective fashion. Sliding-scale therapy has been associated with more episodes of hyperglycemia, hypoglycemia, and variability in glucose values. Furthermore, it interferes with the establishment of a pattern on which to base prospective adjustments in insulin.

Preventing Renal Disease

Because of the frequency and poor outcome of diabetic nephropathy, special attention should be paid to minimizing the risk that renal disease will develop. This requires attention to controlling blood pressure, using angiotensin-converting enzyme (ACE) inhibitors in patients with microalbuminuria, diet, and glycemic control.

Controlling Blood Pressure

Drug therapy to lower blood pressure is an important factor in preventing diabetic nephropathy. The ADA standards of medical care for treatment of hypertension in diabetes recommends that treatment should begin if blood pressure exceeds 130/85 mmHg. For patients with an isolated systolic blood pressure of 180 mmHg or more, the goal is to lower blood pressure to under 160 mmHg. For those with systolic blood pressures of 160 to 179 mmHg, the goal is a reduction of 20 mmHg. If goals are achieved and blood pressure levels and treatment are well tolerated, further lowering to 140 mmHg may be acceptable.

The ACE inhibitors are the drugs of choice for lowering blood pressure in patients with diabetes. These drugs normalize intraglomerular hypertension and prevent development of glomerulosclerosis. For patients who cannot tolerate ACE inhibitors, calcium channel blocking agents are a good second-line therapy. The dihydropyridine class (e.g., nifedipine) of calcium channel blockers should be avoided, however, since they increase proteinuria. High doses of thiazide diuretics may worsen insulin resistance, glycemic control, and lipid levels, but low doses (e.g., 12.5 mg/day) do not show these effects. Furthermore, diuretics may be essential for blood pressure control in hypoalbuminemic and/or volume-overloaded patients. Other antihypertensive drug choices are addressed in Table 4-3.

ACE INHIBITORS FOR MICROALBUMINURIA

Research suggests that normotensive patients with microalbuminuria also benefit from treatment with ACE inhibitors because these drugs improve intraglomerular hemodynamics. In fact, a consensus report from the National Kidney Foundation recommends that all normotensive and hypertensive diabetic patients with microalbuminuria receive ACE inhibitors to decrease intraglomerular pressures.

PROTEIN-RESTRICTED DIETS

Another important measure in the management of nephropathy is dietary protein restriction. Protein raises the single-nephron glomerular filtration rate and glomerular blood flow. Studies in type 1 diabetes have shown that protein restriction helps to decrease glomerular hypertension, hyperfiltration, microalbuminuria, and the progression to renal failure. The benefit probably extends to individuals with type 2 diabetes. Recommended protein intake is 0.6 to 0.8 (g/kg)/d once macroalbuminuria develops, as long as overall nutritional status is satisfactory.

GLYCEMIC CONTROL

Poor glycemic control shortens the interval between the onset of diabetes and the appearance of clinical proteinuria. The DCCT study showed that strict control in type 1 diabetes reduced the risk of development or progression of nephropathy compared with conventional treatment by 50 to 75 percent. Good control in type 2 diabetes is likely to have a similar beneficial effect.

Concurrent Medications

An important component of diabetes treatment is to avoid using medications that interact with antidiabetic drugs or adversely affect glycemic control or diabetes risk factors. Patients with newly diagnosed type 2 diabetes are likely to be older and to have coexisting medical problems and may be taking medications that interact with diabetes care or outcomes. For example, impaired glucose tolerance is caused by thiazide diuretics and beta blockers, and also by conditions such as diuretic-induced hypokalemia. Beta blockers also mask physiologic responses to hypoglycemia. Alpha blockers can aggravate postural hypotension in patients with neuropathy. Tables 4-13 and 4-14 list medications that may interfere with diabetes management.

Nutrition

Important goals of nutrition therapy for diabetes include maintaining optimal glucose levels by balancing food intake with insulin, oral agents, and activity levels, and achieving or maintaining optimal weight. A further goal is to prevent and treat complications such as nephropathy, hypertension, hyperlipidemia, and cardiovascular disease.

DISTRIBUTION OF DIETARY COMPONENTS

Protein intake should account for about 10 to 20 percent of daily caloric intake, except when nephropathy develops, in which case protein restriction is recommended [(0.6 to 0.8 (g/kg)/d)].

Table 4-13

Drug Interactions in Diabetes That May Cause Hypoglycemia

DRUG	MECHANISM
Alcohol	Impairs gluconeogenesis; increases insulin secretion; disulfiram-like reaction may occur with chlorpropamide, glipizide, and glyburide
Allopurinol	Rare reports of hypoglycemia with sulfonylureas; may increase half-life
Anabolic steroids	Unknown
Beta-adrenergic antagonists	Inhibits glycogenolysis; may mask clinical signs and symptoms of hypoglycemia; may delay recovery from hypoglycemia
Chloramphenicol (Chloromycetin)	May inhibit metabolism of sulfonylureas
Chloroquine (Aralen)	Unknown
Cimetidine	Increases half-life of tolbutamide and glyburide
Clofibrate (Atromid-S)	May enhance activity of sulfonylureas or insulin
Coumadin/Dicumerol	Inhibits hepatic clearance of tolbutamide (Orinase) and chlorpropamide (Diabinese)
Disopyramide (Norpace)	Unknown
Doxepin	Potentiates effect of tolazamide; mechanism unknown
Fenfluramine	Has hypoglycemic effect; may potentiate insulin effects
Fluconazole	Increases tolbutamide levels; minimally significant
Gemfibrozil	Enhances effect of glyburide; may displace glyburide from binding sites
Guanethidine	Potentiates insulin; may improve glucose tolerance long-term
Heparin	May decrease binding of glipizide; minimally significant
Methyldopa	Prolongs half-life of tolbutamide; minimally significant
Monoamine oxidase inhibitors	Potentiates insulin and sulfonylureas
Oxytetracycline	May enhance sulfonylurea action; may increase half-life of insulin or interfere with action of epinephrine
Pentamidine isethionate (NebuPent, Pentam 300)	Release of insulin
Phenylbutazone (Azolid, Butazolidin)	Decreases sulfonylurea clearance
Probenecid	May increase half-life of chlorpropamide and tolbutamide; chlorpropamide and probenecid should not be used in patients with renal impairment
Salicylates	Increase insulin secretion and tissue sensitivity; may alter pharmacokinetics of sulfonylureas, particularly chlorpropamide
Sulfonamides	Alter clearance of sulfonylureas
Tobacco	Decrease insulin absorption

Plate 1 *(Figure 3-2)*
In hypertensive retinopathy, the retina may develop flame, or splinter, hemorrhages (seen in the upper part of the photo) and cotton wool spots (light-colored areas), which represent infarction of the nerve fiber layer of the retina. *(Reproduced with permission from AS Fauci et al, eds: Harrison's Principles of Internal Medicine. New York, McGraw-Hill, 1998.)*

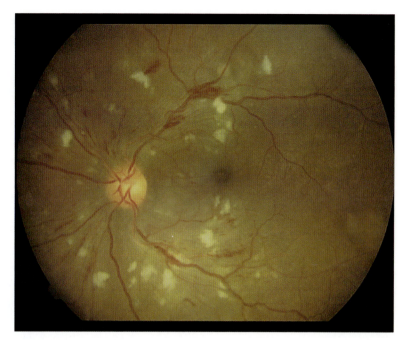

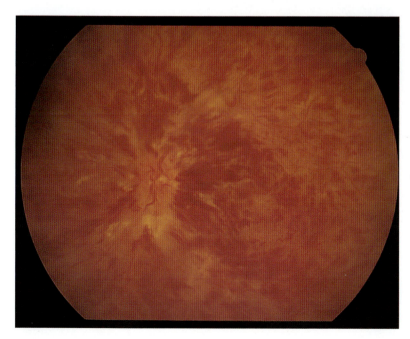

Plate 2 *(Figure 3-3)*
Central retinal vein occlusion can produce massive retinal hemorrhage, retinal ischemia, and visual loss. Its typical appearance, shown in this fundus photograph, is of "blood and thunder." *(Reproduced with permission from AS Fauci et al, eds: Harrison's Principles of Internal Medicine. New York, McGraw-Hill, 1998.)*

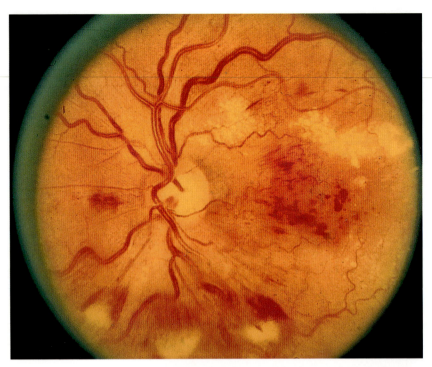

Plate 3 *(Figure 4-1)*
Nonproliferative diabetic retinopathy. The optic fundus photograph shows nonproliferative diabetic retinopathy with hemorrhages (red areas) and "cotton-wool" spots (pale areas).
(Courtesy of Dr. Ching-Jygh Chen, University of Mississippi School of Medicine.)

Plate 4 *(Figure 4-2A)*
Proliferative diabetic retinopathy. Neovascularization from the disc extends to surrounding retina. Localized tractional retinal detachment is also seen (pale areas).
(Courtesy of Dr. Ching-Jygh Chen, University of Mississippi School of Medicine.)

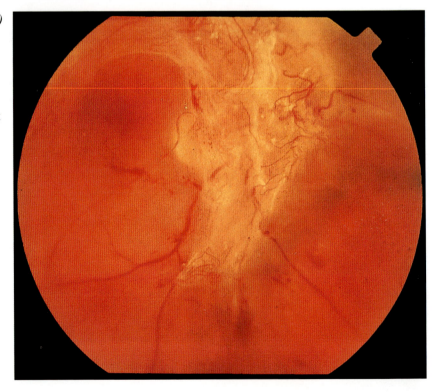

Plate 5 (*Figure 4-2B*)
Advanced proliferative diabetic retinopathy. In more advanced disease, fibrovascular proliferation and preretinal hemorrhages occur. Progressive traction on the retina leads to extensive areas of detachment (pale areas). *(Courtesy of Dr. Ching-Jygh Chen, University of Mississippi School of Medicine.)*

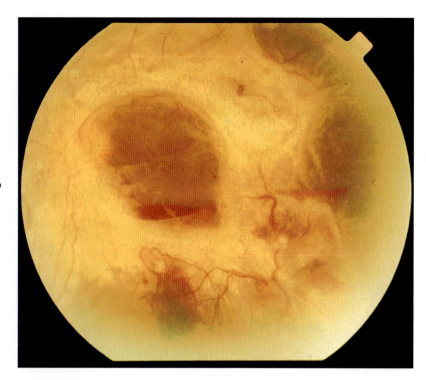

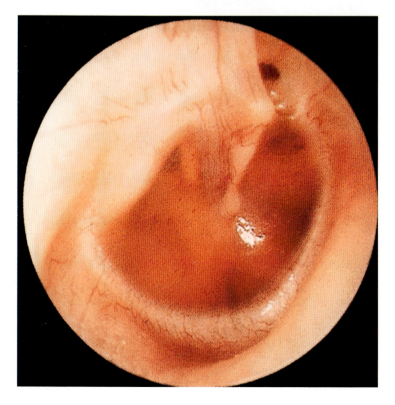

Plate 6 (*Figure 5-1*)
Otitis media with effusion as seen in an otoscopic view of a right tympanic membrane. There are retraction of the central portion of the tympanic membrane and a yellowish discoloration from the serous fluid accumulated in the middle ear behind the membrane. *(Reproduced with permission of Dr. Michael Hawke, Department of Otolaryngology, University of Toronto.)*

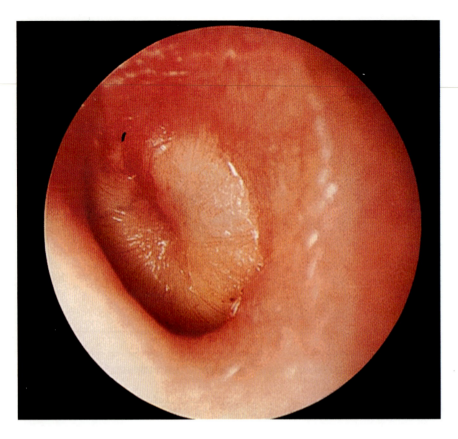

Plate 7 *(Figure 5-2)*
Acute otitis media as seen in an otoscopic view of a left tympanic membrane. Typical findings of acute otitis are present, including redness and bulging of the tympanic membrane.
(Reproduced with permission of Dr. Michael Hawke, Department of Otolaryngology, University of Toronto.)

Table 4-14

Drug Interactions in Diabetes That May Cause Hyperglycemia

DRUG	MECHANISM
Alcohol	Chronic ingestion may increase metabolism of tolbutamide
Asparginase	May inhibit insulin synthesis
Beta-adrenergic agonists	Inhibit insulin secretion
Calcium channel antagonists	Inhibit insulin secretion; impair insulin-mediated glucose transport; may cause insulin resistance by effect on intracellular calcium
Combination oral contraceptives	Unknown
Cholestyramine	Binds and decreases absorption of glipizide and troglitazone
Chlorpromazine	Inhibits insulin release
Diazoxide	Inhibits insulin secretion; may decrease effect of sulfonylureas
Diuretics	Possibly related to hypokalemia; inhibit insulin release
Glucocorticoids	Increase gluconeogenesis; depress insulin action
Glycerol	Unknown
Lithium	May decrease insulin secretion
Niacin	Unknown
Pentamidine	Promotes pancreatic toxicity
Phenytoin sodium	Inhibits insulin secretion
Rifampin	Enhances metabolism of tolbutamide
Sympathomimetics	Increase glycogenolysis and gluconeogenesis; may act synergistically with glucagon to antagonize insulin effect

The remaining 80 to 90 percent of calories should be distributed between dietary fat and carbohydrate. Less than 10 percent of calories should be from saturated fats, up to 10 percent from unsaturated fats, and 60 to 70 percent from monounsaturated fats and carbohydrates. The distribution between fat and carbohydrates is individualized.

Traditional practice has been to avoid simple sugars in favor of complex carbohydrates, based on the assumption that simple sugars caused a greater degree of hyperglycemia. Little scientific evidence supports this assumption, and recent guidelines have focused on the total amount of carbohydrate consumed rather than the source or type of carbohydrate.

Current ADA guidelines also include a moderate increase in monounsaturated fats and a reduced intake of carbohydrates compared with previous guidelines. Examples of monounsaturated fats are those in safflower oil, canola oil, olive oil, avocados, and some nuts.

CARBOHYDRATE COUNTING

The diet exchange lists previously recommended by the ADA are now giving way to more individualized meal plans. Instead of exchange diets, "carbohydrate counting" is now used to provide greater menu flexibility in choices, timing, and quantities. The rationale for carbohydrate counting is that more than 90 percent of ingested carbohydrates are converted to glucose, while this occurs only to a limited degree for ingested fat and protein. Thus, most of the postprandial rise in glucose is attributable to ingested carbohydrates, and so attention should be focused on the total ingestion of carbohydrates.

Most primary care clinicians have neither the time nor the expertise to provide detailed education on the technique of carbohydrate counting. The ADA recommends that patients see a registered dietitian for two to three 45- to 90-min sessions to learn how to properly count carbohydrates.

OTHER DIETARY CONSTITUENTS AND MICRONUTRIENTS

ALCOHOL Moderate alcohol consumption (one to two beverages per day) is acceptable for persons with diabetes if glucose levels are well controlled. Abstinence is advised if there are diabetic complications, a history of substance abuse, or pregnancy. Alcohol increases the risk of hypoglycemia for those taking insulin or oral agents, and patients should be forewarned about this possibility. Alcohol should be consumed only with meals.

FIBER Fiber intake recommendations are the same as for the general population. About 20 to 35 g of fiber should be ingested each day from a variety of food sources.

SODIUM Recommendations regarding sodium intake vary. Most authorities recommend restriction to less than 2.4 g/d for those with hypertension or nephropathy.

VITAMINS AND MINERALS Antioxidant therapy (e.g., vitamins C, E, and β-carotene) for diabetes is still under investigation. Research thus far indicates that it has benefits in decreasing atherogenesis. Potassium intake should be supplemented or restricted, depending on blood pressure, renal function, and concurrent medications.

Hypomagnesemia has been reported in as many as 25 percent of outpatients with diabetes and has been associated with poor control in patients with type 2 diabetes regardless of type of therapy. Hypomagnesemia has also been correlated with insulin resistance in nondiabetic elderly patients. While there is no clear relationship between magnesium and glycated hemoglobin levels, magnesium supplementation may be prudent in patients with diabetes and cardiovascular disease due to their high frequency of hypomagnesemia and its consequences in high-risk groups.

Exercise

Exercise is important for any individual to achieve and maintain cardiovascular and overall fitness and weight control. Maintenance of desirable body weight is particularly important in type 2 diabetes. In addition, physical exercise—especially regular vigorous exercise but also, to a lesser degree, less-frequent nonvigorous physical activity—improves insulin sensitivity in patients with type 2 diabetes. In terms of improving diabetic control, those who respond best to exercise are those who have mild glucose intolerance and hyperinsulinemia.

Patients beginning an exercise program should do so under a clinician's guidance after an appropriate preexercise evaluation. This preexercise evaluation should include cardiovascular, neurologic, musculoskeletal, and ophthalmologic assessment to guide the exercise prescription. For patients over age 35, an exercise stress test should be performed as part of the assessment.

Ideally, patients should increase daily activity and achieve acceptable glycemic control before beginning an exercise program. To reduce the risk of foot infections, patients should wear proper footwear and inspect the feet after exercise. Those with peripheral neuropathy should avoid high-impact exercises. Persons with diabetes should avoid exercise in extremes of ambient temperature and during periods of poor glycemic control. Exercise should be accompanied by close monitoring of blood sugar to avoid exercise-induced hypoglycemia; patients should be prepared to self-treat hypoglycemia if it occurs.

Education

Reassurance

Clinicians must consider the emotional effect of the initial diagnosis of diabetes on patients and their families. Reactions to the diagnosis vary. Patients may feel uncertainty about the immediate short-term outcome for their health, and may feel shock or anger. Many patients feel a sense of helplessness, anxiety, and loss of control, and they may fear departure from normal diet and activity. The diagnosis of diabetes also carries implications for employment and insurance coverage.

Denial is a common reaction. Type 2 patients are particularly prone to denial because at the time of diagnosis they often have no symptoms of diabetes. Denial may adversely affect a patient's ability or willingness to comply with treatment recommendations.

Clinicians must offer reassurance that, with new methods of treatment, a patient can live an almost normal life. Primary care clinicians are in an ideal position to establish a supportive relationship, negotiating with the patient regarding life-style changes.

Teaching the Patient and the Family

A team approach is essential to optimal management of diabetes. The team should include members of the patient's family, especially the person responsible for food selection and preparation. If such resources are available, the involvement of a nurse educator, a dietitian, a social worker, and/or a psychologist will facilitate the education and support of the patient and family. Important goals for education of patients with diabetes are listed on Table 4-15.

Immediate educational needs for newly diagnosed diabetics include a basic explanation of the diagnosis and nature of diabetes, along with simple instructions for monitoring, medications, and diet. Other important issues include guidelines for driving, traveling, missing meals, and responding to hypoglycemia.

As patients learn more about diabetes, they should be given more detailed instructions about achieving glycemic control. Long-term issues include prevention of vascular complications through control of hypertension and hyperlipidemia, and prevention of renal complications through medications and low-protein diets. Because of the synergism of diabetes and smoking in the development of atherosclerosis, patients should be advised not to smoke.

Table 4-15

Important Educational Topics for Patients with Diabetes

Understanding medications actions and regimens
Individualized nutrition recommendations
Life-style changes
How to monitor blood glucose levels
Ophthalmologist visit (1) upon diagnosis of diabetes, then annually, or (2) if visual symptoms occur
Foot problems are serious. Education about prevention and surveillance of foot problems is essential, and includes instruction in foot self-examinations and wearing appropriate shoes.
Arrangements for follow-up, initially as often as necessary to achieve control and patient competence. Contact may be made daily or weekly when initiating or changing an insulin regimen, and weekly when initiating or changing an oral agent. Visits should then be made at least quarterly until all goals are achieved, and then quarterly or semiannually.
Instructions on when and how to contact the health care team
Importance of dental hygiene

SOURCE: Adapted with permission from American Diabetes Association: Standards of medical care for patients with diabetes mellitus (position statement).

Benefit of Patients' Education

Although intuitively the education of patients seems important for management of diabetes, limited information is available to show that it has a beneficial effect on diabetes outcomes. One study has shown a relationship between poor diabetes control and patients having a passive, dependent approach to their condition. Other studies have demonstrated benefits from selected educational interventions. For example, a brief office-based intervention using a touch-screen computer in conjunction with follow-up phone calls and video instruction has been shown to facilitate dietary self-management. After the intervention, there were significant differences in dietary behavior measures, serum cholesterol levels, and patients' satisfaction with diabetes care. However, glycated hemoglobin levels—arguably the most important outcome measure—did not improve.

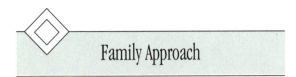

Family Approach

From the outset, clinicians must involve the patient's family. Patients' families report greater satisfaction in seeing the results of their efforts when they are involved from the beginning. Family education and involvement are particularly important when patients are elderly or mentally or physically disabled. The family's role in management, which includes achieving glycemic control, preventing complications, and, in particular, recognizing signs and symptoms of hypoglycemia, is crucial. Responsibilities of each party should be clearly defined.

Patients' and families' education should be initiated early, rather than after problems develop. During the early period following diagnosis, the support of a social worker or psychologist may be helpful. The clinician should ask about stressors at home and also assess the patient's and family's health care beliefs, educational level, and cultural background. Family support systems and financial circumstances, as well as life-styles and eating habits, are important issues.

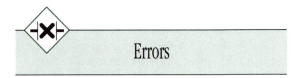

Errors

Common errors in management are failure to (1) seek tight control by prescribing multiple-daily insulin injections rather than once-daily injections, (2) employ self-glucose monitoring, (3) screen for microalbuminuria, and (4) measure and monitor lipids and glycated hemoglobin levels. Other common errors include omission of diet and exercise counseling, and many clinicians fail to perform routine funduscopic and foot examinations. Finally, sliding-scale therapy remains commonly used but should be avoided, as discussed earlier.

These deficiencies in management have been demonstrated in multiple studies in a variety of settings. For example, one survey published in the late 1990s showed that only about half of patients on insulin used multiple daily injections. In addition, only a quarter of type 2 patients taking insulin monitor their glucose levels daily, and the corresponding figure for those not taking insulin is 5 percent. This study also showed a low rate of visits to ophthalmologists, podiatrists, nutritionists, and diabetic education classes.

Another study of adherence to the ADA clinical practice guidelines by primary care physicians showed that, while over 75 percent said that they recommended glycated hemoglobin testing, only about 50 percent of patients had billings records demonstrating that the test had been performed. All physicians stated that they recommended annual eye examinations, but only 43 percent of patients said that their primary care physician recommended such examinations.

A third study in five Medicare managed-care plans determined adherence to ten quality indicators and found that the care of only 5 percent of patients met nine or ten of the indicators. Adherence to only two standards was found for more than 60 percent of patients: blood pressure measurement (98 percent) and foot examination (62 percent). Two standards (urine testing for microalbuminuria and use of ACE inhibitors) were achieved in less than one-third of patients.

Finally, another study assessed practice patterns of rural family physicians based on ADA standards of care. A chart review for compliance with ADA parameters demonstrated only 66 percent compliance with dietary counseling, 33 percent with exercise counseling, 66 percent with funduscopic examination, and 64 percent with foot examination. Seventy percent of charts documented that a urinalysis had been performed, but only 45 percent contained evidence that lipids had been measured, and only 15 percent had documentation of glycated hemoglobin tests.

These studies provide evidence that diabetic patients across the US, seen in a variety of specialties and practice settings, do not receive the care they should receive to maximize outcomes. It is not clear why these errors occur. Lack of compliance with guidelines reflects possible deficiencies in clinicians' knowledge, problems implementing recommended care, lack of belief in or awareness of guidelines, or patient compliance problems. Whatever the reason, these studies indicate the need for large-scale improvement in the way diabetes care is provided.

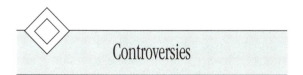

Controversies

Diet

The recommended composition of the diet of patients with diabetes is an ongoing subject of controversy. For example, new insights into adverse health correlates of hyperinsulinemia (which may be more marked following ingestion of simple sugars) is generating controversy about current dietary guidelines that focus only on total carbohydrates, instead of on the nature and speed-of-absorption of ingested carbohydrates. And, although low-fat diets may improve lipid profiles, high-carbohydrate diets may worsen lipoprotein levels. Further studies are needed to determine the optimal proportions and types of macronutrients.

In addition, the role of chromium in diabetes control has not been clarified. As a trace element, chromium is essential for normal carbohydrate and fat metabolism. Some authors have proposed that chromium may improve insulin efficiency because it improves glycemic control in those who are chromium-deficient. However, there have been no large controlled studies in the United States, and research elsewhere has yielded conflicting results. Thus, while there is a need to clarify the role of this nutrient in outcomes in patients with diabetes, at this point there is not even a recommended daily allowance for chromium. A dose of up to 200 μg/d apparently is safe but is not routinely recommended for treatment of diabetes.

Practicality of Tight Control

Some authors have questioned whether the tight diabetic control demonstrated in the DCCT and similar studies is feasible in routine clinical practice. The DCCT involved a large-scale investigative effort with close follow-up of study participants. In reality, clinicians care for many patients in whom tight glycemic control is impossible because of motivation, socioeconomic issues, and logistical factors. In fact, in a recent study in a health maintenance organization, over 8500 type 2 diabetics were treated with a variety of insulin regimens; at the end of 3 years, most patients had not achieved glycemic control, despite higher health care costs and resource utilization than among those not treated with insulin. Thus, while the dramatic reduction in complications of diabetes reported in research under tightly controlled conditions makes it seem desirable to attempt to achieve normoglycemia all patients, the investment of time and resources required for such an attempt may not yield the desired outcomes in real-life situations.

Fetal Tissue Harvesting

Preliminary research suggests that islet cells transplanted from fetal pancreas into living diabetic patients can restore glycemic control. However, fetal tissue harvesting for islet cell transplantation is investigational and extremely controversial. It has generated considerable ethical debate that is unlikely to be resolved quickly.

Emerging Concepts

"Smart Pump"

For many years, selected patients (mostly in investigational settings) have controlled glucose values successfully with the use of an insulin pump. Insulin pumps administer a continuous infusion of regular or lispro insulin, and the patient makes adjustments in the infusion rate based on self-monitoring of blood glucose.

Development has been under way on a device that would not only deliver insulin but also monitor glucose and automatically make appropriate adjustments in the insulin infusion rate. Such a device has not yet been perfected, but it is likely that it will be available for clinical use in coming years.

New Medications

Amylin is a peptide that is synthesized and secreted, along with insulin, by pancreatic beta cells. Amylin slows gastric emptying and gas-

trointestinal glucose absorption, thereby decreasing postprandial glucose levels. Investigations are ongoing to develop synthetic analogues of amylin.

Glucagon-like peptide-1 potentiates glucose-induced insulin secretion. It may reduce the postprandial increase in blood glucose by delaying gastric emptying. It is likely to have a future role in the treatment of diabetes.

Pancreas Transplantation

Pancreatic transplantation is performed to restore an effective insulin-secreting organ to an insulin-deficient diabetic patient. The most common type of pancreas transplantation is a simultaneous pancreas and kidney (SPK) transplantation performed from a single cadaver donor. The next most common is pancreas transplantation after successful kidney (PAK) transplantation. A few centers are performing pancreas transplantation alone (PTA) in diabetic recipients without renal disease but with significant complications of diabetes. The overall results for pancreatic transplantation show 1-year graft survival of 75 percent for SPK transplantation and 48 percent for PAK and PTA transplantation. The principal use of pancreas transplantation, however, is for patients with type 1 diabetes.

Computer Programs

In the future, diabetes management will be facilitated by computer technology. Even now, a few computer programs, which can be downloaded from the Internet, are available to guide clinicians through care of diabetic patients.

Bibliography

Aiello LP, Cavallerano J, Bursell S: Diabetic eye disease: Chronic complications of diabetes. *Endocrinol Metab Clin North Am* 25:271, 1996.

American Diabetes Association: Guide to diagnosis and classification of diabetes mellitus and other categories of glucose intolerance (position statement). *Diabetes Care* 20:S21, 1997.

American Diabetes Association: Hospital admission guidelines for diabetes mellitus. *Diabetes Care* 20:S52, 1997.

American Diabetes Association: Nutrition recommendations and principles for people with diabetes mellitus (position statement). *Diabetes Care* 20:S14, 1997.

American Diabetes Association: Standards of medical care for patients with diabetes mellitus (position statement). *Diabetes Care* 20:S1, 1997.

Anderson RA, Cheng N, Bryden NA, et al: Elevated intakes of supplemental chromium improve glucose and insulin variables in individuals with type 2 diabetes. *Diabetes* 46:1786, 1997.

Brancati FL, Whelton PK, Randall BL, et al: Risk of end-stage renal disease in diabetes mellitus: A prospective cohort study in men screened for MRFIT. *JAMA* 278:2069, 1997.

Camilleri M: Gastrointestinal problems in diabetes. *Endocrinol Metab Clin North Am* 25:361, 1996.

Campbell RK, Campbell LK, White JR: Insulin lispro: Its role in the treatment of diabetes mellitus. *Ann Pharmacother* 30:1263, 1996.

Diabetes Control and Complications Trial Research Group: The effect of intensive treatment of diabetes on the development and progression of long-term complications in insulin-dependent diabetes mellitus. *New Engl J Med* 329:977, 1993.

Diabetes: 1996 Vital Statistics. Alexandria, VA, American Diabetes Association, 1996.

Fuller JH: When to treat the hypertensive diabetic patient. *Diabetes Complications* 10:144, 1996.

Gautier JF, Beressi JP, Leblanc H, et al: Are the implications of the Diabetes Control and Complications Trial (DCCT) feasible in daily clinical practice? *Diabetes Metab* 22:415, 1996.

Gearhart JG, Duncan J, Replogle B, et al: Efficacy of sliding scale insulin therapy: A comparison with prospective methods. *Fam Pract Res J* 14:313, 1994.

Gearhart JG, Forbes RC: Initial management of the patient with newly diagnosed diabetes. *Am Fam Phys* 51:1953, 1995.

Glasgow RE, Toobert DJ, Hampson SE: Effects of a brief office-based intervention to facilitate diabetes dietary self-management. *Diabetes Care* 19:835, 1996.

Gorman C, Looker J, et al: A clinically useful diabetes electronic medical record: Lessons from the past; pointers toward the future. *Eur J Endocrino* 134:31, 1996.

Groggel GC: Diabetic nephropathy. *Arch Fam Med* 5:513, 1996.

Hayward RA, Manning WG, Kaplan SH: Starting insulin therapy in patients with type 2 diabetes: Effectiveness, complications, and resource utilization. *JAMA* 278:1663, 1997.

Lawler FH, Viviani N: Patient and physician perspectives regarding treatment of diabetes: Compliance with practice guidelines. *J Fam Pract* 44: 369, 1997.

LoGerfo FW, Gibbons GW: Vascular disease of the lower extremities in diabetes mellitus. *Endocrinol Metab Clin North Am* 25:439, 1996.

Marshall CL, Bluestein M, et al: Outpatient management of diabetes mellitus in five Arizona Medicare managed care plans. *Am J Med Qual* 11:87, 1996.

Mayer-Davis EJ, D-Agostino R, Lartner AJ, et al: Intensity and amount of physical activity in relation to insulin sensitivity. *JAMA* 279:669, 1998.

Mazze RS, Etzwiler DD, Strock E, et al: Staged diabetes management. *Diabetes Care* 17:S56, 1994.

Mogensen CE: Management of early nephropathy in diabetic patients. *Annu Rev Med* 46:79, 1995.

Nilsson P: Diabetes and syndrome X in hypertension: Population aspects. *J Hum Hypertens* 10:S81, 1996.

Noble SL, Johnston E, Walton B: Insulin lispro: A fast acting insulin analog. *Am Fam Phys* 57:279, 1998.

O'Conner PJ, Rush WA, Peterson J, et al: Continuous quality improvement can improve glycemic control for HMO patients with diabetes. *Arch Fam Med* 5:502, 1996.

Ohdubo Y, Kishikawa H, Araki E, et al: Intensive insulin therapy prevents the progression of diabetic microvascular complications in Japanese patients with non-insulin dependent diabetes mellitus: A randomized, prospective 6-year study. *Diabetes Res Clin Pract* 28:103, 1995.

Queale WS, et al: Glycemic control and sliding scale insulin in medical inpatients with diabetes mellitus. *Arch Intern Med* 157:545, 1997.

Skyler JS: Diabetic complications: The importance of glucose control. *Endocrinol Metab Clin North Am* 25:243, 1996.

Tosiello L: Hypomagnesemia and diabetes mellitus: A review of clinical complications. *Arch Intern Med* 156:1143, 1996.

White JR: Combination oral agent/insulin therapy in patients with type II diabetes mellitus. *Clin Diabetes* 15:102, 1997.

Zoorob RJ, Mainous AG III: Practice patterns of rural family physicians based on the American Diabetes Association standards of care. *J Community Health* 21:175, 1996.

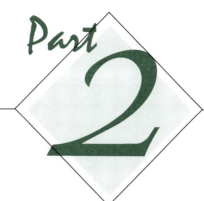

Part 2

Respiratory Problems

Evan W. Kligman

Chapter

5

Earache

How Common Is Earache?

Earache caused by otitis media is one of the most common conditions treated by primary care clinicians. In fact, otitis media accounts for more than 30 million outpatient visits annually in the United States and is the most frequent diagnosis given to children under 15 years of age. Furthermore, treatment of acute otitis media accounts for 42 percent of all antibiotics prescribed for children. The cost for outpatient management of otitis media in the United States exceeds $1 billion per year, and almost $2 billion more is spent on surgical treatments such as tympanostomy tube placement (the most common minor surgical procedure performed in the United States).

The incidence of otitis media is highest in children between age 6 months and 3 years of age, and it becomes uncommon after age 7. Most children will have at least one ear infection before age 3, and more than one-third of all children have three ear infections by that age. Otitis media is more common in males than in females, and its incidence rises in the winter months and decreases during the summer. It is interesting to note that the prevalence of recurrent otitis media has increased by almost 50 percent over the last 5 years. This rise is believed to be a result of increased use of day care and a higher prevalence of childhood allergies.

Earache caused by otitis externa is also common in primary care practice, with a prevalence of between 3 and 10 percent in the general population. In contrast to otitis media, however, otitis externa is seen more frequently in adults than in children.

Principal Diagnoses

Earache may be caused by an infection of the middle ear or external auditory canal. Otitis

media, or inflammation of the middle ear, is now generally divided into two major diagnostic entities: acute otitis media (suppurative) and otitis media with effusion (serous). Otitis externa is infection of the external canal. These three conditions (acute otitis media, otitis media with effusion, and otitis externa) are the principal diagnoses to consider in patients presenting with earache.

Although not reviewed in this chapter, several conditions unrelated to the ear can cause apparent earache. The most common of these conditions include dental problems, angina pectoris, arthropathy of the temporomandibular joint, and herpes zoster. When history and physical examination fail to identify an ear-related cause for ear pain, these alternative diagnoses should be considered if appropriate to a patient's clinical presentation.

Acute Otitis Media

Acute otitis media is inflammation of the middle ear with signs of infection. It is the most common cause of earache. A pus accumulation develops in the middle ear, usually with rapid onset of one or more of the following symptoms: otalgia, ear pulling, otorrhea, fever, irritability, anorexia, vomiting, or diarrhea. Typically, the tympanic membrane is bulging and/or opaque, and it has abnormal mobility. Erythema of the tympanic membrane is common, but may or may not be present.

As noted above, more than half (about 60 percent) of all children will have at least one episode by age 3. By age 7, over 90 percent of children will have had one or more episode. Acute otitis media is uncommon in adolescents and young adults, and rare in older adults.

PATHOPHYSIOLOGY

Acute otitis media usually results from eustachian tube dysfunction, which impairs effective clearance of fluid from the middle ear.

Eustachian tube dysfunction occurs via one or both of two mechanisms. Most commonly, a viral upper respiratory tract infection or allergic rhinitis causes congestion, inflammation, and obstruction of the eustachian tube, preventing drainage of middle ear fluid from the middle ear into the nasopharynx. The other mechanism is delayed innervation of the tensor veli palatini muscle, which results in abnormal eustachian tube patency and reflux of nasopharyngeal fluid into the middle ear.

Through either mechanism, fluid accumulates in the middle ear and becomes a "culture medium" for bacterial and viral pathogens. The common pathogens involved in acute otitis media are listed in Table 5-1. The presence of bacteria and accumulated fluid in the middle ear leads to a cytokine-mediated inflammatory response, resulting in the clinical syndrome of acute otitis media.

The risk of bacterial colonization is highest in infants, who have shorter and more horizontal eustachian tubes. The risk decreases with age as the eustachian tube lengthens and becomes less horizontal, and as innervation of the tensor veli palatini muscle becomes fully developed.

RISK FACTORS

An infant's risk of developing acute otitis media is increased by being fed in the prone position, especially during the first 4 months of life. A family history of atopy, group day care attendance, male gender, and having a sibling with a history of recurrent otitis media also increase risk. Exposure to environmental tobacco smoke is another factor that may increase a child's susceptibility to acute otitis media. In addition, certain ethnic groups (Native Americans, including Alaskan and Canadian Inuits) have a higher incidence of acute otitis media, as do children with various craniofacial anatomic anomalies. These anomalies include intranasal or postnasal atresia, open or submucosal cleft palate, bifid uvula, and structural abnormalities that occur in trisomy 21. Finally,

there is contradictory evidence about whether breast feeding decreases the incidence of acute otitis media.

Otitis Media with Effusion

Otitis media with effusion, formerly known as serous otitis media, is defined as the presence of serous fluid in the middle ear without clinical signs or symptoms of infection. If the effusion persists longer than 2 to 3 months, the condition is considered chronic. Symptoms may include inflammation, otalgia, irritability, poor feeding, and restlessness.

Otitis media with effusion can occur de novo in healthy children but usually develops after an episode of acute otitis media. In fact, 3 months after treatment of acute otitis media, approximately one-quarter of children have a persistent serous effusion. Otitis media with effusion occurs most often in children between the ages of 1 and 3 years. It is more prevalent in winter and in cold climates.

PATHOPHYSIOLOGY AND RISK FACTORS

Otitis media with effusion usually occurs after an episode of acute otitis media when, in the presence of eustachian tube obstruction, suppurative middle ear fluid is reabsorbed into the circulation, leaving negative pressure within the middle ear chamber. This negative pressure results in transudation of serous fluid from the middle ear mucosa into the middle ear. The serous effusion in the middle ear then causes conductive hearing loss, which is usually temporary, and it also serves as a culture medium for recurrent infection. Risk factors for serous otitis media with effusion are similar to those for acute otitis media.

Otitis media with effusion has traditionally been thought not to represent an active infectious process because bacterial organisms have not been detected in the middle ear fluid. However, recent research indicates that, with

Table 5-1

Common Pathogens in Otitis Media

PATHOGEN	COMMENTS
Bacterial	
Streptococcus pneumoniae (29%)	All ages; most common cause of bacterial mastoiditis
Haemophilus influenzae (20–25%)	Predominant in preschool-aged children and children up to age 8 (in as many as 40% of cases, organism may produce β-lactamase, which hydrolyzes amoxicillin and some cephalosporins)
Moraxella catarrhalis (10–15%)	Increased incidence in infants under 6 months of age; up to 90% of cases may be β-lactamase positive
Group A beta-hemolytic streptococcus (2%)	
Staphylococcus aureus (2%)	Up to 10% of neonatal otitis media
Other bacteria (2%)	
Escherichia coli (rare)	Neonates
Group B streptococcus (rare)	Neonates
Pseudomonas aeruginosa (rare)	Neonates or adults
Pneumocystis carinii	May be associated with acquired immunodeficiency syndrome
Mycoplasma pneumoniae	
Chlamydia trachomatis	
Nonbacterial	
Viral, alone or combined with bacteria (8–25%)	
Influenza A virus	
Respiratory syncytial virus	
Coxsackievirus	
Adenovirus	
Parainfluenza virus	
Candida (rare)	
Sterile or rare pathogens (25–70%)	

SOURCE: Adapted from Kligman with permission from the January 1992, vol 45, no 1, issue of *American Family Physician*. Copyright by the American Academy of Family Physicians. All rights reserved.

such highly sensitive techniques as polymerase chain reaction assay, the presence of bacteria can be detected in the middle ear fluid of nearly one-third of patients undergoing tympanostomy tube placement for otitis media with effusion. While the significance of this finding for clinical practice is still uncertain, it raises the possibility that infectious processes are involved in otitis media with effusion.

Otitis Externa

Otitis externa is inflammation or infection of the external auditory canal that sometimes extends to involve the auricle. Acute diffuse otitis externa is the most common form. The severity of this condition ranges from a mild inflammation to a life-threatening disorder. Milder, superficial inflammation is the norm. Typical signs and symptoms of otitis externa include itching, plugging of ear, otalgia, periauricular adenitis, erythematous canal, purulent discharge, and eczema of the pinna.

The overall incidence of otitis externa is unknown, but the prevalence in the population may be as high as 10 percent. The condition occurs in individuals of all ages and both genders, and is more frequent in the summer months.

Pathophysiology and Risk Factors

In both acute and chronic otitis externa, there is desquamation of the superficial epithelium of the external auditory canal. About 90 percent of otitis externa involves bacterial infection, and approximately two-thirds of these bacterial infections are caused by *Pseudomonas aeruginosa*. Other bacterial pathogens include staphylococcus, streptococcus, and gram-negative rods. Otomycosis (fungal otitis externa) accounts for about 10 percent of otitis externa in the United States, and *Aspergillus* is responsible for 80 to 90 percent of these fungal infections. Other fungal pathogens include *Phycomycetes*, *Rhizopus*, *Actinomyces*, *Penicillium*, and yeast.

Risk factors for acute otitis externa include trauma to the external canal, such as from removal of cerumen, in which case bacterial or fungal infection is a secondary process. Swimming ("swimmer's ear") and hot humid weather are additional risk factors, since moisture in the external auditory canal can impair the integrity of underlying tissue and raise pH, thereby decreasing resistance to infection. Elderly persons are at particular risk for otitis externa, often related to use of hearing aids, debilitating or chronic diseases (including diabetes), and diminished or absent cerumen (which normally plays an antimicrobial role).

Why Is Earache Important?

In addition to causing pain, otitis media and externa are important because they can cause chronic and acute complications, including hearing loss, a variety of problems within the temporal bone, intracranial complications, and complications of therapy. Complications develop by one or more of several mechanisms, including infection with aggressive microorganisms, bacterial resistance to or toxic actions of antibiotics, obstructed lymphatic or middle ear drainage, and/or spread of infection by direct extension via the lymphatic or circulatory systems. The most important complications are described here.

Complications of Otitis Media

Hearing Loss

Temporary hearing loss is common with acute otitis media, exceeding 10 dB in 45 to 75 percent of infections. The hearing loss usually involves higher frequencies and is probably due to infection-related microtoxins and hypoxia, in addition to alterations of the stiffness of the cochlear partition.

Temporary hearing loss of 25 to 35 dB can occur when effusion is present, and persistent effusion may cause long-term hearing loss. In very young children, this hearing loss may lead to delays in development of both receptive and expressive language. In older children, the hearing loss is commonly manifest as behavioral problems, often mislabeled as attention deficit hyperactivity disorder. Other behavioral manifestations of chronic hearing loss in older children include decreased responsiveness, social withdrawal, and disturbed sleep. Children who have otitis media with effusion persisting longer than 3 months and children under age 3 years with three or more episodes of acute otitis media within a 6-month period should be referred for evaluation of speech and language development.

DAMAGE TO THE TYMPANIC MEMBRANE AND OSSICULAR CHAIN

The most common complication within the temporal bone is chronic perforation of the tympanic membrane. Chronic perforation causes conductive hearing loss and may lead to formation of cholesteatoma, which generally requires surgical intervention. Otitis media can also cause disruption or fixation of the middle ear ossicular chain, both of which result in conductive hearing loss.

MASTOIDITIS AND RELATED COMPLICATIONS

Inflammation of the middle ear can spread to the mastoid air cells, resulting in mastoiditis. Mastoiditis is uncommon due to the widespread use of antibiotics for ear infections, but when it occurs, it is most common in children under the age of 6 years. Diagnosis is usually made by history and physical examination. Usually the patient is febrile with a prolonged, purulent episode of acute otitis media, has pain and tenderness in the mastoid region, and may or may not have tympanic membrane perforation and drainage. Magnetic resonance imaging and/or computerized tomography are not always necessary to confirm the diagnosis but are helpful when more extensive infections are suspected (e.g., petrositis or extradural or subperiosteal abscess). Treatment of mastoiditis requires parenteral antibiotics and often surgery (myringotomy followed by mastoidectomy) to establish drainage.

FACIAL NERVE PARALYSIS

Since the advent of antibiotics, facial nerve paralysis occurs following only about 0.16 percent of otitis media episodes. Facial nerve paralysis is caused by a combination of osteitis, bone erosion, and compression or direct infection and inflammation of the nerve. Patients with facial nerve paralysis often have a concomitant cholesteatoma. To eradicate the infection, parenteral antibiotics and transcortical mastoidectomy and myringotomy are often necessary.

LABYRINTHITIS

Labyrinthitis usually presents with a progressive high-frequency sensorineural hearing loss, along with unsteadiness, vertigo, and nystagmus; fever may or may not be present. Patients with labyrinthitis usually require hospitalization and parenteral antibiotics. Intracranial abscess or meningitis may accompany labyrinthitis. When these conditions are suspected, lumbar puncture and magnetic resonance or computerized tomographic imaging should be performed to confirm the diagnosis.

INTRACRANIAL COMPLICATIONS

Intracranial complications of otitis media include meningitis, extradural or subdural abscess, brain abscess, and lateral sinus thrombophlebitis. Hydrocephalus may develop subsequent to any of these complications. Since the widespread availability of antibiotics, these intracranial complications are uncommon. Meningitis, however, accompanies otitis media with sufficient frequency to warrant consideration of meningitis in every febrile child with acute otitis media.

MENINGITIS   When it accompanies acute otitis media, meningitis is usually the result of hematogenous spread of organisms from the infected middle ear. The most common organism is *Streptococcus pneumoniae*, although *Haemophilus influenza* and other gram-negative meningeal infections also occur.

In chronic otitis media, infection may spread to the meninges through the bone and dura, or through the inner ear via fistulas caused by a cholesteatoma. Multiple organisms, usually gram-negative rods, are frequently identified in meningitis following chronic otitis and require broad-spectrum parenteral antibiotic coverage. Mortality rates from meningitis complicating chronic otitis media have been reported to be as high as 31 percent.

BRAIN ABSCESS Incidence of brain abscess has declined with widespread antibiotic treatment for otitis media. The condition still occurs, however, primarily in infants and young children, and the mortality rate exceeds 10 percent. Abscesses usually originate from venous thrombophlebitis in the temporal bone. They are typically polymicrobial, with streptococcus, staphylococcus, and *Proteus* species the most common. Treatment includes multiple parenteral antibiotics and surgical drainage.

LATERAL SINUS THROMBOSIS Although it is a rare complication of otitis media, lateral sinus thrombosis has a mortality rate as high as 36 percent. The sigmoid sinus is most commonly involved, with infection in the adjacent temporal bone resulting from spread of otitis media. Patients usually suffer from fever, headache, pain in the mastoid area, and increased intracranial pressure with papilledema. Diagnosis is made by magnetic resonance imaging. Treatment includes parenteral antibiotics, mastoidectomy, and surgical exploration of the dura of the sigmoid sinus.

Complications of Otitis Externa

The principal complication of otitis externa is necrotizing infection with spread to adjacent structures. In necrotizing otitis externa, the infection can spread from the ear canal into deep surrounding tissues and then to contiguous bone and nervous system structures. The result is cellulitis and/or osteomyelitis, abscess, or meningitis. These complications are rare in children, but they are seen in adults, especially those with diabetes mellitus. Acute otitis externa can also

spread to the pinna, causing infection of the ear cartilage (chondritis).

Complications of Antibiotic Therapy

Various agents used to treat otitis media and externa have ototoxic properties. These agents include the vehicles that carry active medication (e.g., propylene glycol, alcohol, and benzalkonium chloride) as well as the active medications themselves. Antibiotics with ototoxic properties include chloramphenicol, colistin, gentamicin, tobramycin, neomycin, polymyxin B, and several other antifungals. Nonantibiotic medications with potential ototoxicity include acetic acid, povidone-iodine, and hydrocortisone. Several medications, however, have no known ototoxicity, even in animal studies, and they should be considered for treatment of patients who have preexisting hearing loss. These nonototoxic agents include nystatin, amphotericin B, clotrimazole, tolnaftate, sulfacetamide, ciprofloxacin, triamcinolone, and dexamethasone.

Typical Presentation

In primary care practice, the usual presentation of acute otitis media is earache following an upper respiratory infection. The respiratory symptoms are usually still present, and complaints of fever, anorexia, and irritability are common. However, fever and even ear pain are absent in about one-half of children with acute otitis media. Conversely, one-half of children with earache do not have an acute infection. Primary care clinicians typically see patients with earache soon after onset, prior to development of any complications, including otitis media with effusion.

Otitis externa most typically presents as an acute diffuse infection. The common symptoms are itching, tenderness, and pain in the ear. Some patients also complain of hearing loss and a sensation of fullness in the ear.

In contrast to the presentation of earache in primary care practice, when patients present to otolaryngologists for otitis media, it is more often for multiple or recalcitrant infections, to consider surgical interventions, for audiometric testing, or for evaluation and treatment of complications. For otitis externa, otolaryngologists are more likely to see necrotizing infections than are primary care clinicians.

Key History

In evaluating patients with ear pain, the objectives are to (1) distinguish otitis media from otitis externa, (2) distinguish acute otitis media from otitis media with effusion, and (3) identify complications. These tasks may be difficult because patients with both acute otitis media and otitis media with effusion may lack differentiating symptoms. Nonetheless, the history may provide clues to the diagnosis.

Patients who are symptomatic with fever, ear pain, and respiratory symptoms are more likely to have acute otitis media. The onset of ear pain and other symptoms is often sudden; the ear pain may be unilateral or bilateral. The absence of such symptoms, combined with a recent acute ear infection and complaints of hearing loss, are more suggestive of otitis media with effusion. Alternatively, patients who have otitis media with effusion may have only mild symptoms, such as fullness in the ear, decreased attentiveness, irritability, or a sleep disturbance.

The typical history in persons with otitis externa includes itching in the ear or pain and tenderness near the outside of the ear. Patients may also report ear drainage, although this can

also be present in otitis media if the tympanic membrane has been perforated.

To identify complications, clinicians should ask about ear drainage, pain in the temporal bone, impaired speech and language, fever and associated headache, facial paralysis, vertigo, nystagmus, and unsteady balance or gait. The history should also include questions about immunocompromising conditions, such as diabetes, since such conditions predispose patients to invasive complications, especially necrotizing otitis externa.

Physical Examination

Adequate diagnosis of ear pain requires inspection and palpation of the external ear, visualization of the tympanic membrane and external canal with an otoscope, and examination to detect complications or nonaural conditions if suggested by the history and initial physical examination.

External Ear

In examining the external ear, the clinician should seek evidence of otitis externa, such as redness or inflammation, eczema of the skin, or discharge from the ear canal. Discharge, of course, can also be caused by otitis media with a perforated tympanic membrane. Widespread redness, swelling, and tenderness of the pinna suggest the possibility or cellulitis or chondritis.

Otoscopic Examination

The first step is to examine the external auditory canal for erythema, swelling, or discharge. If erythema and/or swelling is present, otitis externa is the likely diagnosis. Discharge, as noted above, may indicate either otitis media or otitis externa. In the absence of fever, inflammation of the tympanic membrane, or tympanic membrane perforation, otitis externa is the likely cause of discharge.

Next, the tympanic membrane is examined. It is important to have a sufficiently strong light bulb (100 footcandles or greater) to assure adequate visualization. If the tympanic membrane is convex or retracted, there is a 70- or a 79-percent chance, respectively, that otitis media with effusion is present. In addition, the tympanic membrane in otitis media with effusion is usually opaque or translucent, and amber or bluish fluid may be seen behind the membrane [Fig. 5-1 (Plate 6)]. Sometimes, air bubbles or an air-fluid level can be seen.

If erythema, bulging, and loss of normal light reflection are noted, acute otitis media is diagnosed [Fig. 5-2 (Plate 7)]. However, if a child

Figure 5-2 (Plate 7)

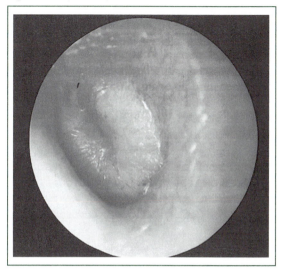

Acute otitis media as seen in an otoscopic view of a left tympanic membrane. Typical findings of acute otitis are present, including redness and bulging of the tympanic membrane. *(Reproduced with permission of Dr. Michael Hawke, Department of Otolaryngology, University of Toronto.)*

Figure 5-1 (Plate 6)

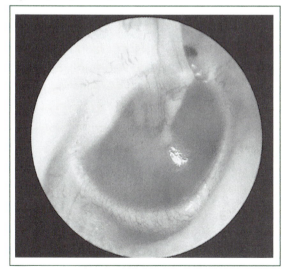

Otitis media with effusion as seen in an otoscopic view of a right tympanic membrane. There is retraction of the central portion of the tympanic membrane and a yellowish discoloration from the serous fluid accumulated in the middle ear behind the membrane. *(Reproduced with permission of Dr. Michael Hawke, Department of Otolaryngology, University of Toronto.)*

is crying during the examination, the same findings may be noted. Therefore, testing for tympanic membrane mobility is important, since mobility is not generally affected by crying.

A pneumatic otoscope is required to check tympanic membrane mobility; it should be fitted with an appropriate-sized otoscope speculum to assure a satisfactory air seal. While puffing air through the insufflator, the clinician should observe the mobility of the membrane. Good mobility argues against a diagnosis of acute otitis media or otitis with effusion.

Examination of the ear of an infant or a young child presents a significant challenge and requires experience and skill. In addition to tympanic membrane erythema caused by crying, the examination may also be hindered by cerumen in the external auditory canal. To remove cerumen, the child must be properly positioned (and calmed or restrained) to prevent injury from the cerumen curette. A flexible curette should be used, although some clinicians remove cerumen by irrigating the canal with water. Irrigation is an acceptable method, but it may cause temporary erythema of the tympanic membrane. If irrigation is used, therefore, time must be permitted for erythema to resolve before proceeding with the examination. Some clinicians also use hydrogen peroxide or commercial solutions (e.g., Debrox) to soften cerumen prior to irrigation or removal.

Ancillary Tests

A variety of ancillary diagnostic tests are available for evaluating patients with ear pain. These tests are rarely needed for routine diagnosis in primary care practice. Rather, they are usually reserved for patients who are not responding to initial treatment or who are suspected of developing a complication.

Tympanometry

When the diagnosis is in question, tympanometric studies are helpful in documenting the presence of middle ear fluid. Tympanometers can be purchased for office use, but they require staff training and careful attention to technique.

Tympanometry measures movement of the tympanic membrane in response to application of positive and negative pressure to the ear canal, thereby providing an indirect measure of pressure within the middle ear. A "type A" tympanogram curve is generated when middle ear pressure is normal and equilibrated with external (ambient) pressure. A "type C" curve is usually associated with middle ear effusion (Fig. 5-3).

Figure 5-3

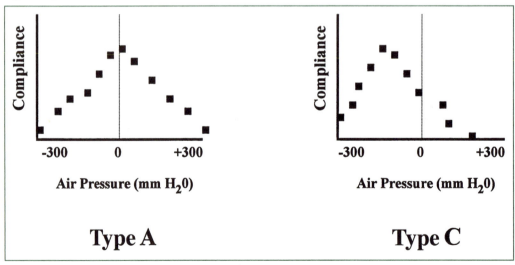

Tympanography involves applying varying degrees of positive and negative pressure to the external ear canal while measuring compliance of the tympanic membrane. In patients with a normally ventilated eustachian tubes, ambient pressure and middle ear pressures are equal, leading to maximal compliance when no pressure is applied. This is illustrated on the left in the type A schematic tympanogram. In otitis media with effusion, there is a negative pressure within the middle ear, and therefore compliance is maximal when a negative pressure is applied to the ear canal, as shown on the right in the type C schematic tympanogram.

The positive predictive value of a type C tympanogram for otitis media with effusion can range from 49 to 99 percent. In other words, half or more of patients with an abnormal type C tympanogram will have otitis media with effusion. The negative predictive value of tympanometry exceeds 90 percent, meaning that most ears with a normal tympanogram are indeed normal, without an effusion.

Audiometry

Audiometric (hearing) tests can be helpful in assessing the need for surgical intervention in otitis media with effusion. A hearing evaluation should be performed when bilateral otitis media (acute or with effusion) has been present for more than 3 months. Audiometric studies are probably not needed earlier, since surgical interventions would not be undertaken until effusion has persisted for 3 months or more.

Tympanocentesis

Tympanocentesis with culture of aspirated middle ear fluid is indicated for acute otitis media in a hospitalized newborn or in a child with compromised host resistance. Tympanocentesis with culture of middle ear fluid also is appropriate for selected patients with acute otitis media who fail treatment with multiple courses of antibiotics. Tympanocentesis can also be useful for pain relief in patients with persistent, painful bullae of the tympanic membrane unresponsive to analgesic measures.

In usual office practice, however, culture of middle ear fluid is rarely practical or necessary, and antibiotic treatment is usually guided by the known epidemiologic and microbiologic features of otitis media. In patients who have not responded to antibiotic therapy, cultures of the throat, nares, or nasopharynx are sometimes used to make presumptive identification of the infecting organism. This approach is unreliable, however, since organisms isolated from middle ear

infection by tympanocentesis do not consistently correspond to isolates from the nose and mouth.

Tuning-Fork Tests

Tuning-fork tests (the Weber and Rinne tests) are often recommended to distinguish conductive from sensorineural hearing loss. However, tuning fork tests cannot be used with young children. In other age groups, tuning-fork tests have not been sufficiently studied in otitis media to support a recommendation for use.

Acoustic Reflex Measurement (Acoustic Reflectometry)

Sound waves reflected from the tympanic membrane can be used to detect a middle-ear effusion, because sound-wave reflection is increased in the presence of effusion. Increased reflectivity is positively correlated with conductive hearing loss and is 90-percent sensitive and 86-percent specific for diagnosing middle-ear effusion. The U.S. Agency for Health Care Policy and Research (AHCPR), in its guideline for managing otitis media with effusion, did not recommend acoustic reflex testing for diagnosis of this condition. However, the technique may be useful for diagnosis of otitis media in infants.

Algorithm

The algorithm (Fig. 5-4) shows that in most cases a history and physical examination are all that is needed to make the distinction between otitis media and otitis externa, and between acute otitis media and otitis media with effusion. Tympanograms can be helpful when otitis media with effusion is suspected but cannot be confirmed on physical examination.

Figure 5-4

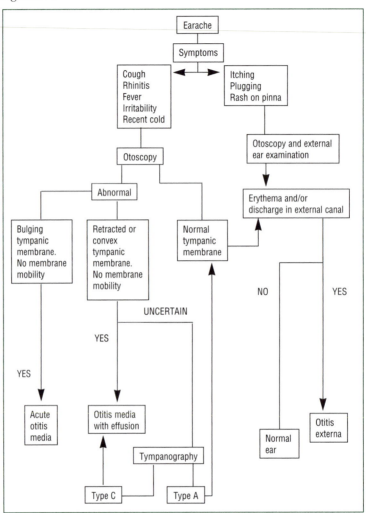

Algorithm for earache.

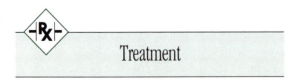

Treatment

Standard treatment of otitis media and otitis externa involves antibiotics, anti-inflammatory agents, and surgical procedures. As discussed later, however, there is considerable controversy about the need for antibiotics in the treatment of otitis media.

Acute Otitis Media

Acute otitis media is often painful and may be associated with fever. Therefore, general measures for treating acute otitis media typically include antipyretics and analgesics. Acetaminophen and nonsteroidal anti-inflammatory drugs are the usual medications for these indications. Aspirin should be avoided in children because of the risk of Reye's syndrome. Clinicians also frequently prescribe antihistamine-decongestant medications, but there is no substantial evidence that they have value for treating acute otitis media.

ANTIBIOTICS FOR ACUTE INFECTION

Bacteria cannot be identified in 20 to 30 percent of cases of acute otitis media studied by middle ear fluid culture, and many cases resolve spontaneously. Nonetheless, most clinicians treat acute otitis media with antibiotics with the intent of shortening the duration of symptoms and preventing complications.

Rational selection of antibiotics is based on awareness of pathogens commonly infecting the middle ear (Table 5-1). The most common bacterial pathogen in all age groups is *S. pneumoniae*, which can be cultured from up to 40 percent of middle ear infections. The next most common bacterial pathogens are nontypable *H. influenzae*, found in about 20 percent of cases, and

Moraxella catarrhalis, which occurs in 10 to 15 percent of cases.

Based on the likelihood of infection with these organisms, the first-line antibiotic for patients without penicillin allergy has been thought to be amoxicillin. However, other antibiotics are being used more frequently because of concerns about otitis media pathogens being resistant to amoxicillin. Specifically, infections with β-lactamase-producing *H. influenzae* and penicillin-resistant *S. pneumoniae* are increasingly common. Thus, traditional "second-line" antibiotics, such as amoxicillin-clavulanate, erythromycin-sulfisoxazole, and especially trimethoprim-sulfamethoxazole, are frequently prescribed as first-choice therapy. Amoxicillin-clavulanate is often considered the "gold standard" treatment because of its high efficacy in clinical trials. "Third-line" antibiotics include broader-spectrum agents, such as cefaclor, cefixime, ceftriaxone, cefuroxime axetil, clarithromycin, and azithromycin. Table 5-2 lists

Table 5-2

Antibiotics for Otitis Media

ANTIBIOTIC	ANTIMICROBIAL SPECTRUM FOR OTITIS MEDIA PATHOGENS					DOSE FOR CHILDREN
	P	H	M	S	E	
FIRST CHOICE						
Amoxicillin	X	X			x	40 mg/kg/d q8h
Trimethoprim-sulfamethoxazole*	X	X	X	X	x	8/40 mg/kg/d q12h
SECOND CHOICE						
Erythromycin-sulfisoxazole	X	x	X	x	x	50/150 mg/kg/d q6–8h
Ampicillin-clavulanate	X	X	X	X	x	40 mg/kg/d q8h
THIRD CHOICE						
Cefaclor	X	X	X	X	x	40 mg/kg/d q8h
Cefuroxime axetil	X	X	X	X	x	40 mg/kg/d q12h
Cefixime	X	X	X		x	8 mg/kg/d q24h
Clarithromycin	X	X	X	X		7.5 mg/kg/d q12h
Azithromycin	X	X	X	X		5 mg/kg/d q24h (10 mg/kg first day)

ABBREVIATIONS: P, pneumococcus (*Streptococcus pneumoniae*); H, *Haemophilus influenzae*; M, *Moraxella catarrhalis*; S, *Staphylococcus aureus*; E, Enterobacteriaceae; X, pathogen usually sensitive to this antibiotic; x, pathogen may or may not be sensitive to this antibiotic; *, many experts consider this drug a first-line treatment.

antibiotic choices, their spectra of activity, and doses for children.

DURATION OF TREATMENT Oral antibiotics are routinely prescribed for 10 to 14 days. However, several studies show that shorter treatments (5 days) may be just as effective. When infection persists beyond the typical 10- to 14-day treatment period, once-a-day "pulsed-dose" antibiotic therapy may be efficacious, thus obviating the need for continued administration of multiple daily antibiotic doses.

A recent trial with children age 3 months to 3 years has showed that a single intramuscular injection of ceftriaxone was as effective as a 10-day course of trimethoprim-sulfamethoxazole. The benefits of this single-dose treatment include increased compliance, decreased cost, and reduced opportunities for resistant organisms.

TOPICAL THERAPY FOR TYMPANIC MEMBRANE PERFORATION

If acute infection is accompanied by perforation of the tympanic membrane, a topical therapy is usually administered to the external ear canal. The combination of neomycin sulfate, polymyxin b, and hydrocortisone is often used (Cortisporin Otic Suspension).

PROPHYLAXIS

Antibiotic prophylaxis should be considered for children who have three or four documented episodes of acute otitis media within a 6-month period or 4 episodes within 12 months. Also, children with frequent ear infections in relation to seasonal allergies or seasonal respiratory infections may be given antibiotic prophylaxis to prevent acute otitis media during allergy or winter "flu" season. Amoxicillin 20 mg/kg/d for 3 to 6 months, or until the end of the winter or allergy season, is a common prophylactic regimen. Alternative prophylactic antibiotics are sulfisoxazole or trimethoprim-sulfamethoxazole. When given as a single bedtime dose at one-half

the usual daily treatment dose, these agents are safe and effective.

Chronic prophylaxis may lead to emergence of resistant bacterial strains, leading some experts to advocate tympanostomy tubes to prevent recurrences of acute otitis media. In fact, recent decision analyses suggest that, for some children with recurrent acute otitis media, tympanostomy tubes may be the preferred approach, depending on parental attitudes and the severity of infections.

In patients over the age of 2 years who are prone to having recurrent episodes of otitis media, it has long been known that the frequency of ear infections may be reduced with pneumococcal vaccine. A new conjugated pneumococcal vaccine containing about 85 percent of the strains that cause acute otitis media may offer more substantial protection than prior versions of the vaccine. It should be considered for patients with recurrent ear infections.

Otitis Media with Effusion

A variety of treatments have been recommended for otitis media with effusion including antibiotics, steroids, antihistamines and decongestants, and surgery. The diversity of treatments, often applied to patients with identical clinical presentations, was a principal reason why the AHCPR developed guidelines for standardized management of otitis media with effusion.

ANTIBIOTICS

As noted earlier, sensitive polymerase chain reaction assays have detected the presence of bacteria in nearly one-third of patients undergoing tympanostomy tube placement for otitis media with effusion. Despite this, amoxicillin promotes resolution of effusion in only 10 to 15 percent of cases, and cessation of symptoms is usually transient, returning after antibiotics are discontinued. Thus, antibiotics for otitis media with effusion are not recommended as a sole therapy.

STEROIDS

Based on a meta-analysis conducted by the AHCPR, the AHCPR guidelines did not recommend steroids for treatment of otitis media with effusion. However, there is now a growing literature to support the benefits of steroids for this condition, especially with concurrent use of oral antibiotics. Specifically, there is evidence that oral prednisone (1 mg/kg/d) can hasten resolution of persistent effusion when prescribed in combination with a 30-day course of trimethoprim-sulfamethoxazole. Similarly, concurrent use of steroids and antibiotics for a short course of 7 to 10 days appears to prevent the eventual need for tympanostomy tube placement in as many as 25 percent of patients. Oral steroids may be particularly effective in children aged 4 to 10 years who do not have enlarged adenoids. However, the potential adverse effects of long-term (i.e., greater than 1-month) steroid therapy mandate caution in using steroids repetitively for treatment of otitis media with effusion.

ANTIHISTAMINES AND DECONGESTANTS

Most cases of otitis media with effusion follow upper respiratory infections, not nasal allergies. Thus, there is limited rationale for treatment with antihistamines and decongestants. Nonetheless, patients with pollen allergies may benefit from antihistamine-decongestant medications or nasal steroid inhalers to prevent nasal and eustachian tube obstruction if they have frequent acute otitis media or and/or otitis media with effusion in association with allergic rhinitis. Because evidence to support this strategy is limited, the AHCPR guidelines did not recommend routine use of these agents.

SURGICAL TREATMENTS

Surgical procedures for persistent otitis media with effusion include placement of tympanostomy tubes and tonsillectomy-adenoidectomy. Tympanostomy tube placement, as noted, is the most common minor surgical procedure performed in the United States.

TYMPANOSTOMY TUBES   Tympanostomy tubes are placed into the tympanic membrane through a myringotomy incision (Fig. 5-5). Their purpose is to permit ventilation of the middle ear in order to eliminate the negative pressure that contributes to persistent effusion.

Over 1 million children in the United States undergo tube placement annually. This treatment is over five times more costly than medical management. To avoid placing tympanostomy tubes unnecessarily, the AHCPR guidelines recommend that tube placement be performed only when effusion has persisted for at least 3 months despite appropriate medical management and follow-up observation, *and* if there is documented bilateral hearing loss of greater than 20 dB. Tube placement is also recommended for children with more than 4 to 6 months of effusion and bilateral hearing loss, regardless of adequacy of prior medical management. Based on these guidelines, tubes are not recommended in children with only unilateral hearing loss and are inappropriate for patients with no hearing loss.

Despite these well-defined indications, many experts recommend surgical placement of tympanostomy tubes in other situations. These

Figure 5-5

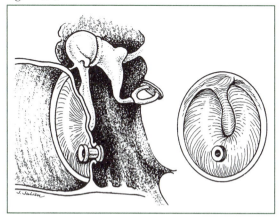

Tympanostomy tubes, also known as middle ear ventilation tubes, are placed through the tympanic membrane and act as an artificial eustachian tube. *(Reproduced with permission from TM Davidson: Clinical Manual of Otolaryngology. New York, McGraw-Hill, 1992.)*

include (1) otitis media with effusion persisting for at least 3 months despite a total of 3 months of treatment with at least two different antibiotics, even without hearing loss; (2) acute otitis media recurring at least three times within a 6-month period despite preventive efforts, including antibiotic prophylaxis for at least 3 months; (3) symptomatic conductive hearing loss with persistently high negative middle ear pressure on tympanometric testing; and/or (4) persistent symptoms of disequilibrium (vertigo or ataxia).

Tympanostomy tubes remain functional for an average of 10 to 12 months, after which time they are spontaneously extruded from the tympanic membrane into the external ear canal. Their major chronic complication is tympanosclerosis. Permanent tympanic membrane perforation may also occur, but this is relatively rare. Children with tubes in place may bathe normally and may swim if earplugs are used to prevent water from passing through the tube into the middle ear.

ADENOIDECTOMY AND TONSILLECTOMY Some patients with indications for tube placement also have significant nasopharyngeal obstruction from adenoidal hypertrophy. In addition to leading to otitis media, adenoidal enlargement is also associated with obstructive sleep apnea. For individuals who have otitis media with effusion, hearing loss, and adenoid-related nasopharyngeal obstruction or sleep apnea, tonsillectomy and adenoidectomy are appropriate surgical treatments. However, tonsillectomy and adenoidectomy are not recommended for patients who have only otitis media with effusion, without evidence of adenoidal obstruction. In fact, there is no evidence that tonsillectomy and adenoidectomy are effective when effusion is the only indication for surgery; therefore, the risks associated with anesthesia and postoperative bleeding outweigh any potential benefits in this situation. Furthermore, recent evidence suggests that prolonged antibiotic treatment (1 month of therapy with amoxicillin clavulanate) in children with chronic adenotonsillar hypertrophy can result in a substantial reduction in the need for tonsillectomy and adenoidectomy.

Otitis Externa

When substantial amounts of debris are present in the ear canal of patients with otitis externa, treatment usually begins with débridement of the canal. This procedure is performed by carefully suctioning with a Frasier suction tip or by mechanical débridement with a small cotton- or Dacron-tipped metal applicator. Topical otic or ophthalmic drops or hydrogen peroxide can help with the removal of debris or crusted discharge from the canal. These same drops can then be instilled three to four times daily to continue with the cleansing.

For treatment of infection, antibiotic preparations are available with and without steroids, and as both solutions and suspensions. Steroids decrease the inflammation and edema, thereby decreasing pain. In general, antibiotics with corticosteroids are recommended, typically for 10 days, usually combined with an antifungal agent and sometimes combined with a 2% acetic acid solution. Commercially available Neosporin otic preparations contain these medications and are widely used for treating otitis externa.

Occasionally, oral medications are indicated for otitis externa if there is spread of the infection beyond the auditory canal. In such situations, cultures should be obtained to guide the appropriate antibiotic therapy. Diabetics with early otitis externa should receive a 2-week course of oral ciprofloxacin (500 mg bid) for antipseudomonal coverage. More serious infections ("malignant" otitis externa) require hospitalization for parenteral antibiotics (including amphotericin B). Consultation with a specialist should be considered for most patients with malignant otitis and is almost always in order if there is no satisfactory response to treatment within 48 to 72 h or if there is a complicated course due to diabetes or other immunocompromised conditions.

Alternative Therapies

There are several reports of using chiropractic manipulation, osteopathic craniosacral manipulation, and acupuncture for treating otitis media with effusion. Various herbal treatments with purported antimicrobial or immune-enhancing function also have been used. These methods include aromatherapy using locally applied oils of lavender, chamomile, and evening primrose; and ayurvedic techniques, such as massage of periauricular lymph nodes complemented with a drink made from the herb amala. Chinese herbs used to treat otitis media include skullcap, alisma, plantain, bupleurum, and licorice. Western herbal therapies to enhance immune function include echinacea, chamomile, and goldenseal. Homeopathic remedies for the early stages of inflammation include aconite, belladonna, chamomile, and pulsatilla.

None of these nontraditional treatments has been studied in randomized controlled trials. Thus, the benefit of these treatments remains untested.

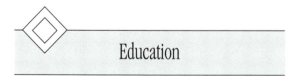

Education

Patients and their families should be educated about prevention of ear infections, options for diagnosis and treatment, and expected outcomes. Information about prevention is perhaps most important, because it permits families and patients to implement measures that might reduce the incidence of subsequent ear problems.

Prevention

Parents of infants with middle ear problems should understand that feeding infants in the supine position may increase the risk of ear infection. Clinicians should tell parents about the association between childhood ear infections and parental cigarette smoking and about the lower incidence of ear infections in breast-fed infants. As discussed later, however, there is no firm evidence that modifying these behaviors will change the incidence of ear infections in a given patient.

To prevent otitis externa, patients should be educated to avoid prolonged exposure to moisture, which can macerate the skin of the ear canal. This information is of greatest importance for patients in warm and humid climates and those participating in water sports. The ear canal can be dried after water exposure by blow-drying with a hair dryer on a low setting. Similarly, 70% ethyl alcohol drops can be used as a drying agent. Self-inflicted trauma to the external canal, such as from overzealous ear cleaning with Q-tips and fingernails, should also be discouraged. Finally, conditions of the auricle that impair skin integrity, such as eczema, should be treated before secondary infection occurs.

Diagnosis and Treatment

Patients and parents of children with ear infection should have a basic understanding of how ear problems are diagnosed, the difference between middle and external ear problems, and the difference between middle ear infections and effusions. Some clinicians provide otoscope training to parents of children with frequent ear infections, to permit diagnosis by parents without need for an office visit. However, the accuracy of parentally diagnosed otitis media is not known.

The range of treatment options for otitis media should be reviewed, from observation without treatment to antibiotics to surgery. Clinicians should explain the advantages and disadvantages of each treatment under consideration. The need to minimize unnecessary antibiotic use to decrease the problem of antibiotic resistance should be emphasized. In selected children with extremely frequent infections, it may be necessary to develop plans for treating ear infections that might occur while traveling. Finally, when children with frequent ear problems are moving or using multiple sources of health care, it is important that parents have a detailed record of the frequency and treatment of infections.

Expected Outcomes

Patients (or their parents) should be advised that the majority of acute infections will respond to first-line antibiotic therapy, usually within 2 to 3 days. However, as many as 15 percent of infections are caused by antibiotic-resistant bacteria. Therefore, failure to improve substantially within 72 h should prompt patients to recontact their clinician. Improvement without full resolution of symptoms is common, however, and resistant strains may produce symptoms for up to 3 months.

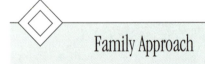

Family Approach

In addition to providing general education to patients and parents and discouraging family members from smoking, clinicians should be prepared to deal with changes in family dynamics that may take place when ear infections occur in a family member, who is usually a small child. Two issues are of most concern.

The first concern is pain relief, because individuals with otitis media may have considerable ear pain. Children, in particular, may be difficult to console, and their crying may cause disruption of family sleep and other activities. Clinicians should be cognizant of this concern and provide parents with effective methods for dealing with pain.

The second issue is that children with hearing loss from chronic middle ear effusions may develop school or behavioral problems that cause stress or disruption in the family. In some cases, these behavioral problems are the presenting symptoms of persistent middle ear effusion. Clinicians should recognize the possibility that behavioral problems and middle ear effusions are linked, and explore this possibility when appropriate.

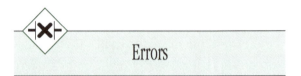

Errors

Primary care clinicians make several errors in the diagnosis and treatment of ear problems. These include both diagnostic and treatment errors.

Diagnostic Errors

One of the most common errors is diagnosing the nature of a middle ear infection without aid of a pneumatic otoscope. As noted earlier, without assessment of tympanic membrane mobility, it may not be possible to distinguish middle ears containing effusions from those that do not. A related problem is diagnosing acute otitis media solely on the basis of symptoms without examining the ear. As noted earlier, about half of all children with earache have no diagnosable ear problem, and otalgia may be the result of many nonotic conditions.

The other common, though sometimes unavoidable, error is incorrectly distinguishing acute otitis media from otitis media with effusion. The signs and symptoms of these conditions frequently overlap, and the examination can be difficult, especially in small children. In addition, clinicians frequently "overcall" otitis media, making the diagnosis and providing treatment when none is indicated. This may contribute to the growing problem of antibiotic resistance.

Treatment Errors

Without doubt, the most common treatment error made by primary care clinicians is prescribing unnecessarily broad-spectrum (and often expensive) antibiotics for uncomplicated acute otitis media. First-line or inexpensive second-line agents are almost always preferred. With nearly 25 million antibiotic prescriptions written each year in the United States for otitis media, prescribing patterns for otitis probably have an important influence on nationwide antibiotic sensitivity patterns. Avoiding second- and third-line agents and using amoxicillin for most infections probably can reduce the emergence of antibiotic-resistant bacterial strains. In fact, concerns about increasing antibiotic resistance have led some experts to advocate short-course antibiotics, or even no antibiotics, for routine treatment of uncomplicated otitis media.

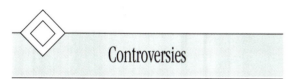

Controversies

The Role of Antibiotics

A major current controversy in management of otitis media revolves around the role of antibiotics for treatment. A meta-analysis of 33 randomized clinical trials of antibiotic therapy for acute otitis involving over 5000 children found that overall, fewer than 15 percent of children benefit from treatment, and for most the benefit is only a shorter duration of symptoms or effusions. In the Netherlands, practice guidelines developed by the Dutch College of General Practitioners specify that children over 6 months of age should not routinely receive antibiotics unless pain or fever continue for more than 3 days. Children treated by this protocol have similar outcomes to those of patients in other industrialized nations where antibiotics are widely used. It is interesting to note that antimicrobial resistance of common otitis media-causing

organisms in the Netherlands is less frequent than in neighboring countries, suggesting that limiting antibiotic use may reverse or minimize the development of bacterial resistance, an important issue, given the emergence of penicillin-resistant *S. pneumoniae*.

However, many clinicians are uncomfortable with the notion of not treating acute otitis media. Therefore, evidence of good treatment outcomes with short-course oral antibiotics or single-dose intramuscular antibiotics provides treatment alternatives that may be more acceptable to these practitioners. A recent meta-analysis indicated that for children 2 years old or older, a 5-day course of antibiotics is just as effective as longer treatment for uncomplicated otitis media. Such short-course regimens offer the opportunity to minimize children's exposure to antibiotics, perhaps decreasing the prevalence of antibiotic-resistant organisms. Studies of short-course antibiotics in infants and children younger than 2, however, suggest that resolution of ear problems is more likely with 10 to 14 days of therapy than with short-course therapy.

Prevention

There are inadequate data to support the concept that removing otitis-prone children from day care settings or exposure to tobacco smoke results in a decreased incidence or prevalence of acute otitis media or otitis media with effusion. Similarly, there is no solid evidence that the incidence of otitis can be lowered in an individual child by having the child breast feed. Ear infections and effusions are multifactorial in origin, and it is not clear that any one intervention can influence the likelihood of infection in a given patient.

Tympanostomy Tubes

As discussed above, while the AHCPR guidelines were intended to reduce variation in the indications for tympanostomy tube placement, indications still vary in practice, and there is considerable controversy about inconsistencies in the guidelines. For example, the AHCPR guidelines state that persistent unilateral hearing loss is not an indication for tube placement, yet evidence is lacking that unilateral loss has no significant sequelae. If there were evidence that unilateral hearing loss was without harm, then one could argue that antibiotic therapy is not necessary for unilateral otitis media. Finally, with the emergence of resistant strains of microbes, tube placement as a strategy to prevent recurrent otitis may prove more desirable than antibiotic prophylaxis. Thus, it is likely that the role of tympanostomy tubes will be reconsidered in the future.

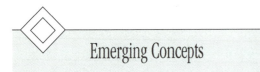

Emerging Concepts

Over the next decade, vaccines are likely to be developed to prevent the microbial infections that commonly cause ear infections. However, vaccine development combined with widespread alterations in antibiotic resistance patterns may lead to changes in the organisms that cause otitis media. Short-course and single-dose treatments will probably see more general use.

With the public's growing interest in self-care, initial diagnosis of otitis media in the home with an otoscope may occur more frequently. Simultaneously, with the increasing popularity of alternative and complementary therapies, combined with concerns about antibiotic overuse and questions about antibiotic benefit, it is likely that more patients will seek and use nonconventional treatments for otitis media.

Bibliography

Barnett ED, Teele DW, Klein JO, et al: Comparison of ceftriaxone and trimethoprim-sulfamethoxazole for acute otitis media: Greater Boston Otitis Media Study Group. *Pediatrics* 99:23, 1997.

Bergus GR, Lofgren MM: Tubes, antibiotic prophylaxis, or watchful waiting: A decision analysis for managing recurrent acute otitis media. *J Fam Pract* 46:304, 1998.

Berman S, Grose K, Nuss R, et al: Management of chronic middle ear effusion with prednisone combined with trimethoprim-sulfamethoxazole. *Pediatr Infect Dis J* 9:533, 1990.

Berman S, Roark R, Luckey D: Theoretical cost effectiveness of management options for children with persisting middle ear effusions. *Pediatrics* 93:353, 1994.

Boccazzi A, Careddu P: Acute otitis media in pediatrics: Are there rational issues for empiric therapy? *Pediatr Infect Dis J* 16:S65, 1997.

Bojrab DL, Bruderly T, Abdulrazzak Y: Otitis externa. *Otolaryngol Clin North Am* 29:761, 1996.

Cohen R: The antibiotic treatment of acute otitis media and sinusitis in children. *Diagn Microbiol Infect Dis* 27:35, 1997.

Culpepper L, Froom J: Routine antimicrobial treatment of acute otitis media: Is it necessary? *JAMA* 278:1643, 1997.

Editors of Time-Life Books: *The Medical Advisor: The Complete Guide to Alternative and Conventional Treatments.* New York, Time-Life Books, 1996, pp 642–643.

Fireman P: The role of antihistamines in otitis. *J Allergy Clin Immunol* 86:638, 1990.

Froom J, Culpepper L, Grob P, et al: Diagnosis and treatment of acute otitis media: Report from International Primary Care Network. *BMJ* 300:582, 1990.

Klein JO, Bluestone CD, McCracken GH Jr (eds): New perspectives in management of otitis media. *Pediatr Infect Dis J* 13:1029, 1994.

Kligman, EW: Treatment of otitis media. *Am Fam Physician* 45:242, 1992.

Kozyrskyj AL, Hildes-Ripstein E, Longstaff SEA, et al: Treatment of acut otitis media with a shortened course of antibiotics. A meta-analysis. *JAMA* 279:1736, 1998.

Mandel E, Casselbrandt M, Rockette H, et al: Efficacy of 20- versus 10-day antimicrobial treatment for acute otitis media. *Pediatrics* 96:5, 1995.

Nissen AJ: Complications of chronic otitis media. *ENT J* 75:284, 1996.

Paap CM: Management of otitis media with effusion in young children. *Ann Pharmacother* 30:1291, 1996.

Paradise JL: Treatment guidelines for otitis media: The need for breadth and flexibility. *Pediatr Infect Dis J* 14:429, 1995.

Paradise JL: Short-course antimicrobial treatment for acute otitis media: Not best for infants and young children. *JAMA* 278:1640, 1997.

Pelton SI: New concepts in the pathophysiology and management of middle ear disease in childhood. *Drugs* 52(suppl 2):62, 1996.

Podoshin L, Fradis M, Ben-David Y, et al: The efficacy of oral steroids in the treatment of persistent otitis media with effusion. *Arch Otolaryngol Head Neck Surg* 116:1404, 1990.

Poehlman GS: Chronic otitis media with effusion. *Primary Care* 23:687, 1996.

Rayner MG, Zhang Y, Gorry MC, et al: Evidence of bacterial metabolic activity in culture-negative otitis media with effusion. *JAMA* 279:296, 1998.

Rohn GN, Meyerhoff WL, Wright CG: Ototoxicity of topical agents. *Otolaryngol Clin North Am* 26:747, 1993.

Rosenfeld RM, Vertrees JE, Carr J, et al: Clinical efficacy of antimicrobial drugs for acute otitis media: Meta-analysis of 5400 children from thirty-three randomized trials. *J Pediatr* 1124:355, 1994.

Sclafanai A, Ginsburg J, Shah M, et al: Treatment of symptomatic chronic adenotonsillar hypertrophy with amoxicillin/clavulanate potassium: Short and long-term results. *Pediatrics* 101:675, 1998.

Stanway A: *The New Natural Family Doctor.* Berkeley, North Atlantic Books, 1995.

Stool S, Berg A, Berman S, et al: *Managing otitis media with effusion in young children: Quick Reference Guide for Clinicians*, AHCPR publication no 94-0623. Rockville, MD, Agency for Health Care Policy and Research, Public Health Service, U.S. Department of Health and Human Services, 1994.

Swanson JA, Hoecker JL: Otitis media in young children. *Mayo Clin Proc* 71:179, 1996.

Weiss JC, Yates GR, Quinn LD: Acute otitis media: Making an accurate diagnosis. *Am Fam Physician* 53:1200, 1996.

David R. Brown
Kay A. Bauman

Chapter 6

Sore Throat and Nasal Congestion

How Common Are Sore Throats and Nasal Congestion?

Sore throats and nasal congestion, together or individually, are among the most common complaints in primary care practice. Upper respiratory infections (URIs), which include the common cold, pharyngitis, ear infections, and sinusitis, are the most common infectious problems worldwide. Various reports, including the National Ambulatory Medical Care Survey, the U.S. Army Ambulatory Care Data Base, and surveys by the National Center for Health Statistics, rank URIs in the top three reasons why patients seek care from family physicians and general internists.

Children, on average, have six to eight URIs per year, but the rates may be much higher for children in day care. The typical adult has three to four URIs per year. Morbidity from URIs accounts for nearly half the time lost from work by adults and the great majority of time lost from school by children.

Upper respiratory symptoms frequently represent a URI, but they may also be noninfectious. The most common form of non-infectious upper respiratory symptoms is allergic rhinitis. Allergic rhinitis affects up to one-fifth of the U.S. population, making it the sixth most common chronic condition in the United States.

Principal Diagnoses

The principal diagnoses to consider in patients with sore throat and/or nasal congestion are URIs and allergic rhinitis. *Upper respiratory infection* is a general term for infections affecting structures of the respiratory tract above the larynx, even though many of these illnesses actually affect both upper and lower portions of the respiratory tract. The URIs may be subdivided further to specify the anatomic area that is infected, leading to a diagnostic nomenclature that includes the common cold (also termed nasopharyngitis or rhinosinusitis), sore throat (pharyngitis or pharyngotonsillitis), sinus infection (sinusitis), and ear infection (otitis media). Otitis media is not considered in this chapter because it is reviewed in Chap. 5. Laryngitis, epiglottitis, and bronchitis are often discussed in the context of URIs, but they are actually lower respiratory tract processes.

Common Cold

Common cold refers to mild, self-limited infections of the upper respiratory tract. The common cold is not a single entity. Rather, it is a group of similar diseases caused by a variety of microorganisms, most of which are viruses. The most common cause of colds in adults and children is rhinovirus infection, which accounts for 20 to 30 percent of all colds; coronaviruses account for another 5 to 20 percent. Other viruses that cause colds include parainfluenza virus, respiratory syncytial virus (RSV), influenza virus, and adenovirus (Table 6-1).

Peak incidence for colds is during winter months. Crowding (in the home, military barracks, school, or day care center) leads to an increased incidence of colds as viruses are passed from person to person. In addition, adults living with children have a greater frequency of colds than those who do not.

The pathophysiology of colds appears to be simple viral infection of the mucous membranes of the upper respiratory tract. Immune mechanisms (e.g., infiltration of the submucosa with inflammatory cells) are responsible for some of the symptoms. Viral infection also causes mucus production, impairment of ciliary function, and,

Table 6-1

Viruses That Cause Common Colds

Virus	Percent of Colds	Epidemiology	Incubation Period	Duration of Illness	Comments
Rhinovirus	20–30	Children and adults	2–4 days	3–21 days	Most common cause of colds worldwide, can cause exacerbations of asthma and other lung diseases
Coronavirus	5–20	Children and adults	2–4 days	2–18 days	Syndrome similar to that caused by rhinovirus, may exacerbate asthma and other lung conditions
RSV	<5	Children and elderly; winter epidemics	4–6 days	1–2 weeks	Causes bronchiolitis in small children, may exacerbate chronic lung conditions
Parainfluenza virus	5–20	More common in children	2–6 days	5 days	Also causes croup, bronchiolitis, and pneumonia in children
Adenovirus	<5	Most common in infants, children, and adolescents	4–5 days	3–5 days	Usually indistinguishable from colds caused by other viruses
Influenza	<5	Winter epidemics	1–2 days	1–3 weeks	Often causes a systemic, febrile illness; in children, may present as a simple cold
Coxsackievirus	<5	Sporadic or epidemic	3–6 days	3–6 days	May have prominent gastrointestinal symptoms, can cause epidemics in military populations

Abbreviation: RSV, respiratory syncytial virus.

in severe infections, possible sloughing of mucosal epithelial cells. These alterations in the local defenses (i.e., ciliary dysfunction and mucosal sloughing) may lead to bacterial superinfection with development of otitis media, mastoiditis, sinusitis, peritonsillar abscess, periorbital cellulitis, or bronchitis. These complications typically occur later in the course of illness, rather than with the onset of cold symptoms.

Pharyngitis/Tonsillitis

Pharyngitis (sore throat) is defined as inflammation of the pharynx and posterior oral cavity. When inflammation of the associated lymphoid tissue (tonsils) occurs, tonsillitis is also present. Most commonly, pharyngitis and tonsillitis occur together. The normal anatomy of the posterior oral cavity is shown in Fig. 6-1.

Sore throats are most common during the colder months in temperate climates. They are usually caused by a virus and may be associated with common colds or influenza. Like the common cold, sore throats are generally self-limited and do not cause serious morbidity. Important viruses that cause pharyngotonsillitis include rhinovirus (which causes about 20 percent of cases), coronavirus (5 percent), adenovirus (5 percent), herpes simplex virus (4 percent), influenza (2 percent), and parainfluenza virus (2 percent).

Figure 6-1

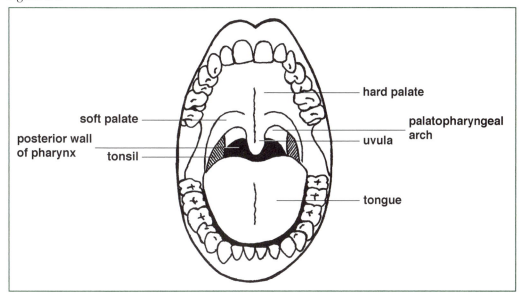

The oral cavity. The normal anatomical structures of the mouth and oropharynx are noted. *(Illustration by Liza Brown.)*

Sore throats can also be caused by bacteria, specifically, group A beta-hemolytic streptococcus, which causes 15 to 30 percent of pharyngitis. Other, less common manifestations of pharyngitis, each responsible for fewer than 1 percent of cases, include herpangina due to coxsackievirus, infectious mononucleosis with sore throat due to Epstein-Barr virus (EBV) or cytomegalovirus, and sore throats due to *Neisseria gonorrhea*, *Mycoplasma pneumoniae*, diphtheria, *Arcanobacterium haemolyticum*, beta-hemolytic streptococci (groups B, C, and G), and mixed anaerobic bacteria.

The pathogenesis of pharyngitis varies with the infectious agent involved. Most organisms invade the mucosa and cause release of inflammatory mediators, leading to edema and hyperemia. Group A beta-hemolytic streptococci release a number of specific factors that lead to inflammation, tonsillar hemorrhage, and exudates. Exudates may also occur with adenovirus or EBV. Vesicles or ulcers may be present with herpes simplex virus or coxsackievirus infec-

tions. *Corynebacterium diphtheria* infection can lead to the formation of a pseudomembrane composed of bacteria, white blood cells, and necrotic epithelial cells.

Clinically, it is usually unimportant to identify the specific virus or bacteria responsible for sore throat in an individual patient. The only exception to this is identification of group A beta-hemolytic streptococci or *N. gonorrhea*, because these infections require specific treatment.

MICROBIOLOGY OF SORE THROAT: COMMON CAUSES

A variety of bacteria and viruses cause sore throats. Many of them also cause common colds, which may occur concomitantly with sore throat.

STREPTOCOCCUS Streptococci cause a wide range of human infections, of which pharyngitis is perhaps the most common. Streptococci are categorized by their ability to hemolyze sheep blood agar completely (beta hemolysis), partially (alpha hemolysis), or not at all (gamma hemolysis). Beta-hemolytic streptococci are further differentiated into groups A, B, C, D, and G based on saccharide antigens on the bacterial surface.

Group A beta-hemolytic streptococcus is the agent that causes classic "strep throat" and its most important sequela, acute rheumatic fever. There are more than 80 distinct serotypes of group A beta-hemolytic streptococci, some that are specific for respiratory tract infection and others that cause skin or soft tissue infections. Only certain serotypes, called "rheumatogenic," are associated with rheumatic fever. Although groups C and G streptococcus may also cause symptomatic pharyngitis, they are more commonly nonpathogenic colonizers of the respiratory tract, and they do not cause rheumatic fever.

Epidemiology   Acute streptococcal pharyngitis is most common in children. Transmission of streptococcal pharyngitis is by respiratory secretions, with an incubation period of about 2 to 5 days. Close interpersonal contact is considered an important factor in the spread of streptococcal pharyngitis. Thus, children in child care centers or schools are at particular risk, as are families in crowded living conditions and young adults in military barracks or college dormitories. The course of untreated disease is approximately 3 to 5 days.

Streptococcal pharyngitis is most common in school-aged children, and this is also the group at highest risk for progression of streptococcal pharyngitis to acute rheumatic fever. During strep throat epidemics involving rheumatogenic strains, up to 3 percent of school-aged children with untreated streptococcal pharyngitis will develop rheumatic fever. At other times and in other age groups, the rate of rheumatic fever is considerably lower.

Approximately 5 to 20 percent of school-aged children are asymptomatic carriers of group A beta-hemolytic streptococci, although these carrier rates vary from community to community. Adults have a lower carrier rate than do children. In general, carriers do not transmit disease and do not have virulent strains that progress to rheumatic fever. They do, however, test positive for group A beta-hemolytic streptococcus on throat cultures. As many as 15 to 20 percent of positive throat culture results obtained in children with sore throat are due to asymptomatic carriage, rather than acute streptococcal infection.

Clinical Manifestations   The symptoms of streptococcal pharyngitis are variable. In the "classic" case, children are febrile and have throat pain with tonsillar enlargement, and purulent exudate appears on the tonsils and posterior pharynx. Tender anterior cervical lymphadenopathy is also common. Some patients develop a typical erythematous sandpaper-like rash, most prominent in the flexural areas of the arms and on the abdomen. When such a rash is present, the patient is said to have scarlet fever, and the rash is "scarlatiniform." However, not all patients present with these classic findings, and in some cases the symptoms and signs are relatively mild.

Streptococcal pharyngitis can cause a number of suppurative and nonsuppurative complications. Suppurative complications include otitis media, sinusitis, peritonsillar or retropharyngeal abscess, peritonsillar cellulitis, and cervical adenitis. On rare occasions, group A beta-hemolytic streptococcal disease can cause necrotizing fasciitis (referred to in the lay press as infection with "flesh-eating bacteria"). The important nonsuppurative complication of streptococcal pharyngitis is acute rheumatic fever, and the principal reason for detecting and treating strep throat is to prevent rheumatic fever.

Rheumatic Fever

Rheumatic fever is thought to result from an immune response to a streptococcal antigen that has similarities to an antigen in patients' cardiac tissues. This immune response damages cardiac tissue, leading to valvular heart disease, which is responsible for the majority of the morbidity, mortality, and economic burden of the rheumatic fever. Diagnosis of rheumatic fever is based on a diagnostic scheme known as the "modified Jones criteria" (Table 6-2).

High frequencies of rheumatic fever are still reported in nonindustrialized countries, where large numbers of young patients have disabling valvular heart disease. In fact, rheumatic heart disease is the most frequent cause of heart disease and death worldwide among 5- to 30-year-olds.

In industrialized nations, the incidence rheumatic fever has decreased substantially in recent decades. The decrease in rheumatic fever began prior to the widespread use of antibiotics to treat acute streptococcal throat infections and has been attributed to improved socioeconomic con-

Table 6-2

Modified Jones Criteria for Diagnosis of Acute Rheumatic Fever

MAJOR CRITERIA
Carditis (usually cardiac valvular or conduction-system disease)
Migratory polyarthritis
Erythema marginatum
Chorea
Subcutaneous nodules

MINOR CRITERIA
Fever
Arthralgia
Previous rheumatic fever
Elevated acute-phase reactants (erythrocyte sedimentation rate or C-reactive protein)
Prolonged P-R interval on electrocardiogram

EVIDENCE OF PRECEDING STREPTOCOCCAL INFECTION, BASED ON ANY OF THE FOLLOWING:
Elevated titer of anti-streptolysin O (ASO)
Elevated streptococcal anti-DNase B
Recent positive throat culture or rapid streptococcus antigen test result

NOTE: According to these criteria, rheumatic fever is diagnosed if there is evidence of a preceding streptococcal infection plus the presence of either two major criteria or one major and two minor criteria.
SOURCE: Adapted with permission from AS Dajani et al: *JAMA* 268:2069–2073, copyright 1992, American Medical Association.

ditions with less crowded housing. In the late 1980s and early 1990s, however, there were several small outbreaks of rheumatic fever in the United States related to regional epidemics of rheumatogenic strains of group A beta-hemolytic streptococci. These mini-epidemics of rheumatic fever occurred in middle-class populations, not in low-income groups with crowded housing conditions. This suggests that the epidemiology of rheumatic fever may be changing, but more research is needed to clarify the nature and implications of this change.

COXSACKIEVIRUS The Coxsackie group of RNA enteroviruses has many subtypes that produce different clinical syndromes, including exudative pharyngitis, herpangina, hand-foot-and-mouth disease, and a variety of exanthems, as well as more serious infections involving the pericardium, myocardium, or central nervous system. Herpangina is a mild, self-limited pharyngitis, lasting 1 to 2 weeks and characterized by papules or vesicles on the pharynx, tonsils, and posterior palate. Hand-foot-and-mouth disease, also a mild and self-limited illness, primarily affects children, causing small vesicles on the oral mucosa and distal extremities.

EPSTEIN-BARR VIRUS Infectious mononucleosis is caused by EBV, a DNA virus that is a member of the herpesvirus group. The clinical triad of pharyngitis, fever, and lymphadenopathy may follow prodromal symptoms of malaise, anorexia, and chills. Hepatomegaly and splenomegaly are common. In some cases, severe pharyngitis is what causes the patient to seek medical attention. The symptoms and signs of infectious mononucleosis pharyngitis are often similar to those of streptococcal pharyngitis, and, due to the high rate of asymptomatic streptococcal carriage in the general population, a positive streptococcal culture result does not exclude the diagnosis of infectious mononucleosis.

The incubation period for EBV infectious mononucleosis is 30 to 50 days. It is transmitted primarily in saliva, although it can be transmitted by blood transfusion. Approximately 50 percent of individuals have a primary EBV infection during childhood. A second wave of seroconversions occurs during adolescence and young adulthood. Duration of symptoms is variable. Most patients are well enough to return to school or work within 3 to 4 weeks, but fatigue and malaise may continue for months.

HERPES SIMPLEX VIRUS   Oral herpes simplex infections occur worldwide. They often are contracted in the first few years of life, but some individuals have their first (primary) oral herpes infection in adulthood. Incubation period is 2 to 12 days, and the virus is usually spread directly by oral secretions. Oral infections with this virus (herpes stomatitis) can present with fever, irritability, and vesicles or ulcers of the mucous membranes of the mouth. However, herpes stomatitis can present with what appears to be a straightforward pharyngitis for which streptococcal infection may be a diagnostic consideration because of the associated systemic signs and pharyngeal inflammation. This presentation is particularly common in toddlers and young children.

MYCOPLASMA PNEUMONIAE   *M. pneumoniae* is a major cause of respiratory infections in school-aged children and young adults. Although the lower respiratory tract is the usual site of infection, patients may present with sore throat, fever, malaise, and headache. Cough is usually prominent. The incubation period is 2 to 3 weeks. Otitis media in children and sinusitis in adults may complicate mycoplasma pharyngitis.

ARCANOBACTERIUM HAEMOLYTICUM   This gram-positive pleomorphic bacillus, previously named *Corynebacterium haemolyticum*, has been identified as a cause of pharyngitis, primarily in adolescents and young adults. It is commonly associated with a rash that may appear scarlatinaform or urticarial. Common throat culture techniques may not identify this bacterium; thus, the infection usually goes unidentified. *Arcano-bacterium* pharyngitis generally resolves without treatment. However, it has been suggested that treatment with erythromycin may shorten the course, although clinical trials have not been performed to confirm the benefit of erythromycin. Rare complications, such as peritonsillar abscess, endocarditis, or meningitis, may occur.

MICROBIOLOGY OF SORE THROAT: UNCOMMON BUT SERIOUS CAUSES

A number of serious or life-threatening conditions may present with sore throat. While uncommon, they should always be considered when evaluating patients who have what appears to be a straightforward pharyngitis.

DIPHTHERIA   Diphtheria, caused by the bacterium *C. diphtheria*, is a serious bacterial infection in which patients develop a pharyngeal membranous exudate that may obstruct the airway. Although the membranous exudate can cover the entire posterior pharynx, including the uvula and tonsils, the initial onset of diphtheria may include only inflammation of the pharynx indistinguishable from common pharyngitis. The infection is usually associated with a low-grade fever. Although diphtheria is rare in industrialized nations because of universal immunization with diphtheria toxoid, countries of the former Soviet Union experienced approximately 4,000 deaths from this disease during the early part of the 1990s.

CANDIDA   Oral infections with various *Candida* species, such as *Candida albicans*, manifest as "thrush" on the buccal mucosa and are common in young infants. Oral *Candida* may also be found in healthy adults who are taking antibiotics.

With these two exceptions (young children and patients on antibiotics), oral *Candida* is an unusual infection and, if present, may indicate impairment of the immune system. With the increasing number of patients who have immunosuppressing conditions, such as HIV infection, cancer, or transplant chemotherapy, oral candidal infection should always be considered as a possible cause of pharyngitis.

Classic candidal infections present with a white exudate that can be scraped off the buccal mucosa, posterior tongue, or pharynx. *Candida* can also present with an inflammatory pharyngitis that is visually indistinguishable from streptococcal and viral pharyngitis. However, both classic thrush and candidal pharyngitis will show pseudohyphae on a potassium hydroxide wet mount of buccal mucosal scrapings, while other forms of pharyngitis will not.

GONORRHEA Orogenital sex can be a route of infection with *N. gonorrhea*. Orally acquired infection frequently is accompanied by only minimal symptoms, but it may present with symptomatic sore throat indistinguishable from that caused by other organisms. Thus, it is important to consider gonorrhea in the differential diagnosis of sore throat and to obtain an adequate sexual history and cultures when appropriate. Pharyngeal infection can be treated with the same antibiotic regimens used for uncomplicated gonorrheal urethritis or vulvovaginitis.

EPIGLOTTITIS Epiglottitis is a life-threatening infection that can occur in both children and adults. It often presents initially as a sore throat. In children, *Haemophilus influenzae* has been a principal cause of epiglottitis. With the advent of a vaccine against this bacterium, however, epiglottitis in children is now relatively uncommon.

In adults, epiglottitis is caused by gram-positive organisms such as *Streptococcus pneumoniae* and *Staphylococcus aureus*. Adults with epiglottitis typically present with fever, dysphagia, hoarseness, and loss of voice. Clues to the diagnosis are fever and symptoms of severe sore throat with minimal evidence of pharyngitis on visual inspection of the pharynx.

In infants and children, a lateral x-ray film of the neck may reveal an enlarged epiglottis. In adults, x-rays and fiberoptic examinations are used for diagnosis.

PERITONSILLAR ABSCESS This serious infection of the peritonsillar space is usually preceded by a group A beta-hemolytic streptococcal infection, even though organisms cultured from the abscess itself usually include mostly anaerobes. Patients with a peritonsillar abscess will present with severe throat pain, high fever, and occasionally drooling, trismus, severe hoarseness, or inability to speak. Clinical examination reveals a markedly swollen and inflamed tonsillar area with displacement of the uvula to the side opposite the abscess and trismus. Antibiotics and incision and drainage or aspiration are usually required, and occasionally hospitalization is indicated.

Sinusitis

EPIDEMIOLOGY

Sinusitis is an inflammatory process of the paranasal sinuses. It may be classified as either acute (10 to 30 days' duration), subacute (31 to 90 days' duration), or chronic (more than 90 days' duration). Acute sinusitis develops as a complication of 0.5 percent of URIs, and its occurrence generally follows the seasonal patterns of URIs. Sinusitis may also be a complication of allergic or nonallergic rhinitis, adenoidal hypertrophy, nasal obstruction due to polyps, septal deviation, foreign bodies or tumors in the nose or nasopharynx, ciliary motility abnormalities (cystic fibrosis), or immunodeficiency states. When sinusitis is associated with pain in the upper teeth, dental infection may be the primary factor, with spread of anaerobic bacteria from the teeth to the maxillary sinus.

DEVELOPMENTAL ANATOMY

Small maxillary and ethmoid sinuses are present at birth and enlarge during childhood. The other sinuses appear and develop throughout infancy and childhood. The sphenoid sinus appears at 3 years of age and develops further until adolescence. The frontal sinuses develop from the ethmoids starting at age 6 to 8 years and develop further until adolescence. By early adolescence, all of the sinuses have reached adult proportions. These dating parameters are important because they determine the age at which infection may first occur in a particular sinus. For example, frontal sinusitis cannot occur until the frontal sinuses appear, usually after age 6.

The anatomic relationships of the maxillary, frontal, ethmoid, and sphenoid sinuses are shown in Figs. 6-2 and 6-3. The sinuses are air-filled cavities with bony walls lined by ciliated respiratory mucosa. Ciliary activity helps drain the sinuses through individual openings into the nasal cavity. The anterior ethmoid, frontal, and maxillary sinuses drain into a common region in the superiolateral part of the nasal cavity known as the osteomeatal complex. It is in this area that obstruction of sinus drainage most commonly

occurs. The maxillary sinuses, in particular, drain into this area from openings in the highest part of their medial walls through a narrow bony channel known as the infundibulum. The narrow caliber of the infundibulum and its location (which requires ciliary motion to drain against gravity) predispose the maxillary sinus to the highest incidence of sinusitis.

MICROBIOLOGY AND PATHOGENESIS

Bacteria and viruses can be cultured by puncture and aspiration of the sinuses. In some studies, bacteria are found in normal sinuses, but the quantity of bacteria in normal sinuses is small. Bacterial isolates from normal sinuses are similar to the oropharyngeal floral and include

Figure 6-2

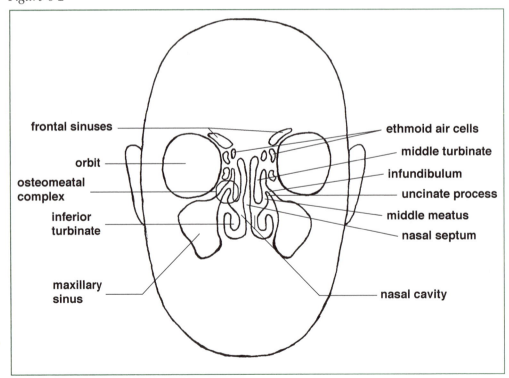

Paranasal sinuses. Coronal section through the paranasal sinuses. The ethmoid, frontal, and maxillary sinuses all drain into the osteomeatal complex, which is the site of nasal obstruction in many patients with sinusitis. *(Illustration by Liza Brown.)*

Figure 6-3

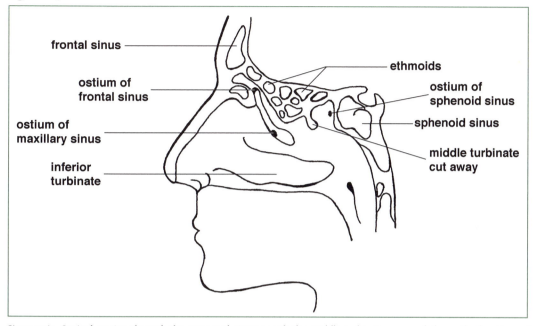

Sinus ostia. Sagittal section through the paranasal sinuses with the middle turbinate removed shows the locations of the ostia through which several of the paranasal sinuses drain into the nasal cavity. *(Illustration by Liza Brown.)*

S. pneumoniae, H. influenzae, alpha- and beta-hemolytic streptococci, *S. aureus,* and a variety of anaerobes.

Acute sinusitis is usually caused by infections with viral or bacterial organisms, which may be classic pathogens or normal oropharyngeal flora. Mechanisms by which sinus inflammation develops include capsular virulence factors (*H. influenzae and S. pneumoniae*) and toxin production (*S. aureus* and Enterobacteriacae). It is often unclear, however, to what extent acute bacterial infections are the cause or result of impaired sinus drainage. Chronic sinusitis, in contrast, is more often related to structural problems affecting sinus drainage, with superinfection as a secondary process.

ACUTE SINUSITIS   In acute sinusitis, the most commonly isolated bacteria are *H. influenzae, S. pneumoniae,* and *Moraxella catarrhalis. Staphylococcus aureus,* group A beta-hemolytic streptococci, Enterobacteriacae, and anaerobic bacteria may also be present. Viruses (rhinovirus, influenza virus, parainfluenza virus, and adenovirus) have been isolated from 4 to 23 percent of sinus puncture specimens in patients with acute sinusitis.

CHRONIC SINUSITIS   A variety of microorganisms have been found in chronic sinusitis. They include normal oropharyngeal flora, typical viral or bacterial respiratory tract pathogens, and anaerobes of uncertain significance. On rare occasions, fungi have been isolated from the sinuses of patients with chronic sinusitis. As noted previously, structural problems affecting sinus drainage may be more important than microorganisms in the genesis of chronic sinusitis.

NOSOCOMIAL SINUSITIS   Nosocomial sinusitis most commonly occurs in hospitalized patients who have had nasotracheal or nasogastric tubes in place, in which case sinusitis is due to obstruction of sinus drainage by the tube. Organisms isolated from sinuses of these patients include typical hospital-acquired pathogens such as Enterobacteriaceae or *Pseudomonas aeruginosa.*

COURSE AND COMPLICATIONS

Acute sinusitis resolves spontaneously within 1 month in up to 75 to 80 percent of patients. Of those cases that persist beyond 1 month, up to 70 percent resolve without treatment within an additional 6 weeks. Serious complications are rare but include periorbital or orbital cellulitis or abscess, osteomyelitis, bacterial meningitis, brain abscess, and cavernous sinus thrombosis. Sinusitis may also lead to exacerbations of asthma.

Noninfectious Rhinitis

In addition to URIs and sinusitis, primary care clinicians often see patients with nasal congestion and coryza caused by noninfectious processes. These include allergic rhinitis, nonallergic rhinitis with eosinophilia, vasomotor rhinitis, rhinitis medicamentosa, nasal foreign bodies, and several other conditions.

ALLERGIC RHINITIS

Allergic rhinitis is an acquired syndrome of immune-mediated hyperresponsiveness to inhaled (or, rarely, ingested) environmental allergens. Symptoms can include nasal blockage, rhinorrhea, anosmia, sneezing, pharyngitis, conjunctivitis, nasal voice, and recurrent infections of the sinuses or ears. Allergic symptoms in the eye (allergic conjunctivitis), such as itching, tearing, and vascular injection, frequently accompany allergic rhinitis. Symptoms may be seasonal as in "hay fever" due to wind-borne pollens of weeds, grasses, and trees. Symptoms may also be perennial, from exposure to house dust, molds, or animal dander.

Allergic rhinitis affects 5 to 22 percent of people worldwide. The prevalence increases during childhood, peaks in adolescence and young adulthood, and diminishes with aging. Affected persons generally are "atopic," with a genetic predisposition to form IgE antibodies on exposure to certain environmental substances. Atopic individuals may have allergy to one or multiple allergens and may also suffer from eczema, asthma, and urticaria.

Allergens are proteins with a molecular weight between 10,000 and 100,000 daltons. They are water-soluble components of the larger airborne substances (e.g., pollens) from which they are derived. Once allergens reach the nasal mucosa, they diffuse into the epithelium and stimulate IgE production by plasma cells (increased IgE levels can be measured in the blood) and proliferation of mucosal eosinophils (which can be detected on stained smears of nasal secretions). The IgE antibodies stimulate basophils and mast cells to release histamine and other inflammatory mediators. These inflammatory agents lead to a variety of changes in the nasal cavity, including increased mucus production, alterations in vascular tone, increased vascular permeability, inflammatory infiltration of the mucosa, and pruritus. In susceptible patients, inflammatory mediators may also cause bronchospasm.

The chronic sequelae of allergic rhinitis can have a major effect on the quality of life for sufferers. There may be swelling of mucous membranes, polyp formation, and obstruction of drainage of the sinuses and eustachian tubes. These sequelae, in turn, may lead to sinusitis, otitis media with effusion, resultant speech abnormalities and learning difficulties, sleep apnea, sleep disturbances, or exacerbations of asthma.

NONALLERGIC RHINITIS WITH EOSINOPHILIA

Nonallergic rhinitis with eosinophilia is similar in presentation to perennial allergic rhinitis, including the presence of eosinophilia on nasal smears. However, serum IgE concentrations are not elevated, and no specific allergy or allergen can be identified.

VASOMOTOR RHINITIS

Vasomotor rhinitis is a poorly understood condition of nasal hyperreactivity to inhaled irritants. Eosinophils are not seen on nasal smear, and no allergic component has been identified. A manifestation of vasomotor rhinitis that is familiar to many individuals is the runny nose that occurs on exposure to cold air or cigarette smoke. Others experience rhinitis with exercise.

RHINITIS MEDICAMENTOSA

Rhinitis medicamentosa results from chronic use of topical nasal decongestants, such as neosynephrine and oxymetazolone. These agents cause vasoconstriction of the nasal mucosal circulation. With prolonged use, tolerance develops and rebound vasodilatation occurs, leading to congestion of the nasal airway and coryza. Patients then increase the frequency of decongestant use in an attempt to diminish symptoms, and a cycle of repeated application and rebound develops.

NASAL FOREIGN BODY

Children frequently insert foreign objects into their nose. Common objects include pebbles, beads, raisins, peas, and other food particles. Typically, symptoms after the foreign body is first introduced are minimal and may include only mild discomfort, sneezing, and local obstruction. Persistence of the foreign object in the nose subsequently leads to mucosal swelling and signs of local obstruction, including obstruction of sinus drainage. Eventually, infection occurs and the child will develop a purulent, malodorous, or bloody discharge coming from one nostril. These unilateral findings are the clue to the diagnosis.

OTHER CAUSES OF RHINITIS

In addition to nasal decongestants, other medications can cause rhinitis in certain patients. These medications include beta-adrenergic block-ing agents, oral contraceptives, and thyroid hormones. The basis for rhinitis with these medications is not clear.

Aspirin sensitivity is linked to a syndrome of "triad asthma," or "nasal polyp syndrome," which consists of asthma, nasal polyps, and aspirin sensitivity. Nasal polyps cause these patients to complain of nasal congestion. If aspirin is given to a patient with nasal polyps and the patient has this syndrome, the result will be an acute episode or exacerbation of asthma.

Nasal congestion and rhinitis are also associated with hypothyroidism and pregnancy. The mechanisms for these associations have not been elucidated.

SERIOUS OR LIFE-THREATENING CAUSES OF RHINITIS

In the vast majority of cases, patients with rhinitis have colds, noninfectious rhinitis, or perhaps complicating conditions such as sinusitis. In a small percentage of patients, however, upper respiratory symptoms may be indicative of serious or life-threatening disorders. Primary care clinicians should be alert to the possibility of three such conditions: Wegener's granulomatosis, nasopharyngeal tumors, and cerebrospinal fluid rhinorrhea.

WEGENER'S GRANULOMATOSIS Wegener's granulomatosis is a rare necrotizing vasculitic disorder of unknown cause. It presents in adulthood, often with severe upper respiratory tract symptoms of sinus pain and drainage, and purulent or bloody nasal discharge that may not initially be recognized as something other than a straightforward nasal or sinus problem. As the condition progresses, nasal mucosal ulceration and nasal septum perforation may occur. Generally, these upper respiratory abnormalities are accompanied by lower respiratory tract findings of cough, hemoptysis, dyspnea, chest discomfort, and infiltrates on x-ray. Renal, eye, and skin disease can also occur. Diagnosis is made by demonstrating necrotizing granulomatous vasculitis on biopsy of involved tissue.

NASOPHARYNGEAL TUMOR While rare, persistent bloody rhinorrhea should alert clinicians to the possibility of a tumor in the nasal or nasopharyngeal cavity. Similarly, in patients with chronic recalcitrant sinus problems, consideration should be given to the possibility that symptoms are caused by a nasopharyngeal tumor obstructing sinus drainage.

CEREBROSPINAL FLUID RHINORRHEA When evaluating patients with head trauma, clinicians should be alert for the possibility of the leakage of cerebrospinal fluid through the cribiform plate into the nose. Leakage is manifested as a clear or bloody nasal discharge. The diagnosis is typically suggested by the clinical context (i.e., head injury). Presumptive confirmation can be made by measuring the glucose level in the nasal drainage. Cerebrospinal fluid has a glucose level similar to that in blood, whereas normal nasal secretion does not.

Typical Presentation

Common Cold

Patients with viral URIs present with relatively acute symptoms of rhinitis, which may be clear or purulent. In addition, they may have nasal congestion, sneezing, sore throat, and occasionally cough and hoarseness. Mild headache, fever, and malaise may also be present. With these symptoms, it is impossible to reliably differentiate among the various viruses that cause URIs, but marked systemic signs might suggest influenza virus, prominent cough could suggest parainfluenza virus or RSV, and gastrointestinal symptoms suggest coxsackievirus.

Pharyngitis

It is also impossible to reliably distinguish among the various viral and bacterial causes of pharyngitis based on presentation alone, although several clinical clues may be present. For example, when pharyngitis is associated with prominent clear rhinitis, rhinovirus, RSV, parainfluenza virus, coronavirus, coxsackievirus, or adenovirus may be suspected. *Mycoplasma pneumoniae* generally presents with concomitant lower respiratory tract symptoms. Adenovirus, coxsackievirus, EBV, and streptococcal pharyngitis may all present with (or without) exudate.

STREPTOCOCCAL PHARYNGITIS

It is important to emphasize that, while there are "classic" findings attributed to streptococcal pharyngitis, these findings are neither necessary nor sufficient to make the diagnosis. The classic presentation includes sudden onset of the triad of exudative pharyngotonsillitis, fever, and tender anterior cervical adenopathy. However, this triad of findings is not always present in patients with streptococcal pharyngitis, and only about a third of patients with acute streptococcal pharyngitis have tonsillar exudate or fever greater than 38.3°C (101°F). In fact, children can be infected with group A beta-hemolytic streptococcus and have no symptoms at all. Furthermore, many patients with the triad do not have streptococcal pharyngitis and are instead infected with coxsackievirus, EBV, or other viral pathogens.

In addition to the abovementioned signs, other signs and symptoms that may occur in group A streptococcal pharyngitis include pain on swallowing; palatal petechiae; red, swollen uvula; scarlatinaform rash; headache; malaise; anorexia; nausea; vomiting; and abdominal pain. None of these signs and symptoms, however, either singly or in combination, is diagnostic of strep throat. Patients with strep throat typically do not have laryngitis, hoarseness, conjunctivitis, marked cough or rhinitis, diarrhea, anterior stomatitis, or discrete ulcerative lesions.

Infants and toddlers with strep pharyngitis generally present, not with sore throat, but, rather, with fever, rhinitis, and irritability. Young children (i.e., under 1 year of age) have a very low risk of progression to rheumatic fever, but they may have a protracted clinical course. Peritonsillar abscess may present with severe throat pain, trismus, high fever, drooling, and severe hoarseness or inability to speak.

EPSTEIN-BARR VIRUS PHARYNGITIS

Epstein-Barr virus pharyngitis, like sore throat due to group A beta-hemolytic streptococcus, may present with exudative pharyngitis, fever, and adenopathy. In contrast to streptococcal pharyngitis, however, the onset may be more insidious, and the "mononucleosis" syndrome may also include prominent malaise, fatigue, nausea, and abdominal pain. Associated signs of EBV infection include palatal petechiae and hepatosplenomegaly. The posterior cervical nodes are prominently affected, and generalized adenopathy is also common. A maculopapular rash is common, particularly in patients inadvertently treated with ampicillin or amoxicillin.

COXSACKIEVIRUS PHARYNGITIS

As discussed earlier, coxsackievirus has many presentations. Children may present with a straightforward sore throat, or they may have syndromes such as herpangina or hand-foot-and-mouth disease. They may also present with fever, headache, backache, vomiting, aseptic meningitis, a variety of rashes, myalgia, orchitis, epididymitis, hepatitis, carditis, pericarditis, or nephritis.

OTHER VIRUSES

Adenovirus often presents with prominent rhinitis, but sore throat, cough, and cervical adenopathy may be prominent as well, mimicking streptococcal pharyngitis. The associated pharyngitis may be exudative, and the patient may be febrile. Adenovirus sore throat may or may not be accompanied by a bilateral conjunctivitis.

Herpes simplex virus commonly presents with vesicular lesions in the anterior portion of the oral mucosa. However, a first episode of herpes simplex stomatitis may involve only the pharynx, and exudate may be present, mimicking the presentation of strep throat.

Sinusitis

Patients with acute sinusitis typically present following a URI that almost resolves and then persists or worsens. Symptoms include fever, purulent rhinorrhea, facial pain, maxillary toothache, and/or foul smell from the nose. Less-specific symptoms include sneezing, nasal congestion, decreased sense of smell, cough, or exacerbation of asthma. When these symptoms persist for 30 to 90 days, the condition is termed *subacute sinusitis*. The majority of cases of subacute sinusitis probably represent slowly resolving acute sinusitis.

By definition, symptoms of chronic sinusitis persist longer than 3 months. The symptoms of chronic sinusitis are similar to those of acute sinusitis, but they are less pronounced. Pain is often less prominent, although a dull frontal headache may be present.

Allergic Rhinitis

Allergic rhinitis commonly presents with nasal congestion, rhinorrhea, sneezing, paranasal headache, pruritis, and itching or watery eyes. Patients may also present with hoarseness, chronic pharyngitis, recurrent sinusitis, or otitis media. The symptoms may be seasonal (hay fever) or perennial.

Key History

When evaluating patients with nasal congestion or sore throat, the history is directed at determining whether the condition is infectious or noninfectious. If it is infectious, one must determine the site of infection (e.g., rhinitis versus pharyngitis versus sinusitis). When the infectious process includes pharyngitis, the clinician must determine whether the sore throat is caused by a streptococcal infection. If the condition is non-infectious, the goal is to decide whether the problem is allergic.

Infectious or Noninfectious?

The most important question for determining whether a patient's problem is infectious is whether the patient has been febrile. A history of fever in the presence of upper-respiratory symptoms almost always indicates an infectious process. Similarly, a history indicating that other household members or close friends have similar syndromes, especially if accompanied by fever, suggests contagion and the likelihood of infection.

However, fever and a history of contagion are not always present in patients with URIs. In this situation, other historical clues must be used. For example, a history of rhinorrhea, nasal congestion, and sneezing, with or without conjunctivitis, could be either the common cold or allergic rhinitis. However, when such symptoms have been present for less than a week and there is nothing to strongly suggest allergy, the symptoms should be presumed to be caused by a viral URI. Similarly, it is useful to determine whether the symptoms are part of an ongoing problem or whether they represent a discrete (though possibly recurrent) episode. Discrete or recurrent episodes are the rule in URIs, since both adults and children suffer multiple colds per year. More persistent symptoms, on the other hand, suggest allergic rhinitis or sinusitis.

Sinusitis or Rhinitis?

The timing of symptoms is important for localizing the site of infection. The common cold may last up to 2 weeks in one-quarter to one-third of patients, but if symptoms seem to improve and then worsen (a two-phase illness, or "double sickening") and persist longer than 2 weeks,

sinus infection should be considered. It is important to remember, however, that viral URIs are 20 to 200 times more common than sinusitis and that fever, nasal congestion, facial pressure, and colored nasal discharge may be present in either. Signs and symptoms positively associated with sinusitis include two-phase illness, purulent secretions seen in the nasal cavity on physical examination, unilateral facial pain, maxillary tooth pain, and poor response to decongestants.

Bacterial or Viral?

If infection is suspected and the patient has a sore throat, the key question is whether the sore throat is bacterial or viral—that is, "Is it strep?" Key historical factors increasing the likelihood of group A beta-hemolytic streptococcal pharyngitis include sudden onset of sore throat, fever greater than 38°C, pain on swallowing, abdominal pain, nausea and vomiting, scarlatinaform rash, recent group A streptococcal disease in a close contact, age 5 to 15 years, and past history of acute rheumatic fever. Factors indicating a lower likelihood of group A streptococcal pharyngitis include the presence of rhinitis, laryngitis, cough, diarrhea, and conjunctivitis.

Unfortunately, the sensitivity, specificity, and predictive values of these various symptoms are not sufficient to permit an accurate determination of whether a patient has streptococcal pharyngitis. This is particularly important when rheumatic fever is epidemic in a community (implying an increased prevalence of rheumatogenic strains), and extra caution in searching for group A beta-hemolytic streptococcal pharyngitis would be warranted in such a situation.

Is It Allergy?

If the symptoms clearly occur in association with exposure to an identifiable allergen, the diagnosis of allergy is easy. Other factors suggestive of allergy include itchy mucous membranes, clear rhinorrhea, itchy or watery eyes, or a previous history of atopy (such as asthma, eczema, nasal polyps, hay fever, or recurrent "sinus" problems). Relief of symptoms with antihistamines or nasal steroids also suggests an allergic basis for the patient's symptoms.

If a parent is atopic, there is a 30 percent chance that his or her child is atopic. If both parents are atopic, the figure rises to 50 to 70 percent. In children, other symptoms suggestive of atopy include a history of colic, food allergies, multiple formula changes, recurrent otitis, or sinusitis.

Is It Allergic Rhinitis or Sinusitis?

A history of ongoing sinus problems may represent chronic allergic rhinitis and/or sinusitis, because many patients misinterpret allergic symptoms as "sinus problems." However, differentiating chronic allergic sinusitis from allergic rhinitis by history may be quite difficult, since each condition is associated with nasal blockage, rhinorrhea, sneezing, coughing, and facial pressure or pain. Unilateral symptoms (i.e., unilateral discharge or pain) suggest sinusitis.

Physical Examination

In evaluating patients with upper respiratory symptoms, the physical examination is directed at confirming impressions formed by the history and localizing the site and nature of the patient's problem. Some examination findings suggest infection with specific microbial agents.

Common Cold

The physical findings in the common cold may be minimal or absent, or they can include inflamed nasal and/or pharyngeal mucosa with a watery or purulent nasal discharge. Slight fever and a mild cough may also be present. Severe cough points to infection with influenza virus or *M. pneumoniae.*

Pharyngitis

An inflamed pharynx always warrants consideration of group A beta-hemolytic streptococcal infection. This is true regardless of whether the pharyngitis is accompanied by exudate, cervical adenopathy, or fever, and regardless of whether the patient has associated rhinitis or lower respiratory involvement. Nonetheless, exudate, adenopathy, and fever are somewhat more typical of streptococcal pharyngitis, although they also occur in EBV infectious mononucleosis and coxsackievirus infection.

Various other findings associated with sore throat also suggest specific infectious organisms. A scarlatinaform rash may be seen with group A streptococcus or with *A. haemolyticum.* Other (non-scarlatinaform) rashes may also be seen with *A. haemolyticum,* coxsackievirus, or EBV infection. Associated conjunctivitis is commonly seen with viral pathogens, especially adenovirus. Gonorrheal pharyngitis is usually mild. The physical findings of splenomegaly, hepatomegaly, or other lymphadenopathy may be present in EBV mononucleosis. Vesicular or ulcerative oral mucosal lesions may be seen in coxsackievirus or herpesvirus infections. With severe pharyngitis, clinicians should be alert to the possibility of peritonsillar abscess. If throat pain is severe but pharyngeal inflammation is minimal, epiglottitis should be considered.

Sinusitis

When sinusitis is suspected, the nasal cavity should ideally be examined with a nasal speculum. However, a short, wide ear speculum attached to an otoscope is a reasonable alternative. The physical finding that best correlates with sinusitis is unilateral purulent nasal discharge. If topical decongestants are applied, it may be possible to visualize pus coming out of the sinus from below the middle meatus.

Transillumination may also be helpful, using a special transilluminator light attached to an otoscope handle and performing transillumination in a dark room. To examine the maxillary sinus, the light is placed against the hard palate in the patient's closed mouth; transillumination of a normal maxillary sinus will be seen as a glow on the patient's cheek. The frontal sinus is transilluminated at the supraorbital ridge. Asymmetric findings suggest fluid or pus within the less-illuminated sinus. Otorhinolaryngologists regularly use transillumination as a diagnostic technique. Its accuracy in the hands of primary care clinicians has not been demonstrated.

Other signs of sinusitis are neither sensitive nor specific, but, in combination with the appropriate history, they may help the clinician make a diagnosis of sinusitis. These findings include fever, purulent nasal discharge, cough, worsening of asthma, and tenderness over one or both maxillary sinuses or of the maxillary teeth. Septal deviation or nasal polyps may provide an alternative reason for nasal congestion, or they may contribute to the development of sinusitis by blocking drainage of the sinuses.

Allergic Rhinitis

When allergic rhinitis is suspected, it is useful to directly inspect the nose with a nasal speculum or otoscope. Although the mucosa may simply be red, the classic finding in allergic rhinitis is a pale or bluish, boggy, congested mucosa. Polyps may be seen within the nasal cavity.

The eyes of patients with allergic rhinitis may show inflammation or hypertrophy of the conjunctiva. Dark circles ("allergic shiners") may be seen under the eyes due to chronic congestion with blood. A horizontal crease above the tip of the nose is caused by the "allergic salute"—the wiping of the nose in an upward direction with the palm of the hand. The lips may be chafed from chronic mouth breathing, the skin may show evidence of eczema, and the wheezes of asthma may be present.

Bloody Rhinorrhea

Bloody rhinorrhea is a finding that warrants special attention. If present, it should elicit a careful assessment for the possibility of more serious problems, such as Wegener's granulomatosis or nasopharyngeal tumors.

Ancillary Tests

Testing for Group A Beta-Hemolytic Streptococcus

When a patient presents with pharyngitis, the key question facing clinicians is whether the pharyngitis is caused by group A beta-hemolytic streptococcus. Repeated studies have shown that, while certain history and physical examination findings increase the likelihood of streptococcal infection, it is not possible to reliably diagnose strep throat based on the history and physical examination alone. Specific laboratory testing, as outlined below, is necessary to diagnose or exclude streptococcal pharyngitis.

THROAT CULTURES

The blood agar throat culture is considered the "gold standard" for diagnosis of streptococcal infection. However, even throat cultures results can be falsely negative. Studies in which two cultures are obtained simultaneously from the same patient demonstrate that, in up to 10 percent of cases, group A beta-hemolytic streptococci will be isolated from only one of the two cultures. It is likely that many of these false-negative test results occur in patients who are chronic streptococcus carriers, rather than in those who have acute clinical infections, because chronic carriers typically have low-level colonization with the organism, and therefore their cultures may not always be positive.

Since the advent of the U.S. Clinical Laboratory Improvement Act (CLIA), many clinicians no longer perform throat cultures in their offices. Instead, they rely on outside laboratories to perform these tests. The cost of a throat culture ranges from $30 to $50.

RAPID STREP TESTS

Many "rapid strep tests" are available for testing patients suspected of having streptococcal pharyngitis. As a CLIA-waivered test, most U.S. clinicians can perform these tests in their offices. The cost to clinicians for rapid strep kits is approximately $3 to $4.

Rapid strep tests use enzyme immunoassay techniques to detect streptococcal antigens. The tests take only about 5 min to complete and are easy to perform. These rapid strep tests have a high positive predictive value, exceeding 95 percent. Thus, the diagnosis of streptococcal pharyngitis can be made with confidence in the presence of a positive rapid strep test result. However, the negative predictive value is less than optimal, with false negative rates between 10 and 30 percent.

Rapid tests are most useful for patients who are markedly symptomatic for whom there might be benefit from immediate diagnosis, because symptoms may be reduced by treatment within the first 24 to 36 hours of symptoms. For other patients—those with less severe symptoms or those seen several days into the course of illness—it is reasonable to rely on a throat culture alone, withholding treatment until and unless culture results are positive.

Many authorities recommend performing a throat culture if the rapid test result is negative, to exclude the possibility that the rapid test failed to detect a streptococcal infection. Such follow-up cultures are particularly important when the risk of rheumatic fever is higher, such as in children between 5 and 15 years of age and in communities at higher-than-average epidemio-logic risk for rheumatic fever. In other age groups and in areas with a low prevalence of rheumatic fever, some experts consider follow-up cultures to be optional.

Highly accurate "optical immunoassay" rapid tests have been described in the literature. These or similar tests would make it unnecessary to obtain cultures following negative rapid test results. Such tests are not yet routinely available, and in some studies their sensitivity is similar to that of current rapid step tests.

Finally, it should be noted that there is no indication for follow-up culture or rapid testing for asymptomatic persons following antibiotic therapy for streptococcal pharyngitis.

Testing for Infectious Mononucleosis

The Monospot test is a slide aglutination test used for diagnosis of acute EBV infectious mononucleosis. Testing is appropriate when infectious mononucleosis is suspected in children or young adults with a persistent severe sore throat and negative results on tests for group A beta-hemolytic streptococcal pharyngitis. It is also useful as an initial test in patients with acute pharyngitis accompanied by significant lymphadenopathy or hepatosplenomegaly.

Diagnostic Imaging of the Sinuses

Diagnostic imaging of the sinuses is not routinely recommended in the diagnosis of colds, allergic rhinitis, or acute sinusitis. The reason is that sinus abnormalities on computerized tomographic (CT) scans are found in as many as 25 percent of asymptomatic individuals and 85 percent of patients with uncomplicated colds. Thus, radiographic abnormalities of the sinuses are common and often clinically meaningless.

Sinus imaging is appropriate for patients with the symptoms of chronic sinusitis who have not responded to therapy. Sinus x-rays, CT scans of the sinuses, and sinus ultrasound studies have all been advocated in this situation. With each of these imaging methods, opacification of a sinus and the presence of an air-fluid level are the findings most strongly related to the presence of bacteria and fluid in the sinus (Fig. 6-4). Computerized tomographic scans are generally felt to be the most accurate tests, and the prices of limited CT scanning of the sinuses are frequently comparable to those of a full sinus x-ray series.

Allergy Testing

The diagnosis of allergic rhinitis is predominantly based on the history, with confirmation by the physical examination. Allergy testing is warranted if environmental control measures and therapy with medications are insufficient to control symptoms. In these cases, allergy testing can confirm or refute the diagnosis of allergic rhinitis and provide additional information about specific substances to which a patient is allergic,

Figure 6-4

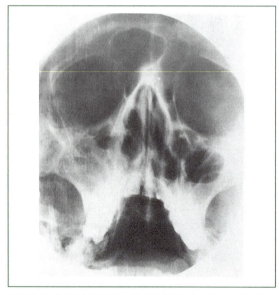

Maxillary sinusitis. This radiograph of the sinuses uses a Water's view and demonstrates maxillary sinusitis. The key findings are opacification of the right maxillary sinus and an air-fluid level in the patient's left maxillary sinus. *(Reproduced with permission from TM Davidson: Clinical Manual of Otolaryngology, 2d ed. New York, McGraw-Hill, 1992.)*

thereby guiding environmental control measures or immunotherapy. Intradermal and skin-prick testing are the techniques most commonly employed by allergists. In vitro allergy testing, such as measurement of serum IgE levels against specific allergens, can be used if skin testing is unavailable or contraindicated.

Algorithm

The algorithm in Fig. 6-5 outlines an initial general approach to patients with sore throat and/or nasal congestion. The first step is to identify clues to problems that might warrant special intervention or investigation. For example, chronic topical decongestant use indicates the possibility of rhinitis medicamentosa, and bloody nasal discharge may indicate a nasopharyngeal tumor or Wegener's granulomatosis. If such clues are not present, the next step is to determine whether the patient has an infection. If not, allergic syndromes are most likely—either rhinitis or sinusitis. If infection is present and symptoms include pharyngitis, streptococcal pharyngitis should be excluded, particularly in the 5- to 15-year-old child. Complications of infectious URIs, such as sinusitis or otitis media, should also be sought. Patients with atypical symptoms or findings may warrant special evaluation.

Treatment

Common Cold

Treatment of viral URIs is symptomatic (Table 6-3). No curative treatments are available, and antibiotics are ineffective in shortening the course or reducing symptoms of viral URIs.

Figure 6-5

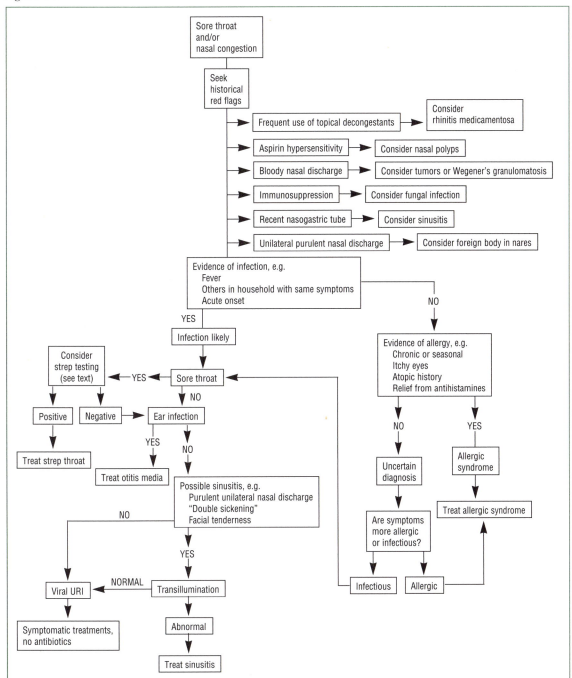

Algorithm outlining a general approach to a patient with sore throat and/or nasal congestion.

Table 6-3

Effectiveness of Medications for the Common Cold

	EFFECTIVENESS	
MEDICATION	CHILDREN	ADULTS
Antipyretics	+	+
Antihistamines	−	±
Decongestants (oral)	±*	+
Decongestants (nasal)	+	+
Ipratropium (nasal)	?	+
Alternative medication (*Echinacea*)	?	±
Zinc gluconate (oral lozenge)	−	±

NOTE: +, effective at relieving cold symptoms; −, ineffective at relieving cold symptoms; ±, evidence of effectiveness equivocal; ?, effectiveness has not been studied.
*There is no evidence that oral decongestants are effective in children under 5 years of age.

ANTIPYRETICS

Antipyretics and analgesics, such as acetaminophen and nonsteroidal anti-inflammatory drugs, may be used to treat fever. In most cases, acetaminophen is the medication of choice. Aspirin should be avoided as an antipyretic in children because of evidence that using salicylate with certain viral infections, such as influenza, increases the risk of developing Reye's syndrome.

ANTIHISTAMINES AND DECONGESTANTS

Prescription and nonprescription antihistamines and decongestants, either individually or in combination, are frequently prescribed to relieve symptoms of URIs. However, there is no evidence supporting the use of antihistamines for common colds in children. In adults, evidence that antihistamines are effective for relieving URI symptoms is contradictory at best. Thus, clinicians should not consider antihistamines as an essential or effective part of URI treatment.

On the other hand, there is evidence that oral decongestants, such as oral pseudoephedrine and phenylpropanolamine, can decrease nasal blockage associated with viral URIs. Oral decongestants are generally safe. However, because they are alpha-adrenergic agonists, these agents increase contraction of smooth muscle, including vascular smooth muscle. It is this action that mediates the drug's beneficial effect through vasoconstriction in nasal mucous membranes. This same action, however, can raise blood pressure through systemic vasoconstriction; thus, these medications should not be prescribed for persons with poorly controlled hypertension. Oral decongestants are safe, however, for short-term use in patients with hypertension that is well-controlled. Alpha-adrenergic-induced smooth muscle contraction can also cause constriction of the urethral sphincter. Therefore, oral decongestants should not be given to individuals with urinary outlet obstruction, such as from prostate enlargement.

INTRANASAL THERAPY

Intranasal therapy is effective for coryza. Marked symptomatic relief can be achieved with decongestant nasal sprays and drops, such as neosynephrine or oxymetazolone. Decongestant sprays and drops should not be used for longer than 3 days, however, to avoid rhinitis medicamentosa. In addition, an anticholinergic prescription medication, nasal ipratropium bromide (0.06%), is effective in decreasing the quantity of nasal discharge and carries no risk of rhinitis medicamentosa. Normal saline or hypertonic (2%) saline nose spray, on the other hand, does not improve nasal symptoms.

ALTERNATIVE MEDICINE

ECHINACEA   Practitioners of alternative medicine often recommend echinacea (*Echinacea angustifolia*) to relieve symptoms of URI. *Echinacea* is a member of the daisy family and is also known as "purple coneflower," "snakeroot," and "hedgehog." Its purported mechanism of action is to stimulate the immune system; it has no specific antibacterial or antiviral properties. *Echinacea* is administered as capsules, drops made from the juice of the plant, or an intramuscular injection. There is some evidence from a double-blind, placebo-controlled German study that this herbal medication can reduce the severity and duration of cold and flu symptoms.

ZINC   Oral zinc therapy is also widely used as a cold remedy. Zinc gluconate lozenges have been shown in some studies to decrease the duration of URI symptoms in adults by up to 40 percent. Other studies have shown no benefit. The mechanism of action is proposed to be a specific action of zinc on viral replication. The doses that have been studied are 23.7 mg eight times per day and 13.3 mg 6 times per day.

Studies of zinc for treatment of URIs in children have yielded contradictory results. A recent randomized controlled trial showed no benefit.

Pharyngitis

There are two primary considerations in the treatment of pharyngitis. The first is antibiotic treatment, which is only necessary for streptococcal pharyngitis or when complications (e.g., peritonsillar abscess) are present. The second consideration is symptomatic treatment of discomfort associated with sore throat, which is applicable to both streptococcal and nonstreptococcal pharyngitis.

ANTIBIOTIC TREATMENT OF STREPTOCOCCAL PHARYNGITIS

BENEFITS OF TREATMENT   Antibiotic treatment of group A beta-hemolytic streptococcal pharyngitis has four objectives. The first and primary purpose of treatment is to decrease the risk of developing rheumatic fever. The second is to shorten the course of symptomatic disease, possible only if treatment is begun within about 24 h of the onset of symptoms. However, even with such early treatment, the course of the disease was shortened by only about 1 day in some studies and not at all in others. The third objective is to shorten the length of time that patients shed streptococcal bacteria. Typically, contagion is eliminated within 24 to 36 h after starting antibiotic treatment. The fourth objective of antibiotic treatment is to decrease the risk of developing such suppurative complications as mastoiditis, brain abscess, and so on. Because these complications are rare, this benefit of treatment is limited at best.

RISKS OF TREATMENT   Antibiotic treatment carries several risks. The most important is the risk of allergic reactions, including life-threatening or fatal anaphylaxis. Another risk suggested in the literature is that patients may fail to develop immunity to streptococcal infection when treatment is begun early, but the significance and magnitude of this risk has not been determined. Finally, antibiotic use carries the risk of generating bacterial resistance; this is a risk for individual patients and for society in general.

INDICATIONS FOR TREATMENT   In general, antibiotic treatment is warranted for any patient with a documented group A beta-hemolytic streptococcal pharyngitis, primarily for the prevention of rheumatic fever. Infection can be documented with a positive throat culture or rapid strep test result. In contrast to rapid tests, however, cultures usually require 24 to 72 h to confirm the presence of streptococcal pharyngitis. It is preferable to wait for a positive test result before starting antibiotics, because antibiotic treatment is effective in preventing rheumatic fever even if begun up to 9 days after onset of symptoms. If streptococcal pharyngitis is suspected, the patient suffers from severe symptoms (e.g., high fever, severe pain, or dysphagia), and rapid testing is not available, many clinicians have recommended beginning antibiotic treatment while awaiting culture results. This practice should be discouraged due to the worldwide development of antibiotic resistance.

TREATMENT REGIMENS Streptococcal pharyngitis can be treated orally or parenterally. The first-choice oral treatment is 10 days of penicillin V. Traditionally, oral penicillin has been given four times per day, but in the last decade it has become clear that, for children, twice-daily oral penicillin is as effective as penicillin given three- or four-times per day. Oral penicillin therapy is inexpensive (the cost to the pharmacist is approximately $2), and life-threatening anaphylaxis is less likely with oral than with parenteral therapy. A concern about oral therapy, however, is that, because symptoms usually last less than 10 days, some patients may discontinue treatment when symptoms resolve and thereby fail to receive adequate protection against rheumatic fever.

If compliance with treatment is of concern, an alternative treatment is injectible benzathine penicillin G. Benzathine penicillin is highly effective and has been used successfully to eliminate rheumatogenic strains of streptococci during rheumatic fever epidemics in military populations. The major risk of injectible penicillin is the higher likelihood of serious anaphylactic reactions in comparison to oral therapy. In addition, benzathine penicillin injections are painful.

For persons who are allergic to penicillin, erythromycin (cost $10 to $11 for 10 days) is the first-choice alternative therapy. As de-

scribed later, there is little rationale for using broader-spectrum antibiotics (e.g., amoxicillin, cephalosporins, fluoroquinolones, etc.) to treat uncomplicated streptococcal pharyngitis.

TREATING CARRIERS Some individuals are asymptomatic carriers of group A beta-hemolytic streptococci. The carrier rate varies greatly by age and is different in every community. As a rule, it is unnecessary to detect carriers and eradicate streptococci from their oropharynx or nasopharynx, because asymptomatic carriage is generally not contagious, and it does not lead to suppurative complications or rheumatic fever. The only situations in which clinicians might attempt to eradicate the carrier state would be in households where other individuals have or have had recurrent streptococcal pharyngitis, acute rheumatic fever, or rheumatic heart disease.

SYMPTOMATIC TREATMENT FOR ALL FORMS OF PHARYNGITIS

As with the common cold, the primary treatment for pharyngitis is symptomatic. A variety of lozenges and topical anesthetic agents containing menthol, phenol, benzocaine, or combinations thereof are available without prescription. While certainly not essential therapy, these remedies may provide symptomatic relief for some individuals with sore throats. Acetaminophen may also be used to control pain and is an appropriate therapy for fever.

Some patients, such as those with streptococcal, EBV, or coxsackievirus infections, may develop severe sore throat with edema, profuse exudate, and/or ulcerations. In such individuals, it may occasionally be appropriate to use lidocaine oral solutions or gargles, or lidocaine gel or ointment applied topically to painful areas with a cotton applicator. These treatments provide excellent pain relief but carry the risk of impairing protective airway and swallowing reflexes. Thus, topical lidocaine should be used with caution, and patients should not eat or drink when their pharynx has been anesthetized with lidocaine. Patients with symptoms severe enough to consider oral lidocaine should be examined carefully for the presence of peritonsillar abscess.

Finally, patients with severe pharyngitis and tonsillar enlargement associated with EBV mononucleosis can receive substantial symptomatic relief from therapy with oral prednisone. The mechanism of action is decreased pharyngeal inflammation and shrinkage of lymphoid (tonsillar) tissue.

Sinusitis

ANTIBIOTICS

Antibiotic therapy has been the mainstay of treatment for acute bacterial sinusitis. However, evidence to support this therapy is limited and equivocal. Several randomized, placebo-controlled trials of acute, subacute, and chronic sinusitis have found no benefit from antibiotic therapy, but subjects in these studies did not have fever or other symptoms suggestive of significant bacterial infection. Another study of patients with acute maxillary sinusitis did show a beneficial effect of antibiotic treatment using amoxicillin and penicillin, with the duration of sinusitis decreasing from 17 days in the placebo group to 9 (amoxicillin) or 11 (penicillin V) days in the active treatment groups. Based on this research, it appears that many, if not most, cases of sinusitis will resolve spontaneously (usually within 2 to 4 weeks) without antibiotic treatment, especially in patients without systemic symptoms of infection.

If antibiotics are to be used, clinicians must decide which of the many available antimicrobial agents is appropriate. Clinical investigations have compared penicillins, trimethoprim-sulfamethoxazole, cephalosporins, tetracyclines, and newer macrolides; none of these agents has been shown to have superior efficacy. Furthermore, a study comparing 3 versus 10 days of therapy

with trimethoprim-sulfamethoxazole in acute maxillary sinusitis found no difference in outcome between the two treatment regimens. The lack of difference among so many treatment regimens could reflect an overall lack of benefit from treating sinusitis with antibiotics, or it could simply reflect the fact that these various treatments are equally effective.

Because no clinical research has clearly established one antibiotic regimen as superior, selection of antibiotic therapy is usually based on the microbiologic characteristics of acute sinusitis. In addition to *S. pneumoniae* and *S. aureus*, *H. influenzae* and *M. catarrhalis* are common bacterial isolates from acute sinusitis, and both may produce beta-lactamase. Thus, while amoxicillin has been a traditional first-line agent for sinusitis, it may be more logical to use trimethoprim-sulfamethoxazole as the antibiotic of choice. It has activity against all of these common bacterial causes of sinusitis, including beta-lactamase-producing organisms, and short-course (3-day) treatment appears to be effective.

For treatment failures following first-line therapy, there is little evidence available to support a specific recommendation for treatment. Most clinicians recommend either a second-generation cephalosporin or amoxicillin-clavulanate, both being appropriate because of their effectiveness against beta-lactamase-producing bacteria. In addition, amoxicillin-clavulanate is also effective against anaerobes. Treatment failures and/or chronic sinusitis are usually treated for longer than 7 to 10 days, but there is no evidence in the primary care literature that defines an optimal length of therapy.

NASAL STEROIDS

A small number of randomized, placebo-controlled trials have evaluated the use of inhaled nasal steroids in acute or chronic sinusitis. These studies have shown both a statistically and a clinically significant benefit. Nasal steroids can be considered in any patient with sinusitis, but particularly in those with history or symptoms suggestive of allergies.

ALLERGY IMMUNOTHERAPY

Immunotherapy should be considered in patients with chronic sinusitis who have failed management with antibiotics and topical steroids. However, immunotherapy should only be used in those with a clinical history suggestive of allergy that is confirmed by allergy testing and for whom a specific allergen extract is available. It is reasonable to provide a trial of immunotherapy before considering surgical management.

SURGERY

Surgical therapy is generally reserved for patients with chronic sinusitis who have failed to respond to antibiotics, nasal steroids, and (if indicated) immunotherapy. Many authors have suggested that, with appropriate medical therapy, surgery is rarely necessary.

A variety of surgical procedures have been used, and the choice of procedures remains controversial. "Minimal sinus surgery," consisting of inferior meatal antrostomy, myringotomy, and adenoidectomy, has been used in young children. Functional endoscopic sinus surgery (FESS) is a relatively new procedure with high success rates reported in case series. Two studies have compared FESS with the traditional Caldwell-Luc surgical drainage procedure, and both studies found FESS to provide better outcomes.

ANCILLARY THERAPIES

A number of ancillary therapies have been recommended for the treatment of sinusitis without demonstrated benefit in clinical trials. Decongestants, either topically (nasally) or systemically administered, are frequently prescribed. They may give symptomatic relief but have not been shown to hasten recovery. Guaifenesin has been recommended because of its theoretical abil-

ity to thin mucous, but any benefit from guaifenesin is purely speculative. Antihistamines are discouraged in sinusitis because their drying effect may thicken and decrease sinus drainage. Saline nasal irrigation; saline nose spray; steam inhalation; hot, dry air; mentholated vapor; and spicy foods (e.g., garlic and horseradish) have all been offered to patients and described in the literature, but there are no clinical trials examining their use.

Allergic Rhinitis

There is a vast array of treatment options for allergic rhinitis. Environmental control is an important intervention, but it frequently is insufficient as the sole therapy. Nasal steroids are the most effective drug treatment, but antihistamines, antihistamine-decongestant combinations, topical antihistamines, mast-cell stabilizers (cromolyn), and anticholinergic agents (ipratropium bromide) are all effective. Immunotherapy is useful for those who do not wish to use daily medications or in whom pharmacotherapy does not provide sufficient relief. An individual treatment plan must be established based on the preference of the patient, cost, and convenience.

ENVIRONMENTAL CONTROL

Elimination of offending allergens is the most obvious method of controlling the symptoms of allergic rhinitis. This approach is discussed later in this chapter (see Education).

STEROIDS

NASAL SPRAYS Nasal sprays containing corticosteroids (e.g., beclomethasone, budesonide, dexamethasone, flunisolide, fluticasone, and triamcinolone) are the most effective pharmacologic treatments for allergic rhinitis and are generally considered the treatment of choice. Intranasal steroid sprays are effective treatments for the entire symptom complex of allergic rhinitis, including nasal blockage, rhinitis, sneezing, and eye symptoms. If symptoms are not completely controlled, oral antihistamines or other medications may be added. Side effects of nasal steroids may include nasal irritation, nosebleed, and, rarely, mucosal yeast infection.

OPHTHALMIC DROPS While ophthalmic steroids are effective for relieving eye symptoms (e.g., itchiness and tearing) that accompany allergic rhinitis, they also carry substantial risk, such as corneal scarring, which may result from unrecognized herpes keratoconjunctivitis. Most experts in primary care and ophthalmology recommend that primary care clinicians not use ophthalmic steroids for treatment of allergic rhinitis and conjunctivitis or other eye disorders without first consulting an ophthalmologist.

SYSTEMIC STEROIDS Some clinicians treat allergic symptoms with oral prednisone or intramuscular injections of long-acting corticosteroids, such as triamcinolone. While effective for relieving allergic symptoms, the chronic and recurrent nature of allergic rhinitis often requires repetitive steroid therapy, thereby exposing patients to the risk of chronic steroid side effects. Most experts in primary care recommend against using systemic steroids, in either oral or injectable form, for treatment of allergic rhinitis.

ANTIHISTAMINES

ORAL ANTIHISTAMINES Before the availability of nasal steroids, oral antihistamines (H_1 receptor blockers) were the first-line therapy for allergic rhinitis. Now, with the availability of nasal steroids, the role of oral antihistamines is less clear. In general, antihistamines are still useful when symptoms are mild or if patients do not like using a nasal spray. Oral antihistamines are effective for controlling symptoms of sneezing, itching, rhinorrhea, and itchy, watery eyes, but they do not decrease nasal congestion or blockage.

The older antihistamines (e.g., brompheniramine, chlorpheniramine, clemastine, cyprohep-

tadine, diphenhydramine, and hydroxyzine) can cause significant sedation. Therefore, they are often prescribed in combination with decongestants such as pseudoephedrine, which decrease nasal congestion and cause mild central nervous system stimulation that counteracts antihistamine-induced sedation.

Newer antihistamines, such as loratadine, fexofenadine, and astemizole, cause minimal or no sedation. Caution is needed when prescribing astemizole, however, because of QT-interval prolongation and serious ventricular arrhythmias that may occur when this drug is taken in combination with macrolide antibiotics (erythromycin and clarithromycin) or azole antifungals (ketoconazole and itraconazole), or in patients with hepatic dysfunction. Terfenadine, a drug related to astemizole, was withdrawn from commercial availability because of the same problem with QT-interval prolongation. Other nonsedating antihistamines, such as loratadine or fexofenadine, are generally preferable because they do not appear to induce cardiac arrhythmias.

Most older antihistamines are available without prescription and are relatively inexpensive. Most of the newer antihistamines require a prescription, and they can be costly. To decrease the cost of treatment, some clinicians recommend combined therapy, with an older antihistamine (e.g., chlorpheniramine) before bed and one of the newer antihistamines during the day—so-called "AM/PM dosing." While this approach reduces cost, carry-over sedation from the nighttime antihistamine may still occur.

NASAL ANTIHISTAMINES Nasal antihistamines became available in the late 1990s in the form of azelastine and are effective at decreasing the nasal symptoms of allergic rhinitis. Like systemic antihistamines, intranasal antihistamines have the potential to cause sedation, but this side effect may be of more theoretical than clinical concern. Research is needed to determine the role of nasal antihistamines in relation to oral antihistamines, inhaled nasal steroids, and other treatments for allergic rhinitis.

OPHTHALMIC ANTIHISTAMINES Ophthalmic antihistamine drops are effective in controlling ocular symptoms of itching and tearing (allergic conjunctivitis), which frequently accompany allergic rhinitis. The prototypical agent is levocarbastine, the first ophthalmic antihistamine available in the United States. At this point, its role as a first-line therapy for allergic symptoms in unclear.

DECONGESTANTS

Oral decongestants, such as pseudoephedrine, phenylephrine, and phenylpropanolamine, are used to decrease nasal congestion and blockage. As noted above, these agents have a stimulant effect and are commonly combined with antihistamines. Topical decongestants, such as oxymetazolone and phenylephrine, are effective at decreasing nasal congestion but should not be used for longer than 3 successive days due to the risk of rhinitis medicamentosa. Because allergic rhinitis tends to be a chronic condition, topical decongestants are often inappropriate for allergic rhinitis.

CROMOLYN SODIUM

NASAL CROMOLYN Cromolyn sodium is a mast-cell stabilizer that prevents the release of histamine from mast cells after allergen challenge. Nasal cromolyn, which is available without prescription, is useful for controlling the nasal symptoms of allergic rhinitis. It is not as effective as nasal steroids or antihistamines, but the only side effects that have been described with cromolyn are transient stinging or sneezing. Thus, for patients who experience side effects from antihistamines or nasal steroids, nasal cromolyn is a useful treatment.

OPHTHALMIC CROMOLYN Ophthalmic cromolyn sodium is useful for controlling the ocular symptoms of allergic rhinitis. This medication is par-

ticularly attractive because it is both effective and extremely safe. The only side effect is transient eye discomfort.

OTHER MEDICATIONS

IPRATROPIUM BROMIDE Ipratropium bromide nasal spray is an anticholinergic agent that is effective in controlling the rhinorrhea of allergic, nonallergic, and infectious rhinitis. The 0.03% formulation is indicated for allergic rhinitis, while the 0.06% strength is used for rhinitis associated with URIs.

OPHTHALMIC NON-STEROIDAL ANTI-INFLAMMATORY DRUGS Ophthalmic non-steroidal anti-inflammatory drugs, such as ketorolac, reduce ocular itching associated with allergic rhinitis and conjunctivitis. Their role in relation to the many drugs listed above, such as ophthalmic cromolyn and ophthalmic antihistamines, is unclear. Cromolyn preparations are probably preferred.

IMMUNOTHERAPY

Immunotherapy ("allergy shots") involves frequent injections of small amounts of allergen. IgG antibody develops in response to the allergen. This antibody blocks IgE-mediated interactions with the allergen and allergic pathways.

Immunotherapy is effective for reducing symptoms of allergic rhinitis. It is most appropriate for patients whose symptoms persist despite pharmacotherapy or in patients who cannot or will not use daily medications. Immunotherapy should only be provided to patients whose clinical history of allergy is confirmed by allergy testing and for whom a specific allergen extract is available. Furthermore, because immunotherapy can cause serious allergic reactions, including anaphylaxis, it should be administered by clinicians and in facilities prepared for and experienced in managing serious allergic reactions. Immunotherapy injections should never be self-administered by patients in an unsupervised non-medical setting.

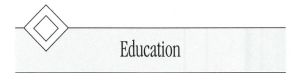

Education

Upper Respiratory Infections

Many patients do not understand the difference between viral and bacterial infections. Clinicians should teach patients that nearly all URIs are viral, will resolve spontaneously, and require no antibiotic treatment. If possible, clinicians should educate their patients about the growing problem of antibiotic resistance and its relationship to excessive and unnecessary use of antibiotics.

Clinicians should also educate patients about situations in which antibiotics might be necessary for URIs. For example, patients should seek care if they experience symptoms consistent with complications of URI, such as prolonged illness with purulent rhinorrhea, fever, and facial pain; isolated sore throat with fever; stridor or dyspnea; productive cough with fever or dyspnea; or the subjective feeling of a severe illness. In the absence of such symptoms, patients should understand that their URI symptoms usually require no treatment at all, or perhaps oral decongestants or ipratropium nasal spray to decrease nasal congestion and coryza. In young infants or elderly individuals, symptoms such as irritability, behavior change, decreased feeding, or somnolence are reasons to seek medical attention because these symptoms indicate the possibility of a bacteremic complication.

To prevent transmission of a viral illness to others, patients should be advised to stay out of school or work while they are symptomatic. This advice is often ignored, leading to epidemics of viral URIs in the workplace, schools, and day-care centers. It is also helpful to provide information about non-prescription remedies for which there is limited or no evidence of efficacy in URIs (e.g., antihistamines and guaifenesin), so that patients can avoid purchasing products not likely to improve symptoms.

Pharyngitis

Patients with streptococcal pharyngitis must be advised that a complete 10-day course of antibiotics is necessary to prevent rheumatic fever, particularly in children 5 to 15 years of age. It may help to specifically remind them that antibiotics should be finished even if sore throat symptoms resolve.

Anyone who has had rheumatic fever must understand the significant risk of recurrent illness. A throat culture should be obtained with every sore throat, and prophylactic antibiotics must often be taken until adulthood. Those with rheumatic valvular heart disease will need to take antibiotic prophylaxis prior to many dental, surgical, and diagnostic procedures.

Sinusitis

Acute sinusitis is generally a much longer illness than a common cold or pharyngitis. Patients should be told that, while the average duration of sinusitis is about 9 to 11 days from the start of treatment, in some cases sinusitis may last as long as 4 weeks.

Allergic Rhinitis

The three most important education topics for patients with allergic rhinitis are (1) the chronic recurrent nature of the disease, (2) the importance of self-management, and (3) the potential benefits of environmental control. Instructions regarding self-management include information on the proper use of nasal steroids.

For environmental control, patients should understand that, although allergens vary with areas of the country and climate, certain antigens are universally common. Dust mites, household pets (particularly cats), cockroaches, and molds are the most common allergens in perennial rhinitis, while outdoor pollens are the most frequent offenders in seasonal rhinitis. Minimizing reservoirs of mites, molds, and pet allergens in the patient's bedding, upholstered furniture, and household carpeting is an important environmental control measure. Decreasing household humidity, if possible, and adding high-efficiency air filters to air-ducts and vacuum cleaners are frequently recommended for reducing exposure to molds. Encasing mattresses and pillows in plastic and weekly washing of bedding in hot water are also appropriate to decrease exposure to allergens.

If pets cannot be eliminated from the house, they should not be allowed in the room of the allergic family member, and the pet should be bathed weekly to decrease the quantity of shed dander. Mold may grow on houseplants; it should be treated with appropriate fungicides, or the plants removed from the house. Closing windows helps to keep out pollen and decrease the amount of dust. Although cigarette and cigar smoke are not technically allergens, they can be powerful irritants to patients whose nasal mucosae are already hypersensitive and inflamed because of exposure to allergens; smoking by or in the presence of individuals with allergic respiratory symptoms should be avoided.

Family Approach

Spread of Infection

Sore throat and URIs, whether viral or bacterial in etiology, are contagious within families. Unaffected family members can attempt to decrease the likelihood of acquiring infection through such measures as good hand washing and avoidance of sharing glasses and towels. There is limited evidence, however, that these precautions can actually reduce the spread of URIs and sore throats among family members living together. However, if immunosuppressed or elderly persons reside in the home, it would be prudent to institute such infection-control measures to minimize the risk of contagion to these individuals, who may suffer adverse health consequences even from common viral or bacterial respiratory infections.

Streptococcal Pharyngitis in Family Members

Once streptococcal pharyngitis has been identified in a family, other family members who develop sore throat should be brought to a clinician's attention. Most clinicians feel it is appropriate to diagnose streptococcal pharyngitis in the newly symptomatic family member without obtaining bacteriologic confirmation. If the secondary patient is not suspected of having a marked febrile or complicated illness, it is often reasonable to treat the secondary case by prescribing antibiotics over the phone.

Antibiotic treatment of streptococcal pharyngitis stops bacterial shedding in 24 to 36 h. Therefore, if a patient is minimally symptomatic or asymptomatic, he or she can return to work, school, and family activities without concern for contagion after 1 day of antibiotic therapy.

Family Dynamics in Allergic Rhinitis and Chronic Sinusitis

Allergic rhinitis and chronic sinusitis, like other chronic illnesses, may interfere with family dynamics as the sufferer takes on the sick role. In addition, family members will be affected by the efforts required to achieve environmental control through measures such as removing the family pet to outdoors, control of dust, and other interventions that may be perceived as undesirable by unaffected family members.

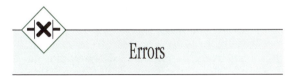

Errors

Inappropriate Use of Antibiotics

Without doubt, the most common error in management of URIs is the inappropriate prescribing of antibiotics. A recent study involving insurance claims for 50,000 patients found that 60 percent of outpatient visits for URI resulted in an antibiotic prescription being filled. The result was that antibiotics—a completely ineffective therapy—accounted for 23 percent of the total cost of medical care for URIs.

The increasing prevalence of penicillin-resistant pneumococci and other antibiotic-resistant bacteria has been linked to the excessive and inappropriate prescribing of antimicrobial drugs. In fact, several years ago researchers in Finland reported that up to 13 percent of group A beta-hemolytic streptococcal isolates were resistant to erythromycin. After introducing a nationwide program to reduce inappropriate use of antibiotics, the rate of erythromycin resistance decreased substantially, suggesting that reducing improper antibiotic prescribing can influence antimicrobial resistance patterns.

Clinicians often attribute prescribing of non-indicated antibiotics to patients' expectations for receiving antibiotics for all infections. Two studies have questioned this premise. Cowen studied satisfaction of patients in a family practice office who were seeing a physician because of URI symptoms. There was little difference in satisfaction among patients who received antibiotic prescriptions, those who were advised to take non-prescription medications, and those given no medications at all. Parents of small children

generally only wanted the clinician to exclude serious disease, not prescribe antibiotics. Fewer than 5 percent of patients were dissatisfied because they did not receive antibiotics, and a similar percentage were dissatisfied because they received unwanted medications.

In a larger trial of primary care patients seen for sore throat, 716 patients were randomized to receive 10 days of oral penicillin, no prescription, or a delayed prescription for antibiotics if symptoms did not resolve within 3 days. There was no difference in the proportion of patients in the three groups who were satisfied with their care. In addition, the proportion of patients whose symptoms had resolved in 3 days did not differ significantly among the three groups, nor did the duration of time off from work or school. However, patients who initially received antibiotics were more likely to believe that antibiotics were effective for their illness and planned to visit a clinician again if a similar illness occurred. The conclusions of the study were that use of antibiotics did not improve outcomes, but it "medicalized" the illness by promoting a belief that antibiotics were helpful.

Inappropriate Diagnosis and Treatment of Pharyngitis

Many clinicians make a presumptive diagnosis of streptococcal pharyngitis and institute antibiotic treatment based on clinical findings alone. As discussed earlier, it is not possible to reliably diagnose streptococcal pharyngitis on clinical grounds. Rather, the diagnosis of strep throat should be based on throat cultures and rapid antigen tests. Treating for streptococcal pharyngitis without bacteriologic confirmation results in the unnecessary use of antibiotics and the risk of drug allergy.

In addition to using antibiotics for non-streptococcal pharyngitis, another common error in treating pharyngitis is the use of unnecessarily broad-spectrum antibiotics. Streptococcal pharyngitis should be treated with an antibiotic narrowly focused for activity against group A beta-hemolytic streptococci, such as penicillin. Unnecessary use of broad-spectrum antibiotics contributes to development of antibiotic resistance and is generally more expensive.

Inaccurate Diagnosis of Sinusitis and Allergic Rhinitis

Clinicians often incorrectly diagnose sinusitis in patients who have such symptoms as nasal congestion and headache. This occurs so frequently that some experts believe the majority of patients diagnosed with sinusitis in primary care practice do not, in fact, have sinusitis. Rather, many of these patients have chronic or perennial allergic rhinitis. The diagnosis of and antibiotic treatment for acute sinusitis should be reserved for patients who have fever, unequivocal sinus tenderness, and/or a purulent nasal discharge, and transillumination may be desirable to confirm the diagnosis. Inaccurately diagnosing sinusitis results in repeated treatment with antibiotics, rather than effective treatment of allergic rhinitis with nasal steroids or antihistamines.

Controversies

Diagnosis and Treatment of Pharyngitis

IS IT NECESSARY TO DETECT AND TREAT STREP THROAT IN ALL AGE GROUPS?

Acute rheumatic fever as a complication of streptococcal pharyngitis occurs predominantly in children aged 5 to 15. Infants and toddlers up to age 2 to 3 have essentially no risk of rheumatic fever, and 3 to 4-year-old children are at extremely low risk. Adults, like children under 5, have a much smaller risk of acute rheumatic fever following streptococcal pharyngitis than do

children between age 5 and 15. Furthermore, suppurative complications are less frequent in adults.

Thus, one topic of controversy is whether antibiotic treatment of streptococcal sore throat to prevent rheumatic fever is necessary in persons younger than 5 or older than 15 years. In these age groups, streptococcal pharyngitis has a relatively short clinical course that would not benefit from the marginal illness-shortening benefit of antibiotic treatment. In addition, early treatment of streptococcal pharyngitis may lead to decreased immunity and more frequent recurrences. Finally, less use of antibiotics might decrease the rate of emergence of drug-resistant organisms. Thus, detection and treatment of streptococcal pharyngitis may not provide significant benefit in any patients other than children 5 to 15 years old and the most severely symptomatic individuals outside that age group. Some argue that if rheumatic fever is non-existent within one's community or country, it may not even be necessary to treat strep throat in 5 to 15-year-olds.

On the other side of the controversy, however, is the resurgence of rheumatogenic streptococcal strains in the United States during the late 1980s and 1990s. If rheumatic fever is prevalent in a community or population, children aged 5 to 15 years potentially benefit from diagnosis and treatment of strep throat. In addition, because streptococcal infections are transmissible within families and social groups, it is also important to identify and treat strep throat in toddlers and older adults who have contact with individuals age 5 to 15. Thus, from this point of view, there is strong rationale for routinely treating strep throat.

Resolution of this controversy will probably depend on future trends in the prevalence of rheumatic fever. The higher the rate of rheumatic fever, the greater the benefit of treatment.

For persons with a previous history of rheumatic fever, however, the risk of recurrent streptococcal infection is substantial, and the benefits of detection and treatment are undisputed. The same rationale justifies the detection and treatment of strep infection in family members of those affected by rheumatic fever, regardless of their ages.

SHOULD ALL SORE THROATS BE TREATED WITH ANTIBIOTICS?

Some experts argue that all patients with possible strep throat should receive antibiotic treatment, without any attempt to confirm the presence of streptococci. The rationale is based on cost. The wholesale cost of 10 days of oral penicillin is only about $2, and the retail cost to patients is usually less than $10. In contrast, the wholesale cost to physicians of a rapid strep test is $3 to $4, and the cost of a throat culture is $30 to $50. In purely economic terms, therefore, patients and society would realize substantial savings if physicians simply treated all patients with presumptive streptococcal pharyngitis and reserved bacteriologic testing for cases in which the diagnosis is less clear or firm bacteriologic diagnosis is essential.

This approach, however, would lead to over-treatment of most (up to 80 percent of) patients with sore throats, while failing to accurately identify some less-symptomatic individuals who actually have a streptococcal infection. It also ignores the risk of developing resistant bacteria and the risks to patients of allergic reactions to antibiotics prescribed without indication.

SHOULD BROAD-SPECTRUM ANTIBIOTICS BE USED FOR STREPTOCOCCAL PHARYNGITIS?

Shorter courses of a variety of expensive and broader-spectrum antibiotics have been found effective in eradicating group A beta-hemolytic streptococci from the pharynx. These antibiotics include the newer macrolides, such as azithromycin, and cephalosporins, such as cefadroxil, cefixime, cefuroxime, cefprozil, ceftibuten, and others. Some clinicians argue that the shorter course of therapy possible with these broad-spectrum antibiotics would improve patients'

compliance with treatments, thereby further reducing the risk of rheumatic fever. They recommend these antibiotics as first-line treatment for strep throat.

Most experts, however, argue against using these antibiotics as first-line treatments. One reason is that there is now evidence that streptococci can be successfully eradicated with shorter courses of standard anti-streptococcal antibiotics. In particular, 5 days of erythromycin estolate provides results similar to those provided by 10 days of penicillin V in children, with no significant difference in rates of eradication of the streptococci, adverse effects, or recurrence. No data are available, however, on the effectiveness of this regimen in adults or on the effectiveness of short-course penicillin regimens.

Other reasons to avoid routine use of broad-spectrum antibiotics as first-line treatments are cost and the potential for increasing antibiotic resistance. The wholesale cost to the pharmacist (in 1998) for a short course of broad-spectrum antibiotics typically ranges from $25 to $38, and the cost to patients is even higher. In contrast, as noted earlier, penicillin V costs the pharmacist only about $2. Finally, use of broad-spectrum antibiotics is associated with the development of multi-drug resistant bacteria. Given that penicillin resistance is rare with group A beta-hemolytic streptococcus and given the lower cost of penicillin and erythromycin, penicillin remains the clear drug of choice, with erythromycin an alternative for penicillin-allergic patients.

Indications for Tonsillectomy and Adenoidectomy

A significant concern of primary care providers is whether or when to refer patients for tonsillectomy. There is relative consensus that tonsillectomy should be performed in children in whom tonsillar enlargement causes persistent difficulty with swallowing or breathing. Tonsillectomy with adenoidectomy is also indicated in children with obstructive sleep apnea. However, the consensus ends there. Controversy remains about the indications for tonsillectomy in patients with recurrent pharyngitis, peritonsillar abscess, and chronic sinusitis. Furthermore, recent evidence indicates that a prolonged course of antibiotics (e.g., 30 days of amoxicillin clavulanate) can eliminate the need for surgery in a third or more of children being considered for tonsillectomy. This new finding suggests that the indications for tonsillectomy will continue to evolve.

RECURRENT PHARYNGITIS

Recurrent pharyngitis (or pharyngotonsillitis) is the usual indication for tonsillectomy, and tonsillectomy is effective in reducing the rate of recurrent streptococcal pharyngitis. Those undergoing tonsillectomy have an average of 40 percent fewer infections in the year following tonsillectomy, and the lower rate of infection persists for several years.

However, there is no agreement on definition of "recurrent." Definitions in the literature include three infections per year for 3 years, five infections per year for 2 years, or seven infections in 1 year, all of which must be either probable or confirmed streptococcal pharyngitis. The American Society of Otolaryngology and Head and Neck Surgery, on the other hand, suggests that three episodes of tonsillitis is an indication for tonsillectomy, regardless of the time interval during which the episodes occur.

The lack of consensus about indications for tonsillectomy for recurrent tonsillitis takes on even more meaning when one considers that the recurrence rates for streptococcal pharyngitis diminish over time, with or without treatment. Thus, even without tonsillectomy, most patients will experience fewer episodes of tonsillitis. Currently, the most prudent recommendation is that the risks and benefits of surgery should be considered on a case by case basis, with the greatest benefit to those with the most frequent and severe recurrences.

PERITONSILLAR ABSCESS

Peritonsillar abscess is another indication for tonsillectomy, but the timing of surgery is controversial. Some surgeons recommend tonsillectomy in patients who have had only a single episode of peritonsillar abscess, while others recommend the procedure only for recurrent peritonsillar abscess. To complicate matters, recurrences of peritonsillar abscess are uncommon in children without a history of recurrent pharyngotonsillitis. Thus, it is unclear whether tonsillectomy is appropriate for children with a single abscess and no history of recurrent infections. Additional controversy exists as to whether it is preferable to perform tonsillectomy after the abscess has resolved or whether it should be performed during the acute abscessed stage. There is limited evidence with which any of these controversies can be resolved.

CHRONIC SINUSITIS

The symptoms of adenoidal hypertrophy may mimic the symptoms of sinusitis. Therefore, some surgeons recommend adenoidectomy for children with chronic sinusitis. It is not clear whether this is appropriate therapy, since controlled studies have not been performed to demonstrate the benefit of this treatment.

Emerging Concepts

Penicillin-Resistant Pneumococcus

Streptococcus pneumoniae (pneumococcus) is an important cause of sinusitis. In the 1980s, the rate of penicillin resistance to pneumococci in the United States and most other countries was less than 1 percent. Recent surveillance studies from the Centers for Disease Control and Prevention, performed in laboratories throughout the United States, have found intermediate penicillin resistance in 14 percent of pneumococcal isolates, full penicillin resistance in 3 percent, and multiple drug resistance in 25 percent. Similar results have emerged from other studies in the United States and abroad. In U.S. day-care centers, penicillin resistance rates may be as high as 40 percent. The increasing prevalence of penicillin-resistant pneumococci has repeatedly been linked to the excessive prescribing of antibiotics. The eventual clinical significance of the increase in penicillin and multi-drug resistance is unclear but will probably influence how sinusitis and other respiratory tract infections are treated.

Etiology of Sinusitis

Researchers are reconsidering the pathophysiology of sinusitis. The normal sinus cavities have traditionally been considered sterile. As noted earlier, however, new research has shown that bacteria are present in normal sinuses and in the sinuses of individuals with simple URIs, suggesting that the presence of bacteria is not the inciting event in sinusitis. Rather, evidence is building that the primary factor in the development of sinusitis is improper sinus drainage, due to interference with ciliary function by a viral infection, allergy, structural problems in sinus drainage, or immunodeficiency states. Bacterial infection may thus be a secondary process related to improper drainage. It is likely that future treatment of sinusitis will emphasize improvement of sinus drainage with nasal steroids or decongestants, rather than antibiotic therapy.

New Treatments and Prevention for URIs

Vaccine development to prevent common colds is an elusive goal because so many different viruses cause URIs and because there is substantial antigenic variation with each virus category. Thus, no single vaccine is likely to be effective in preventing viral URIs.

Instead, research has focused on other mechanisms for prevention and treatment of colds. For example, rhinoviruses enter nasal mucosal cells by attaching to receptor proteins on the cell surface. One unique approach to URI prevention and treatment is development of receptor analogues that can be sprayed into the nose. In essence, these analogues provide "decoy" receptors to which viral particles attach, instead of attaching to cell receptors on a patient's nasal mucous membranes. This and similar approaches are likely to result in future availability of novel treatments and preventive measures for URIs.

Bibliography

Adam P, Stiffman M, Blake RL: A clinical trial of hypertonic saline nasal spray in subjects with the common cold or rhinosinusitis. *Arch Fam Med* 7:39, 1998.

Adams D, Scholz H: 5 days of drythromycin estolate versus 10 days of penicillin V in the treatment of group A streptococcal tonsillar pharyngitis in children. Pharyngitis Study Group. *Eur J Clin Microbiol Infect Dis* 15:712, 1996.

Arason VA, Kristinsson KG, Sigurdsson JA, et al: Do antimicrobials increase the carriage rate of penicillin resistant pneumococci in children? Cross sectional prevalence study. *Br Med J* 313:387, 1996.

Blaunt BW, Hart LG, Ehreth JL: A comparison of the content of army family practice with nonfederal family practice. *J Am Board Fam Pract* 7:395, 1994.

Calderon E, O'Neal ML, Fox RW, et al: Chronic sinusitis in children. *J Invest Aller Clin Immunol* 6:5, 1996.

Cauwenberge PV, Ingels K: Effects of viral and bacterial infection on nasal and sinus mucosa. *Acta Otolaryngol (Stockh)* 116:316, 1996.

Cowen PF: Patient satisfaction with an office visit for the common cold. *J Fam Pract* 24:412, 1987.

Dajani A, Taubert K, Ferrieri P, et al: Treatment of acute streptococcal pharyngitis and prevention of rheumatic fever: A statement for health professionals. *Pediatrics* 96:758, 1995.

Deutsch ES: Tonsillectomy and adenoidectomy: Changing indications. *Pediatr Clin North Am* 43: 1319, 1996.

Doern GV, Brueggemann A, Holley HP Jr et al: Antimicrobial resistance of *Streptococcus pneumoniae* recovered from outpatients in the United States during the winter months of 1994–1995: Results of a 30-center national surveillance study. *Antimicrob Agents Chemother* 40:1208, 1996.

Dohlman AW, Hemstreet MPB, Odezin GT, et al: Subacute sinusitis: Are antimicrobials necessary? *J Allergy Clin Immunol* 91:1015, 1993.

Gwaltney JM Jr, Philips CD, Miller RD, et al: Computer tomographic study of the common cold. *New Engl J Med* 330:25, 1994.

Kay GG, Plotkin KE, Quig MB, et al: Sedating effects of AM/PM antihistamine dosing with evening chlorpheniramine and morning terfenadine. *Am J Managed Care* 3:1843, 1997.

Kreher NE, Hickner JM, Barry HC, et al: Do gastrointestinal symptoms accompanying sore throat predict streptococcal pharyngitis? *J Fam Pract* 46:159, 1998.

Lindbaek M, Hjortdahl P, Johnsen UL-H: Randomised, double blind, placebo controlled trial of penicillin V and amoxycillin in treatment of acute sinus infection in adults. *Br Med J* 313: 325, 1996.

Little P, Gould C, Williamson I, et al: Open randomised trial of prescribing strategies and managing sore throat. *Br Med J* 314:722, 1997.

Macknin ML, Piedmonte M, Calendine C, et al: Zinc gluconate lozenges for treating the common cold in children. A randomized controlled trial. *JAMA* 279:1962, 1998.

Mainous AG, Hueston WJ: The cost of antibiotics in treating upper respiratory tract infections in a Medicaid population. *Arch Fam Med* 7:45, 1998.

Malone DC, Lawson KA, Smith DH, et al: A cost of illness study of allergic rhinitis in the United States. *J Allergy Clin Immunol* 99:22, 1997.

Meltzer EO, Orgel A, Backhaus JW, et al: Intranasal flunisolide spray as an adjunct to oral antibiotic therapy for sinusitis. *J Allergy Clin Immunol* 92:812, 1993.

Muller JL, Clauson KA: Pharmaceutical considerations of common herbal medicine. *Am J Managed Care* 3:1753, 1997.

Otten HW, Antvelink JB, De Wildt HR, et al: Is antibiotic treatment of chronic sinusitis effective in children? *Clin Otolaryngol* 19:215, 1994.

Paradise JL, Bluestone CD, Bachman RZ, et al: Efficacy of tonsillectomy for recurrent throat infection in severely affected children. *New Engl J Med* 310:674, 1984.

Qvarnberg Y, Kantola O, Salo J, et al: Influence of topical steroid treatment of maxillary sinusitis. *Rhinology* 30:103, 1992.

Sclafani AP, Ginsburg J, Shah MK, et al: Treatment of symptomatic chronic adenotonsillar hypertrophy with amoxicillin/clavulanate potassium: Short- and long-term results. *Pediatrics* 101:675, 1998.

Seppala H, Klaukka T, Vuopio-Varkila J: The effect of changes in the consumption of macrolide antibiotics on erythromycin resistance in group A streptococci in Finland. *New Engl J Med* 337:441, 1997.

Stempel DA, Thomas M: Treatment of allergic rhinitis: An evidence-based evaluation of nasal corticosteroids versus nonsedating antihistamines. *Am J Managed Care* 4:89, 1998.

van Buchem FL, Knottnerus JA, Schrijnemaekers VJJ, et al: Primary-care-based randomised placebo-controlled trial of antibiotic treatment in acute maxillary sinusitis. *Lancet* 349:683, 1997.

Williams JW Jr, Holleman DR Jr, Samsa GP, et al: Randomized controlled trial of 3 vs 10 days of trimethoprim/sulfamethoxazole for acute maxillary sinusitis. *JAMA* 273:1015, 1995.

Williams JW Jr, Simel DL: Does this patient have sinusitis? *JAMA* 270:1242, 1993.

William J. Hueston

Cough

How Common Is Cough?

Conditions that present with a cough are among the most common reasons why patients seek care from primary care clinicians. Data from a variety of sources show that acute bronchitis, one of the major causes of cough, consistently ranks among the top 10 reasons for visits to family physicians. Other respiratory problems, including upper respiratory infections, allergic rhinitis, and asthma, are also frequently accompanied by cough and account for an estimated 200 to 800 million episodes of illness in the United States each year.

Data from several sources indicate that visits for cough-related conditions are increasing in frequency. In England and Wales, for example, visits for acute asthma have risen nearly threefold since the late 1970s. Over the same time frame, visits for acute bronchitis increased by over 40 percent. The increase has been most pronounced among children.

Among adults, the frequency of chronic bronchitis, an important cause of cough that occurs in chronic obstructive pulmonary disease (COPD), has also increased (by nearly a third over the past decade). Almost 14 million American adults are affected by COPD, which is the fourth most common cause of death in the United States.

In addition to occurring with bronchitis and upper respiratory problems, cough almost always accompanies pneumonia. More than one of every 100 persons in the United States develops pneumonia each year, and over 5 million of these individuals die. Most pneumonia-related deaths occur in older adults, in whom the hospitalization rate for pneumonia is almost 12 times that of young adults and for whom the length of each hospitalization is nearly double.

Principal Diagnoses

Coughing is usually the result of either acute or chronic external insults to the respiratory tract, but it can also be caused by internal stimuli or by drugs. The four primary mechanisms that cause cough are (1) inflammation of the respiratory tract, as seen with infections, asthma, and chronic exposure to toxic substances such as tobacco smoke; (2) mechanical insults to the respiratory tract, such as with aspiration of particulate matter or pressure on the bronchial tree; (3) chemical insults that accompany inhalation of gases; and (4) thermal stimuli, such as very hot or cold air.

The pathophysiologic mechanism of cough is a complex interaction between the airway, glottis, diaphragm, and respiratory muscles. Stimulation of the airway's sensory nerves causes closure of the glottis and contraction of the respiratory muscles to increase the intrathoracic pressure. Once intrathoracic pressure reaches a critical level, the glottis reopens, with a subsequent release of the intrathoracic pressure and expulsion of any material that may be present in the respiratory tract. Because of the need to generate large intrathoracic pressures to achieve expulsion of respiratory irritants, persons with impaired neuromuscular function or diminished pulmonary compliance often have ineffective coughing that predisposes them to aspiration or respiratory infections.

Normal Cough

Not all coughs are pathologic. Cough can be voluntary. In addition, many healthy individuals cough out of habit with no apparent underlying pulmonary or cardiac disorders. In a recent study of healthy children, it was observed that nearly all children cough every day, with the average child coughing 11 times daily, nearly always when awake. Thus, one of the challenges facing primary care clinicians when evaluating patients with cough is to determine whether the cough is normal, whether it represents a benign self-limited condition, or whether it is indicative of a more serious pathologic condition.

Pathological Cough

Cough has a multitude of causes (Table 7-1). While the differential diagnosis of cough is vast, only a few disorders are responsible for the overwhelming majority of cases of cough seen in primary care practices. These disorders are described in the following paragraphs.

UPPER RESPIRATORY TRACT INFECTIONS AND RHINITIS

Upper respiratory tract infections, including the common cold, and post-nasal drip from allergic rhinitis or sinusitis, account for the largest proportion of patients who come to primary care clinicians for cough. These problems were addressed more extensively in Chap. 6 and are not discussed in detail here.

LOWER RESPIRATORY TRACT INFECTIONS

Lower respiratory infections account for another large percentage of patients with cough. Acute bronchitis and pneumonia are the two most common lower respiratory infections seen in primary care practice. As discussed below, the presentation and physical findings are similar in these two conditions, and it is often difficult to distinguish between them without a chest x-ray.

ASTHMA

Asthma, including exercise-induced asthma, is also a frequent cause of cough. In children,

Table 7-1
Causes of Cough

Upper respiratory tract
    Acute rhinitis/pharyngitis (common cold)
    Allergic rhinitis
    Sinusitis
    Tracheolaryngitis (croup)
    Epiglottitis
Lower respiratory tract
    Infectious
        Acute bronchitis
        Pneumonia
        Tuberculosis
        Pneumocystis carinii
        Bronchiectasis
        Lung abscess
    Noninfectious
        Asthma
        Chronic bronchitis
        Allergic aspergillosis
        Bronchogenic neoplasms
        Sarcoidosis
        Pulmonary fibrosis
        Chemical or smoke inhalation
Cardiovascular
    Congestive heart failure/pulmonary edema
    Enlargement of left atrium
Gastrointestinal tract
    Reflux esophagitis
    Esophageal-tracheal fistula
Other
    Medications, especially ACE inhibitors
    Psychogenic cough
    Foreign body aspiration

cough-variant asthma is common and may go unrecognized if confused with recurrent bronchitis or allergies. Asthma having its onset in adults can also present as cough, although this is less common. As discussed later, there is some evidence that asthma in adults may be linked to previous infection with *Chlamydia pneumoniae.* This observation may make it important to differentiate adult-onset asthma from other causes of cough, so that appropriate anti-chlamydial therapy can be prescribed.

CHRONIC BRONCHITIS

Chronic bronchitis is a common cause of cough in adults. It is one of the principal syndromes of COPD and is usually defined as a cough with sputum production that persists for at least 3 months in a row over a 2-year time period. The pathophysiology of chronic bronchitis involves long-standing inflammation from external irritants, typically tobacco smoke, causing irreversible changes in bronchial wall structure and mucous glands in the lungs. The thickened bronchial walls and excessive mucus production result in a chronic cough, typically accompanied by shortness of breath and daily production of sputum.

In patients with chronic bronchitis, cough can change in character and become acutely worse when patients develop acute viral upper respiratory tract infections or lower respiratory infections such as bronchitis and pneumonia. Since patients with COPD already have compromised pulmonary function, any change or worsening of a chronic bronchitic cough is cause for concern, because it may presage further deterioration of respiratory status.

LUNG CANCER

Pulmonary neoplasms should be suspected, especially in older persons, when cough occurs in association with a history of cigarette smoking, asbestos exposure, or exposure to other carcinogenic substances. Hemoptysis or constitutional signs of cancer (e.g., weight loss) should further increase the suspicion of cancer.

NONRESPIRATORY CAUSES OF COUGH

Numerous nonrespiratory conditions commonly cause cough seen in primary care prac-

tice. For example, gastroesophageal reflux disease or other conditions associated with chronic aspiration may cause bronchial inflammation resulting in a chronic nonproductive cough. Reflux-induced cough may occur in both adults and small children. Cardiac causes of cough include congestive heart failure with interstitial lung edema or compression of the bronchus by an enlarged atrium.

One of the more common non-respiratory causes of cough in primary care practice is use of angiotensin-converting enzyme (ACE) inhibiting drugs for treatment of hypertension or cardiac failure. The ACE inhibitors cause cough because, in addition to their cardiovascular effects, these drugs also inhibit the ACE-dependent breakdown of bradykinin, a cough-inducing inflammatory mediator.

Typical Presentation

Most patients present to primary care clinicians with a cough of brief duration, typically caused by an acute self-limiting condition such as upper respiratory infections or acute bronchitis. Nearly half of all patients with uncomplicated acute viral bronchitis will cough for more than 2 weeks; 25 percent will cough for more than a month. Cough lasting for more than a month may be the presenting symptom of a chronic or serious respiratory tract disorder, such as cancer, tuberculosis, or COPD.

Key History

Duration of cough is an important factor in determining the likely cause. Brief episodes of cough are very common and mostly represent self-limited conditions such as upper respiratory infections or acute bronchitis. When cough has been present for a longer period of time (over 3 weeks), it is characterized as a chronic cough, which has a different differential diagnosis than acute, short-term cough (see below).

Acute Cough

In acute (short-duration) cough, a variety of symptoms may be useful in identifying the cause. These symptoms include fever, dyspnea, sputum production, hemoptysis, and the character and timing of the cough.

FEVER

Fever is an important historical factor in determining the cause of cough. Conditions such as upper respiratory infections and acute bronchitis usually have either no fever or a low-grade fever. A high fever, especially if accompanied by prostration, poor appetite, and other constitutional symptoms, raises the likelihood of pneumonia. Conditions such as cancer, asthma, gastroesophageal reflux, and cardiac causes of cough are rarely associated with fever.

DYSPNEA

Dyspnea is another important symptom in the evaluation of cough. Respiratory infections such as acute bronchitis and pneumonia may be accompanied by dyspnea on exertion or at rest, especially in older individuals and persons with underlying COPD or other lung disorders. Congestive heart failure is also associated with dyspnea, but in heart failure, shortness of breath may be of fairly sudden onset and accompanied by orthopnea or paroxysmal nocturnal dyspnea. However, orthopnea can also occur in patients with COPD, and in those with COPD complicated by bronchitis or pneumonia, making orthopnea relatively less useful for determining the cause of cough.

SPUTUM PRODUCTION

The presence or absence of sputum can be useful in evaluating the cause of a cough. Upper respiratory infections or allergic rhinitis may produce only small quantities of mucus or sputum, often representing posterior nasal discharge that drips into the oropharynx, supraglottic area, or upper airway. Most non-infectious causes of cough, such as asthma, chemical or smoke inhalation, ACE inhibitor use, sarcoidosis, and pulmonary fibrosis, rarely cause excessive sputum production.

On the other hand, cough in acute lower-tract infections, such as pneumonia and acute bronchitis, is likely to produce sputum, sometimes in large amounts. It should be noted, however, that *Pneumocystis carinii* pneumonia is only rarely associated with sputum production; most patients with *P. carinii* report a dry cough and increasing shortness of breath.

While the production and quantity of sputum may be helpful in differential diagnosis, contrary to popular myth the color of sputum is not helpful in differentiating viral infections from bacterial infection. In fact, the use of antibiotics based solely on whether sputum appears purulent produces no better results than does treatment with placebo.

HEMOPTYSIS

Hemoptysis can occur with a variety of pulmonary conditions. In primary care practice, acute or recent-onset hemoptysis is most commonly associated with uncomplicated acute bronchitis. Subacute hemoptysis, manifest as "rust-colored" sputum, is also a frequently mentioned sign of pneumococcal pneumonia. However, hemoptysis may also be a symptom of a variety of other conditions (Table 7-2), some of which are serious. When hemoptysis occurs, most clinicians will institute a search for some of the more common serious conditions, such as lung cancer and tuberculosis.

Table 7-2

Conditions Associated with Hemoptysis

Inflammatory disorders of the lung
   Acute bronchitis
   Bronchiectasis
   Tuberculosis
   Lung abscess
   Pneumonia, especially *Klebsiella*
Neoplastic conditions
   Lung cancer
   Benign bronchial adenomas
Cardiac disorders
   Pulmonary embolism
   Left ventricular heart failure
   Mitral stenosis
Trauma
   Pulmonary contusion
   Foreign-body aspiration with bronchial
   trauma
Primary pulmonary hypertension
Pulmonary vasculitis
   Wegener's vasculitis
   Goodpasture's syndrome
Bleeding disorder

CHARACTER AND TIMING

The character and timing of a cough may be useful in elucidating the cause of the patient's problem (Table 7-3). Laryngeal inflammation that accompanies croup or epiglottitis often produces a "barking" cough. Tracheal irritation or large-airway inflammation causes a brassy or hornlike cough. A "tight" or wheezing cough is seen in asthma and acute or chronic bronchitis. Patients with asthma, chronic bronchitis, esophageal reflux, and congestive heart failure may complain of a cough that is present or worse at night. Several infections classically produce paroxysms of uncontrollable coughing: pertussis, mycoplasma, and chlamydia.

Table 7-3

Characteristics of Cough that Suggest Specific Diagnoses

TYPE OF COUGH	DIAGNOSTIC CONSIDERATION
Barking cough	Croup
	Epiglottitis
	Laryngeal tumor
Brassy cough	Tracheitis
	Tracheal tumor
Wheezy cough	Acute bronchitis
	Asthma
Worsening at night	Asthma
	Chronic bronchitis
	Congestive heart failure
	Gastroesophageal reflux
Paroxysmal cough	Pertussis
	Chlamydia
	Mycoplasma
	Asthma
Honking cough	Psychogenic

When patients have bizarre or honking coughs, psychogenic factors should be considered as the cause. Psychogenic cough should also be considered for a cough that is present only when patients are aware that others are nearby and that disappears when patients think they are alone.

Chronic Cough

When cough has been present and not improved for more than 3 to 4 weeks, other historical factors are of increased importance. Some of these factors are similar to those of importance with acute cough, but their significance is different in chronic cough.

SPUTUM PRODUCTION

As with acute cough, sputum production in patients with chronic cough suggests lower respiratory tract disease. Chronic bronchitis, chronic pneumonia due to bronchial obstruction, and bronchiectasis all produce purulent sputum. It is usually produced in great quantity, with production increased when bending over or lying down. The sputum with bronchiectasis may be putrid-smelling due to overgrowth of anaerobic bacteria in the lung cavity; therefore, patients with bronchiectasis may have chronic halitosis.

When patients have been coughing for 3 weeks or more without sputum production, noninfectious conditions are more likely. The most common of these seen in primary care practice are bronchial neoplasms, asthma, and gastroesophageal reflux.

HEMOPTYSIS

Chronic hemoptysis is almost always indicative of a serious underlying disorder. In primary care practice, the most important conditions to consider are cancer and tuberculosis. Other causes of hemoptysis are listed in Table 7-2.

SYSTEMIC SYMPTOMS

Chronic constitutional symptoms are important because they signal the possibility of serious disease. Weight loss, lethargy, and poor appetite can signal tuberculosis or lung cancer. Isolated chronic cough with constitutional symptoms in patients with persistent radiographic evidence of pneumonia is a sign of malignancy obstructing a bronchus.

IMMUNODEFICIENCY

In patients with chronic cough, clinicians should also consider the possibility of immunodeficiency. In primary care practice, the most common immunodeficient conditions are those related to chronic corticosteroid use, cancer, and HIV infection. While steroid use and cancer may be readily diagnosed, it is necessary to question patients with chronic cough about risk factors for HIV disease. This is particularly true if typical HIV-related pulmonary infections are found to be the cause of the cough, such as tuberculosis, atypical mycobacterial infections, or *P. carinii* pneumonia. If no risk factors for HIV are present, assessment of HIV status is still indicated if the diagnosis remains elusive.

Physical Examination

Patients presenting with cough require a thorough examination of the nose, ears, throat, and neck, as well as a chest and cardiac examination. In addition, vital signs including temperature, respiratory rate, and pulse should be measured.

Nose, Ears, and Throat

Key features to evaluate in the nose are the character and color of the nasal mucosa. Pale and boggy nasal mucosa or the presence of nasal polyps suggests allergy-related post-nasal drip as the cause of the cough. If the mucosa is erythematous with exudate, infection is more likely to be causing the symptoms.

Evidence of sinusitis and/or ear infection would also suggest that post-nasal drip is the cause of the cough. However, physical examination provides few findings that are sensitive and specific for sinusitis. Tenderness over the sinuses or inability to transilluminate the sinuses is often thought to differentiate sinusitis from other respiratory illnesses, but neither of these signs alone is highly correlated with sinusitis diagnosed by computerized tomographic scan. The best predictors of acute sinusitis are a combination of signs and symptoms, as outlined in Chap. 6. In addition, the ears should be examined because patients (especially children) with upper respiratory tract problems and cough often have concomitant ear infections.

The throat should be examined for the presence of post-nasal drip from either infection or allergic rhinitis. In one series, almost 40 percent of patients evaluated in a specialty clinic for chronic cough had post-nasal drainage as their problem. The neck examination should include palpation of the anterior cervical lymph nodes to detect enlargement or tenderness, which would suggest upper respiratory infection. Supraclavicular lymph nodes should be examined for enlargement, which could signify lymphoma or lung cancer.

Heart and Lungs

Auscultation of the chest is performed to detect differences in breath sounds between the left and right lungs, as well as rales, wheezing, or a pleural rub. Localized decreases in breath sounds will be noted when lung consolidation or pleural effusion is present. Rales may indicate fluid accumulation in the alveolar spaces from congestive heart failure or pneumonia, or they can be heard with interstitial changes that accompany pulmonary fibrosis.

Bilateral wheezing is present with asthma and acute bronchitis. Wheezing may not be heard at rest but can sometimes be elicited by having the patient forcibly exhale, or it can be heard by listening to a forced exhalation while the patient is in a recumbent position. Unilateral wheezing can be present with either asthma or bronchitis, but it also raises the possibility of aspiration of a foreign body or obstructing tumor. Recurrent wheezing on the right side should raise suspicion of gastroesophageal reflux with aspiration because aspirated material is more likely to drain into the right main-stem bronchus.

The evaluation of cough should also include a cardiac examination. Signs of congestive heart failure include an S_3 heart sound and a displaced point of maximal impulse that may be diffuse. Irregular heartbeat, indicative of acute or chronic arrhythmia, may also cause congestive heart failure with auscultatory signs of pulmonary vascular congestion.

Ancillary Tests

In primary care practice, only a few ancillary tests are regularly used to evaluate the cause of cough. The most common tests are radiographic imaging, including x-rays of the chest and/or paranasal sinuses. For some patients, pulmonary function tests and sputum examinations are appropriate. Infrequently, such invasive tests as esophageal pH monitoring and bronchoscopy are needed to identify the cause of a cough.

Chest X-rays

Chest x-rays are not needed for most patients with acute cough. However, if a patient appears ill or if rales are present and the individual is at risk for pneumonia or aspiration, a chest x-ray is appropriate to confirm the presence of pneumonia (Fig. 7-1). In addition, complete blood counts, blood cultures, and other tests are in order if a patient with pneumonia is being considered for hospitalization. Chest x-rays are also needed for patients in whom foreign-body aspiration is a possible explanation for a cough.

Patients with a cough that persists more than a month usually require a more thorough evaluation than do patients with an acute cough. If the history and physical examination do not clearly point to a non-pulmonary cause for the cough (e.g., ACE-inhibitor use), a posterior-anterior and lateral chest x-ray should be performed to detect occult pneumonic infiltrate, a lung mass or hilar adenopathy, pulmonary fibrosis, or interstitial edema suggestive of congestive heart failure. Chest x-rays can also detect differences in aeration between lung fields that could suggest an obstruction from either a foreign body or proximal bronchial lesions. Computerized tomography or magnetic resonance imaging of the chest may be needed to further characterize abnormalities found on chest x-rays.

Figure 7-1

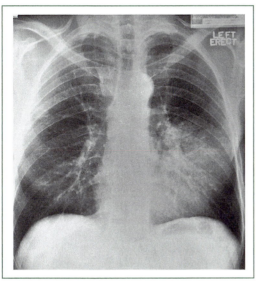

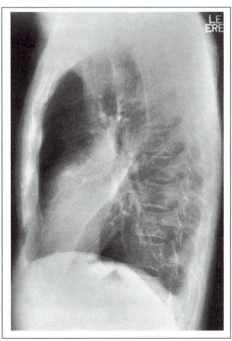

A   **B**

Radiographic appearance of pneumonia. Posterior-anterior and lateral x-rays of the chest show a pulmonary infiltrate in the lingula of the upper lobe of the left lung. The patient was a 57-year-old man who presented with fever and cough productive of purulent sputum. Cultures grew *Streptococcus pneumoniae.* (*Reproduced with permission from MYM Chen, TL Pope, DJ Ott: Basic Radiology. New York, McGraw-Hill, 1996.*)

Sinus X-rays

Although sinusitis can cause post-nasal drainage with cough, sinus x-rays are neither sensitive nor specific for diagnosing sinusitis. They are rarely of use in evaluating acute cough.

Pulmonary Function Tests

If the chest x-ray is normal, pulmonary function tests can be useful to detect mild or intermittent pulmonary obstruction. The most commonly used tests are spirometric measurement of the forced expiratory volume in the first second (FEV_1) and the forced vital capacity, and use of a peak flow meter to measure peak expiratory flow rate. Pulmonary function can be measured before and after administration of a bronchodilator to determine whether airflow obstruction is fixed or reversible.

For patients with nighttime cough, exercise-induced cough, or other symptoms suggestive of asthma, a methacholine challenge test may be added to standard pulmonary function tests to detect occult asthma if other testing is not diagnostic. Pulmonary function testing can also be useful for detecting restrictive lung changes that accompany fibrotic lung disease. Finally, diffusion studies, such as measurement of carbon dioxide diffusion capacity, can help determine whether significant interstitial lung disease is present.

Gram's Stain and Culture

In the hospital setting, Gram's stain and culture of sputum are sometimes helpful in distinguishing bacterial pneumonia from pneumonia caused by non-bacterial organisms. In bacterial pneumonia, Gram's staining of sputum will reveal a predominant bacterial organism, and presumptive morphologic identification of this organism can be used to guide initial therapy. The presence of polymorphonuclear leukocytes in the sputum, along with the relative absence of squamous cells, indicates that the sputum specimen is of satisfactory quality. Culture may then confirm the morphologic diagnosis.

However, Gram's staining and culture of sputum are rarely practical in an office setting. Many patients with pneumonia are unable to produce a satisfactory sputum specimen, and others may have a non-productive cough. Sputum production may be induced with inhalation of nebulized saline solution, but this is generally impractical in office practice. Furthermore, the high rate with which Gram's staining and culture produce no diagnosis further limits their use. Thus, Gram's stains and cultures are generally not performed when evaluating pneumonia in office practice.

Invasive Tests

Even with patients who are referred to specialists for the evaluation of chronic cough, invasive testing is rarely needed. However, invasive testing may be appropriate for patients with severe pneumonia unresponsive to therapy or when malignancy, airway obstruction, or gastroesophageal reflux is suspected. Two invasive tests, esophageal pH monitoring and bronchoscopy, are particularly relevant to primary care clinicians.

For patients with histories suggestive of gastroesophageal reflux with aspiration, esophageal pH monitoring can confirm reflux of acidic material into the upper gastrointestinal tract during sleep. While documented gastroesophageal reflux does not definitively prove that the cough is due to aspiration, it is highly suggestive that the cough is reflux-induced, especially if other testing has found no other cause for the cough.

Bronchoscopy is useful when there is suspicion that the cough is due to neoplastic lesion, aspiration of a foreign body, or chronic interstitial lung diseases. Older individuals who have smoked cigarettes for many years, or who have constitutional symptoms or hemoptysis, should be considered for bronchoscopy to exclude the presence of a neoplasm. Debilitated or very young patients with unilateral wheezes or signs of obstructions should undergo bronchoscopy to confirm or exclude the presence of an aspirated foreign body, chronic aspiration of gastric contents, or lesions obstructing a bronchus. Bronchoscopy is also useful for aspiration of obstructing bronchial secretions, and for obtaining culture or biopsy specimens in difficult-to-diagnose pulmonary infections.

Algorithms

Algorithms for the evaluation of cough are presented in Figs. 7-2, 7-3, and 7-4. The most useful first step is to differentiate acute from chronic cough. For patients with acute cough, in the absence of constitutional signs, high fever, or other signs of severe illness, physical examination can be used to identify the likely cause and select empiric therapy. If the patient appears ill, or if abnormalities are detected on percussion or auscultation, chest x-ray is appropriate to help detect pneumonia or other intrathoracic processes. If the x-ray is normal, empiric treatment for acute bronchitis is usually indicated. When

Figure 7-2

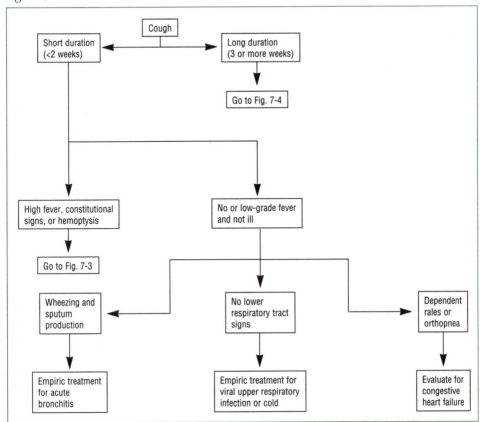

Initial evaluation of patients with cough.

pneumonia or a mass is present on the x-ray, further investigation is needed.

Patients with chronic cough require additional evaluation. History and physical examination to identify causes of post-nasal drip (allergies, chronic sinusitis, etc.) should be the first step because post-nasal drip is the most common cause of chronic cough. Evaluation for risk factors of HIV is also important. Further radiologic and invasive testing should be used when history and physical examination fail to reveal the cause of the cough.

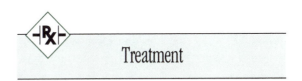

Treatment

This section discusses the treatment of three common causes of cough: acute bronchitis, pneumonia, and exacerbations of chronic bronchitis. Treatment of upper respiratory infections, the most common cause of cough, is discussed in Chap. 6, and treatment of gastroesophageal reflux disease is discussed in Chap. 15. Cough-variant asthma is treated with standard asthma

Figure 7-3

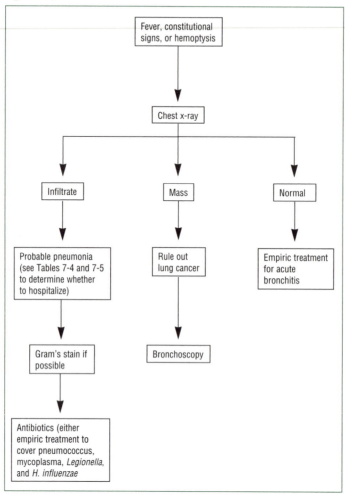

Evaluation of cough accompanied by fever, constitutional symptoms or hemoptysis.

medications, including inhaled steroids or other anti-inflammatory agents, along with inhaled bronchodilators and other drugs as indicated. A full discussion of asthma treatment, for which cough is usually not the most predominant symptom, is beyond the scope of this chapter.

Acute Bronchitis

In the overwhelming majority of cases, acute bronchitis is caused by a viral infection. Despite evidence that acute bronchitis is caused by viruses, however, multiple studies have shown that clinicians inappropriately prescribe antibiotics to treat most cases of acute bronchitis.

ANTIBIOTICS

There is little evidence that antibiotics are of any use in treating acute bronchitis. Several studies using a variety of antibiotics have failed to demonstrate significant improvement of patients with acute bronchitis who are given antibiotics

Figure 7-4

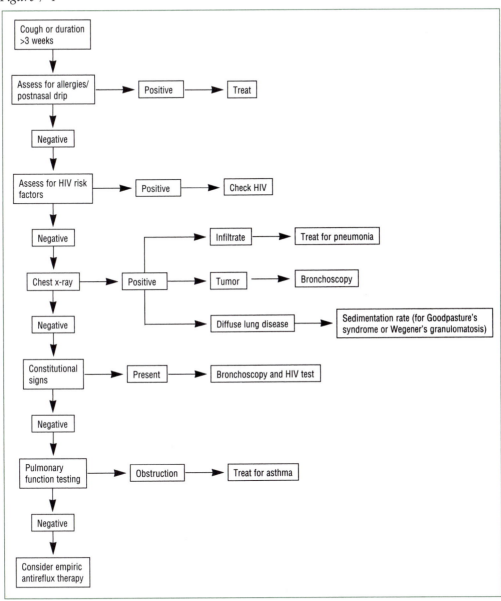

Evaluation of chronic cough.

in comparison to those given a placebo. These studies have included most common antibiotics, such as erythromycin, doxycycline, and trimethoprim-sulfamethoxazole. Although a few studies have showed some improvement in selected outcomes in patients treated with antibiotics, the results have not been dramatic. The lack of consistent findings from multiple studies suggests that antibiotics are not effective for acute bronchitis.

Interest in antibiotic treatment of acute bronchitis was renewed, however, when some studies suggested a causative role for *Mycoplasma pneumoniae*, especially in younger populations, such as college students or military recruits. One recent study even demonstrated the presence of *M. pneumoniae* in 25 percent of adults seen for acute bronchitis. It is unknown, however, whether *M. pneumoniae* was the cause of bronchitis in these patients or whether patients were simply colonized with or chronic carriers of the organism. When antibiotic (erythromycin) therapy was prescribed to patients in whom *M. pneumoniae* was identified, patients improved no faster with antibiotic treatment than with placebo. This suggests that *M. pneumoniae* is not a common causative agent of acute bronchitis.

BRONCHODILATORS

Multiple studies have shown that the bronchospasm and cough associated with acute bronchitis can be successfully treated with bronchodilators. The rationale for using bronchodilators to treat acute bronchitis is based on evidence that the bronchial changes, including abnormal pulmonary function test results, seen in acute bronchitis are similar to those in patients with asthma, and that patients with bronchitis are at higher risk for subsequently developing asthma. Rather than being chronic in nature, as in asthma, however, bronchospasm and airflow obstruction in acute bronchitis are short-lived and dissipate with resolution of the acute infection.

The similarities in pulmonary function between acute bronchitis and mild to moderate asthma led investigators to test beta-agonist agents for the treatment of acute bronchitis. A British study using oral fentolol showed improvement in pulmonary function studies and symptoms in patients with acute bronchitis. Two studies in the United States using oral or inhaled albuterol also showed clinical improvement in treated patients. Individuals who were given albuterol were more likely to stop coughing within 7 days and returned to work earlier than did those treated with placebo. As might be expected, patients treated with oral albuterol had more side effects than those treated with metered-dose inhalers; however, the effectiveness of albuterol was the same with both oral and inhaled drug.

While albuterol has a benefit for acute bronchitis, there appears to be little benefit when given to patients with undifferentiated cough. Thus, cough due to colds, sinusitis, or other upper respiratory tract illnesses should be distinguished from acute bronchitis, since bronchodilator therapy is not appropriate for these conditions.

The dose of albuterol or other bronchodilators is similar to that used for asthma. A typical starting dose might be two puffs of albuterol from a metered-dose inhaler up to four times per day on an as-needed basis.

ADJUNCTIVE TREATMENTS

Antitussive agents, such as dextromethorphan and codeine-containing cough suppressants, are effective for reducing the severity of cough. There is concern, however, that cough suppression in patients with acute bronchitis will interfere with clearance of sputum from the airway. Thus, many clinicians do not recommend cough suppression for patients with coughs that produce sputum.

Finally, patients with acute bronchitis who smoke cigarettes should be encouraged to stop smoking or at least reduce their cigarette consumption. Cigarette smoke interferes with normal muco-ciliary clearance of the bronchial tree, and smoking cessation allows more efficient clearance of mucous and debris from the bronchial system and may reduce symptoms. In addition, the toxic effects of cigarette smoke may delay healing of the inflamed bronchial epithelium.

TREATING POST-BRONCHITIC COUGH

Up to one-quarter of patients with acute bronchitis will develop a cough that lasts more than a month after resolution of the acute illness. In some individuals, this "post-bronchitic" cough can last up to 6 months. Post-bronchitic cough is thought to be due to delayed healing of the bronchial epithelium.

Treatment of post-bronchitic cough may include albuterol or similar beta-mimetic agents to relieve symptoms until the injured bronchial epithelium is healed. However, in patients with risk factors for lung cancer (e.g., cigarette smoking or asbestosis), prolonged or chronic cough following acute bronchitis should prompt a search for causes other than simple post-bronchitic cough.

Pneumonia

Clinicians must make two important decisions before beginning treatment for pneumonia. The first is whether to treat the patient in or out of the hospital. The second decision is selecting the proper antimicrobial treatment. In general, cough suppression is inadvisable in patients with pneumonia because it may interfere with clearance of sputum from the respiratory tract.

HOSPITAL VERSUS OUTPATIENT TREATMENT

The decision on whether pneumonia requires in-hospital treatment depends on patients' clinical condition, as well as their age, underlying health, and social situation. In general, this decision can be guided by whether a patient has risk factors for poor outcomes (Table 7-4).

Fine and colleagues developed an algorithm (Fig. 7-5) to guide the decision regarding hospitalization for pneumonia. The algorithm is based on risk factors for poor outcomes in community-acquired pneumonia. Based on this algorithm, patients under the age of 50 with pneumonia who have no evidence of neoplastic, cardiac, cerebrovascular, renal, and hepatic comorbidity; who have a normal mental status, pulse, blood pressure, and respiratory rate; and who have a temperature under 40°C (104°F) are at very low risk of death or needing admission to the hospital. Such individuals generally do well with outpatient antibiotic therapy.

For patients over 50 years old, Fine and colleagues developed a scoring system that can be used to stratify patients by risk (Table 7-5). Individuals with fewer than 70 points (which generally include patients over 50 with no risk factors) have a pneumonia-related mortality rate of less than 1 percent. Such individuals can usually be treated out of the hospital with minimal risk. Patients with scores between 70 and 90 have a slightly higher overall mortality rate, but still less than 3 percent. Home treatment with orally-administered antibiotics may be an option for these patients. Patients with risk scores over 90 should be admitted to and treated in a hospital

Table 7-4

Risk Factors for Death from Pneumonia

Age >65
Altered mental status
Tachycardia >140 beats/min
Hypotension (systolic BP <90)
Tachypnea (respiratory rate >30 breaths/min)
Underlying neoplastic disease
High-risk pathogen, such as *Pseudomonas*

Figure 7-5

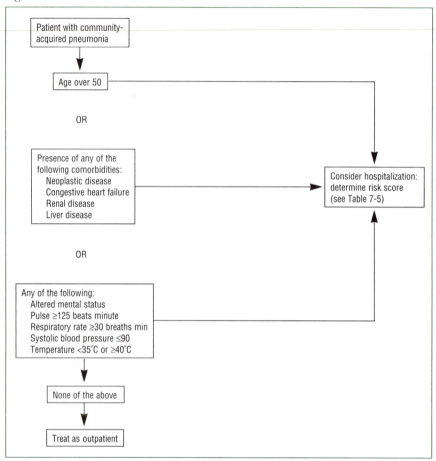

Algorithm for initial decision on hospitalizing patients with pneumonia. (*Reprinted with permission from Fine, Auble, Yearly, et al.*)

because mortality rates are much higher in these patients.

ANTIBIOTICS

It is difficult to distinguish bacterial pneumonia from viral pneumonia or from pneumonia caused by other non-bacterial pathogens. Therefore, antibiotics are prescribed for nearly all patients with pneumonia. As described below, the choice of antibiotics for pneumonia (Table 7-6) should be guided by the age and health of the patient, the relative prevalence of various infectious agents, and local antibiotic resistance patterns.

In addition, for patients in any age group, influenza virus should be considered as a cause of pneumonia during influenza outbreaks. Unless another cause for pneumonia is identified, individuals who are at high risk for complications of influenza should be treated with an anti-viral agent active against influenza, particularly if they have not received an influenza immunization. High-risk patients include the elderly; persons with such chronic respiratory conditions as asthma, chronic bronchitis, and

Table 7-5

Risk Scoring System for Hospitalization of Patients with Pneumonia

SCORE	MORTALITY RATE	
<70	Low risk for death (<1%)	
71–90	Moderate–low risk for death (1–3%)	
>90–129	Moderate risk for death (8–13%)	
>130	High risk for death (>25%)	

RISK FACTOR		SCORE
Age		
Men		+ Age in years
Women		+ Age in years − 10
Nursing home resident		+ 10
Comorbidities		
Cancer		+ 30
Liver disease		+ 20
Congestive heart failure		+ 10
Cerebrovascular disease		+ 10
Renal disease		+ 10
Physical findings		
Altered mental status		+ 20
Respiratory rate ≥30 breaths/min		+ 20
Systolic blood pressure ≤90		+ 20
Temperature ≤35° or >40°C		+ 10
Pulse ≥125 beats/min		+ 10
Laboratory/radiographic findings		
Arterial pH <7.35		+ 30
Blood urea nitrogen ≥30 mg/dL		+ 20
Sodium ≤130 mmol/L		+ 20
Glucose ≥250 mg/dL		+ 10
Hematocrit <30%		+ 10
Partial pressure of arterial O_2 <60		+ 10
Pleural effusion present		+ 10

SOURCE: Reprinted with permission from Fine, Auble, Yearly, et al.

emphysema; and those with diabetes who develop pneumonia during influenza epidemics. Either amantadine or rimantadine is an appropriate anti-viral medication. There has not yet been extensive experience using rimantadine in older persons, however, although the incidence of nervous system side effects is probably lower with rimantadine than amantadine.

CHILDREN, ADOLESCENTS, AND YOUNG ADULTS For children, adolescents, and healthy young adults, viruses and so-called "atypical" organisms such as *M. pneumoniae* and *Legionella pneumophilia* are the most common causes of pneumonia. *Streptococcus pneumoniae* (pneumococcus) is also frequent. *Haemophilus influenzae*, formerly a common cause of pneumonia in children, has

Table 7-6

Antibiotics for Empiric Treatment of Pneumonia in Selected Clinical Situations

AGE GROUP/CONDITION	LIKELY CAUSES	TYPICAL ANTIBIOTIC REGIMENS
Young children (1 month–5 years)	Viruses, pneumococcus, *Hemophilus*, or staphylococcus	Ceftriaxone or cefotaxime for inpatient; cefaclor, trimethoprim-sulfamethoxazole, or ampicillin-clavulanate for outpatient
Older children and adults (outpatient treatment)	Viruses, pneumococcus, mycoplasma, *Legionella*, or *Hemophilus*	Erythromycin, azithromycin, or clarithromycin
Older adults, no chronic illness and not severely ill, community acquired (inpatient treatment)	Viruses, pneumococcus, mycoplasma, *Legionella*, or chlamydia	Erythromycin, azithromycin, clarithromycin, levofloxacin, doxycycline
Older adults, community acquired, with chronic illness and not severely ill, (inpatient treatment)	Pneumococcus, *Legionella*, gram negatives, mycoplasma, or chlamydia	Macrolide + either second- or third-generation cephalosporin; or macrolide + ampicillin + β-lactamaseinhibitor; or levofloxacin

been less common since the advent of an immunization against this organism. For otherwise healthy younger patients with community-acquired pneumonia, the recommended treatment is usually a macrolide antibiotic, such as erythromycin, clarithromycin, or azithromycin (Table 7-6).

OLDER PATIENTS For treatment of older patients with community-acquired pneumonia, broad-spectrum antibiotics should be used because of the higher prevalence of gram-negative infections. These gram-negative organisms include *H. influenzae* and, in persons with chronic health problems, coliform bacteria. *Legionella pneumophilia* and *Staphylococcus aureus* infections may also occur. However, the most common cause of pneumonia in older patients is *S. pneumoniae*.

While broad-spectrum antibiotic coverage is needed for pneumonia in older patients, the high prevalence of pneumococcus requires that the treatment regimen almost always include agents active against pneumococcus. Ideally, the selected agent should be active against pneumococcus, *L. pneumophilia*, *H. influenzae*, and coliforms bacteria. For patients admitted to the hospital who are likely to have bacterial pneumonia, therapy with a second- or third-generation cephalosporin plus a macrolide will provide coverage.

For outpatient therapy, oral alternatives include erythromycin/sulfamethoxazole, azithromycin, and clarithromycin, although the activity of non-erythromycin macrolides against *L. pneumophilia* has not been conclusively demonstrated in clinical trials. Newer quinolones, such as levofloxacin, sparfloxacin, and trovafloxacin, have activity against all of these common agents.

However, given the rapid development of resistance that has occurred with other quinolones, widespread use of levofloxacin for pneumonia may be undesirable because it could hasten the development of resistance to this antibiotic.

HOSPITAL-ACQUIRED PNEUMONIA The relative frequency of organisms causing pneumonia contracted while in a hospital or nursing home is typically different than those causing community-acquired pneumonia. While pneumococcus is still a frequent cause, gram-negative infections are also common. In addition to the high prevalence of gram-negative infections, patients who contract institutionally acquired pneumonia are at higher risk of complications and death due to debilitation from age or disease. Thus, patients with hospital- or nursing-home-acquired pneumonia typically require aggressive therapy with broad-spectrum agents that cover a range of gram-negative organisms. Third-generation cephalosporins are first-line therapy. Depending on the severity of infection, other agents may also be appropriate, such as aminoglycosides and broad-spectrum penicillins.

ALCOHOLISM Another special population is persons who abuse alcohol. Pneumonia in alcoholics is more likely to be caused by *Klebsiella pneumoniae*. Therefore, treatment for pneumonia in alcoholic individuals should provide antimicrobial activity against *Klebsiella* in addition to pneumococcus and other organisms that typically cause pneumonia in the patient's age group. For patients who are not seriously ill, a second-generation cephalosporin is usually appropriate therapy for *Klebsiella* infection and provides reasonable coverage for pneumococcus.

PENICILLIN-RESISTANT PNEUMOCOCCUS Patients at high risk for infection with penicillin-resistant pneumococcus should generally be treated with vancomycin. Risk factors for and management of this increasingly common pathogen are discussed later in this chapter.

Chronic Bronchitis

Treatment of chronic bronchitis has two goals. The first goal is to deal with the chronic symptoms of sputum production and dyspnea that are the hallmarks of chronic bronchitis. The second goal is the effective management of acute exacerbations of bronchitis.

MANAGEMENT OF CHRONIC SYMPTOMS

SMOKING CESSATION Smoking cessation is the most important intervention for the treatment of chronic bronchitis and other manifestations of COPD. The Lung Health Study demonstrated that discontinuation of smoking resulted in improved pulmonary function during the first year of abstinence, followed by stable function thereafter. In contrast, patients who did not stop smoking had a continued deterioration in lung function.

BRONCHOSPASM AND BRONCHIAL INFLAMMATION The pathologic changes in chronic bronchitis include bronchial inflammation and excessive mucous production, both of which are also seen in asthma. Thus, therapy for chronic bronchitis includes many of the treatment strategies used for asthma, including bronchodilators and steroids. Antibiotics also have a role in treating chronic bronchitis.

Bronchodilators Patients with chronic cough that is mild and intermittent will benefit from occasional use of beta-agonist inhalers. Individuals who require more frequent treatment may benefit from aerosols or inhalers containing anticholinergic agents such as ipratropium. Compared to beta-agonists, ipratropium may be more effective than beta-agonists at reducing the symptoms of dyspnea and cough, has fewer side effects, and has a longer duration of action. However, ipratropium's onset of action is also slower than that of beta-agonists. Therefore, ipratropium is recommended for chronic use, with beta-agonists being reserved for intermittent treatment of acute dyspnea and cough. While ipratropium is effective for relieving the symptoms of chronic bronchitis, it has no long-term effect on pulmonary function.

For patients with moderate symptoms, theophylline can be added to ipratropium. In addition to its modest bronchodilatory effects, theophylline enhances diaphragmatic muscle function. Improved diaphragmatic function can decrease the muscle work that is responsible for the sensation of breathlessness and also improve clearance of thickened secretions. For improvement in diaphragmatic activity, theophylline levels of 8 to 12 mg/dL are adequate; when treating patients with chronic bronchitis with theophylline, clinicians should titrate doses to achieve serum values within these levels, rather than the 10- to 20-mg/dL range sometimes recommended for asthma.

Corticosteroids Unlike chronic treatment for asthma, in which inhaled corticosteroids are considered the mainstay of long-term therapy and short-course oral steroids are used for most exacerbations, steroid treatment for chronic bronchitis is generally used only for severe cases or exacerbations. Inhaled and/or oral corticosteroids can be used chronically with patients who have unremitting symptoms of chronic bronchitis while on anticholinergic and theophylline therapy, or used intermittently to treat exacerbations. However, because individuals with COPD are generally older and have multiple chronic medical conditions, they are at increased risk for the long- and short-term side effects of steroids. Therefore, clinicians should limit chronic steroid treatment to the lowest doses that are effective. When used for exacerbations, oral steroid bursts should be employed to ensure that an adequate amount of drug is given immediately, and then quickly tapered and discontinued if possible.

Antibiotics Antibiotics can be considered for exacerbations of chronic bronchitis. Data from several small trials have yielded conflicting results, resulting in controversy about the benefits of antibiotic treatment. However, a meta-analysis of nine placebo-controlled trials that examined the effects of antibiotics on chronic bronchitis did show a small, but statistically significant, beneficial effect. Studies demonstrating improved pulmonary function all used tetracycline analogues, amoxicillin, or trimethoprim-sulfamethoxazole. Thus, antibiotic treatment for exacerbations of chronic bronchitis should use these drugs instead of more-expensive alternatives, since there has been no evidence that newer or broader-spectrum agents offer any advantage. When antibiotics are used in chronic bronchitis, Gram's stain and culture of sputum are not useful in guiding therapy because patients with COPD usually have numerous bacteria colonizing their respiratory tract.

Education

Smoking Cessation

The most important educational intervention is addressing the issue of cigarette smoking with patients who smoke. Office visits for cough often represent a "teachable moment," in which patients may be more receptive to education about smoking cessation. Smokers who present with a cough may be worried that the cough represents a serious condition, such as cancer, and clinicians can take advantage of this concern to encourage smoking cessation. In addition, clinicians can point out that acute cough is likely to resolve more quickly if patients do not smoke. Clinicians can cite data on the reduction frequency of respiratory infections in individuals who have stopped smoking as evidence that smoking cessation will be beneficial. In fact, individuals who stop smoking have been found to have a 50-percent reduction in the incidence of respiratory problems compared to those who continue to smoke. Finally, it is important to point out that the longer one smokes and the more one smokes, the less benefit is ultimately derived from smoking cessation.

Therefore, patients should be advised to stop smoking now, because the benefit will be greater now than if they wait until the future. Techniques for smoking cessation are discussed in Chap. 1.

Unnecessary Treatments

Clinicians should teach patients that antibiotics are generally not necessary for acute cough problems, such as upper respiratory infections and acute bronchitis, since there is little evidence that antibiotics are beneficial for these conditions. Increasing public awareness about the growing problem of antibiotic resistance has made many patients receptive to the notion that avoiding antimicrobial therapy may be advantageous.

Similarly, clinicians should teach patients that there is no clear benefit to antitussive medications for acute cough or for cough accompanied by production of purulent sputum, and antitussives may even be undesirable. A more complete discussion of the effectiveness of cough suppression for acute upper respiratory infections is presented in Chap. 6.

Follow-up for Failure to Improve

The importance of follow-up for a cough that does not improve is an important facet in the care of the coughing individual. While a substantial percentage of patients with uncomplicated acute bronchitis cough for more than 2 weeks, a cough that persists for more than 2 to 3 weeks, especially if the cough is not improving, warrants further evaluation. In addition, if a chronic cough changes in character, especially if hemoptysis develops, patients should seek further evaluation.

Pneumococcal and Influenza Immunizations

A final teaching point for patients who present with cough is prevention of pulmonary infections, especially for those whose cough is related to chronic respiratory problems, such as COPD-related chronic bronchitis. High-risk patients should be advised to have yearly influenza vaccinations and a pneumococcal vaccination.

Persons considered candidates for influenza vaccination include all individuals over age 65; those aged 6 months or older with any chronic respiratory condition, such as asthma or emphysema; those with chronic cardiac disease, diabetes mellitus, hemoglobinopathies, immunosuppression, or chronic renal disease; and those living in institutions, such as prisons or chronic care facilities. Influenza vaccination is also indicated for family members of, or health care workers exposed to, high-risk individuals.

Pneumococcal immunization is indicated for persons over age 65 and those 2 years of age or older with diabetes mellitus, with chronic pulmonary or cardiac disease, and for those without a spleen. In addition, people in certain high-risk populations, such as Native Americans (including Alaskan natives) and those people over age 50 living in chronic-care facilities, should be immunized. Immunosuppressed patients, including those with HIV, alcoholism, cirrhosis, chronic renal failure, sickle cell disease, or multiple myeloma, may benefit from pneumococcal immunization, but the evidence is less convincing.

Clinicians should advise patients that the duration of protection from pneumococcal immunization is uncertain. For those at particularly high risk of mortality from pneumococcal pneumonia, such as patients over age 75 and those with chronic pulmonary disease or lacking a spleen, revaccination every 5 years may be beneficial, but firm data on which to base this recommendation are not available.

Family Approach

Cough is a common problem most often resulting from self-limited conditions. Simply because the condition is self-limited, however, does not reduce the anxiety and concern of patients and their families. Thus, reassurance should be provided, when appropriate, that a patient's cough is not caused by a serious underlying problem. In some cases, use of antitussive agents for treatment of non-productive cough may have a beneficial effect on the quality of family life, even if the cough would have resolved spontaneously with time.

Smoking by family members of patients with respiratory diseases is also an important issue. Exposure to "second-hand" smoke may worsen bronchial diseases such as asthma and acute or chronic bronchitis. In addition, support from family members is essential for patients with respiratory illnesses who are trying to stop smoking. Family members who continue smoking may sabotage the efforts of individuals who are trying to stop. Thus, all household members should appreciate the effort required to help a patient stop smoking.

Common Errors

Unnecessary Antibiotic Use

As noted earlier, antibiotics are of limited benefit for empiric treatment of acute cough unless the cough is caused by pneumonia. The over-prescribing of antibiotics is not only expensive and may result in side effects, but it may promote the development of antibiotic resistance. In fact, many experts believe that over-prescribing of antibiotics for upper respiratory infections and acute bronchitis has been a major factor in the development of penicillin-resistant pneumococcus (see below).

Data from several studies, however, demonstrate that clinicians prescribe antibiotics for about 30 percent of patients with upper respiratory infections, and for 60 to 80 percent of patients with acute bronchitis. This occurs despite clinicians' knowing that antibiotics are of little value for most patients with these conditions.

Clinicians often justify the use of antibiotics by stating that they are simply meeting patients' expectations that antibiotics be prescribed. However, research on patients' expectations does not support clinicians' belief that patients expect antibiotics. In fact, a study by Hamm and colleagues showed that, even among patients who did come into a clinical encounter expecting antibiotics, those who did not receive them were just as likely to be satisfied with their care as those who did, provided clinicians explained the rationale for not prescribing antibiotics. In reality, most patients are content to have their symptoms explained and receive reassurance that their cough or other symptoms do not constitute a serious problem, such as lung cancer.

Inadequate Evaluation

A second common error is failure to evaluate patients with chronic cough in a thorough manner. Patients who have been coughing for over 3 weeks with little improvement are less likely to have an uncomplicated acute bronchial infection. Empiric antibiotic or antitussive therapy for these individuals, or repeated prescription of broad-spectrum antibiotics, is likely to delay the diagnosis of a more serious problem. Further evaluation of patients with prolonged cough should be undertaken and typically includes chest imaging, tests for less common infections (e.g., tuberculosis), and pulmonary function tests.

Controversies and Emerging Concepts

Several important and controversial issues have emerged in the past decade: (1) the development of penicillin-resistant pneumococcus, (2) a potential association between chlamydial bronchitis and subsequent development of adult-onset asthma, and (3) the role of *Bordetella pertussis* as a cause of persistent cough in adults.

Penicillin-Resistant Streptococcus Pneumoniae

In recent years, laboratory surveillance has revealed the emergence of *S. pneumoniae* strains that are resistant to penicillin. Given that pneumococcus is among the most common causes of bacterial pneumonia, the development of antibiotic resistance is a great public health concern. These resistant strains were originally observed in Europe and South Africa but were not common in the United States. In the last several years, however, penicillin-resistant pneumococcus has been detected with increasing frequency in the United States.

To date, penicillin-resistant pneumococcus has been primarily a problem of previously hospitalized patients with severe underlying chronic disease. The majority of cases have been hospital-acquired, occurring in patients with malignancy, liver dysfunction, or chronic renal disease who had received β-lactam antibiotics within the previous 3 months. Community acquisition of penicillin-resistant strains has been fairly uncommon, and some have doubted whether penicillin-resistant pneumococcus is of any clinical significance.

Pneumococcal colonization of the nasopharynx is very common, occurring in up to 70 percent of healthy adults. The recent rise in colonization by resistant strains in healthy community-dwelling individuals raises fears that community-acquired penicillin-resistant pneumonia may become more frequent in the future. Research has identified several risk factors for carriage of penicillin-resistant pneumococcal strains, as listed in Table 7-7.

Currently, it is recommended that clinicians maintain awareness of the possibility of penicillin-resistant pneumococcal infections in seriously ill patients with pneumonia, especially if patients have an underlying disease and have been hospitalized recently. Positive sputum cultures results for *S. pneumoniae* should be examined for penicillin resistance. If penicillin-resistance is highly suspected or confirmed, the usual treatment is vancomycin. However, there have now been reports of vancomycin-resistant pneumococcus, raising concern about over-use of vancomycin inducing development of resistant strains. Third-generation cephalosporins may be a suitable alternative treatment if susceptibility is documented by laboratory testing.

Table 7-7

Risk Factors for Colonization with Penicillin-Resistant Pneumococcus

Age <2 or >70
Longer duration of hospitalization for pneumonia
Use of β-lactam antibiotics in last 3 months
Children in day-care settings
Staff in day-care settings

Chlamydia pneumoniae
and Adult-Onset Asthma

Observational studies of chlamydial antibodies in patients with adult-onset asthma have led to the hypothesis that adult-onset asthma may be related to previous or chronic bronchial infection with *C. pneumoniae*. Preliminary evidence from a small case series in a single practice suggests that treatment of adult-onset asthma with a macrolide antibiotic may improve asthmatic symptoms and pulmonary function test results. These observations raise the possibility that, when acute bronchitis is caused by chlamydia, failure to treat with anti-chlamydial antibiotics may have long-term consequences.

There are still several unanswered questions that must be addressed before the role of anti-chlamydial therapy in bronchitis or asthma is defined. The first important question is that of causation. Simply identifying past chlamydial infection in individuals with adult-onset asthma does not constitute proof that chlamydia caused the asthma. Rather, it could be that patients with abnormal pulmonary function are at greater risk of contracting chlamydial infections. At this time, there is insufficient evidence to infer causality between chlamydia and adult-onset asthma.

A second question is how often chlamydia is involved in acute bronchitis. Since the prevalence of chlamydial infection in acute bronchitis is unknown, it is difficult to justify universal treatment of acute bronchitis with antibiotics. At present, there are no inexpensive, accurate tests for office use that can distinguish patients in whom bronchitis might be caused by chlamydia from patients in whom bronchitis is virus-induced, the more common situation. Thus, there currently is no basis for the rational prescribing of antichlamydial therapy for patients with bronchitis.

A third important question is whether there would be benefit from anti-chlamydial treatment for patients with acute bronchitis or adult-onset asthma. As noted above, a preliminary study did demonstrate improvement in asthma when patients were treated with antibiotics. However,

this study included no control group; thus, it is unclear whether the apparent benefit was due to treatment effects or to a coincidental improvement in symptoms over time. In addition, even if antibiotic therapy is effective in the short term, it is not clear that the improvement will be sustained over time. Moreover, there is little evidence regarding the value of early treatment (i.e., treatment of acute bronchitis) versus waiting until (or waiting to see whether) a patient develops asthma. Thus, while it is intriguing to believe that treatment of acute chlamydial bronchitis might prevent adult-onset asthma, available evidence does not yet support this belief. Further research is needed to clarify the relationship between chlamydial infection and subsequent development of asthma.

Bordetella pertussis
and Chronic Cough

Several investigators have reported that *Bordetella pertussis*, the causative agent of childhood whooping cough, may be a cause of persistent cough in adults—even in those who were immunized against pertussis during childhood. In one large health maintenance organization, 12 percent of adults with coughs lasting 2 weeks or more had evidence of pertussis infection. In an emergency room setting, the prevalence of acute adult pertussis infection causing persistent cough may exceed 20 percent. Pertussis can be diagnosed by culturing a nasopharyngeal aspirate for *B. pertussis* or by polymerase chain reaction or direct fluorescent antibody testing of nasal secretions. At present, however, it is unclear whether the possible role of *B. pertussis* should lead to a change in the diagnostic and therapeutic approach to persistent cough.

Bibliography

Areno JP, San Pedro GS, Campbell GD: Diagnosis and prognosis in community-acquired pneumonia: When and where should the patient be treated. *Semin Respir Crit Care Med* 17:231, 1996.

Bariffi F, Sanduzzi A, Ponticello A: Epidemiology of lower respiratory tract infections. *J Chemothe* 7:263, 1995.

Bavastrelli M, Midulla M, Rossi D, et al: *Chlamydia trachomatis* infection in children with wheezing simulating asthma. *Lancet* 339:1174, 1992.

Caputo GMM, Appelbaum PC, Liu HH: Infections due to penicillin-resistant pneumococci: Clinical, epidemiologic, and microbiologic features. *Arch Intern Med* 153:1301, 1993.

Emre U, Roblin PM, Gelling M, et al: The association of *Chlamydia pneumoniae* infection and reactive airway disease in children. *Arch Pediatr Adolesc Med* 148:727, 1994.

Fine MJ, Auble TE, Yealy DM, et al: A prediction rule to identify low-risk patients with community-acquired pneumonia. *New Engl J Med* 336:243, 1997.

Fine MJ, Smith DN, Singer DE: Hospitalization decision in patients with community-acquired pneumonia: a prospective cohort study. *Am J Med* 89:713, 1990.

Hahn DL: Treatment of *Chlamydia pneumoniae* infection in adult asthma: A before-after trial. *J Fam Pract* 41:345, 1995.

Hamm RM, Hicks RJ, Bemben DA: Antibiotics and respiratory infections: are patients more satisfied when expectations are met? *J Fam Pract* 43:56, 1996.

Hueston WJ: A comparison of albuterol and erythromycin for the treatment of acute bronchitis. *J Fam Pract* 33:476, 1991.

Hueston WJ: Albuterol metered-dose inhaler in the treatment of acute bronchitis. *J Fam Pract* 39:437, 1994.

Kanner RE for the Lung Health Study Research Group: Early interventions in chronic obstructive pulmonary disease: A review of the Lung Health Study results. *Med Clin North Am* 80:523, 1996.

King DE, Williams WC, Bishop L, et al: Effectiveness of erythromycin in the treatment of acute bronchitis. *J Fam Pract* 42:601, 1996.

Klugman KP: The clinical relevance of in-vitro resistance to penicillin, ampicillin, amoxycillin and alternative agents, for the treatment of community-acquired pneumonia caused by *Streptococcus pneumoniae*, *Haemophilus influenzae* and *Moraxella catarrhalis*. *J Antimicrob Chemother* 38 (suppl A):133, 1996.

Krzyzanowski M, Robbins DR, Lebowitz MD: Smoking cessation and changes in respiratory symptoms in two population followed for 13 years. *Int J Epidemiol* 22:666, 1993.

Littenberg B, Wheeler M, Smith DS: A randomized controlled trial of albuterol in acute cough. *J Fam Pract* 42:49, 1996.

Mainous AG III, Zoorob RJ, Hueston WJ: Current management of acute bronchitis in ambulatory care: The use of antibiotics and bronchodilators. *Arch Fam Med* 5:79, 1996.

Melbye H, Aasebo U, Straume B: Symptomatic effect of inhaled fenoterol in acute bronchitis: A placebo-controlled double-blind study. *Fam Pract* 8:216, 1991.

Mello CJ, Irwin RS, Curley FJ: Predictive values of the character, timing, and complications of chronic cough in diagnosing its cause. *Arch Intern Med* 156:997, 1996.

Meza RA, Bridges-Webb C, Sayer GP, et al: The management of acute bronchitis in general practice: results from the Australian Morbidity and Treatment Survey, 1990–1991. *Aust Fam Physician* 23:1550, 1994.

Munyard P, Bush A: How much coughing is normal? *Arch Dis Child* 74:531, 1996.

Nenning ME, Shinefield HR, Edwards KM, Black SB, et al: Prevalence and incidence of adult pertussis in an urban population. *JAMA* 275:1672, 1996.

Orr PH, Scherer K, Macdonald A, et al: Randomized placebo-controlled trials of antibiotics for acute bronchitis: A critical review of the literature. *J Fam Pract* 36:507, 1993.

Saint S, Bent S, Vittinghoff E, et al: Antibiotics in chronic obstructive pulmonary disease exacerbations: A meta-analysis. *JAMA* 273:957, 1995.

Sparfloxacin and levofloxacin. *Med Lett* 39:41, 1997.

Statistical Abstract of the United States, 1994, 114th ed. Washington, U.S. Bureau of the Census, 1994, p 95.

U.S. Preventive Services Task Force: *Guide to Clinical Preventive Services*, 2d ed. Baltimore, Williams & Wilkins, 1996.

Vinson DC, Lutz LJ: The effect of parental expectation on the treatment of children with a cough: A report from ASPN. *J Fam Pract* 37:23, 1993.

Williams JW, Simel DL: Does this patient have sinusitis? Diagnosing acute sinusitis by history and physical exam. *JAMA* 2790:1242, 1993.

Williamson HA: A randomized, controlled trial of doxycycline in the treatment of acute bronchitis. *J Fam Pract* 19:481, 1984.

Wright SW, Edwards KM, Decker MD, et al: Pertussis infection in adults with persistent cough. *JAMA* 273:1044, 1995.

Behavioral Problems

Michael K. Magill

Chapter

8

Depression

How Common Is Depression?

Principal Diagnoses

Depression is among the most common problems seen in primary care practice. In some studies, half or more of patients in primary care offices report symptoms of depression on self-administered written tests. While many of these are false-positive results, other research indicates that 10 to 20 percent of primary care patients suffer from depression. In other words, if the average primary care clinician sees 20 to 25 patients each day, at least 2 to 4 of them can be expected to have depression. If a clinician identifies fewer than 2 to 4 depressed patients per day on a regular basis, it is likely that depression is going unrecognized in some patients and, therefore, that these patients are suffering unnecessarily from a treatable condition.

About half of all patients who receive care for depression do so from primary care clinicians and about half from mental health professionals. This pattern of care follows that for other mental health problems, for which primary care providers are a substantial source of care. According to the National Institutes of Mental Health's epidemiologic catchment area survey, of all persons treated in a 1-year period for mental and addictive disorders, 44 percent are treated only by general medical care providers. Less than 40 percent are seen by specialty mental health services providers; the remainder are seen by both.

For persons over 65 years old, reliance on primary care clinicians is even greater. More than 55 percent of persons in this age group who receive care for mental health problems receive it from primary care clinicians. In fact, only 3 percent of geriatric-aged individuals report ever having received outpatient care from a mental health professional.

The condition commonly known as "depression" actually consists of a variety of depression syndromes. When evaluating patients for depression, each of these syndromes should be considered as a possible diagnosis.

Criteria exist to separate the various recognized psychiatric syndromes from one another. While these criteria can be useful in clinical practice, it should be recognized that they generally were developed in research or referral settings with select populations of patients. The most well accepted of these criteria are set forth by the American Psychiatric Association in its *Diagnostic and Statistical Manual of Mental Disorders*, fourth edition (DSM-IV). The DSM-IV approach to diagnosis requires the patient's syndrome to meet specified criteria and results in categorization of patients into various depressive syndromes.

Unfortunately, the criteria set forth in the DSM-IV do not fully reflect the spectrum of depressive illness encountered in primary care settings. For example, some patients do not meet the formal DSM-IV criteria for depression, yet experience "subsyndromal" levels of depressive symptoms that can be very disturbing or even disabling. Other patients have subsyndromal depressive syndromes that represent more chronic dysthymic disorders that respond to standard treatments for depression. There is also considerable overlap between the DSM-IV definitions of depression and other syndromes, such as anxiety and somatization disorders, all of which are common in primary care practice. Finally, patients with depression in primary care practice are likely to have medical illnesses that can cause or exacerbate depression.

Acknowledging these limitations, it is nonetheless useful to categorize the various depressive syndromes by the standard definitions set forth in the DSM-IV. The principal syndromes of depression seen in primary care practice are (1) major depression, (2) bipolar illness, (3) dysthymia, and (4) depression associated with medical illness. Clinicians must exercise clinical judgment in deciding whether to initiate treatment for depressive syndromes falling short of the DSM-IV definitions.

Major Depression

DEFINITION

According to the DSM-IV, the diagnosis of major depression requires the presence of either depressed mood or loss of interest in normal activities. Most patients with depression experience feelings analogous to the intermittent sadness or discouragement that is a part of the normal life of healthy adults. However, for patients with major depression, the intensity and duration of these feelings exceed those of every day life. The DSM-IV requires the depressed mood or loss of interest to be present for at least 2 weeks and not be accounted for by underlying physical illness, medication, or grief. It should be emphasized that not all patients with major depression experience a sensation of sadness. Loss of pleasure or interest in activities may be the only major symptom, and it qualifies as a defining characteristic of depression in DSM-IV.

In addition to sadness or loss of interest, to meet criteria for major depression, DSM-IV states that the patient must have at least four of the following symptoms:

- sleep disturbance, commonly manifested as loss of sleep with frequent nighttime awakenings, especially towards morning, or as excess sleeping
- appetite and/or weight change; most often loss of appetite or weight, but sometimes increased appetite and weight gain
- fatigue or loss of energy
- psychomotor agitation or retardation

- feelings of guilt
- suicidal ideation

Some patients with depression experience so-called "atypical" symptoms of increased eating or sleep, weight gain, and prominent anxiety. In these patients, depression may be more difficult to recognize and may respond to different medications than "typical" depression.

EPIDEMIOLOGY

PREVALENCE   At any point in time, 2 to 3 percent of men and 4 to 9 percent of women in the United States have major depression. In any 1 year, approximately 10 percent of the adult population experiences a major depressive episode. In a lifetime, around 17 percent of all persons, about 10 to 25 percent of women and 5 to 12 percent of men, experience one or more major depressive episodes. These figures probably underestimate the true incidence and prevalence of depression because people sometimes have difficulty remembering episodes of depression, and, when depressed, they frequently do not report it to health care professionals.

Prevalence of depression is even higher in patients seeking medical care than it is in the general community, with 10 to 20 percent or more of primary care patients meeting research criteria for depression. Depression is also common among patients hospitalized for medical illnesses, occurring in up to 14 percent of inpatients. Despite these high prevalence statistics, however, and despite the fact that depression causes major disability and can be effectively treated, primary care clinicians detect depression in less than half of the patients with this illness.

Persons with family histories of depression, substance abuse (including alcoholism), and suicide are at higher risk of experiencing major depression. Children of individuals with major depression may also have a higher risk of attention deficit/hyperactivity disorder.

NATURAL HISTORY　Patients most often experience their first episode of depression in their twenties. Recurrences are common. About half of patients with one episode of major depression experience a second episode. Of patients experiencing two episodes, about 70 percent have a third. Patients having three episodes have a 90-percent likelihood of a fourth.

Episodes of major depression often resolve spontaneously. One year after onset of symptoms, about 40 percent of patients are free of depression, even without treatment. Unfortunately, however, approximately 40 percent will have had no substantial change in their depression, and the remaining 20 percent will have improved but still experience symptoms of depression. In some studies, as many as 15 percent of persons with major depressive disorder die of suicide.

Patients with depression are high utilizers of health care services and suffer substantial disability. Treatment for depression is a large component of health care costs in the United States. Depression is also a risk factor for development of subsequent illness, such as hypertension.

PATHOPHYSIOLOGY

Current research indicates that depression is caused by alterations of neurotransmitter function in the brain. Antidepressant medications inhibit pre-synaptic reuptake of neurotransmitters or stimulate (or sometimes inhibit) post-synaptic receptors for these neurotransmitters, which include dopamine, serotonin, and norepinephrine. The precise mechanism or mechanisms whereby these neurotransmitters are involved in causing depression is as yet unclear.

Some patients with depression have elevated serum cortisol levels and decreased cortisol suppression in response to infusion of dexamethasone. This abnormality occurs during the depressive episode. With resolution of depression, these endocrine changes revert to normal. In addition to changes in cortisol, electroencephalographic (EEG) changes may also accompany depression. Abnormal sleep EEGs may precede depression and be found after remission of the depressive episode. These endocrine and EEG abnormalities are thought to be markers of the presence of depression in some patients but are probably not the cause of most cases of depression.

Finally, depression can be caused by the central nervous system action of many medications prescribed for other medical problems. These medications are listed in Table 8-1.

Bipolar Illness

DEFINITION

Bipolar illness is characterized by episodes of depression alternating with mania (bipolar I) or hypomania (bipolar II). The episodes of mania or hypomania distinguish bipolar illness from major depression, which is also referred to as "unipolar" depression. Clinically, the distinction is critical because of the different medications effective for treating bipolar disorder. In addition, there is a risk of inducing mania or hypomania in bipolar patients if they are treated solely with standard antidepressant medications.

Manic episodes are discrete periods of elevated mood during which the patient may also be irritable and may engage in excessive or risky behaviors, such as extreme sexual activities, uncontrolled gambling, spending sprees, or similar activities. The patient may sleep very little for days or weeks, feeling no fatigue or need to sleep. Hallucinations and delusions may occur. Hypomanic episodes involve similar behaviors, but they are less severe.

EPIDEMIOLOGY

Men and women are equally likely to experience bipolar disorder, with a lifetime prevalence of 0.4 to 1.2 percent in the U.S. population. First-degree relatives of persons with bipolar I disor-

Table 8-1
Medications That Can Cause or Precipitate Depression

CENTRAL NERVOUS SYSTEM	ANTIMICROBIALS	CARDIOVASCULAR AND ANTIHYPERTENSIVES	HORMONES	OTHERS	ANTIINFLAMMATORY AGENTS AND ANALGESICS
Amantadine	Cycloserine	Clonidine	ACTH	Antineoplastic agents	Indomethacin
Amphetamine and derivatives	Ethambutol	Digitalis	Corticosteroids	Cimetidine	Pentazocine
Barbiturates	Selected gram-negative antibiotics	Diuretics	Estrogen	Disulfuram	Phenacetin
Carbamazepine	Sulfonamides	Guanethidine	Melatonin	Organic pesticides	Phenylbutazone
Chloral hydrate		Hydralazine	Progesterone	Physostigmine	
Chlordiazepoxide		Indapamide			
Cocaine		Methyldopa			
Diazepam and other benzodiazepines		Propranolol			
Ethanol		Prazosin			
Fluphenazine and other phenothiazines		Reserpine			
Haloperidol		Procainamide			
Levodopa					
Succinimide derivatives					

NOTE: ACTH, adrenocorticotropic hormone.
SOURCE: Adapted with permission from S Saklad: Pharmacoeconomic issues in the treatment of depression. *Pharmacotherapy* 15:774, 1995.

der have a 12-percent lifetime risk of bipolar I disorder, a 12-percent risk of recurrent major depression, and a 12-percent risk of dysthymia or other mood disorders.

Dysthymic Disorder

DEFINITION

The third common syndrome of depression in primary care is dysthymic disorder, also referred to as dysthymia. Dysthymia may be thought of as "mild" but chronic depression. Despite the lesser severity of symptoms, however, patients with dysthymia suffer considerable disability. Previously considered more a personality trait than a psychiatric syndrome responsive to medication, it is now recognized as treatable with antidepressant drugs.

According to DSM-IV, the key criterion for dysthymia is presence of depressed mood most of the time for a minimum of 2 years. In addition, the patient must also have at least two of the following symptoms: appetite change, sleep disturbance, fatigue, poor self-esteem, difficulty with concentration or decision-making, or hopelessness.

EPIDEMIOLOGY

In the general population, the prevalence of dysthymia at any point in time is about 3 percent, but 5 to 15 percent of patients in primary care practice have dysthymia. About 5 percent of adults experience dysthymia each year, and it is more common in women than in men.

Dysthymia is often associated with other psychiatric disorders. Up to 70 percent of individuals with dysthymia experience superimposed major depression (so-called "double depression"). Many patients also suffer from personality disorders. Specifically, up to 50 percent may have borderline personality disorder, and as many as 15 percent have social phobia (see Chap. 9).

Depression Associated with Medical Illness

DEFINITION

Patients with chronic medical illnesses often experience depression. Despite the presence of a medical disorder, however, major depression should be diagnosed if the patient's symptoms meet DSM-IV criteria for a major depressive episode.

The depression may be caused directly by the medical illness and improve with control of the underlying problem. However, if depression fails to resolve with control of the medical illness or within 1 month of control (whichever comes first), the depression should be treated directly. Patients with diabetes and depression, however, should not have treatment for depression delayed while the diabetes is being brought under control, since these two conditions in the same patient are generally unrelated. In dealing with depressed patients who have concomitant medical illnesses, it is important to keep in mind that many medications prescribed for the medical illness can cause depression (Table 8-1).

EPIDEMIOLOGY

Depression associated with medical illness is quite common. Up to 27 percent of patients with stroke experience major depressive episodes within 2 months of their stroke; and up to 40 percent experience lesser degrees of depression. More than half of patients with myocardial infarction become depressed. As many as 40 percent of patients with dementia experience depression. Apparent cooccurrence of dementia and depression can pose a challenging diagnostic problem, since symptoms similar to dementia may be a manifestation of depression. Patients may also have depression in association with many other physical illnesses, including thyroid and parathyroid disease, congestive heart failure, chronic obstructive pulmonary disease, acquired immune deficiency syndrome, rheumatoid arthritis, systemic lupus erythematosus, pernicious anemia, and chronic pain.

Typical Presentation

There are important differences between the presentation of depression in primary care practice and that in psychiatric practice. In primary care practice, depressive symptoms are likely to be relatively "undifferentiated" or "subsyndromal" and more likely to include somatic complaints. In fact, patients with "sub-threshold" or subsyndromal depression or dysthymia are 25 to 30 percent more likely to be seen by primary care clinicians than by mental health specialists. Although such individuals have a lesser intensity of depressive symptoms, they nonetheless have disability comparable to that seen in patients with chronic somatic illnesses. Individuals with atypical depression and personality disorders are also more likely to seek care from primary care clinicians.

Unlike subsyndromal or dysthymic depression, other depressive syndromes are relatively less common in primary care practice than in the practices of mental health professionals. In particular, primary care patients are less likely to be experiencing depression as part of bipolar illness or to have a schizoaffective disorder.

Somatic Complaints

As mentioned earlier, a critical difference between depression seen in primary care and that seen in psychiatric practice is that, typically, primary care patients with depression present for evaluation of somatic complaints, rather than because of affective or emotional symptoms. These somatic complaints include an array of vague physical complaints, the most common of

which are shown in Table 8-2. Patients may present with somatic symptoms because such symptoms are common manifestations of depression, because they do not recognize their somatic complaints as symptoms of depression, or perhaps because of a preference to attribute symptoms to medical illness because of social stigma associated with a diagnosis of depression.

For each the symptoms listed in Table 8-2, the likelihood that a patient with the specified symptoms has depression (i.e., the positive predictive value of the symptom) exceeds 33 percent in primary care practice. Symptoms of depression warranting special comment, including sleep disturbances, fatigue, and pain, are discussed in the paragraphs that follow.

SLEEP DISTURBANCE

Insomnia is a common presenting complaint of patients who are depressed. Classically, patients with depression can fall asleep without difficulty but then awaken during the night. The nighttime awakenings may simply be frequent awakenings, or patients may awaken towards the end of the night and not be able to return to sleep. A smaller number of patients with depression, especially those with anxiety as a prominent manifestation of depression, may have difficulty falling asleep at bedtime. Other patients with depression may experience excess sleeping.

Corresponding to the clinical complaints of insomnia, patients with depression exhibit early onset of rapid eye movement sleep and decreased duration of levels III and IV ("deep") sleep. They frequently complain of not feeling refreshed by sleep and of persistent fatigue during the day.

FATIGUE

Complaints of fatigue are common in patients with depression. Certainly, individuals complaining of fatigue should be evaluated for organic

Table 8-2

Positive Predictive Value of Physical Symptoms for Depression in Adult Patients Seen in a Primary Care Internal Medicine Practice

SYMPTOM	POSITIVE PREDICTIVE VALUE, PERCENT
Sleep disturbance	61
Fatigue	60
Three or more somatic complaints	56
Nonspecific musculoskeletal complaints	43
Back pain	39
Shortness of breath	39
Chest pain	35
Gastrointestinal complaints	34

NOTE: *Positive predictive value* refers to the percentage of patients with the specified presenting complaint who score in the depressed range on a written symptom checklist for depression.
SOURCE: Modified with permission from Gerber, Barrett, Barrett, et al.

causes, such as hypothyroidism, other endocrine disease (e.g., diabetes), and anemia. Consideration should also be given to other physical illnesses, such as vitamin B_{12} deficiency, renal disease, chronic infections, or malignancy as a cause of the fatigue. Despite the need to consider medical causes of fatigue, however, clinicians should keep in mind that among patients with prolonged (e.g., longer than 6 months) complaints of fatigue, depression is the most likely cause.

PAIN

Various forms of pain are common in persons suffering from depression. Patients with depression may present with complaints of headache, chest pain, abdominal pain, back pain, or other, less common pain syndromes. In many of these patients, pain is a symptom of some other problem, such as muscle tension headache, chest pain due to panic disorder, irritable bowel syndrome, or mechanical low back pain. However, even in these situations, pain may still be exacerbated or made less tolerable by the concomitant depression. Pain also may fail to respond to

appropriate specific treatment if the clinician does not identify clues that the depression is also present and simultaneously treat the depression.

Not only is pain a manifestation of depression, but as many as 50 percent of patients with chronic pain syndromes become depressed. While pain syndromes alone may be appropriately treated with low-dose tricyclic antidepressants, chronic pain patients who develop depression should be treated with full doses of antidepressant medication.

Psychological and Behavioral Complaints

DEPRESSION

Occasionally, patients will present with a straightforward complaint of depression. Generally, these patients have been previously diagnosed and treated for depression. Once patients have experienced the symptomatic improvement from treatment of depression, they more easily recognize early symptoms of recurrence.

Some patients with a chief complaint of depression have a family history of depression or are brought to the clinician by family members who suspect the patient is depressed. Clinical experience suggests that these family members' observations are often accurate.

For some patients, a suicide attempt will be the first clinically recognized sign of depression. Many, but not all, patients with suicide attempts are experiencing major depressive episodes. Some are suffering from other disorders, such as substance abuse, borderline personality disorder, or adjustment disorder. For this reason, although depression is a major cause of suicide, patients with suicide attempts should be evaluated carefully for psychiatric illnesses other than depression.

ANXIETY

Anxiety is a common symptom among patients seen in primary care practice. While anxiety is often a symptom of anxiety disorders or somatic illnesses such as hyperthyroidism, anxiety can also be the presenting complaint of depression. It is not uncommon for depression to be confused with anxiety disorders because, in addition to overt anxiety, depressive syndromes can also include anxiety-related symptoms, such as psychomotor agitation, or sleep disturbances, such as difficulty falling asleep.

Patients with depression also have a higher prevalence of concomitant anxiety syndromes, such as panic attacks. Patients with depression and anxiety or panic disorder should be treated for the depression in addition to the anxiety symptoms. Benzodiazepines, for example, are useful and appropriate for patients who have anxiety disorders in combination with depression but can worsen depression if used without concomitant antidepressant therapy in depressed patients.

BEHAVIORAL AND COGNITIVE PROBLEMS

Younger and older patients with depression are more likely than others to present with behavioral or cognitive problems rather than depressive mood changes. Adolescents may demonstrate problems with school, friends, sexual behavior, or substance abuse as the main symptoms of depression. Older patients with depression may present with memory difficulties ("pseudodementia"). Diagnosis of depression in the elderly can also be challenging because of concomitant somatic symptoms, medical illnesses, medication effects, true dementia, and anxiety.

Key History

Somatic Symptoms

Because somatic complaints are such common manifestations of depression in primary care practice, it is essential to inquire about depressive symptoms when patients present with somatic complaints such as insomnia, fatigue, or any of the other symptoms listed in Table 8-2. The history should include questions to discover causes for these symptoms other than depression. For example, before initiating treatment for depression for patients with insomnia, the clinician should inquire about other causes of poor sleep, such as cardiorespiratory problems, sleep-related movement disorders, and excess caffeine ingestion.

Because benzodiazepines can cause or aggravate depression, it is inappropriate to prescribe such medication for any cause of insomnia without first excluding depression as the cause of insomnia. When in doubt about whether the insomnia may be caused by depression, it is preferable to initiate a therapeutic trial of antidepressant medication rather than a benzodiazepine.

Depression Symptoms

Clinicians should ask about the full range of symptoms of a major depressive episode outlined in the DSM-IV. This inquiry may need to be direct and specific, especially because depressed patients with psychomotor retardation may provide few details of their history. Others may not volunteer their symptoms due to the stigmatization of the problem of depression. However, when clinicians ask about specific depressive symptoms, patients are typically relieved and reassured to know, both that their symptoms are expected or not unusual, and that their clinician is comfortable dealing with those symptoms.

One recent study demonstrated that two simple questions, directed at the key DSM-IV criteria for depression, are particularly useful: "During the past month, have you often been bothered by feeling down, depressed, or hopeless?" and "During the past month, have you often been bothered by little interest or pleasure in doing things?" A "yes" answer to either of these questions was 96-percent sensitive for detecting major depression.

In addition, it is useful to inquire about sad feelings, tearfulness, sleep disturbance, appetite and weight change, difficulty concentrating, fatigue, psychomotor retardation or agitation, guilty feelings or thoughts, and suicidal ideation. Patients should also be asked about alcohol and other drug use (including prescription, non-prescription, and illicit drugs) that might be causally or secondarily associated with depression.

Past History

Key past history includes previous episodes of depression or mania, prior treatment for depression, and prior suicide attempts. If the patient received a particular medication for depression in the past, successful treatment in the past predicts repeated success with the same medication. Patients should also be asked about past or current history of other chronic illnesses, and should be asked specifically about current symptoms suggesting underlying chronic illnesses that

commonly cause depression (e.g., hypothyroidism or cardiorespiratory disease).

Family History

Family history should focus on family members with depression, bipolar illness, alcoholism or drug abuse, and suicide. If family members have been treated for depression, it is helpful to learn what medication worked for them, since this may predict a higher likelihood of response by the patient to the same medication.

Suicidal Ideation

Suicidal ideation is one of the DSM-IV criteria for depression, and every patient with suspected depression should be asked about suicidal ideation. Questioning about suicide can be introduced indirectly, such as by asking patients if they ever think about death or giving up, or if they wish they were dead. It can be also done directly, by asking patients if they have thought of hurting themselves or ending their life.

It is important to understand that asking about suicidal ideation does not cause patients to consider suicide when they otherwise have not. On the contrary, direct inquiry can be effective in engaging the patient in a discussion about suicide, thereby decreasing the risk that it will occur.

Several findings raise the risk that the patient may attempt suicide and should lead the clinician to consider hospitalization or psychiatric consultation. First, certain demographic factors are associated with a higher risk of successful suicide, including older age, male gender, alcohol or drug abuse, and living alone. Age and gender are particularly important, as the suicide rate among white males over 85 is six times that in the general population.

Second, patients expressing suicidal thoughts should be asked about plans or ideas they have as to how the suicide would be accomplished. Those with more specific plans and the means to complete them (e.g., planning to shoot themselves and possessing a gun) are at higher risk.

Third, giving away possessions may be a clue that a patient is contemplating suicide. Patients may do this without stating the reason for giving things away or may simply comment that "I won't be needing these any more."

Finally, clinicians should be alert to the fact that patients are at high risk of completing suicide during the early recovery phase from depressive illness. It is during this time that patients may still feel the psychological pain of the depression but are beginning to recover from the indecision, fatigue, or psychomotor retardation of the most severe phase of the illness. Thus, they are more able to conceive of and follow through with specific plans for suicide and are motivated to do so if they continue to suffer emotionally from depression.

Bipolar Symptoms

Other symptoms of concern are those suggesting that depression is a part of bipolar, rather than unipolar, depression. Patients with a history of hypomanic or manic episodes, or with a "mixed" depressive-manic picture, should be evaluated carefully for bipolar illness. If bipolar patients are treated with antidepressants alone (i.e., without anti-manic agents such as lithium and or valproate), this can precipitate a hypomanic or manic episode.

Psychotic Symptoms

Another worrisome group of symptoms are those suggesting psychosis. The typical positive symptoms of psychosis are hallucinations, delusions, and paranoid ideation. Patients with psychotic depression should be hospitalized and considered candidates for early treatment with electroconvulsive therapy (ECT).

Cognitive Dysfunction

The final worrisome symptom complex is apparent memory disturbance or dementia. Especially in the elderly, depression can present with a primary symptom of forgetfulness. History may help distinguish this "pseudodementia" of depression from true dementia, in that patients with depression, when asked questions testing memory, may tend to reply "I don't know." Demented patients, on the other hand, are more likely to respond with incorrect answers. However, the distinction between dementia and depression may not be so clear in individual patients, and formal psychometric testing may be needed to clarify the situation.

Also, early in the course of dementing illness, many patients become depressed. For example, patients diagnosed with early Alzheimer's dementia may become depressed because they understand the prognosis of their condition. In other illnesses, such as Parkinson's disease, patients are at high risk for both depression and dementia. In any case, when there is doubt about relative contributions to the symptom complex from depression and dementia, a therapeutic trial of antidepressant treatment is often appropriate.

 Physical Examination

Depressed mood, decreased variability of affect, tearfulness, psychomotor retardation, or agitation may be the only physical examination findings of depression. Negative findings for specific organic illness also are consistent with the diagnosis of depression. However, the presence of other illnesses does not exclude the concomitant presence of depression, since depression frequently coexists with medical disorders.

Ancillary Tests

No specific ancillary tests are routinely indicated to support or refute the diagnosis of depression. The only laboratory abnormalities specifically linked with depression, such as abnormal EEGs and decreased suppression of cortisol following a dexamethasone challenge, are insufficiently sensitive and specific to use for diagnostic purposes.

Instead, ancillary tests are indicated to exclude concomitant medical illnesses in patients for whom history and/or physical examination suggest specific medical problems. Laboratory tests, such as hemograms, chemistry panels, and thyroid function tests, should be considered for (1) patients who have symptoms that rarely occur in straightforward depression, (2) geriatric patients, (3) patients who are experiencing their first episode of depression after age 40, and (4) patients whose depression does not respond fully to standard treatment.

Thyroid Function Tests

Women over age 50 have an approximately 10-percent prevalence of unrecognized hypothyroidism. This rate is the same for patients with and without depression. Because of the high prevalence of undetected hypothyroidism in this age group, some experts recommend screening all women over age 50 for the serum thyroid-stimulating hormone level, regardless of symptoms. The U.S. Preventive Services Task Force, however, found insufficient evidence to recommend for or against screening for thyroid disease among asymptomatic persons. The task force did recommend that clinicians be alert to subtle signs of hypothyroidism, including fatigue, concentration difficulties, and depressive symptoms. Thus, it is reasonable to consider and test for hypothyroidism as part of the evaluation of depression, particularly among older patients and those with fatigue, difficulty concentrating, or other symptoms of hypothyroidism.

Clinicians should be aware that thyroid testing in patients with fatigue alone does not yield a higher than expected rate of abnormal test results. However, thyroid function abnormalities are more likely if patients have symptoms of hypothyroidism in addition to fatigue, such as weight gain, difficulty concentrating, skin or hair changes, hoarseness, and so on. In patients with more than five symptoms of thyroid disease, there is as much as a 50-percent likelihood of having demonstrable hypothyroidism on blood testing. Thus, if such symptoms occur in patients with fatigue and depression, thyroid testing is warranted.

Clinicians should also keep in mind that, in addition to occurring in hypothyroidism, depressive symptoms can be a manifestation of *hyper*thyroidism. This typically occurs in older patients with hyperthyroidism, who sometimes manifest "apathetic" symptoms, such as fatigue and depression, instead of the classic stimulatory hyperthyroid symptoms. Thus, older patients with depression and symptoms suggesting apathetic hyperthyroidism should also have thyroid function measured.

Screening Instruments

It has been repeatedly demonstrated that primary care clinicians fail to recognize depression in about half of the patients who have this problem. This failure is probably due to an array of factors that make detection and diagnosis of depression in primary care difficult in comparison to diagnosis in offices of behavioral health specialists. These factors include the somatic presentation of patients with depression, the multiple medical problems the primary care clinician may be managing in addition to depression, and the limited time available for assessment of the patient in primary care practice. On the other hand, primary care clinicians have several advantages in diagnosing and managing depression. These advantages include the ability to incorporate depression into the differential diagnosis and evaluation of vague somatic complaints, continuity of relationships with patients and their families, and the ability to adapt depression treatment to interact favorably with any medical illnesses the patient may have.

Many have suggested that diagnosis of depression, and, therefore, benefit to patients from treatment of depression, may be increased by routine use of depression screening instruments. In clinical investigations, use of such instruments has increased the rate of recognition and treatment of depression. However, this increased detection and earlier treatment has not been shown to improve outcomes compared to beginning treatment after symptoms are recognized clinically. Therefore, the U.S. Preventive Services Task Force pointed out that the benefits to patients of such screening have not been clearly demonstrated, and it was concluded that evidence is insufficient to recommend either for or against such screening.

If used, screening test results indicating depression should alert clinicians to the need for more in-depth assessment. No screening test results should be considered diagnostic of depression without additional clinical evaluation of the patient, because some patients will test in the depressed range but not have depression.

Many screening instruments are available to clinicians choosing to use them, either to routinely screen for unsuspected depressive symptoms, to quantitate changes in depressive symptoms once the problem is diagnosed and under treatment, or to help distinguish dementia from depression. These instruments include the Beck Depression Inventory, the Zung Self-Rating Depression Scale, the Geriatric Depression Scale, the Hamilton Depression Scale, the Duke Anxiety-Depression Scale, the Primary Care Evaluation of Mental Disorders, and the Qualitative Evaluation of Dementia.

BECK AND ZUNG TESTS

The Beck and Zung instruments are probably the best known and most widely used. The Beck Depression Inventory is a brief, self-administered questionnaire that is convenient for patients to complete while waiting to see their clinician (Fig. 8-1). The Zung Self-Rating Depression Scale is also a self-administered instrument that has

Figure 8-1

The Beck Depression Inventory: Sample Questions.

DIRECTIONS: Some groups of statements are given below. Please read each group of statements carefully, then circle the number beside the one statement in each group which *best* describes the way you have been feeling in the *past week, including today.* If several statements in the group seem to apply equally well, circle each one. *Be sure to read all the statements in each group before making your choice.*

I do not feel sad 0
I feel sad 1
I am sad all the time and I can't snap out of it 2
I am so sad or unhappy that I can't stand it 3

I do not feel like a failure 0
I feel I have failed more than the average person 1
As I look back on my life, all I can see is a lot of failures 2
I feel I am a complete failure as a person 3

been used in many studies of depression. In contrast to the Beck inventory, which detects the presence of depression, the Zung scale also gives an estimate of the severity of depression. However, while the Zung test has been used in depression screening studies, it was not designed to detect depression in previously undiagnosed individuals.

GERIATRIC DEPRESSION SCALE

The Geriatric Depression Scale is also widely used. It was specifically developed for depression screening of elderly patients and is used in research and in practice. It is available in both a long (30-question) and short (15-question) form, and it can be self-administered or administered verbally by an interviewer. All responses are simple yes-or-no answers (Fig. 8-2).

HAMILTON AND DUKE SCALES

The Hamilton scale differs from the Beck test, the Zung test, and the Geriatric Depression Scale, in that it must be administered by a trained interviewer. It is therefore less practical for use in primary care practice than are self-administered tests. Other, newer scales have also been developed. For example, the Duke Anxiety-Depression Scale was developed as a screening instrument to detect patients with a high likelihood of having either one of these two syndromes. While it does not distinguish between them, its use is based on recognition that depression and anxiety frequently overlap in primary care.

QUALITATIVE EVALUATION OF DEMENTIA

The Qualitative Evaluation of Dementia is a 2-min checklist that distinguishes cognitive impairment with cortical features (e.g., Alzheimer's disease) from cognitive impairment with subcortical features, such as occur in depression. The instrument has 98-percent sensitivity and 88-per-

cent specificity for distinguishing Alzheimer's disease from subcortical cognitive impairment.

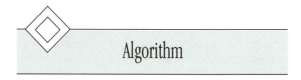

Algorithm

An algorithm for diagnosis and treatment of depression is presented in Fig. 8-3. While this algorithmic approach can be useful in dealing with depressed patients, readers should be aware that, in clinical practice, primary care clinicians actually use three major approaches to the diagnosis of depression.

One approach is to base the diagnosis on positive findings in the history. In this approach, depression becomes a positive, affirmative diagnosis, rather than a diagnosis of exclusion. This is the approach most often used by mental health professionals, and it is also widely used by primary care clinicians when there are clear symptoms of depressive illness.

The second approach is to evaluate physical complaints first, and then diagnose depression by exclusion. This approach is useful when various aspects of the history, physical examination, and indicated laboratory tests suggest somatic illness. However, this approach can disrupt the clinician-patient relationship if the clinician pursues an extended search for somatic illnesses and then tells a depressed patients at the end of a (negative) workup that he or she is well and that the problem is psychological or "all in your head." Such explanations are interpreted as rejection by patients and may lead to patients changing clinicians in a fruitless quest to find an obscure organic illness, thereby interfering with early effective treatment for depression.

A third approach is the "synergistic approach," in which both physical and mental health concerns are addressed simultaneously. This approach is most appropriate when doubt exists as to whether symptoms are related to

Figure 8-2

The Geriatric Depression Scale.

Choose the best answer for how you felt over the past week.

1.	Are you basically satisfied with your life?	Yes/No
2.	Have you dropped many of your activities and interests?	Yes/No
3.	Do you feel that your life is empty?	Yes/No
4.	Do you often get bored?	Yes/No
5.	Are you hopeful about the future?	Yes/No
6.	Are you bothered by thoughts you can't get out of your head?	Yes/No
7.	Are you in good spirits most of the time?	Yes/No
8.	Are you afraid that something bad is going to happen to you?	Yes/No
9.	Do you feel happy most of the time?	Yes/No
10.	Do you often feel helpless?	Yes/No
11.	Do you often get restless and fidgety?	Yes/No
12.	Do you prefer to stay at home, rather than going out and doing new things?	Yes/No
13.	Do you frequently worry about the future?	Yes/No
14.	Do you feel you have more problems with memory than most?	Yes/No
15.	Do you think it is wonderful to be alive now?	Yes/No
16.	Do you often feel downhearted and blue?	Yes/No
17.	Do you feel pretty worthless the way you are now?	Yes/No
18.	Do you worry a lot about the past?	Yes/No
19.	Do you find life very exciting?	Yes/No
20.	Is it hard for you to get started on new projects?	Yes/No
21.	Do you feel full of energy?	Yes/No
22.	Do you feel that your situation is hopeless?	Yes/No
23.	Do you think that most people are better off than you are?	Yes/No
24.	Do you frequently get upset over little things?	Yes/No
25.	Do you frequently feel like crying?	Yes/No
26.	Do you have trouble concentrating?	Yes/No
27.	Do you enjoy getting up in the morning?	Yes/No
28.	Do you prefer to avoid social gatherings?	Yes/No
29.	Is it easy for you to make decisions?	Yes/No
30.	Is your mind as clear as it used to be?	Yes/No

Critical responses:

Yes: Items 2, 3, 4, 6, 8, 10, 11, 12, 13, 14, 16, 17, 18, 20, 22, 23, 24, 25, 26, 28.

No: Items 1, 5, 7, 9, 15, 19, 21, 27, 29, 30.

Scoring: ≥11 critical responses raises a question of depression.

(Reprinted from J Yesavage, T. Brink, T. Rose, et al: Development and validation of a geriatric depression screening scale: A preliminary report. J Psychtr Res 17:37, 1983, with permission from Elsevier Science.)

Figure 8-3

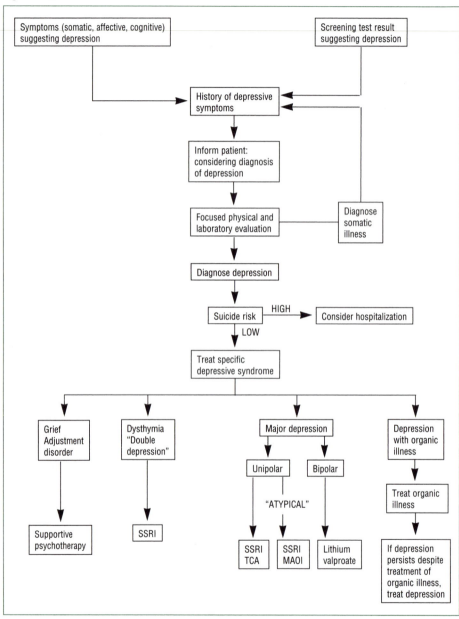

Algorithm showing the key steps in the diagnosis and management of depression in patients seen in outpatient primary care settings.

depression or physical illness. The patient is informed at an early occasion (preferably during the first visit at which depression is considered) that the symptoms may result from a medical illness but that depression is also a likely diagnosis. The patient should then be told that depression is a treatable disease and that the results of testing for other problems will be used to decide whether to treat another problem first or to treat depression first.

Treatment

Self-Treatments

SELF-DIRECTED EFFORT

Before seeking professional care, many patients try to deal with depression on their own. It is a common expectation of persons with sad feelings that they can and should "pull themselves out of it" and start behaving normally.

Patients with depression affect the lives of others in their home, work, or social environment. Family members, for example, are likely to have experienced the patient's irritability or social withdrawal for weeks or months before the patient comes to medical attention. They may not have recognized the patient's behavior as a sign of depression, however, and may have attempted unsuccessful interventions, such as telling the patient to "snap out of it" or responding angrily to the patient's inability to fulfill usual social or emotional roles. Family members may become frustrated or depressed themselves in response to the patient's depression.

Thus, the most common self-treatment is likely to be failed attempts by patients and those around them to overcome the symptoms of depression by acts of will. An important role of the clinician is to educate the patient and others

that patients are not able to overcome depression by effort alone.

SUBSTANCE ABUSE

The next most common self-treatment is use of drugs or alcohol. When this occurs, depression may be complicated by substance abuse. In general, the patient must stop using the substance (e.g., stop drinking alcohol) for a few weeks before the clinician can clarify whether the depression will clear following removal of the offending substance. If the depression persists after the substance abuse stops, then the patient's depression should be treated directly.

HERBAL REMEDIES

In recent years, there has been growing interest in using extracts of *Hypericum perforatum* (St. John's Wort), usually as a tea, for treatment of depression. In vitro studies have shown that *Hypericum* extract inhibits the uptake of several neurotransmitters, including serotonin, norepinephrine, and dopamine, and that it also inhibits the action of monoamine oxidase.

The extent to which this herb is used by the public to treat depression is unknown, but there is evidence that it may be effective. A recent meta-analysis of studies involving 1757 outpatients with mild or moderately severe depressive disorders found *Hypericum* extracts to be significantly superior to placebo and as effective as standard tricyclic antidepressants, but with a much lower side-effect rate than drug treatment. More research is needed, however, to clarify the role, dose, and ideal candidates for this treatment.

Conventional Treatments

The major treatment options for depression include antidepressant medication, psychotherapy, and ECT. Most patients treated in primary care settings are treated principally with antidepressant medication. Formal psychotherapy without medication is an effective option for patients with mild to moderate depression. More severely depressed patients should receive medication or ECT. Patients with severe depression for whom medication is contraindicated should also receive ECT, as should patients with psychotic depression.

A combination of psychotherapy and medication is especially appropriate for patients who respond only partially to an adequate trial of either therapy alone and for patients with a history of chronic depression (dysthymia) in addition to an acute depressive episode ("double depression").

Selection of antidepressant treatment for patients with coexisting medical illnesses can present a special challenge. Treatment should be adapted to patients' medical illnesses to avoid side effects that will aggravate the medical problem. Some patients with concomitant medical illness can most safely be treated with ECT, rather than medication.

Whatever initial treatment is chosen, it should be continued with sufficient duration to identify a response before the treatment is changed. Medication usually leads to partial remission by 4 to 6 weeks, psychotherapy by 6 to 8 weeks. Either may be expected to lead to nearly complete improvement by 10 to 12 weeks. Thus, an initial trial of 6 weeks' treatment is usually sufficient to identify whether the patient will respond. If partial improvement is identified, the treatment should be continued for another 6 weeks. If no improvement is evident after the initial 6 weeks or only partial improvement is seen by 12 weeks, then the treatment should be changed. Generally, if psychotherapy was the initial treatment, the second option is to begin medication. If medication was the initial treatment, the patient should either be switched to a different medication or the first medication should be augmented with a second.

ANTIDEPRESSANT MEDICATION

Medication is almost always effective for major depressive disorders, and primary care clinicians should consider it the first-line treatment for depression. The most commonly used medications are selective serotonin reuptake inhibitors (SSRIs) and tricyclic antidepressants (TCAs). Monoamine oxidase inhibitors (MAOIs) and a variety of newer antidepressant medications are also available, such as bupropion, venlafaxine, mirtazapine, and maprotiline. These other medications are rarely used as first-line therapy for treating depression in primary care practice. The various antidepressant medications, their therapeutic doses, and their side effects are shown in Table 8-3.

Patients should be seen every 1 to 2 weeks for the first 6 to 8 weeks of medication treatment and may be seen less frequently (every 4 to 12 weeks) once remission is achieved. If remission is achieved, full-dose treatment should be continued for 4 to 9 months after the patient is clinically well to avoid risk of relapse. After this time, antidepressants may be discontinued.

If depression recurs after discontinuing treatment, patients should be restarted on the same treatment to which they initially responded. Patients with three or more episodes of depression have a 90-percent rate of recurrence and should be considered for long-term antidepressant treatment at the dosage that led to remission. In fact, some experts are now advocating long-term, and even life-long, treatment for patients whose depression recurs after one course of treatment. Patients with dysthymia or with major depression plus a history of dysthymia may show only partial improvement with treatment and should be continued on the initial effective treatment for at least 2 to 3 years.

When discontinuing antidepressants, it is important to remember that these medications should be tapered to avoid withdrawal reactions and to monitor for relapse of depression. Both

Table 8-3
Antidepressant Medications

ANTIDEPRESSANTS	ADULT DOSAGE RANGE, MG/D*	CARDIAC SIDE EFFECTS	ORTHOSTATIC HYPOTENSION	SEDATION	WEIGHT GAIN
TRICYCLICS (TERTIARY)					
Amitriptyline	25–300	+++	++++	++++	+++
Clomipramine	25–250	+++	+++	++	++
Doxepin	25–300	++	++++	++++	+++
Imipramine	25–300	+++	+++	++	+++
Trimipramine	25–300	+++	+++	++++	+++
TRICYCLICS (SECONDARY)					
Amoxapine	50–600	++	++	++	+
Desipramine	25–300	++	++	+	
Nortriptyline	25–250	++	+	++	+
Protriptyline	15–60	+++	++	+	
MISCELLANEOUS					
Buproprion	100–450	0	0	0	0
Maprotiline	50–225	++	+++	+++	++
Mirtazapine	15–45	++	++	++	
Nefazodone	200–600	0/+	+++	+++	+
Trazodone	50–600	0/+	+++	+++	+
Venlafaxine	75–375	0/+	0	0	
SELECTIVE SEROTONIN REUPTAKE INHIBITORS					
Fluoxetine	20–80	0	0	0	0
Fluvoxamine	50–300	0	0/+	0/+	0
Paroxetine	20–50	0	+	+	0
Sertraline	50–200	0	0/+	0/+	0
MONOAMINE OXIDASE INHIBITORS					
Phenelzine	45–90	0	+	+	++
Tranylcypromine	30–60	0	0/+	0/+	+

NOTE: 0, none; +, low; ++, moderate; +++, moderate to high; ++++, high.

*Lower doses are recommended for adolescents and elderly patients. Sexual dysfunction may also occur with most antidepressants. Medications may be prescribed in single or divided doses, except bupropion, venlafaxine, phenelzine and tranylcypromine prescribed in divided doses, and mirtazapine, fluvoxamine, paroxetine, and sertraline in single dose.

SOURCE: From Bhatia and Bhatia, adapted with permission from the April 1997, vol 55 issue of *American Family Physician*, published by the American Academy of Family Physicians.

SSRIs and TCAs cause withdrawal reactions, but such reactions are more common with TCAs, occurring in up to 80 percent of patients. The most common withdrawal symptoms from TCAs are gastrointestinal distress, sleep disturbances, movement disorders, and activation of mania. Symptoms begin within 2 days after discontinuing medication and can last for as long as 2 weeks. Withdrawal reactions to SSRIs are less common (35 percent with paroxetine, 3 to 4 percent with sertraline, and less than 1 percent with fluoxetine). The most common SSRI-withdrawal symptoms are dizziness, parasthesias, anxiety, nausea, and sleep disturbances. Symptoms can last for 1 to 2 weeks and are more common following prolonged SSRI use.

SELECTIVE SEROTONIN REUPTAKE INHIBITORS The SSRIs are the newest class of antidepressants and have rapidly become the most frequently prescribed medications for depression. Most experts consider them the drugs of choice for treating major depression because of their ease of administration, low rate of side effects, and relative safety when taken in overdose. In addition, SSRIs lack significant anticholinergic effects, making them highly preferable for treating depression in older individuals. They also have few or no cardiac side effects.

The SSRIs are generally well tolerated by most patients. However, sexual dysfunction, notably difficulty reaching orgasm in women and delayed ejaculation in men, has been noted as a troublesome side effect of SSRIs for some patients.

The SSRIs are more expensive than the older antidepressant medications (i.e., TCAs and MAOIs). However, their cost is offset by the lower rate of side effects, which leads to a higher rate of continuing therapy and a resultant lower overall cost for medical and psychiatric care and hospitalizations, and a lower suicide rate. The SSRIs have therefore replaced the older antidepressants for first-line use in primary care.

TRICYCLIC ANTIDEPRESSANTS The TCAs are well-established, effective treatments for depression. Their cost is relatively low compared to that of SSRIs, but TCAs have higher side effect rates and, therefore, higher discontinuation rates due to side effects. If TCAs are used, clinicians should be cognizant of the fact that secondary amine forms (e.g., nortriptyline) generally have lower rates and lesser severity of side effects than do the tertiary amines (e.g., amitriptyline) from which they are derived. Nonetheless, side effects are still of concern with the secondary amine TCAs, especially for patients with ischemic heart disease, of whom 10 to 20 percent experience undesirable cardiac effects, such as increased heart rate.

The TCAs should generally be used at dosages in the mid-range of those shown in Table 8-3 for at least 6 weeks before a treatment failure is declared and the medication changed. However, to reduce the severity of side effects, patients are often started on lower doses and gradually increased to the target therapeutic dose (e.g., 150 mg/d of desipramine or 75 mg/day of nortriptyline) over the course of the first week or two of therapy. The timing of a 6-week clinical trial begins from the time that the full therapeutic dose is achieved. Because of their high toxicity and the risk of death when taken in overdose (e.g., when used for suicide attempts), TCAs should be prescribed in limited amounts, generally not over a total of 1000 mg per prescription, until the clinician is confident the patient is at low risk of suicide.

MONOAMINE OXIDASE INHIBITORS The MAOIs are not often prescribed by primary care clinicians because of the potentially fatal interaction with high-tyramine foods and the safety and efficacy of alternative medications. However, MAOIs are effective for patients with major depression with so-called "atypical" features (increased eating or sleep, weight gain, and anxiety).

COUNSELING AND PSYCHOTHERAPY

Formal psychotherapy is an effective alternative to medication for patients with mild to moderate depression who prefer this treatment option. However, it is more expensive, may be logistically more difficult, and is not effective as a long-term treatment to prevent remission. Few primary care clinicians have schedules or training that permit them to undertake prolonged psychotherapy for depression.

ELECTROCONVULSIVE THERAPY

Despite its negative public image and the stigmatization of patients who undergo it, ECT is an effective and safe treatment for depression. However, it is expensive, requires hospitalization, and leads to amnesia for events around the time of the ECT. It is therefore reserved for patients with severe or psychotic depression, those unresponsive after trials of several medications, and those for whom antidepressant medication is contraindicated.

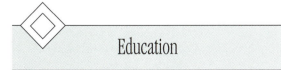

Education

The Nature of Depression

All depressed patients should receive appropriate basic education about the nature of their condition. Adherence to therapy and, therefore, likelihood of earlier improvement in symptoms of depression are increased with appropriate education. Education should include vocabulary at the patient's level of understanding; most patients and their families will understand the concept that an altered balance of chemicals in the brain causes depression.

Such education can relieve much of the guilt and anger felt by patients and by the friends and family members who are needed to help the patient recover. In addition, the patient and family members should be encouraged not to make major life decisions, such as changing jobs, moving, or divorcing, in the midst of a depressive episode. Depressed patients' judgment for such decision making can be adversely affected by the illness, and family members need to recognize that patients are "not themselves" during a major depressive episode.

It is essential to explain that depression may be something to which a patient is genetically predisposed, and it is not the result of moral or other failings. Furthermore, as discussed earlier, it should be explained that depression is not something the patient can resolve by an act of will.

Dealing with Depression until Treatment Is Effective

Feelings of hopelessness are common in depression. As a result, it is often difficult for patients to imagine that they can feel better with treatment. It is therefore often useful for the clinician specifically to acknowledge that the patient may not believe that any treatment will work. The clinician should point out that this belief may be a symptom of the illness itself and that the patient may need to rely on the clinician's experience and confidence from having seen other patients in similar circumstances improve dramatically. Patients sometimes report that, while they were unable to believe such a message at the time they were most depressed, they were able to understand it and rely on it as they waited for treatment to become effective.

Patients should be told about treatment options, expected time course of treatment, and possible side effects. Patients should be told that treatment for depression is usually very effective, but it may take several weeks to be so. It is especially important to inform patients of the need for an adequate trial of the initial treatment and to tell them that, if it does not lead to resolution of the depression, other treatment options are available that still have a high likelihood of success.

Patients may see acceptance of treatment as a personal failure. It is helpful, therefore, to label treatment as the patient's opportunity to "take control back" from the illness. Patients who adhere to antidepressant medication treatment are more likely to say their clinician told them five basic points: (1) take the medicine every day as prescribed; (2) expect beneficial effects of the medicine to be delayed up to 2 to 4 weeks; (3) do not stop taking the medicine without speaking first with the clinician; (4) if you are feeling better, keep taking the medicine; and (5) contact the clinician if you have questions.

Written and Internet Information

Written materials about depression, dysthymic disorder, and ECT are available for the education of patients. The Internet also has a wealth of sources of education. Many of the Internet sites offer self-help or support contacts for persons with depression. Some high-quality professionally-developed Internet sites are listed in Table 8-4. Written materials and Internet sites may be especially helpful for patients who have trouble concentrating on words from the clinician.

Family Approach

Family Involvement before Diagnosis

Families of depressed individuals are deeply involved in the problem of depression long before diagnosis. Most will have noticed that the affected family member has not been interacting

Table 8-4

Internet Sites for Educational Material for Patients About Depression

> http://www.mentalhealth.com/dis/
>   p20-md01.html
> http://www.psycom.net/depression.central.html
> http://www.cmhc.com/guide/depress.htm
> http://text.nlm.nih.gov/ahcpr/dep/www/
>   depptxt.html

with them normally, has altered or given up usual interests, and is exhibiting depressed or irritable affect. If the depressed family member is using alcohol or illicit drugs, the effect of this substance abuse on the patient's behavior further disrupts family relationships. Family members may have developed conflicts with the patient due to any of these effects or due to frustration surrounding misguided attempts to "talk the patient out of" his or her symptoms. Family members may also have gradually developed inappropriate roles (e.g., children filling a parenting role) due to the patient's withdrawal from normal activities and family responsibilities.

Family Reaction to Diagnosis and Treatment

Families commonly react with relief and renewed optimism when informed that their family member's altered behavior is the result of a treatable illness. In fact, families, friends, and coworkers may recognize improvement in the patient before the patient recognizes such improvement. Indeed, patients may be "the last to know" they are recovering from the depression. Reporting such observed improvement to the patient while acknowledging that recovery is not yet complete can be helpful to encourage continued adherence to treatment.

Errors

Underrecognition

The most common error in management of depression in primary care is underrecognition. As discussed earlier, multiple studies have shown that primary care clinicians recognize only about half of the depressed patients seen in the outpatient setting. This apparent problem may represent the fact that diagnostic categories of the DSM-IV are inadequate to describe the range of depressive problems seen in primary care practice, or that clinicians may have difficulties finding time to identify depression in busy practice settings. Clinical policies and guidelines on depression are based on research in relatively rarified settings of academic health centers, and they frequently translate poorly to the real world of clinical practice. Thus, while recognition of depression in primary care needs to be improved, a great deal more work is needed to provide adequate diagnostic support to primary care clinicians.

Undertreatment

There is evidence that, even when patients are recognized as being depressed, therapy is not always initiated. In fact, in up to a third of patients with identified major depression, primary care clinicians do not institute treatment.

When treatment is instituted, primary care clinicians often prescribe inadequate doses of antidepressant medications and/or prescribe them for an insufficient length of time. The TCAs should be used for 6 weeks at full antidepressant dosages before failure to respond is declared and the patient switched to another antidepressant medication. The SSRIs should be used at therapeutic doses for up to month. While it is often appropriate to start treatment at low doses to avoid side effects, especially in older patients, judgment about treatment effect should only be made after full therapeutic doses are reached and continued for an appropriate time interval. For some antidepressants (e.g., some TCAs), blood levels can be measured to ensure that a therapeutic dose has been achieved.

A related error is use of improper medications, such as benzodiazepines, to treat depression. As discussed earlier, sedative-hypnotic drugs are not appropriate as sole treatments for depression.

Controversies

Perhaps the major controversy surrounding treatment of depression in recent years has been the claim in the lay press that SSRIs increase suicide rates. This claim led to reluctance on the part of many patients, and their clinicians, to use antidepressant medication (particularly SSRIs). While suicide is a risk in depression, treatment of the depression does not increase the risk of suicide except in those patients unable to summon the energy or planning required for a suicide attempt until they begin to recover. In addition, there is no evidence that this occurs more frequently with SSRIs than with other classes of antidepressants.

A second important controversy, and one that will probably continue into the future, is the issue of what type of medical professional should treat depression. As discussed above, there are reports that primary care clinicians, as a group, tend to under-diagnose and under-treat depression. In addition, some providers who self-designate themselves as primary care clinicians (e.g., obstetrician-gynecologists) have received minimal training in the treatment of depression. This situation has led to recommendations by some that only mental health professionals, and not primary care physicians, should treat depression. Many managed-care organizations even "carve out" mental health care as a special service to be provided only by mental health professionals. However, this approach may not be effective because, as noted earlier, much of the underdiagnosis of depression probably results from factors such as the varying somatic and subsyndromal presentations of depression that occur in primary care practice.

Emerging Concepts

The major emerging concept in treatment of depression is prolonged treatment with medication. While standard practice, as described earlier in this chapter, involves discontinuing antidepressants after a specified period of time, some patients, especially those with recurrent depression, may benefit from taking antidepressant medication for a lifetime.

Another emerging concept is the growing number of conditions and syndromes for which SSRIs are effective treatments. The SSRIs, with their ease of administration and low side-effect profile, are being increasingly used with success for a range of depressive symptoms, including dysthymia and syndromes such as premenstrual dysphoric disorder. It is likely that accepted indications for SSRIs will continue to broaden.

Finally, depression in particular and mental illness in general remain stigmatized in American society. Such stigmatization can lead to inappropriate job or school discrimination, differential insurance coverage for psychological disorders, and an unwillingness by patients to seek treatment for these treatable conditions. Growing awareness by the public of the scope, prevalence, and treatability of depression and other mental health conditions may lead to more openness by patients in identifying, acknowledging, and seeking treatment for depression.

Bibliography

American Psychiatric Association: *Diagnostic and Statistical Manual of Mental Disorders*, 4th ed. Washington, American Psychiatric Association, 1994.

Banazak D: Electroconvulsive therapy: A guide for family clinicians. *Am Fam Phys* 53:273, 1996.

Beck A, Ward C, Mendelson M, et al: An inventory for measuring depression. *Arch Gen Psychiatry* 4:561, 1961.

Bhatia S, Bhatia S: Major depression: Selecting safe and effective treatment. *Am Fam Phys* 55:1683, 1997.

Burvill P: Recent progress in the epidemiology of major depression. *Epidemiol Rev* 17:21, 1995.

Carney PA, Rhodes LA, Eliassen S, et al: Variations in approaching the diagnosis of depression: A guided focus group study. *J Fam Pract* 46:73, 1998.

Clarkin J, Pilkonis P, Magruder K: Psychotherapy of depression: Implications for reform of the health care system. *Arch Gen Psychiatry* 53:717, 1996.

Depression Guideline Panel: *Depression in Primary Care: Detection and Diagnosis*, vols 1 and 2: Clinical Practice Guideline no 5, AHCPR publication nos 93-0550 and 93-0551. Rockville, MD, US Department of Health and Human Services, Public Health Service, Agency for Health Care Policy and Research 1993.

DeWester J: Recognizing and treating the patient with somatic manifestations of depression. *J Fam Pract* 43:S3, 1996.

Finger W, Lund M, Slagle M: Medications that may contribute to sexual disorders: A guide to assessment and treatment in family practice. *J Fam Pract* 44:33, 1997.

Gerber P, Barrett J, Barrett J, et al: The relationship of presenting physical complaints to depressive symptoms in primary care patients. *J Gen Intern Med* 7:170, 1992.

Hamilton M: A rating scale for depression. *J Neurol Neurosurg Psychiatry* 23:56, 1960.

Howland R: General health, health care utilization, and medical comorbidity in dysthymia. *Int J Psychiatry Med* 23:211, 1993.

Jonas B, Franks P, Ingram D: Are symptoms of anxiety and depression risk factors for hypertension? Longitudinal evidence from the National Health and Nutrition Examination Survey I epidemiologic follow-up study. *Arch Fam Med* 6:43, 1997.

Kessler R, McGonagle K, Zhao S, et al: Lifetime and 12-month prevalence of DSM-III-R psychiatric disorders in the United States: Results from the national comorbidity survey. *Arch Gen Psychiatry* 51:8, 1994.

Linde K, Ramirez G, Mulrow C, et al: St. John's Wort for depression: An overview and meta-analysis of randomised clinical trials. *BMJ* 313:253, 1996.

Mitchell J, Greenberg J, Finch I, et al: Effectiveness and economic impact of antidepressant medications: A review. *Am J Managed Care* 3:323, 1997.

Narrow W, Regier D, Rae D, et al: Use of services by persons with mental and addictive disorders: Findings from the National Institute of Mental Health epidemiological catchment area program. *Arch Gen Psychiatry* 50:95, 1993.

Neese R, Finlayson R: Management of depression in patients with coexisting medical illness. *Am Fam Phys* 53:2125, 1996.

Nutting P: Why can't clinical policies be relevant to practice? *J Fam Pract* 44:350, 1997.

Parkerson G, Broadhead W: Screening for anxiety and depression in primary care with the Duke Anxiety-Depression Scale. *Fam Med* 29:177, 1997.

Regier D, Narrow W, Rae D, et al: The de facto U.S. mental and addictive disorders system: Epidemiologic catchment area prospective 1-year prevalence rates of disorders and services. *Arch Gen Psychiatry* 50:85, 1993.

Roose SP, Laghrissi-Thode F, Kennedy JS, et al: Comparison of paroxetine and nortryptiline in depressed patients with ischemic heart disease. *JAMA* 279:287, 1998.

Rothschild A: The diagnosis and treatment of late-life depression. *J Clin Psychiatry* 57(suppl 5):5, 1996.

Ruoff G: Depression in the patient with chronic pain. *J Fam Pract* 43:S25, 1996.

Sansone R, Sansone L: Dysthymic disorder: The chronic depression. *Am Fam Phys* 53:2588, 1996.

Schmidt LA, Greenberg BD, Holzman GB, et al: Treatment of depression by obstetrician-gynecologists: A survey study. *Obstet Gynecol* 90:296, 1997.

Schulberg HC, Block MR, Madonia MJ, et al: The "usual care" of major depression in primary care practice. *Arch Fam Med* 6:334, 1997.

Whooley MA, Avins AL, Miranda J, et al: Case-finding instruments for depression. *J Gen Intern Med* 12:439, 1997.

Wolfe RM: Antidepressant withdrawal reactions. *Am Fam Phys* 56:455, 1997.

Yesavage J, Brink T, Rose T, et al: Development and validation of a geriatric depression screening scale: A preliminary report. *J Psychiatr Res* 17:37, 1983.

Zung W: A self-rating depression scale. *Arch Gen Psychiatry* 12:63, 1965.

David A. Katerndahl

Chapter

9

Anxiety

How Common Is Anxiety?

Although patients with anxiety disorders rarely present with complaints of "anxiety," the National Ambulatory Medical Care Survey found that anxiety ranked as the sixteenth most-common reason for office visits to physicians in the United States. In other studies, anxiety ranked fifteenth overall among reasons for visits to primary care providers and eighth in inner-city primary care settings. The lifetime prevalence of anxiety disorders in the general population is about 15 percent, and nearly half of individuals who seek medical care for anxiety do so only from a primary care clinician.

When one considers specific anxiety disorders, the prevalence in primary care settings is even more impressive. The prevalence of panic disorder and that of generalized anxiety disorder among patients in family practice settings are 13 and 14 percent, respectively, and although only 1 to 2 percent of primary care patients meet formal diagnostic criteria for obsessive-compulsive disorder, 10 percent have obsessive-compulsive characteristics. Mixed anxiety/depression accounts for an additional 2 percent of patients, although some research indicates that mixed anxiety/depression occurs in up to 8 percent of patients in primary care practice. Among geriatric-aged individuals, anxiety is particularly common, with studies reporting that 10 to 20 percent of older patients experience anxiety symptoms. Thus, anxiety is a common problem in primary care practice, and the various anxiety disorders are common syndromes seen by primary care clinicians.

Principal Diagnoses

Anxiety is a symptom, not a disease, and a number of diagnoses should be considered. The anxiety disorders commonly seen in primary care practice can be divided into several groups. The first group includes anxiety disorders with familial patterns that are mediated through the serotonergic, noradrenergic, or gamma-aminobutyric acid (GABA) systems. The second group includes anxiety syndromes that represent learned phenomena in response to a variety of social and environmental situations. The salient features of the familial and nonfamilial anxiety disorders are shown in Table 9-1.

In addition to the familial and nonfamilial anxiety disorders, anxiety also may be a manifestation of medical conditions (Table 9-2), or it may be associated with depression. The concomitant presence of medical conditions and/or depression must be considered in all patients being evaluated for anxiety. Although certain other anxiety conditions may be seen in primary care patients (e.g., several types of phobias), they rarely cause disability and rarely cause patients to seek help from clinicians. Therefore, they are not discussed in this chapter.

Familial Anxiety Disorders

The common familial anxiety disorders seen in primary care practice include (1) panic disorder, (2) generalized anxiety disorder, and (3) obsessive-compulsive disorder. Each condition is thought to involve abnormalities of one or more neurotransmitter systems. Despite being linked under the common diagnostic rubric of anxiety, however, each condition has quite different clinical manifestations.

Panic Disorder

Of the familial disorders, panic disorder has the most dramatic symptoms. Panic disorder is characterized by episodes of unexpected and intense fear or emotional discomfort. The fear is accompanied by anxiety symptoms that develop abruptly and reach a peak within a few minutes. Some of the most common symptoms are palpi-

Table 9-1

Key Characteristics of the Common Anxiety Disorders in Primary Care Practice

CHARACTERISTIC	ANXIETY DISORDER					
	PANIC DISORDER	GENERALIZED ANXIETY DISORDER	OBSESSIVE COMPULSIVE DISORDER	POSTTRAUMATIC STRESS DISORDER	SOCIAL PHOBIA	ADJUSTMENT DISORDER
Familial	Yes	Yes	Yes	No	No	No
Key symptom	Chest pain, palpitations, and/or dyspnea with rapid onset	Multiple somatic complaints or pain	Obsessions or compulsions, rash, depression	Anger, depression, reliving traumatic event	Fear of humiliation	Nonspecific somatic complaints
Timing of episodes	Sporadic, lasting minutes to hours	On most days for ≥ 6 months	≥ 1 h/d	Onset within 6 months of traumatic event	Related to social or performance situations	Usually lasts < 6 months after termination of stress
Prevalence in primary care practice, %	10–15	6–12	1–2	4–5	13	Uncertain

Table 9-2

Medical Conditions Associated with Anxiety

Cardiopulmonary disorders
  Mitral valve prolapse
  Cardiac arrhythmias
  Chronic obstructive pulmonary disease
  Hypoxemia
  Pulmonary embolus
  Pneumonia
Endocrine disorders
  Hyperthyroidism
  Hypoglycemia
  Menopause
  Pheochromocytoma
  Carcinoid syndrome
Neurologic disorders
  Temporal lobe epilepsy
  Cerebral tumor
  Parkinson's disease
  Vertigo
Sleep Disorders
  Narcolepsy
  Sleep apnea
Drug-related disorders
  Antidepressant or sedative-tranquilizer
    withdrawal
  Stimulant (e.g., caffeine, theophylline,
    cocaine, cannabis, phencyclidine)
  Metronidazole
  L-dopa
  Neuroleptic
  Organic solvent exposure
Miscellaneous
  Wilson's disease
  Acute intermittent porphyria
  Hyperventilation syndrome

tations, sweating, trembling, shortness of breath, a choking sensation, and chest pain. The diagnostic criteria for panic attacks and panic disorder, as specified by the American Psychiatric Association in the *Diagnostic and Statistical*

Manual of Mental Disorders, fourth edition (DSM-IV), are shown in Tables 9-3 and 9-4.

In some cases, panic attacks occur when the patient is exposed to crowds of people or is in crowded places, in which case the panic episodes are classified as "accompanied by agoraphobia,"—or fear of people or crowds (Table 9-4). In other cases, the panic episodes are unrelated to agoraphobia.

EPIDEMIOLOGY   The prevalence of panic disorder among patients in primary care settings may be as high as 13 percent. In addition, up to 9 percent of primary care patients report panic attacks that occur infrequently—too infrequently to

Table 9-3

Diagnostic Criteria for Panic Attack

A discrete period of intense fear or discomfort, in which four (or more) of the following symptoms developed abruptly and reached a peak within 10 min:

1. Palpitations, pounding heart, or accelerated heart rate
2. Sweating
3. Trembling or shaking
4. Sensations of shortness of breath or smothering
5. Feeling of choking
6. Chest pain or discomfort
7. Nausea or abdominal distress
8. Feeling dizzy, unsteady, lightheaded, or faint
9. Derealization (feelings of unreality) or depersonalization (being detached)
10. Fear of losing control or going crazy
11. Fear of dying
12. Paresthesias (numbness or tingling sensations)
13. Chills or hot flashes

SOURCE: Reproduced with permission from *Diagnostic and Statistical Manual of Mental Disorders*, 4th ed. Washington, American Psychiatric Association, 1994.

Table 9-4

Diagnostic Criteria for Panic Disorder with Agoraphobia

A. Both 1 and 2:
1. Recurrent unexpected panic attacks (see Table 9-3)
2. At least one of the attacks has been followed by 1 month (or more) of one (or more) of the following:
   a. Persistent concern about having additional attacks
   b. Worry about the implications of the attack or its consequences (e.g., losing control, having a heart attack, "going crazy")
   c. A significant change in behavior related to the attacks
B. The presence of agoraphobia
C. The panic attacks are not due to the direct physiological effects of a substance (e.g., a drug of abuse, a medication) or a general medical condition (e.g., hyperthyroidism).
D. The panic attacks are not better accounted for by another mental disorder, such as social phobia (e.g., occurring on exposure to feared social situations), specific phobia (e.g., on exposure to a specific phobic situation), obsessive-compulsive disorder (e.g., on exposure to dirt in someone with an obsession about contamination), posttraumatic stress disorder (e.g., in response to stimuli associated with a severe stressor), or separation anxiety disorder (e.g., in response to being away from home or close relatives).

SOURCE: Reproduced with permission from *Diagnostic and Statistical Manual of Mental Disorders*, 4th ed. Washington, American Psychiatric Association, 1994.

meet DSM-IV criteria for panic disorder. Such individuals are said to have "sub-syndromal" panic.

Panic disorder usually begins in young adulthood and is more common in women. It is often associated with periods of emotional stress and has been linked to a history of childhood sexual abuse.

Panic disorder is familial; first-degree relatives of patients with panic disorder are more than twice as likely as the general population to develop panic disorder. However, it is not clear whether the familial tendency is genetic, due to behavior learned within families, or both. There is no consistent ethnic predisposition to developing panic disorder.

PATHOPHYSIOLOGY Current research indicates that panic disorder involves multiple neurotransmitters, including serotonin, norepinephrine, and GABA. The specific neurobiologic defect

that leads to panic disorder is not fully understood, but the locus ceruleus is believed to play a key role, and it has afferent and efferent connections involving a variety of neurotransmitters. The diversity of neurotransmitters implicated in panic disorder may explain why selective serotonin re-uptake inhibitors (SSRIs), monoamine oxidase inhibitors (MAOIs), tricyclic antidepressants, and benzodiazepines all have a beneficial effect in treating panic disorder.

GENERALIZED ANXIETY DISORDER

Generalized anxiety disorder is characterized by excessive worry out of proportion to any problems that really exist. According to diagnostic criteria of the DSM-IV, the state of worry usually occupies more than half of the individual's time, and it goes on for at least 6 months. The worry is difficult to control, interferes with social or occupational function, and is associated with symptoms such as restlessness, fatigue, irritability, difficulty concentrating, or muscle tension. The full DSM-IV definition of generalized anxiety disorder is shown in Table 9-5.

EPIDEMIOLOGY From 6 to 12 percent of primary care patients have generalized anxiety disorder, and the condition is more common in women. Symptoms often have their onset during adolescence, but they may begin at any age. Generalized anxiety disorder is more common in family members of affected individuals. Although there appears to be no ethnic predisposition to generalized anxiety disorder, familial cultural factors may affect the clinical presentation.

PATHOPHYSIOLOGY Generalized anxiety disorder may be mediated through the GABA system. Gamma-aminobutyric acid acts centrally to produce general inhibition of other neurotransmitters. In generalized anxiety disorder, it is believed that a defect in GABA activity interferes with its normal inhibitory function. This mechanism could explain why benzodiazepines, which act by augmenting GABA activity, are effective treatments for generalized anxiety disorder.

OBSESSIVE-COMPULSIVE DISORDER

Obsessive-compulsive disorder is characterized by the presence of unwanted recurring

Table 9-5

Diagnostic Criteria for Generalized Anxiety Disorder

A. Excessive anxiety and worry (apprehensive expectation), occurring more days than not for at least 6 months, about a number of events
B. The person finds it difficult to control the worry.
C. The anxiety and worry are associated with three (or more) of the following six symptoms (with at least some symptoms present for more days than not for the past 6 months). Only one item is required in children.
1. Restlessness or feeling keyed up or on edge
2. Being easily fatigued
3. Difficulty concentrating or mind going blank
4. Irritability
5. Muscle tension
6. Sleep disturbance (difficulty falling or staying asleep, or restless, unsatisfying sleep)
D. The focus of the anxiety and worry is not about symptoms of another psychiatric disorder, e.g., having a panic attack (as in panic disorder), being embarrassed in public (as in social phobia), being contaminated (as in obsessive-compulsive disorder), being away from home or close relatives (as in separation anxiety disorder), gaining weight (as in anorexia nervosa), having multiple physical complaints (as in somatization disorder), or having a serious illness (as in hypochondriasis), and the anxiety and worry do not occur exclusively during posttraumatic stress disorder.
E. The anxiety, worry, or physical symptoms cause clinically significant distress or impairment in social, occupational, or other important areas of functioning.
F. The disturbance is not due to the direct physiological effects of a substance (e.g., a drug of abuse, a medication) or a general medical condition (e.g., hyperthyroidism) and does not occur exclusively during a mood disorder, a psychotic disorder, or a pervasive developmental disorder.

SOURCE: Reproduced with permission from *Diagnostic and Statistical Manual of Mental Disorders*, 4th ed. Washington, American Psychiatric Association, 1994.

thoughts (obsessions) and/or ritualized behaviors (compulsions; Table 9-6). Some of the most common behaviors include repetitive hand washing, praying, counting, or feeling the need to check on things multiple times. These behaviors can be so severe that they interfere with normal social function or employment. On the other hand, some patients are successful at incorporating their abnormal behaviors into their daily routines and remain quite functional.

EPIDEMIOLOGY Obsessive-compulsive disorder is present in 1 to 2 percent of primary care patients. The onset is usually during adolescence, al-

Table 9-6

Diagnostic Criteria for Obsessive-Compulsive Disorder

A. Either obsessions or compulsions
   Obsessions as defined by 1, 2, 3, and 4:
   1. Recurrent and persistent thoughts, impulses, or images that are experienced, at some time during the disturbance, as intrusive and inappropriate and that cause marked anxiety or distress
   2. The thoughts, impulses, or images are not simply excessive worries about real-life problems.
   3. Patients attempt to ignore or suppress such thoughts, impulses, or images, or to neutralize them with some other thought or action.
   4. Patients recognize that the obsessional thoughts, impulses, or images are a product of their own mind (not imposed from without as in thought insertion).
   Compulsions as defined by 1 and 2:
   1. Repetitive behaviors (e.g., hand washing, ordering, checking) or mental acts (e.g., praying, counting, repeating words silently) that the person feels driven to perform in response to an obsession, or according to rules that must be applied rigidly
   2. The behaviors or mental acts are aimed at preventing or reducing distress or preventing some dreaded event or situation; however, these behaviors or mental acts either are not connected in a realistic way with what they are designed to neutralize or prevent or are clearly excessive.

B. At some point during the course of the disorder, the person has recognized that the obsessions or compulsions are excessive or unreasonable. If, for most of the time during the current episode, the person does not recognize that obsessions and compulsions are excessive or unreasonable, the patient is characterized as having obsessive-compulsive disorder with "poor insight." Criteria pertaining to recognition that obsessions and compulsions are unreasonable do not apply to children.

C. The obsessions or compulsions cause marked distress, are time consuming (take more than 1 h/d), or significantly interfere with the person's normal routine, occupational (or academic) functioning, or usual social activities or relationships.

D. If another psychiatric disorder is present, the content of the obsessions or compulsions is not restricted to it (e.g., preoccupation with food in the presence of an eating disorder; hair pulling in the presence of trichotillomania; concern with appearance in the presence of body dysmorphic disorder; preoccupation with drugs in the presence of a substance use disorder; preoccupation with having a serious illness in the presence of hypochondriasis; preoccupation with sexual urges or fantasies in the presence of a paraphilia; or guilty ruminations in the presence of major depressive disorder).

E. The disturbance is not due to the direct physiological effects of a substance (e.g., drug abuse or a prescription medication) or a general medical condition.

SOURCE: Reproduced with permission from *Diagnostic and Statistical Manual of Mental Disorders*, 4th ed. Washington, American Psychiatric Association, 1994.

though in some cases the condition does not begin until individuals reach their twenties or thirties. Sometimes, symptoms suggesting obsessive-compulsive disorder are present in childhood but are not recognized as such until later in life. The condition is more common in men and is familial, but there is no evidence of a genetic predisposition. It may be, therefore, that cultural factors or familial behaviors lead to all or some of the manifestations of obsessive-compulsive disorder.

PATHOPHYSIOLOGY Obsessive-compulsive disorder may be mediated through the serotonergic system. This conclusion is based on the response to treatment with SSRIs. It is likely that the underlying cause of obsessive-compulsive disorder is decreased activity of central serotonergic neurons. This results in an enhanced sensitivity of serotonin receptors, which is used to therapeutic advantage when SSRIs are prescribed.

NONFAMILIAL (LEARNED OR SITUATIONAL BEHAVIOR) ANXIETY DISORDERS

Anxiety disorders can also develop without a familial tendency as learned behaviors in response to various situational or psychological stressors. The most common learned anxiety disorders seen in primary care are posttraumatic stress disorder, social phobias, and adjustment disorders.

POSTTRAUMATIC STRESS DISORDER

Posttraumatic stress disorder is the most extreme example of a "learned" anxiety behavior. Posttraumatic stress disorder typically follows exposure to an emotionally traumatizing event, such as witnessing or being a victim of a wartime experience, motor vehicle crash, physical violence, or a similar event. However, the emotional stressor may also be a less severe and less physically threatening event, such as observing someone else being robbed.

Typically, symptoms appear within 6 months of the event but may occasionally develop later. Symptoms are typically characterized by recurrent dreams and/or recurrent, intrusive, distressing recollections of the event. In children, these recollections may be associated with nightmares or may be manifested by play in which themes of the event are expressed. The symptoms are associated with an increased state of arousal (e.g., hypervigilance, irritability, or insomnia) and avoidance of stimuli associated with the event. The DSM-IV criteria for posttraumatic stress disorder are shown in Table 9-7.

EPIDEMIOLOGY Posttraumatic stress disorder is present in 4 to 5 percent of primary care patients in the United States. It occurs with equal frequency in men and women, and can develop at any age. Family history and social support may influence the development of posttraumatic stress disorder, although the disorder is not familial per se. Persons living in areas of extreme social unrest or civil conflict (e.g., war or urban violence) are at particularly high risk of developing posttraumatic stress disorder

SOCIAL PHOBIA

Social phobia involves fear and anxiety provoked by certain social situations. The full DSM-IV definition of social phobia is displayed in Table 9-8.

The main symptom of social phobia is a marked and persistent fear of one or more social or performance situations in which the person is exposed to unfamiliar people or to possible scrutiny by others. Although individuals with social phobias recognize that their fear is excessive or unreasonable, they nonetheless worry that they will act in a way that will be humiliating or embarrassing. Ultimately, the fear interferes with the person's normal occupational or academic functioning, or with their social activities or relationships.

Table 9-7

Diagnostic Criteria for Posttraumatic Stress Disorder

A. The person was exposed to a traumatic event in which both of the following were present:
1. The person experienced, witnessed, or was confronted with an event or events that involved actual or threatened death or serious injury, or a threat to the physical integrity of self or others.
2. The person's response involved intense fear, helplessness, or horror. In children, this may be expressed instead by disorganized or agitated behavior.

B. The traumatic event is persistently reexperienced in one (or more) of the following ways:
1. Recurrent and intrusive distressing recollections of the event, including images, thoughts, or perceptions. In young children, repetitive play may occur in which themes or aspects of the trauma are expressed.
2. Recurrent distressing dreams of the event. In children, there may be frightening dreams without recognizable content.
3. Acting or feeling as if the traumatic event were recurring (includes a sense of reliving the experience, illusions, hallucinations, and dissociative flashback episodes, including those that occur on awakening or when intoxicated). Note: In young children, trauma-specific reenactment may occur.
4. Intense psychological distress at exposure to internal or external cues that symbolize or resemble an aspect of the traumatic event
5. Physiological reactivity on exposure to internal or external cues that symbolize or resemble an aspect of the traumatic event

C. Persistent avoidance of stimuli associated with the trauma, and numbing of general responsiveness (not present before the trauma), as indicated by three (or more) of:
1. Efforts to avoid thoughts, feelings, or conversations associated with the trauma
2. Efforts to avoid activities, places, or people that arouse recollections of the trauma
3. Inability to recall an important aspect of the trauma
4. Markedly diminished interest or participation in significant activities
5. Feeling of detachment or estrangement from others
6. Restricted range of affect (e.g., unable to have loving feelings)
7. Sense of foreshortened future (e.g., does not expect to have a career, marriage, children, or a normal life span)

D. Persistent symptoms of increased arousal (not present before the trauma), as indicated by two (or more) of the following:
1. Difficulty falling or staying asleep
2. Irritability or outbursts of anger
3. Difficulty concentrating
4. Hypervigilance
5. Exaggerated startle response

E. Duration of the disturbance (symptoms in criteria B, C, and D) is more than 1 month.

F. Causes clinically significant distress or impairment in social, occupational, or other function

SOURCE: Reproduced with permission from *Diagnostic and Statistical Manual of Mental Disorders*, 4th ed. Washington, American Psychiatric Association, 1994.

Table 9-8

Diagnostic Criteria for Social Phobia

A. A marked and persistent fear of one or more social or performance situations in which the person is exposed to unfamiliar people or to possible scrutiny by others. The individual fears that he or she will act in a way (or show anxiety symptoms) that will be humiliating or embarrassing. In children, there must be evidence of the capacity for age-appropriate social relationships with familiar people, and the anxiety must occur in peer settings, not just in interactions with adults.

B. Exposure to the feared social situation almost invariably provokes anxiety, which may take the form of a situationally bound or situationally predisposed panic attack. In children, the anxiety may be expressed by crying, tantrums, freezing, or shrinking from social situations with unfamiliar people.

C. The person recognizes that the fear is excessive or unreasonable. In children, this feature may be absent.

D. The feared social or performance situations are avoided or else are endured with intense anxiety or distress.

E. The avoidance, anxious anticipation, or distress in the feared social or performance situation(s) interferes significantly with the person's normal routine occupational (academic) functioning, or social activities or relationships. Or there is marked distress about having the phobia.

F. In individuals under age 18 years, the duration is at least 6 months. For adults, duration of symptoms is not a defining diagnostic criterion.

G. The fear or avoidance is not due to the direct physiological effects of a substance (e.g., a drug of abuse, a medication) or a general medical condition, and is not better accounted for by another mental disorder.

H. If a general medical condition or another mental disorder is present, the fear in criterion A is unrelated to it. For example, the fear is not of trembling in Parkinson's disease, or of exhibiting abnormal eating behavior in anorexia nervosa.

SOURCE: Reproduced with permission from *Diagnostic and Statistical Manual of Mental Disorders*, 4th ed. Washington, American Psychiatric Association, 1994.

One familiar manifestation of social phobia is severe performance anxiety (i.e., "stage fright"), such as occurs in the context of making public speeches or giving musical performances. Other, more extreme manifestations of social phobia include fear of eating or writing in public.

Social phobia is different from agoraphobia. Fears in social phobia are restricted to situations in which patients are under scrutiny (or in view) of others, and they have concern about embarrassment or humiliation. By contrast, in agoraphobia the fears are more generalized, unrelated to fears of humiliation, and not always associated with specific events. While patients with agoraphobia typically have an irrational fear of being in public places or in crowds, symptoms may occur even when others are not present.

EPIDEMIOLOGY Because norms of behavior vary among cultural groups, it is sometimes difficult to characterize the prevalence of phobic social behavior in different populations. Current estimates are that social phobias are present in about 13 percent of primary care patients. Social phobias occur in both men and women. They usually begin during adolescence, but may persist into adulthood.

ADJUSTMENT DISORDER

Adjustment disorders, which are often associated with anxiety, are defined as emotional or behavioral symptoms that develop in response to situational stress. In contrast to posttraumatic stress disorder, the stressor in adjustment disorders is not a discrete or violent traumatic event. To qualify as symptoms of an adjustment disorder, the symptoms must cause either (1) marked distress out of proportion to what would be expected from exposure to the stressor or (2) significant impairment of social, occupational, or academic functioning.

Adjustment disorders may be associated with anxiety, in which case the patient experiences a short-lived anxious reaction to a particular stressor. Once the stressor (or its consequences) has terminated, the symptoms do not persist. The DSM-IV definition of adjustment disorder associated with anxiety is shown on Table 9-9.

EPIDEMIOLOGY Adjustment disorders can develop at any age and are seen equally in males and females. Although there is probably no ethnic difference in the prevalence of adjustment disorders, cultural factors can affect the behavioral manifestations, and therefore the measured prevalence of the condition varies among cultural groups.

Anxiety Associated with Medical Problems

Although most patients with anxiety have one of the disorders mentioned above, anxiety can also be caused by nonpsychiatric disorders, and these conditions should be considered in any patient presenting with symptoms of anxiety (Table 9-2). The prevalence with which medical illnesses cause anxiety is unknown, but this situation probably occurs more frequently in elderly individuals. Failure to recognize some of these

Table 9-9

Diagnostic Criteria for Adjustment Disorders

A. The development of emotional or behavioral symptoms in response to an identifiable stressor(s)
B. These symptoms or behaviors are clinically significant, as evidenced by either of the following:
    1. Marked distress that is in excess of what would be expected from exposure to the stressor
    2. Significant impairment in social or occupational (academic) functioning
C. The stress-related disturbance does not meet the criteria for another specific psychiatric disorder and is not merely an exacerbation of a preexisting psychiatric disorder.
D. The symptoms do not represent bereavement.
E. Once the stressor (or its consequences) has terminated, symptoms do not persist for more than an additional 6 months. Specify if:
    Acute: if the disturbance lasts less than 6 months
    Chronic: if the disturbance lasts for 6 months or longer
F. Adjustment disorders are coded based on the subtype, which is selected according to the predominant symptoms:
    With depressed mood
    With anxiety
    With mixed anxiety and depressed mood
    With disturbance of conduct
    With mixed disturbance of emotions and conduct

SOURCE: Reproduced with permission from *Diagnostic and Statistical Manual of Mental Disorders*, 4th ed. Washington, American Psychiatric Association, 1994.

conditions, especially the more serious cardiopulmonary conditions, may have immediate and fatal consequences.

The most common acute life-threatening cardiopulmonary conditions that cause anxiety are myocardial infarction, pulmonary embolism, and pulmonary edema. Cardiac arrhythmias that result in hemodynamic instability can also cause patients to feel anxious. These arrhythmias include supraventricular tachycardia, ventricular tachycardia, heart block with bradycardia, and atrial fibrillation or flutter with a rapid ventricular rate. Other life-threatening causes of anxiety include severe hyperthyroidism (i.e., thyroid storm), stimulant-drug overdoses, withdrawal from sedative-hypnotic drugs, and the other conditions listed in Table 9-2.

Anxiety Associated with Depression

It is important to remember that anxiety can be a symptom of major depression, and depressive symptoms can also occur in anxiety disorders. The association of depression and anxiety makes it essential that clinicians seek and deal with symptoms of depression, including suicidal ideation, in patients who present with anxiety symptoms.

Typical Presentation

Patients with the common anxiety disorders described above most often present to primary care clinicians rather than to mental health professionals. However, such patients usually do not complain of anxiety. Instead, patients with anxiety disorders usually present with vague somatic complaints.

These complaints may be multiple and nonspecific, such as chronic pain or headaches.

However, patients with anxiety may also complain of symptoms that are specifically related to an anxiety disorder. A typical example is chest pain that occurs during panic attacks; panic disorder is present in up to half of patients with unexplained chest pain in primary care practices. Panic disorder is also common in patients who complain of palpitations or syncope, and individuals with panic disorder have higher overall rates of health care utilization than the general population.

The typical presentation of anxiety disorders in specialty practices also involves somatic complaints, but the complaints are usually specific to the clinician's area of specialization. Thus, when patients with generalized anxiety disorder or panic disorder seek help from cardiologists and pulmonologists, it is usually for symptoms like chest pain, palpitations, or dyspnea, often in the setting of emergency care or when repetitive symptoms have eluded diagnosis by primary care clinicians. When otolaryngologists see patients with anxiety disorders, it is often for dizziness. Dermatologists see patients who have chronic dermatitis from repetitive hand washing or alopecia due to trichotillomania, both on the basis of obsessive-compulsive disorder. Patients with obsessive-compulsive disorder may also seek care from plastic surgeons because of an obsession with their appearance and a desire to change it.

Occasionally, individuals with anxiety disorders recognize the psychiatric nature of their symptoms and seek care from mental health specialists. However, these patients often present with complaints related to a concomitant psychiatric condition. For example, patients with obsessive-compulsive disorder may present with symptoms that seem typical of depression but that are really secondary symptoms of their obsessive-compulsive disorder. Similarly, patients with post-traumatic stress disorder may seek help from mental health professionals because of insomnia, depression, substance abuse, and/or uncontrollable anger.

Key History

The diagnosis of anxiety disorders is based solely on the history, using DSM-IV criteria to define and categorize the various anxiety disorders. Thus, clinicians should focus the history on identifying pertinent DSM-IV diagnostic symptoms, rather than asking general or open-ended questions about stress and psychosocial problems. The only exception is the need to ask about stress and psychosocial problems when diagnoses of posttraumatic stress disorder or adjustment disorder are being considered, since stressors are part of the DSM-IV criteria for these conditions.

Symptoms Suggesting Specific Anxiety Disorders

In primary care settings, unexplained somatic symptoms should always suggest the possibility of an anxiety disorder. In addition, certain particular symptoms should suggest the presence of one or more specific anxiety disorders.

PANIC DISORDER

The somatic symptoms most suggestive of panic disorder are chest pain, palpitations, dizziness, or dyspnea, especially if the intensity of symptoms peaks rapidly or is associated with feeling a need to escape. In addition, during a panic attack many patients believe they are having a heart attack, a stroke, or are going crazy.

GENERALIZED ANXIETY DISORDER

In primary care practice, the typical symptoms of generalized anxiety disorder are multiple unexplained somatic complaints, often including unexplained pain. However, in contrast to the rapid escalation of symptom intensity with panic disorder, symptoms in generalized anxiety disorder generally peak over a period of hours or days, and may last days or weeks. Persistent irrational worry also suggests generalized anxiety disorder.

OBSESSIVE-COMPULSIVE DISORDER

Any recurring unpleasant thoughts or repetitive rituals should suggest obsessive-compulsive disorder. However, patients with obsessive-compulsive disorder rarely complain of obsessions or compulsions. Rather, they more often complain of a chronic rash, symptoms related to comorbid anxiety, or depression.

POSTTRAUMATIC STRESS DISORDER

Uncontrollable anger is a key symptom of post-traumatic stress disorder and should always suggest this diagnosis. Patients with post-traumatic stress disorder may complain of depression or of depression-related symptoms such as weight change, fatigue, or late-night awakenings.

SOCIAL PHOBIA

Symptoms that only occur in social situations suggest social phobia, especially if the patient is the center of attention. Sometimes, patients with social phobia may give a straightforward history of performance anxiety.

ADJUSTMENT DISORDER

There are few symptoms that specifically suggest an adjustment disorder. Individuals with adjustment disorder-related anxiety frequently have multiple somatic symptoms, but few will identify a stressful problem associated with their symptoms.

Symptoms Suggesting Medical Conditions

Anxiety caused by psychiatric conditions and that caused by medical conditions can have identical symptoms. For example, substernal chest pressure that is worse with exercise and associated with hypertension suggests coronary artery disease to most clinicians. However, the same symptoms can occur with panic attacks, and it is often impossible to distinguish panic attacks from coronary artery disease based on history. Thus, although anxiety disorders are highly prevalent in primary care settings, when patients have anxiety symptoms that also suggest a medical condition, testing for the medical condition should be pursued.

In particular, symptoms of angina or other acute cardiopulmonary conditions should always lead to an appropriate medical evaluation, particularly (but not only) in patients with risk profiles for such conditions. Symptoms of palpitations generally require evaluation by electrocardiogram or ambulatory cardiac monitoring, and persistent autonomic symptoms, such as diaphoresis and palpitations, require thyroid function tests to exclude hyperthyroidism. Discrete episodes of anxiety-like symptoms accompanied by hypertension, severe headaches, and/or epistaxis should lead to testing for pheochromocytoma. Hallucinations should suggest drug overdose or a psychotic disorder.

Physical Examination

As noted above, the diagnosis of and distinction among anxiety disorders is based solely on the history. No physical finding is specific for any anxiety disorder. Instead, the physical examination should be directed at identifying medical conditions that mimic anxiety disorders. The most important clues to the possibility of a life-threatening condition are abnormal vital signs. In particular, while mild sinus tachycardia and blood pressure elevation may occur in anxiety

disorders (especially panic attacks), an irregular pulse, a heart rate over 160 beats/min, or tachypnea should always suggest the presence of a serous cardiopulmonary or endocrinologic disorder.

Other physical examination findings indicate that a patient's anxiety symptoms might be due to drug use. Such findings include needle injection marks, irritation of the nasal mucosa (from intranasal cocaine), pupillary constriction (from opiates), and erratic behavior. Finally, many of the conditions listed in Table 9-2 have specific physical examination findings. If the history or other clinical circumstances suggest that one of these conditions is present, the physical examination findings associated with the condition should be sought.

Ancillary Tests

Laboratory Tests for Anxiety Disorders

There is no laboratory test for anxiety disorders. Certain tests can induce symptoms of anxiety in research settings, but these tests are not sufficiently sensitive or specific to be used for clinical diagnosis. For example, administration of intravenous sodium lactate (the "lactate infusion test") can provoke a panic attack in patients with panic disorder but will do so only 70 percent of the time. Similarly, results of the dexamethasone suppression test are abnormal for some patients with panic disorder but may be abnormal with other conditions as well.

Questionnaire Tests for Anxiety Disorders

Screening tests have been developed to detect anxiety disorders in primary care settings. Two of the most widely used tests are (1) the Symptom Driven Diagnostic System, which screens for panic disorder, generalized anxiety disorder, and obsessive compulsive disorder; and (2) the Primary Care Evaluation of Mental Disorders (Prime-MD), which screens for panic disorder and generalized anxiety disorder. Although these tests have good specificity for the diagnosis of anxiety disorders, their sensitivities are generally poor, thereby precluding their use as screening tools. The only exception is the Symptom Driven Diagnostic System, which has a sensitivity of 85 to 90 percent for generalized anxiety disorder and therefore can be used effectively to screen for this condition.

Laboratory Tests for Medical Problems

No routine screening laboratory tests are recommended for patients with suspected anxiety disorders unless the history or physical examination suggests the possibility of a medical problem. The tests that are most often useful are thyroid function tests if hyperthyroidism is suspected, pulse oximetric studies in patients with dyspnea or tachypnea, and cardiac monitoring if palpitations are present. In addition, patients presenting with acute chest pain and cardiac risk factors require testing to exclude myocardial infarction or unstable angina, as outlined in Chap. 14.

Echocardiograms are often obtained if auscultatory findings suggest mitral valve prolapse, since the results may be useful if they reveal associated mitral regurgitation that requires endocarditis prophylaxis. However, even though mitral valve prolapse is more common in patients with anxiety, the presence of prolapse does not alter the prognosis of the anxiety disorder or the patient's response to therapy for it.

Urinary drug screening is indicated if substance abuse is suspected as the cause of anxiety symptoms. A variety of other tests can be performed in appropriate clinical circumstances to diagnose the various conditions listed in Table 9-2.

Algorithm

The algorithm shown in Fig. 9-1 provides a suggested approach to diagnosis of anxiety disorders. A variety of symptoms and presentations should lead clinicians to consider anxiety disorders, including multiple or nonspecific somatic complaints, cardiac symptoms such as chest pain and palpitations, overt symptoms consistent with one of the anxiety disorders, or other symptoms discussed above. In such patients, specific diagnostic criteria for anxiety disorders should be actively sought, with questions focused on the DSM-IV definitions of the various anxiety syndromes. If these criteria are met, a diagnosis of anxiety disorder can be made.

If the history or physical examination suggests that a medical illness is causing symptoms that mimic an anxiety disorder, appropriate diagnostic tests should be undertaken to diagnose or exclude such conditions. However, in the absence of symptoms or clues suggesting a medical illness, diagnosis of an anxiety disorder should be a positive affirmative diagnosis based on the presence of DSM-IV criteria, and not a diagnosis of exclusion.

Treatment

If anxiety symptoms are secondary to a medical condition, management should be directed at treating that condition. If no medical condition is suspected or identified and the patient's symptoms meet diagnostic criteria for an anxiety disorder, treatment for that disorder should be instituted. Treatments include diet and exercise, behavioral treatments, and pharmacotherapy.

Although cost-effectiveness studies of treatments for anxiety disorders are lacking, behav-

Figure 9-1

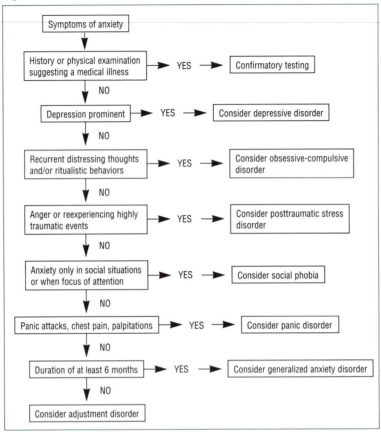

Algorithm for the diagnosis of anxiety disorders.

ioral treatments, such as cognitive behavioral therapy and exposure therapy, described below, are probably the most cost-effective treatment for the majority of patients. The cost-effectiveness of these behavioral treatments is based on the finite duration of treatment and lower long-term relapse rates.

For some patients, however, medication is preferred over behavioral treatments, especially when a rapid response is necessary, the patient cannot comply with or participate in behavioral treatment, or the patient has a coexisting substance abuse problem. In addition, patients with obsessive-compulsive disorder who only have obsessions usually respond best to medication.

When medications are used, SSRIs are generally preferred. While their cost per unit dose is more expensive than other medications, their lack of side effects leads to better compliance with treatment, which ultimately results in better outcomes and lower overall treatment costs. Tricyclic antidepressants and benzodiazepines cost less, but their side effects lead to noncompliance, poorer outcomes, and higher use of health care services.

Diet and Exercise

For all the anxiety disorders, treatment should ideally begin with dietary modifications. In addition, an exercise program is desirable for many patients.

DIETARY MODIFICATIONS

Dietary stimulants should be avoided, including caffeine, chocolate, and tyramine (found in red wines, cheese, almonds, etc). Some patients, particularly those with panic disorder, will already have noted an association between caffeine ingestion and their symptoms, and will have decreased caffeine consumption accordingly.

Dietary inositol may improve, but not eliminate, symptoms of anxiety, especially in panic disorder and obsessive-compulsive disorder. Inositol is found naturally in poultry, fish, and dairy products. For treatment of anxiety disorders, inositol is typically ingested in pill form as a dietary supplement, purchased without prescription at a health food store or pharmacy. The action of inositol is thought to be due to an as yet undefined effect on neurotransmitter synthesis. To be effective, 12 g/d must be taken for panic disorder and 18 g/d for obsessive compulsive disorder. There are no significant side effects. However, due to the inability of inositol to completely resolve anxiety disorders in most patients, its therapeutic role is limited.

EXERCISE

Some studies indicate that exercise can reduce anxiety levels and enable patients to better cope with stress, although this evidence is somewhat limited. Unless exercise is medically contraindicated or is specifically noted to increase panic attacks (which sometimes occurs), patients with anxiety disorders should be encouraged to engage in regular physical exercise.

Behavioral Therapies

General supportive psychotherapy, in which reassurance is offered in response to stress and manifestations of anxiety symptoms, is appropriate for all of the anxiety disorders. In addition, group therapy (in which patients with similar diagnoses discuss their anxiety symptoms) is also useful. Patients with posttraumatic stress disorder should receive in-depth psychotherapy. Two specific behavioral therapies with benefit for anxiety disorders include cognitive therapy and exposure therapy.

COGNITIVE THERAPY

Cognitive therapy is effective for most anxiety disorders. Cognitive therapy is a technique in which a patient's cognitive response to symptoms or thoughts is restructured so that anxiety-provoking interpretations are minimized. In obsessive-compulsive disorder, the focus of cognitive therapy is to restructure patients' fears by showing them the impossibility of their fears' being realized. In generalized anxiety disorder, cognitive therapy is used to change anxious thoughts to positive ones. In panic disorder, symptoms associated with panic attacks—(e.g., dizziness or rapid breathing)—are artificially produced to demonstrate that they need not lead to panic attacks.

EXPOSURE THERAPY

In exposure therapy, patients systematically confront and learn to deal with the objects of their fears. In obsessive-compulsive disorder not complicated by substance abuse, exposure therapy with "response prevention" is the treatment of choice, especially for patients with compulsions. Exposure therapy with response prevention involves having patients expose themselves to stimuli that would normally trigger their compulsions and teaching them to resist performing compulsive behaviors for progressively longer periods of time with each successive exposure. Exposure therapy is also useful for social phobias and panic disorder accompanied by agoraphobia, by desensitizing patients to the situations that cause anxiety.

INEFFECTIVE BEHAVIORAL THERAPIES

Several behavioral treatments are not effective for anxiety disorders. These therapies include formal psychoanalysis, insight therapy (in which counseling is used to assist patients in gaining insight into the causes of their behaviors), and flooding (in which patients are subjected to high levels of anxiety-provoking stress within short periods of time, in an attempt to desensitize them to the stressful stimulus).

Pharmacotherapy

Table 9-10 presents medications used to treat anxiety disorders. With benzodiazepines, response to treatment usually occurs within about 1 to 2 weeks. For other medications, response usually begins in 3 to 4 weeks. After about 1 year of successful therapy, medications are usually discontinued. Their use should be tapered over a period of 2 to 3 months.

CHOICE OF PRIMARY MEDICATION

Several medications are effective for each of the anxiety disorders. Therefore, the choice of medication must be individualized, based on a variety of considerations, including the patient's desires, the clinician's experience with various medications, the presence of concomitant medical or psychiatric conditions, and the goals of therapy.

The first-line therapeutic agents include SSRIs, tricyclic antidepressants, buspirone, and benzodiazepines. The preferred medication for each of the specific anxiety disorders is described below. Most of the first-line drug treatments produce a response in 80 to 90 percent of patients. The only exception is in obsessive compulsive disorder, in which the first-choice medications, SSRIs, are helpful in only about 50 to 70 percent of patients.

Caution should be used in prescribing benzodiazepines because of the potential for developing dependence on this class of drugs. In addition, benzodiazepines should be used with caution in older individuals, since they may impair motor and cognitive function. This is a particular concern with long–half-life benzodiazepines, such as diazepam, clorazepate, and chlordiazepoxide, since these medications have been linked to higher rates of motor vehicle crashes in older persons.

The dosages shown in Table 9-10 represent a range. In general, these medications should be started at the lower end of the dosing range and continued at the lowest dose at which a satisfactory response is achieved.

PANIC DISORDER   In panic disorder, SSRIs are generally the medication of choice. However, if a rapid response is needed, high-potency benzodiazepines are the preferred therapy. Tricyclic antidepressants are the treatment of choice when there are co-morbid medical problems such as migraines or chronic pain syndromes. When either SSRIs or tricyclic antidepressants are used for panic disorder, they should be started at low doses to prevent development of a stimulatory effect.

GENERALIZED ANXIETY DISORDER   In generalized anxiety disorder, buspirone is the treatment of choice. However, benzodiazepines are preferred if there is a history of previous response to these drugs, and tricyclic antidepressants are appropriate for patients with concomitant depression.

OBSESSIVE-COMPULSIVE DISORDER   As noted earlier, exposure therapy is the treatment of choice for obsessive-compulsive disorder when compulsions are present. However, SSRIs are indicated if the patient (1) cannot comply with exposure therapy, (2) is purely obsessional, or (3) has a substance abuse problem.

OTHER ANXIETY DISORDERS   As shown in Table 9-10, few drugs are effective as primary therapy for the common non-familial anxiety disorders

Table 9-10
Medications for Anxiety Disorders

MEDICATION	DAILY DOSE, MG	PANIC DISORDER	GENERALIZED ANXIETY DISORDER	OBSESSIVE-COMPULSIVE DISORDER	POST-TRAUMATIC STRESS	SOCIAL PHOBIA	ADJUSTMENT DISORDER
Tricyclic antidepressants							
Imipramine	25–300	E	A		E		
Desipramine	25–300	E	A				
Clomipramine	25–250	E		E			
SSRIs							
Fluoxetine	20–80	E		E			
Sertraline	50–300	E		E			
Paroxetine	10–60	E		E		E	
Fluvoxamine	50–300	E		E			
Benzodiazepines							
Alprazolam	0.5–9	E	E				A
Lorazepam	2–8	E	E				A
Clonazepam	1–10	E	E				A
Diazepam	2–60		E				A
Chlordiazepoxide	15–100		E				A
Clorazepate	7.5–60		E				A
Oxazepam	30–120		E				A
Prazepam	20–60		E				A
Buspirone	15–30		E	A			A
Propranolol	10–160				A	A	A
MAOIs							
Phenelzine	15–60	E			E		

ABBREVIATIONS: E, effective, drug is effective as primary treatment for the condition; A, augmenting, drug is effective as secondary agent to augment effect of primary drug.

(post-traumatic stress disorder, social phobia, and adjustment disorder). Imipramine and MAO inhibitors have effectiveness for posttraumatic stress disorder, and paroxetine has been used with success for social phobia. None of the standard anti-anxiety medications have demonstrated effectiveness as primary therapy for adjustment disorder.

AUGMENTATION THERAPY

Once a patient's anxiety responds to medication, the medication should be continued. However, if symptoms respond but do not completely resolve, other medications can be added to the regimen to augment the response to the initial agent.

Lithium carbonate can augment the response to SSRIs in obsessive-compulsive disorder and to tricyclic antidepressants in posttraumatic stress disorder. Clonidine and carbamazepine may improve control of hypervigilance, flashbacks, and aggression for patients with posttraumatic stress disorder. It should be noted that neuroleptics (i.e., antipsychotic phenothiazines, butyrophenones, etc.) are not helpful for anxiety disorders and are contraindicated for panic disorder because they may increase the frequency or severity of panic attacks.

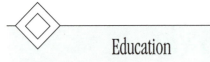

Education

Patients with anxiety disorders often feel they are unusual or peculiar because they have problems with anxiety. They may also feel they are "crazy" or that their problems are "all in my head." For these reasons, education can be beneficial for helping patients to accept their diagnosis and comply with treatments. By informing patients that anxiety disorders are common, clinicians can alleviate patients' sense of being

different. By discussing anxiety in terms of neurotransmitter imbalances, clinicians can dispel the idea that anxiety disorders are somehow controllable by the patient.

It is also reassuring to patients for their problem to be given a label (e.g. "panic disorder") because patients with anxiety disorders have frequently sought care from multiple clinicians without receiving a diagnosis. For similar reasons, patients should be reassured that effective treatments exist, but they should understand that pharmacologic treatments do not take effect for several weeks, and may not produce a full effect for months.

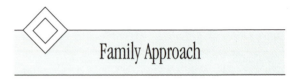

Family Approach

A diagnosis of anxiety disorder may cause a negative reaction in a patient's family members, who may also feel that anxiety is "all in your head" or that it means their relative is either "crazy" or "faking it." In obsessive-compulsive disorder, this reaction may be especially strong because the patient's obsessions and compulsions are often embarrassing to the family, and discussing them openly may represent a family taboo. Thus, family members need the same education as do patients regarding the high prevalence and the biological basis of anxiety disorders.

Treatment of anxiety disorders may also cause changes in the family. For example, marital relations frequently improve when patients with obsessive-compulsive disorder respond to treatment, even when no marital therapy has been offered or provided. Similarly, treatment of social phobias or panic disorder with agoraphobia can have a strong effect on family dynamics, because family members must shift roles in response to changes in the affected family member's behavior. Previously, family members had to adapt to and compensate for the patient's inability to function in a variety of situations. After successful treatment, family members must exchange their old family roles for new ones, and their ability to do this has an effect on whether changes in family dynamics will be positive or negative.

Errors

Practicing clinicians make a variety of errors in dealing with patients who have anxiety disorders. These errors occur in both diagnosis and treatment.

Diagnostic Errors

The most frequent diagnostic error is failure to give primary consideration to anxiety disorders in assessing patients who have multiple and chronic somatic complaints. Instead, many clinicians approach such patients by endlessly seeking physical causes for the patient's symptoms, considering anxiety disorders to be a "diagnoses of exclusion." This approach results in missed diagnoses, delays in beginning treatment, and unnecessary laboratory testing and suffering for patients.

Another common diagnostic error is failure to diagnose a specific anxiety disorder once the presence of anxiety is recognized. This error compromises therapy because various anxiety disorders require different approaches to treatment.

Treatment Errors

FAILURE TO INCLUDE BEHAVIORAL THERAPY

A common error in therapy for anxiety disorders is failure to include behavioral therapy in the treatment regimen. As discussed earlier, non-pharmacological treatments are effective and sometimes produce better long-term results than medication for several of the anxiety disorders, including panic disorders, generalized anxiety disorder, and obsessive compulsive disorder. Thus, failure to provide behavioral therapy deprives patients of potentially beneficial treatment.

USING THE WRONG MEDICATION

Once the decision is made to use drug therapy, the wrong medication is frequently used. For example, beta blockers and buspirone are often prescribed for panic disorder, even though they are not effective for this condition. Similarly, the wrong benzodiazepine may be prescribed for a particular disorder; for example, diazepam may be given for panic disorder when the correct benzodiazepines for this condition are alprazolam, lorazepam, and clonazepam (Table 9-10).

Finally, benzodiazepines are often inappropriately prescribed as a first-choice medication or prescribed when not needed, such as for mild situational anxiety. Because of their side effects and potential for drug dependence, benzodiazepines should be used only with clear indication.

USING THE WRONG DOSE

Dosing errors occur in pharmacotherapy for anxiety, including both doses that are too high and those that are too low. The SSRIs and tricyclic antidepressants are commonly begun at doses that are too high. For example, paroxetine should be started at 10 mg/d and imipramine at 25 mg/d. Benzodiazepines are often started at an inappropriately low dose, when the medication actually needs to be given at levels with which clinicians may be unfamiliar or uncomfortable. For example, in panic disorder, alprazolam may be required at doses as high as 10 mg/d instead of the more common dose of 2 to 4 mg/d.

Finally, it is not uncommon for clinicians to place patients on both benzodiazepines and antidepressants simultaneously with the idea that the benzodiazepine will be discontinued after the antidepressant starts to work. This practice is usually not warranted and often proves to be a problem because benzodiazepines are addictive and patients often resist stopping benzodiazepines once they have been prescribed.

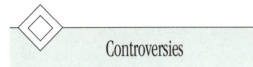

Controversies

The Role of Mental Health Professionals

One source of controversy in the management of anxiety disorders is whether and when patients should be referred to mental health professionals. Although some mental health experts have suggested that all patients with anxiety disorders be referred to mental health providers, this is neither practical nor economically feasible because of the extraordinarily large number of individuals who have anxiety disorders. For most anxiety disorders, primary care clinicians can effectively provide total or partial care. In fact, recognition and treatment of anxiety disorders by a patient's primary care clinician results in a greater likelihood that the patient will receive and accept treatment, and that the duration of illness will be shorter. However, few primary care clinicians are trained in cognitive or other behavioral therapies, nor do they have time to administer them. Thus, patients who are candidates for these behavioral therapies usually must be referred to mental health professionals.

Nearly all health care providers would agree that referral to a mental health professional is also needed when patients with anxiety disorders have suicidal ideation or when a primary care clinician is uncomfortable or inexperienced with an indicated therapy. Referral should also be considered when anxiety disorders occur in the presence of substance abuse. Patients with post-traumatic stress disorder and those with anxiety disorders who have a history of childhood sexual abuse benefit from psychological counseling and should also be referred.

Drugs of Choice

Another controversy is that of "drug-of-choice." Many of the specific anxiety disorders are thought to have specific drugs-of-choice, as outlined earlier in this chapter. However, recommendations of preferred medications are usually based on theoretical considerations or on findings of studies in carefully controlled research settings, not in actual patient care situations. Because primary care clinicians must treat all of their patients' maladies, including concomitant medical problems, a dogmatic approach to choosing medications is unrealistic and not in the best interest of patients. As discussed earlier, therapy should be individualized based upon the patient's desires, medical and psychiatric comorbidity, demographic characteristics, and goals of therapy.

Emerging Concepts

Diagnostic Criteria

Current psychiatric diagnoses and concepts are based on the language and definitions set forth in DSM-IV. These concepts and approaches to diagnosis work well in psychiatric and research settings but are not always useful in primary care practice. The concept of subsyndromal disorders—anxiety disorders that do not quite meet DSM-IV criteria—has been long recognized by primary care clinicians, and it is beginning to be recognized and investigated by psychiatrists and behavioral health researchers. It is likely that, in the future, the definitions used to diagnose anxiety disorders may be expanded to include subsyndromal manifestations. The desirability and choice or treatment for subsyndromal anxiety symptoms, however, has not yet been investigated, so it is not clear whether these patients benefit from the same therapeutic interventions as those whose symptoms meet DSM-IV criteria. Research in this area may change how clinicians diagnose and manage patients with anxiety in primary care settings.

In addition to the concept of subsyndromal disorders, there are other ways in which the current DSM-IV criteria fail to reflect the nature of behavioral disorders seen in primary care practice. The DSM-IV structure inherently suggests that patients' psychological disorders can be classified into well-defined syndromes. However, patients in primary care settings often have anxiety symptoms that overlap DSM-IV-defined syndromes, and many patients meet criteria for multiple disorders.

Furthermore, many different disorders may respond to the same treatment (e.g., panic disorder, obsessive compulsive disorder, and social phobia all respond to SSRIs). These observations suggest the possibility that the various anxiety disorders are really different manifestations of the same underlying neurochemical processes. If true, this could result in a different approach to conceptualizing these disorders and treating the underlying processes.

New Medications and Expanding Indications for Existing Medication

New medications continue to expand treatment options for anxiety disorders. The SSRIs, developed and marketed for treatment of depression, are effective in several anxiety disorders. This finding lends credence to the observations, discussed in the previous paragraph, that many anxiety symptoms are manifestations of the same pathophysiologic processes. If further research finds SSRIs to be effective in all anxiety disorders, it would reduce or eliminate the need for clinicians to diagnose a particular anxiety disorder because treatment would be the same regardless of diagnosis.

Another future development in treatment of anxiety disorder is likely to be the use of selective MAOIs. Traditional non-selective MAOIs, while quite effective for treating several anxiety disorders, have a variety of adverse interactions with foods and medications. These adverse interactions have all but eliminated traditional MAOIs from the prescribing practices of primary care clinicians. The new selective MAOIs have the same spectrum of treatment effects as the traditional MAOIs but do not have the interactions with medications and foods.

Screening Instruments

As noted earlier, several instruments have been developed for use as screening tests for anxiety in primary care practice, but they lack sensitivity for all except generalized anxiety disorder. However, because of concerns that anxiety disorders are under-recognized in primary care settings, it is likely that future research will develop more accurate screening tools for detection of anxiety and other behavioral disorders.

Bibliography

American Psychiatric Association: *Diagnostic and Statistical Manual of Mental Disorders*, 4th ed. Washington, American Psychiatric Association, 1994.

Beitman BD, Kushner MG, Basha I, et al: Follow-up status of patients with angiographically normal coronary arteries and panic disorder. *JAMA* 265:1545, 1991.

Benjamin J, Levine J, Fux M, et al: Double-blind, placebo-controlled, crossover trial of inositol treatment for panic disorder. *Am J Psychiatr* 152:1084, 1995.

Broadhead WE, Leon AC, Weissman MM, et al: Development and validation of the SDDS-PC screen for multiple mental disorders in primary care. *Arch Fam Med* 4:211, 1995.

Butler G, Fennell M, Robson P, et al: Comparison of behavior therapy and cognitive behavior therapy in the treatment of GAD. *J Consult Clinic Psychol* 59:167, 1991.

Carter C, Maddock R, Amsterdam E, et al: Panic disorder and chest pain in the coronary care unit. *Psychosomatics* 33:302, 1992.

Cormier LE, Katon W, Russo J, et al: Chest pain with negative cardiac diagnostic studies. *J Nerv Ment Dis* 176:351, 1988.

Friedin RB: Primary care multidimensional model. *Gen Hosp Psychiatr* 2:10, 1980.

Fux M, Levine J, Aviv A, et al: Inositol treatment of obsessive-compulsive disorder. *Am J Psychiatr* 153:1219, 1996.

Greist JH: Treating the anxiety. *J Clin Psychiatr* 51(suppl):29, 1990.

Hollander E, Kwon JH, Stein DJ, et al: Obsessive-compulsive and spectrum disorders: Overview and quality of life issues. *J Clin Psychiatr* 57(suppl 8):3, 1996.

Insel TR: New pharmacologic approaches to OCD. *Br J Psychiatr* 157:133, 1990.

Katerndahl DA: Relationship between panic attacks and health locus of control. *J Fam Pract* 32:391, 1991.

Katerndahl DA: Panic and prolapse: Meta-analysis. *J Nerv Ment Dis* 181:539, 1993.

Katerndahl DA. Panic attacks and panic disorder. *Am J Psychiatry* 43:275, 1996.

Katerndahl DA, Realini JP: Where do panic attack sufferers seek care? *J Fam Pract* 40:237, 1995.

Katerndahl DA, Trammell C: Prevalence and recognition of panics states in Starnet patients presenting with chest pain. *J Fam Pract* 45:54, 1997.

Katon W, Hall ML, Russo J, et al: Chest pain: Relationship of psychiatric illness to coronary arteriographic results. *Am J Med* 84:1, 1988.

Marks IM, Swinson RP, Basoglu M, et al: Alprazolam and exposure alone and combined in PD with agoraphobia. *Br J Psychiatr* 162:1776, 1993.

Marsland DW, Wood M, Mayo F: A data bank for patient care, curriculum, and research in family practice: 526,196 patient problems. *J Fam Pract* 3:25, 1976.

National Ambulatory Medical Care Survey, publication no 116. Hyattsville, MD, U.S. Department of Health and Human Services, 1994.

Ormel J, Koeter MWJ, van den Brink W, et al: Recognition, management, and course of anxiety and depression in general practice. *Arch Gen Psychiatr* 48:700, 1991.

Realini JP, Katerndahl DA: Factors affecting the threshold for seeking care: The Panic Attack Care-Seeking Threshold (PACT) Study. *J Am Board Fam Pract* 6:215, 1993.

Ried LD, John RE, Gettman DA: Benzodiazepine exposure and functional status in older people. *J Am Geriatr Soc* 46:71, 1998.

Robbins JM, Kirmayer LJ, Cathebras P, et al: Clinician characteristics and the recognition of depression and anxiety in primary care. *Med Care* 32:795, 1994.

Shapiro S, Skinner EA, Kessler LG, et al: Utilization of health and mental health services: Three epidemiologic catchment area sites. *Arch Gen Psychiatr* 41:971, 1984.

Silver JM, Sandberg DP, Hales RE: New approaches in the pharmacotherapy of PTSD. *J Clin Psychiatr* 51(suppl 10):33, 1990.

Spitzer RL, Williams JBW, Kroenke K, et al: Utility of a new procedure for diagnosing mental disorders in primary care. *J Am Med Assoc* 272:1749, 1994.

Tiemens BG, Ormel J, Simon GE: Occurrence, recognition and outcome of psychological disorders in primary care. *Am J Psychiatr* 153:636, 1996.

Zinbarg RE, Barlow DH, Liebowitz M, et al: DSM-IV field trial for mixed anxiety-depression. *Am J Psychiatr* 151:1153, 1994.

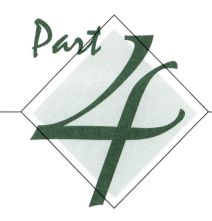

Part

4

Aches and Pains

Anne D. Walling

Chapter

10

Headache

How Common Are Headaches?

Principal Diagnoses

Over 90 percent of adults report at least one headache each year, with the highest prevalence in young- and middle-aged women. Although it has been estimated that less than 15 percent of young men and only 25 percent of young women with headaches ever seek medical care for this problem, headache is still given as the principal reason for nearly 10 million office visits to clinicians each year. This places headache in the top ten reasons why patients seek outpatient medical care. The vast majority of these visits are to primary care clinicians.

If data were available to measure all the telephone calls, emergency room visits, and other contacts in which headache is discussed, the proportion of a clinician's practice devoted to managing headache would rise further. Thus, the abovementioned measures of office visits for headache greatly underestimate the ubiquity of headache in outpatient practice.

Headache is best considered a symptom, not a disease or definitive diagnosis. To diagnose the cause or type of headache, one first must define and classify headaches into a clinically meaningful nomenclature.

There has been considerable confusion over headache terminology, posing a major problem for clinicians and researchers attempting to understand, manage, and study headache. The most widely used system for classification of headache is that of the International Headache Society (IHS), which describes over 80 specific headaches in 13 groups, based on cause or associated conditions (Table 10-1).

In primary care practice, however, making a precise IHS diagnosis for headaches is frequently neither possible nor useful. From the point of view of primary care clinicians, the IHS classification has been criticized for placing too much emphasis on uncommon headache syndromes and headaches caused by major intracranial

Table 10-1

International Headache Society Classification of Headaches

Category	Number of Subtypes	Examples	Occurrence in Primary Care[*]
1. Migraine	7	With aura, Without aura	Common (may be underdiagnosed)
2. Tension	3	Acute, Chronic	Very common (may be overdiagnosed)
3. Cluster	3	Episodic, Chronic	Very Rare
4. Miscellaneous "specific syndromes"	6	Exertional, Coital Cough	Rare
5. Associated with head trauma	2	Acute, Chronic	Variable
6. Associated with vascular disorders	9	Ischemia/stroke Subdural hematoma, Epidural hematoma, Subarachnoid hemorrhage, AVM, Hypertension	Uncommon to present as headache alone
7. Associated with nonvascular intracranial disorders	7	High or low CSF pressure Infection, Neoplasm	Rare
8. Associated with substance abuse	5	Iatrogenesis, Carbon monoxide, Substance/ alcohol withdrawal	Variable/uncommon (may be underdiagnosed)
9. Associated with noncephalic infection	3	Viral/bacterial/other, Systemic/focal	Variable/very common
10. Associated with metabolic disorders	6	Hypoxia, Hypercapnia, Hypoglycemia	Uncommon
11. Associated with structural abnormality of head and neck	7	TMJ, Cervical arthritis Sinus pathology, Glaucoma	Very common
12. Neuralgias and related conditions	8	Neuropathies, Herpes zoster, Trigeminal neuralgia	Uncommon to present as "headache"
13. Not classifiable presentations		"Mixed" and nonclassical presentations	Common

[*]Significance of headache symptoms may vary depending on population served, and on expectations of individual patients and clinicians.

Abbreviations: AVM, arteriovenous malformations; CSF, cerebrospinal fluid; TMJ, temporomandibular joint.

Source: Adapted with permission from *Cephalgia* 8(suppl 7):1–96, 1988. Copyright Scandinavian University Press, as agent for the International Headache Society.

pathology. The vast majority of headaches seen in primary care practice are tension headaches, migraine headaches, or headaches related to common illnesses. Indeed, as few as four per thousand headache patients presenting to primary care clinicians have significant intracranial pathology. Conversely, one study of patients requiring craniotomy for intracranial lesions reported that only 5 to 6 percent of such patients sought medical attention because of headache alone; other problems and diagnostic clues were almost always present.

A useful adaptation of the IHS classification for primary care is to group headaches into six principal categories: (1) migraine headache, (2) tension headache, (3) cluster headaches, (4) uncommon specific headache syndromes, (5) secondary headache, and (6) mixed headaches. These six categories of headaches are the principal diagnoses to consider when evaluating headaches in primary care practice. Each category is discussed below, presented in an order that corresponds to the IHS classification. The discussion of headaches in this chapter does not deal with headaches related to trauma.

Migraine Headache (IHS Group 1)

Migraine is a headache syndrome of which descriptions date back to the ancient Egyptian civilization. The key features of all types of migraine are recurring, episodic attacks, lasting 3 to 72 h, of moderate-to-severe pain that is usually throbbing and unilateral. By definition, the headache is accompanied or preceded by nausea and vomiting and/or photophobia and phonophobia. Migraine headaches can be preceded by a "prodrome" lasting up to 24 h, during which time patients may experience other symptoms, such as food cravings, fatigue, or mood changes.

The IHS definition recognizes several subtypes of migraine, the most important of which is migraine with aura prior to the onset of head pain. Auras are typically either visual or cutaneous. Visual auras consist of symptoms such as

blind spots, flashing lights, or distortions in the size of objects. Cutaneous auras are usually experienced as numbness or tingling of the face or extremities. Auras can last anywhere from a few minutes to an hour, but auras lasting more than 1 hour are not consistent with a diagnosis of migraine headache.

When present, auras can be useful in confirming the diagnosis of migraine headache. In addition, a pre-headache aura permits patients to start treatment early in a migraine attack. However, auras occur in only 20 to 35 percent of migraineurs, and focusing on aura as a defining characteristic of migraine can cause clinicians to under-diagnose migraine. In a small percentage of migraine patients, headaches are accompanied by neurologic symptoms, including hemiparesis, caused by vasoconstriction of the intracranial vascular system.

EPIDEMIOLOGY

The most recent estimates of the prevalence of migraine are that, overall, 23 million people in the United States have migraine headaches, and they occur in 17.6 percent of women and 5.7 percent of men. Migraine is more common in young adult women than any other age group and usually has its onset before age 30. Migraines tend to be familial and inheritable, but the detailed genetic basis for migraine is unclear.

PATHOPHYSIOLOGY

The understanding of the pathophysiology of migraine is progressing rapidly. Current theories attribute migraine to an inherited abnormality in the brain stem that results in decreased activity of the 5-hydroxytryptamine (5-HT) (serotonin) system. Once triggered, this abnormality has several effects, including release of neuropeptides that cause vascular inflammation, stimulation of pain receptors in the intracranial arterial walls, and activation of pain systems mediated through the trigeminal nerve. Cycles of vasoconstriction and vasodilation occur, previously believed to be the primary cause of migraine and other "vascular" headaches, and which account for the throbbing nature of the headache. These changes in vascular activity are currently thought to be secondary to neurogenic (neurotransmitter) abnormalities.

Tension Headache (IHS Group 2)

Tension, or "muscle contraction," headaches are familiar to almost all adults, but they are surprisingly difficult to define. The IHS definition calls for the headache to have at least two characteristics, including sensations of pressure or tightness, bilateral location, mild to moderate intensity, and not aggravated by activity. Classic tension headache begins in the occiput, temple, or upper neck, and may evolve to a band-like distribution around the head. Individual episodes may last from 30 min to several days, and headaches characteristically recur frequently, often on consecutive days. While it may occur, nausea is not a predominant symptom in tension headache. The combination of photophobia and phonophobia is unusual.

EPIDEMIOLOGY

Although described in the literature as either the first or second most-common type of headache encountered in primary care practice, there has been very little systematic study of the epidemiology of tension headache. Only a minute proportion of individuals with tension headache are thought to seek medical care for their headaches. Those who do see a clinician may have particularly severe symptoms, decreased ability to manage symptoms without medical intervention, significant concern about the underlying cause of their headache, or a combination of factors that do not affect the majority of tension headache sufferers. Thus, studies of tension headache conducted in clinicians' offices tell us little about these headaches on a population-wide basis.

Based on telephone interview surveys, about 38 percent of adults have one or more episodic tension headaches each year, and about 2 percent have chronic tension headaches, defined as 15 or more headaches per month. Nearly 10 percent of individuals with tension headaches report absenteeism from work because of headache.

PATHOPHYSIOLOGY

The pathophysiology of tension headache was formerly attributed to contraction of the muscles of the scalp and posterior neck. Emotional stress, in turn, was blamed for this muscle activity. More recent investigations suggest that tension headache has much in common with migraine, possibly involving the same changes in the intracranial neurotransmitter and vascular systems that occur with migraine. Tension headache may thus be a symptom complex resulting from several simultaneous processes (e.g., muscle tension, psychological stress, and neurovascular changes).

CLUSTER HEADACHE (IHS GROUP 3)

Cluster headaches are episodes of intense unilateral pain in the eye or temple accompanied by ipsilateral lacrimation, rhinorrhea, facial sweating, conjunctival injection, and/or Horner's syndrome. Not all patients with cluster headache have all the accompanying symptoms. During a cluster headache, which typically lasts between 5 min and 3 h, patients are restless and distracted by the pain. The term *cluster* refers to the fact that patients have repeated episodes of headaches occurring in time-limited clusters, which may last for days or sometimes for several months. During clusters, these attacks occur at the same time of day or night. They are particularly common upon waking from sleep or following ingestion of alcohol. It is believed that, once a cluster period begins, it will inevitably produce a set number of daily attacks and then terminate. A few unfortunate patients, however, develop continuous or chronic cluster headaches.

EPIDEMIOLOGY

Cluster is a rare form of headache with an estimated prevalence of 69 per 100,000 adults. In contrast to migraine, which is most common in women, cluster headaches are six times more common in males, predominantly affecting middle-aged and older individuals.

PATHOPHYSIOLOGY

The pathophysiology of cluster headaches is believed to originate in the "pacemaker" nuclei of the anterior hypothalamus that control circadian rhythms. Since these areas of the brain are inter-related with the serotonin system and the serotonin system is implicated in the vascular processes of migraine, the vascular and other effects in cluster headache are now believed to be secondary to serotonergic neurologic dysfunction.

Uncommon Specific Headache Syndromes (IHS Group 4)

Several specific headache syndromes have been identified, the most common of which fall into two groups. Unfortunately, the case series on which the understanding of these syndromes is based have not provided sufficient information to clarify their epidemiology or pathophysiology. Patients are usually frightened by these headaches and can be greatly helped by diagnosis (including appropriate investigations to rule out intracranial pathology), explanation, and medications, when appropriate.

The first group of specific headache syndromes may have transient increases in cerebrospinal fluid pressure as a common cause. The transient nature of the spinal fluid hypertension distinguishes these headaches from those caused by the more serious intracranial disorders (e.g., brain tumors), in which elevated cerebrospinal fluid pressure is persistent. In these transient headaches, an intense headache lasting up to a few minutes may follow a Valsalva maneuver, such as cough. These headaches, therefore, are often referred to as "cough headaches" or "exertional headaches." They are most commonly reported by middle-aged and older males who have a history of other types of headache. Orgasm may precipitate a similar headache, a migraine, or a unique, explosive frontal or occipital headache ("coital headache") that lasts for several hours. Although most of these headaches are benign and often respond to indomethacin, investigations to rule out intracranial space-occupying lesions or Arnold-Chiari malformations are usually recommended.

The second group of uncommon headache syndromes is characterized by intense focal "jabbing" pain. The pain occurs in brief attacks multiple times daily, often in middle-aged men, and may be a subset of cluster headache. The pain may also be superimposed on a chronic, dull headache pain. These headaches are sometimes referred to as "chronic paroxysmal hemicrania" and may respond to treatment with indomethacin.

Secondary Headaches (Includes IHS Categories 5–12)

In secondary headaches, pain results from an underlying neurologic or medical condition. Generally, the headache does not resolve until the underlying condition is successfully treated.

Headache may be the presenting feature or included in the symptomatology of a bewildering range of conditions. Some of these are listed in IHS categories 5 through 12, in Table 10-1. These conditions cover a wide spectrum of severity ("from tumor to toothache") and may originate systemically (e.g., from hypoglycemia, fever, or substance abuse) or in the brain. Secondary headaches are diagnosed by the medical history, supported by evidence from physical examination and appropriate diagnostic testing.

Open- and closed-ended questioning about the headache usually reveals a pattern that does not correspond to the typical patterns of well-defined headaches, such as migraine, tension, or specific headache syndromes. The review of symptoms, again using both open-ended and targeted questions, should detect information about co-existing symptoms of the underlying problem.

It has been estimated that the most common causes of secondary headaches in primary care practice are related to respiratory and sinus infections and musculoskeletal problems of the cervical spine. These conditions are at least as prevalent as migraine. Still, both clinicians and patients worry about rare but potentially serious causes of headache, some of which are discussed below. The list of conditions presented below is not all-inclusive, and there are other rare causes of secondary headache that are not discussed. The possibility that these conditions might be causing a patient's headaches often generates the "WHIMS" (What Have I Missed Syndrome) in clinicians. However, it must again be stressed that the vast majority of headaches in primary care practice are of the tension or migraine type or secondary to common, non-life-threatening conditions.

CONDITIONS CAUSING INCREASED INTRACRANIAL PRESSURE

A diverse group of conditions (Table 10-1) can raise intracranial pressure by mass effect and/or obstruction of the normal circulation of cerebrospinal fluid. These include conditions such as tumors, intracerebral hematomas, and central nervous system infections. Each of these conditions has a unique epidemiology and pathophysiology. They are uncommon in everyday practice, and estimates from Britain are that only 1 to 2 intracranial space-occupying lesions are diagnosed every 10 years for each 1000 patients enrolled in a general practitioner's patient panel.

Identifying patients with raised intracranial pressure from all undifferentiated headache pa-

tients depends on the clinician's attention to detail in assessment and tenacity of follow-up. In these secondary headaches, one or more of the classical triad of symptoms (headache, psychological/neurologic symptoms, and nausea/vomiting) is usually the presenting complaint. If headache is the primary complaint, it may be of any type, depending on the size, nature, and location of the lesion. However, the headache is most frequently described as daily, moderately severe, worse at night or in the morning, and exacerbated by exercise or any Valsalva maneuver (e.g., coughing, sneezing, or straining at stool). It usually becomes worse despite adequate use of first-line analgesics, such as acetaminophen or non-steroidal anti-inflammatory drugs (NSAIDs). When the findings upon physical examination are negative and the patient has no other apparent problems, these headaches may be indistinguishable from tension headaches. Only by repeating the history and physical examination at scheduled follow-up visits are clinicians able to make a timely diagnosis.

While headaches from increased cerebrospinal fluid pressure are generally the result of a specific pathologic process, in "benign intracranial hypertension" (pseudotumor cerebri) the rise in intracranial pressure occurs on an idiopathic basis. Pseudotumor cerebri is associated with endocrine abnormalities and use of certain vitamins, hormones, and drugs (especially tetracycline). It is most common in obese young women.

SUBARACHNOID HEMORRHAGE AND INTRACRANIAL VASCULAR CONDITIONS

SUBARACHNOID HEMORRHAGE   Bleeding into the subarachnoid space is usually an acute event that follows rupture of a congenital aneurysm at a bifurcation in the circle of Willis. The condition is rarely encountered in primary care practice (British general practitioners see about 1 case every 8 to 10 years per 1000 enrolled patients). However, the dramatic presentation and often tragic outcome of subarachnoid hemorrhage have earned this condition a well-deserved respect. Approximately 40 percent of patients die, and an additional 10 to 20 percent are significantly disabled.

The severity of the headache, rapid onset of neurologic signs (especially neck stiffness), and progression to coma are characteristic of subarachnoid hemorrhage. Many authorities cite the importance of primary care clinicians recognizing a "warning leak" of the aneurysm, manifested as a transient severe headache that occurs in up to half of patients prior to an overt subarachnoid hemorrhage. In most cases, however, these "warning leaks" are not apparent to patients or clinicians. Given the high prevalence of headaches in the population, the low rate of medical consultation for headaches, the rarity of subarachnoid hemorrhage, and the cost implications of extensively investigating every transient headache, anticipation of subarachnoid hemorrhage is likely and practical only in patients with a family history of subarachnoid hemorrhage or a personal history of polycystic renal disease (in which abnormal vascular structure predisposes to subarachnoid hemorrhage).

INTRACRANIAL VASCULAR CONDITIONS Headache may also be part of the clinical picture in other acute intracranial cerebrovascular events, such as intracerebral hemorrhage, vascular embolism, or thrombosis. In these syndromes, headache may not be severe, but there are often substantial neurological abnormalities. The incidence of all cerebrovascular disease in British general practice has been estimated at 5 to 6 per 1000 enrolled patients per year, but the probability for a specific patient varies with age and risk factors, such as cigarette smoking and hypertension.

Other intracranial vascular problems include arteriovenous malformations and subdural or epidural hematomas. These conditions can produce chronic, increasing headaches due to space-occupying effects and raised intracranial pressure. They can also directly irritate pain-sensitive structures, and arteriovenous malformations can bleed. Persistent headache is the earliest and most characteristic symptom of epidural and subdural hematomas and of thrombosis of the cerebral veins and sinuses.

CENTRAL NERVOUS SYSTEM INFECTIONS

Any condition producing inflammation in the scalp, brain, or central nervous system may produce headache as part of the clinical picture. The type of headache described by the patient depends on several factors, principally the location and type of infection and whether there is an associated increase in intracranial pressure.

The diagnosis of central nervous system infection is usually suspected because the headache is new or different from previous headaches, the patient appears ill, and the overall clinical picture has features indicating toxicity (e.g., fever, tachycardia, and change in consciousness). The physical examination usually reveals nuchal rigidity and may include features of specific conditions, such as the purpuric rash of meningiococcemia.

Classically, bacterial meningitis was the most common central nervous system infection and was suspected whenever signs of meningeal irritation (i.e., nuchal rigidity) were found. The epidemiology of meningitis and cerebral infections has changed due to two developments. One is the introduction of an immunization for *Haemophilus influenzae*, which has markedly reduced the incidence of bacterial meningitis in children. The other is the HIV epidemic, which has resulted in an increased rate of meningitis caused by viruses, fungi, and other non-bacterial agents. Identifying the most likely causative organism of central nervous system infection in an individual patient requires consideration of both common and uncommon organisms (including tuberculosis, syphilis, and parasitic infections) and inquiry about personal, sexual, travel, occupational, and other risk factors. Toxoplasmosis and other parasitic infections (e.g., cysticercosis) are more likely to present as seizure than headaches.

TEMPORAL ARTERITIS

New-onset or changing headache in patients over 50 years of age should raise suspicion of intracranial pathology, such as tumor or other abnormalities described above. It should also prompt consideration of temporal arteritis.

Temporal arteritis is a vasculitis involving the extracranial arteries of the head and sometimes intracranial arteries, such as the ophthalmic artery. Inflammation of the extracranial (temporal) vessels causes headache and pain with mastication, while involvement of the ophthalmic artery can result in blindness. In some patients the condition is part of a more systemic syndrome involving the large intrathoracic arteries (giant cell arteritis) or proximal muscles of the upper and lower extremities (polymyalgia rheumatica).

The headache of temporal arteritis is usually unilateral and of gradual onset. The intensity is variable, and any persistent headache in persons over 50 may represent temporal arteritis. On physical examination, the temporal artery is tender in 70 percent of patients, thickened in 45 percent, and pulseless in 40 percent. Two-thirds of patients report claudication of the jaw upon chewing. Just under half of patients also report visual symptoms and/or symptoms of polymyalgia rheumatica. The erythrocyte sedimentation rate is greater than 50 mm/h in approximately 95 percent of patients but may be normal in some individuals. Temporal artery biopsy confirms the diagnosis. Prompt steroid treatment is necessary to control symptoms and prevent blindness. Steroids may be started before temporal artery biopsy is performed, without influencing histologic interpretation of the biopsy specimen.

ANGLE-CLOSURE GLAUCOMA

Acute angle-closure glaucoma occasionally presents as intense eye pain due to a sudden elevation of intraocular pressure. Angle-closure glaucoma is uncommon (British general practitioner data indicates a prevalence of 1 case per year per 1000 enrolled patients). Since acute glaucoma is often accompanied by nausea and vomiting, it can resemble migraine or cluster headaches. Migraine, however, rarely has its initial onset in older patients, and the continuous, increasing nature of eye pain usually alerts the clinician to ask about visual symptoms, such as seeing colored haloes around lights. Intraocular pressure should be measured immediately when angle-closure glaucoma is suspected, because the condition can cause blindness if not treated promptly.

TRIGEMINAL NEURALGIA

Trigeminal neuralgia ("tic douloureux") usually produces pain in the face and jaw in areas supplied by the maxillary and mandibular divisions of the fifth cranial nerve. Trigeminal neuralgia can also present as headache when the ophthalmic division of the fifth nerve is affected. In this situation, patients experience "electric shocks" of severe pain around the temple and eye. The pain may be precipitated by touch or any activity of facial muscles and may occur continuously for several weeks.

Medications such as carbamazepine and phenytoin provide relief in many cases. Surgical treatment (percutaneous retrogasserian rhizotomy) can be considered if medications fail to control symptoms.

MEDICATIONS AND FOODS

MEDICATIONS A number of widely used medications can cause headache or exacerbate pre-existing migraine. The most common of these drugs include vasodilators (e.g., calcium channel blockers, hydralazine, and nitrates), histamine-$_2$ antagonists, corticosteroids, oral contraceptives, postmenopausal hormone replacement regimens, theophylline, and vitamin A. In addition to these common causes of headache, the package inserts for literally hundreds of prescription and non-prescription drugs list headache as a possible adverse effect.

Paradoxically, analgesics and ergotamines used to treat headache can also cause headache in certain patients. Specifically, indomethacin and other NSAIDS can cause headache. Other analgesics and ergotamine are notorious for "rebound headaches" (i.e., overuse of the medication is followed by exacerbation of headache when the medication is discontinued).

FOODS In susceptible individuals, headaches may be caused by foods that contain nitrites (such as hot dogs) or monosodium glutamate ("Chinese restaurant syndrome"). Alcohol can also induce headache ("hangover headache"). Some individuals experience headaches after eating cold substances ("ice cream headache").

SYSTEMIC ILLNESSES

Medical textbooks list a perplexing array of systemic disorders that may present as headache or include headache in the symptom complex. Probably the most common systemic condition is fever, which is often accompanied by frontal or bi-temporal headache. Hypertension is frequently cited as a cause of headache, but the pain stimulus may actually be a sudden increase in blood pressure, rather than chronically elevated blood pressure. Similarly, headache associated with anemia may be related to sudden falls in hemoglobin or levels below 10g/dL. Any hypoxic state, including carbon monoxide poisoning, can cause headache, as can conditions leading to hypoglycemia. Although less commonly encountered, endocrine conditions such as Cushing's syndrome, Addison's disease, pheochromocytoma, and hypothyroidism may present as headache.

PSYCHIATRIC AND PSYCHOLOGICAL CONDITIONS

Special mention must be made of psychological conditions, such as depression and anxiety, which can cause "secondary headaches." These conditions are more common than any of the other causes of secondary headache listed above. They should be considered as primary diagnostic possibilities in patients with headache, and not just when extensive investigations fail to reveal a specific cause for headaches.

When chronic headache occurs in conjunction with depression, it is unclear whether the distress of headache pain leads to depression, whether headache patients are more vulnerable to depressive illness, or whether depressed individuals are more likely to experience headaches. Regardless of the cause, treatment of depression in these individuals often leads to improvement or elimination of headache. Similarly, various anxiety syndromes, including generalized anxiety disorder and posttraumatic stress disorder, can present as headaches. Headaches may resolve with treatment of the underlying behavioral health problem.

The head is also a frequent site of symptoms in patients with somatization disorder. These individuals may describe unusual headache syndromes, have an affect that seems inappropriate to the clinical picture, and give a history of multiple illnesses or unexplained symptoms in other body systems. Headache may also be a prominent symptom in patients with conversion disorders, those seeking compensation for injuries, and drug seekers. Finally, headache is commonly used as a "ticket of admission" for patients who wish to discuss confidential issues with clinicians without telling the clinician's scheduling staff about the real reason for the visit.

Mixed-Type Headache (IHS Group 13 or Elements of More than One IHS Group)

Mixed-type headaches include those that are unclassifiable (IHS category 13) or that have characteristics of multiple kinds of headaches. Because these headaches, by definition, cannot be clearly classified, selection of treatment is often difficult.

Typical Presentation

The majority of patients with headache are evaluated by primary care clinicians, who encounter four common presentations of headache. The most common presentation of headache in primary care practice is tension headache or secondary headache that has persisted for several days despite appropriate self-treatment with nonprescription analgesics. In this situation, patients may be concerned that their headache is caused by a serious problem, such as a brain tumor.

The next most common presentation is probably that of a patient who has experienced intermittent tension or migraine headaches for several months or years, but who has recently noted a change in the headache pattern or a decreased effectiveness of usual strategies to manage the headache. With this presentation, patients are frequently concerned about deterioration in their ability to cope with chronic headaches.

The third presentation occurs when clinicians ask patients about headaches on review of systems and receive an affirmative response. This is a common scenario and can result in the detection of many previously undiagnosed headaches. Numerous cases of migraine could be detected this way because many migraine sufferers never inform their primary care clinician about symptoms of headaches. In fact, over 60 percent of migraineurs have never been formally diagnosed as having migraine.

The final common presentation is of a patient who arrives in a clinician's office, urgent care center, or emergency room with severe or dramatic headache symptoms. This presentation of headache requires a different diagnostic and management approach than that employed for the other common presentations.

Patients with headache who obtain care from specialists such as ophthalmologists, neurologists, or otolaryngologists often have a different presentation from that of patients in primary care practice. Patients seeking care from subspecialists are more apt to be suffering from headaches refractory to first-line therapy, or to have expectations or prior experiences that lead them to seek consultation with a specific type of specialist. Based on the headache literature, much of which is written by neurologists, patients seen by subspecialty clinicians may have a higher rate of intracranial pathology and more rare forms of headaches than in primary care practice. They may also be less likely to have tension headaches or headaches secondary to common illnesses. This patient selection bias often complicates comparisons of diagnostic and management plans for headaches seen in primary care practice with those seen in subspecialty practices.

Key History

In headache, the history is usually sufficient to make a diagnosis and, therefore, is essential for selecting appropriate therapy. Taking a good history may even have a therapeutic effect, based on one large study that found the strongest predictor of long-term resolution of headache to be patients' perception that their symptoms and concerns had been fully discussed with their clinician.

How to Listen, What to Ask

Obtaining a comprehensive headache history does not take long if a classical combination of open-ended (e.g., "Tell me about your headaches.") and specific closed-ended questions is used to obtain a description of the headache. Perhaps the best advice in taking a history from patients with headache is "watch and listen." Clinicians must maintain a demeanor of interested neutrality to avoid biasing the patient's story. While patients speak, the clinician should observe their facial expressions, gestures, body language, and tone of voice for clues to the severity and the role of psychological factors in genesis of the headache.

Patients must have time to describe their headaches without interruption. Most patients will spontaneously provide a full description of headache frequency, location, severity, associated symptoms, and response to previous treatments within a few minutes. They will also usually convey their principal concerns and expectations of the consultation. The clinician can then use specific questions as needed to further clarify the nature of the headache (Table 10-2). Summarizing

Table 10-2

"Typical" Histories for Different Types of Headache*

QUESTION[†]	TENSION HEADACHE	MIGRAINE HEADACHE	CLUSTER HEADACHE
How bad is pain?	Mild to severe	Severe	Severe to very severe
What does it feel like?	"Squeezing," "pressure," "Nagging"	"Throbbing," "pounding," "knifelike"	"Excruciating," "knifelike"
Which part of the head?	"All over," or bitemporal or occipital	Unilateral eye/temple	Unilateral eye/temple
Does anything bring it on?	Frustration, stress, or nothing	Relief of tension, menstruation, wine, foods, sleeping late	(Sometimes) alcohol, trinitrates
Do you know it is going to start?	"Sometimes just feel it coming on"	Notice energy and appetite changes, (some) flashing lights just before	Same time(s) each day, "regular as clockwork"
How does it start?	"Just there all day, sometimes comes and goes"	Usually starts slowly	Sudden, "wakes me up"
What usually happens?	"Just goes on," "wears me out"	"Pain and symptoms get worse. Then, after a time, I fall asleep."	"Symptoms are really terrible for about 30–45 min, then disappear."
What other symptoms?	Fatigue, irritability, trouble concentrating, ache in shoulders, neck pain, trouble sleeping and wake up tired	Severe nausea, vomiting; intolerant of light, smell, noise; "really ill"	Nose and eye watering, nose stuffed up, restless, red eye
What helps?	Analgesics, exercise, or nothing	Analgesics, antiemetics, sleep, cold compresses, dark quiet room, vomiting, or "nothing helps"	"Nothing" or "going into the cold"
What makes the headache worse?	Stress, noise	Noise, anything to do with food, movement	"It couldn't get worse."
How long does it last?	"Several hours," "on and off all day"	2 h to several days	30 min to 2 h
How often?	Several days per month	From weekly to once or twice per year	Same time(s) each day for several weeks then disappears completely
What do you do?	"Put up with it," "take pills"	"Try to lie still in a dark quiet room," "wait till it goes away"	"Furiously try to get away from the pain; use a lot of paper tissues"
Does anyone in the family have headaches?	Probably	Yes	No

*Secondary and mixed headaches have such wide variations that they cannot be consolidated into a table.
†There is enormous individual variation in the history. In addition, patients may experience different patterns in successive headache episodes. The best information comes from an unprompted question, such as, "Tell me about your headaches?" Questions in this table are then used to clarify and complete the history.

the patient's headache story back to the patient for validation and clarification is useful in assuring the patient that his or her concerns have been heard.

Assessing Effect of the Headache

The conventional history provides sufficient information for developing a diagnosis and formulating a management plan, but it is also useful for establishing the effect of headaches on the patient's life, along with a sense of the patient's expectations for management. The clinical history can take on a completely different perspective when patients are asked specifically about days lost from work, days when normal activities are difficult, quantities of analgesics consumed per week, or the perceptions of families or co-workers. In addition, there is wide variation in how these factors are perceived. For example, some patients believe it quite normal to lose every third weekend to migraine, whereas others are intolerant of any headache requiring more than minimal non-prescription analgesic medication. Similarly, the expectations for treatment may range from "just wanting to check that what I am doing is okay" to demands for cure. A relatively new phenomenon is patients seeking to learn about and obtain new headache medications (especially for migraine) that have been advertised directly to the public. Finally, as already mentioned, patients are frequently concerned about the possibility of brain pathology, and uncovering this fear may require some skill by the clinician.

Interpreting the Symptoms

As shown in Table 10-2, the history is useful in distinguishing the principal types of headache encountered in primary care practice, and patients' responses to specific questions often make the classification of the headache straightforward. Some patients, however, suffer from more than one type of headache and give histories containing elements fitting more than one classification. In addition, the rare but potentially serious causes of secondary headache should be suspected in patients whose headaches are difficult to classify based on Table 10-2.

Serious causes of secondary headache should always be considered in patients over 50 who have new onset of headache. They should also be considered in patients of any age who experience a sudden or significant change in an established headache pattern, headaches that wake them from sleep, any headache accompanied by neurologic signs or symptoms of raised intracranial pressure, or headaches that deteriorate or show no improvement in response to appropriate first-line therapy.

Narcotic drug seeking should be suspected in patients whose pain and related behaviors appear out of proportion to their history and physical findings or that escalate during the assessment. Suspicion should particularly be aroused if patients report "allergy" to or lack of efficacy from nonnarcotic medications and insist that their "usual clinician" or an expert specialist has stated they are always to be treated with narcotic medications. An unknown proportion of headache patients are iatrogenically drug dependent, having been extensively treated with narcotic agents.

Written Headache Inventories

Some authors recommend elaborate written headache inventories to be completed by patients prior to the office visit, but the interactive history provides a more flexible and possibly more valid clinical assessment in a primary care environment. Written questionnaires are useful, however, to record previous medications, results of prior diagnostic tests, and previous diagnoses.

Physical Examination

The Value of the Physical Examination

History is the critical tool in identifying headaches, and physical examination is rarely useful in diagnosis. Most headache patients have normal findings on physical examination, and therefore experts differ on the value of performing a complete physical examination. The examination does provide at least three valuable contributions to the diagnostic and therapeutic process.

First, the examination provides a general assessment of the patient. This assessment should correlate with the most probable diagnosis based on the history. The "hands-on" nature of the physical examination may also lay a foundation for the therapeutic relationship necessary for the management stage, generating confidence in patients that they have been fully evaluated.

Second, the examination permits documentation of pertinent negative findings, particularly in the neurologic and optic fundus examinations. In some patients, the neurologic examination has to be repeated several times over a period of weeks to assure that there are no evolving abnormalities.

Third, the physical examination may be useful if it detects evidence of the underlying cause of the secondary headaches. The search for clues to the cause of secondary headache can be focused based on information obtained from the history.

If a patient appears distressed or ill, physical examination becomes a more important part of assessment. A neurologic assessment should be performed first, often before obtaining a detailed headache history, to exclude any life-threatening causes of headache, such as subarachnoid hemorrhage, meningitis, or stroke. In the absence of abnormal examination findings, however, such diagnoses become quite unlikely. In primary care practice, headaches due to subarachnoid or

intracranial hemorrhage, meningitis, and other serious conditions discussed are present only in about 0.35 percent of new-onset headaches in patients who have normal neurologic examination findings.

Examination Findings in Different Headache Syndromes

MIGRAINE HEADACHE

Most migraine patients present between attacks and have completely normal findings upon physical examination. When seen during an attack, however, the migraine patient is classically curled up in a fetal position with pillows positioned to keep the neck and head still. The room is usually dark, and an emesis basin is nearby. Neurologic examination findings are usually negative, but the patient looks very ill or "hung over." In fact, patients are sometimes accused of being drunk or on drugs during a migraine attack. The retinal funduscopic examination may be difficult because of photophobia. Patients with acute intracranial conditions initially appear very similar to migraineurs but have additional signs specific to their pathologic condition, such as neck stiffness, fever, funduscopic changes, neurologic signs, and usually a deteriorating ability to participate in the assessment.

TENSION HEADACHE

Patients with tension headache may appear similar to those with migraine. Photophobia may be less prominent, however, making it easier to perform a satisfactory funduscopic examination. Some patients with tension headache have tenderness to palpation of the posterior cervical and occipital muscles.

CLUSTER HEADACHE

Patients with cluster headaches are rarely seen during the headache because of the short duration of cluster attacks. If a patient is seen during an attack, the typical findings are unilateral tearing, nasal congestion, and sweating, in addition to the patient's apparently severe reaction to the pain.

SECONDARY HEADACHES

Patients with secondary headaches may have physical examination findings suggesting the underlying conditions responsible for the headache. As noted above, one of the principal benefits of performing a physical examination in patients with headaches is to facilitate identification of these conditions.

Ancillary Tests

Neuroimaging Studies

The most controversial aspect of headache assessment is the role of computerized tomography (CT) and magnetic resonance imaging (MRI) in diagnosis. These highly accurate imaging tests can detect intracranial pathology—if it is present. The controversy surrounding their use in primary care practice is that intracranial pathology is very rare and, even if present, often does not present with an isolated complaint of headache. Both tests are expensive, and MRI, in particular, can be distressing for some patients because of the somewhat claustrophobic conditions of the test. In addition, patents living in areas without CT or MRI availability must travel to obtain the tests. Finally, CT involves radiation exposure and sometimes requires use of contrast agents, thereby exposing patients to the risk of allergy or renal decompensation.

Expert panels and other authorities often stress the importance of obtaining CTs and MRIs in patients with unusual, constant, new-onset, or "severe" headaches. However, even in these selected patients, several studies demonstrate the

very low yield of CT scans for providing useful diagnostic information if neurologic signs are absent. Furthermore, when longitudinal studies have followed patients over time, the value of CT scans becomes even more questionable because a high proportion of the few abnormalities detected by scans are ultimately found to be false-positive results or noncontributory incidental findings. No research has addressed the benefits of reassurance provided by a negative scan, but one estimate is that this may benefit only about 30 percent of patients.

In practice, experienced clinicians appear to be able to select a subset of headache patients for whom further investigation is warranted, but CT and MRI scans are still vastly over-used. They should only be ordered if likely to provide useful diagnostic information (i.e., if there is a strong suspicion of a treatable abnormality based on history or abnormal neurologic findings) or if the benefits of knowing a scan is negative outweigh the costs and risks of the investigation. Definitive evidence-based information on when to obtain imaging studies will require further research, with a focus on primary care practice. The general concepts outlined above—unusual, constant, new-onset, or severe headaches; strong suspicion of a treatable intracranial abnormality; and the benefits of knowing a scan is negative—can be used as guidelines for ordering neuroimaging studies. When imaging is obtained, CT scan is usually the test of choice, while MRI is useful if there is a suspicion of vascular lesions or a lesion in an area that may be obscured by bone (e.g., the posterior fossa).

Finally, it should be emphasized that CT and MRI scans do not substitute for careful history, physical examination, good first-line headache treatment, and diligent follow-up care. Clinicians must avoid disputes with patients over obtaining imaging studies. Discussion with or referral to a neurologist can be a useful strategy for determining whether imaging studies will be helpful, but neurologists may be more apt to order imaging studies because of the higher probability of finding structural intracranial lesions in their referral practices.

Lumbar Puncture

Lumbar puncture is indicated in suspected meningitis to confirm the diagnosis and identify the infecting organism to guide selection of antibiotics. It is also the test of choice for diagnosing pseudotumor cerebri. In addition, lumbar puncture may confirm the presence of subarachnoid or other bleeding into the cerebrospinal fluid when the CT scan does not demonstrate diagnostic findings of fresh bleeding or when several days have passed since the acute event.

Lumbar puncture is either contraindicated or done with extreme caution whenever there is a possibility of raised intracranial pressure. If increased intracranial pressure is suspected, imaging studies should be performed before lumbar puncture to exclude mass lesions in the brain. The only situation in which lumbar puncture is performed in the presence of a suspected increase in cerebrospinal fluid pressure is to diagnose pseudotumor cerebri.

Other Tests

Other tests may be appropriate to confirm diagnostic suspicions in individual patients presenting with what appear to be secondary headaches. For example, determination of the erythrocyte sedimentation rate is in order when temporal arteritis is suspected, sinus x-rays or CT scans may confirm a diagnosis of sinusitis, and tonometric studies can be used to diagnose glaucoma.

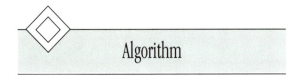

The algorithm shown in Fig. 10-1 outlines the basic approach to evaluating patients who have

headache. For patients who do not appear seriously ill, and in whom the neurologic examination is normal, diagnosis rests heavily on the history.

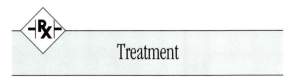

Most headache treatments can be accomplished in the context of good routine care without encouraging patients to become dependent on medications or to overuse health services. In dealing with any headache patient, clinicians should promote the patient's general health and sense of well-being, since increased fitness and reduced levels of emotional stress enable patients to better cope with headache symptoms. Recurrent tension or migraine headaches are rarely completely cured with these interventions, however, but they can assist patients to maintain maximal functional status in spite of their headaches.

Clinicians also need to know what is currently regarded as "the best" headache medication in their community (by talking to patients, pharmacists, and others). It is particularly important to know what treatment might have been given to patients by other clinicians that have seen them in urgent care or emergency room settings.

Self-Treatments

NONPRESCRIPTION MEDICATIONS

Patients presenting with headache should always be asked about self-treatments administered before seeking medical care. Patients frequently take large quantities of nonprescription analgesics, such as aspirin, acetaminophen, ibuprofen, and other NSAIDs, and may have fixed opinions as to which medications are most effective. Specific questioning about which agents are used, and in what frequency and

Figure 10-1

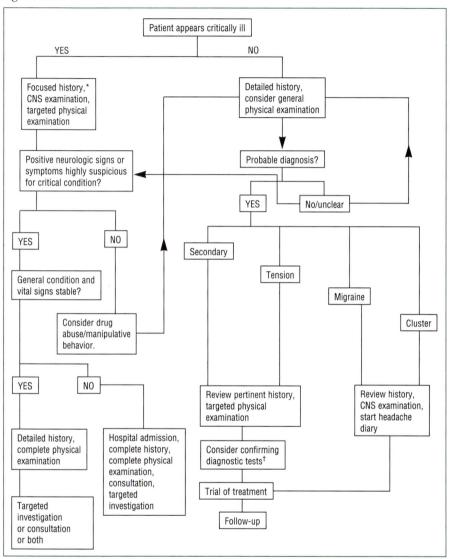

Algorithm for the diagnosis of headache.
*History directed to evidence for diagnosis and factors important in choice of management strategy (e.g., history of peptic ulceration contraindicates NSAIDs).
†Includes laboratory tests, imaging studies, and screening for depression.

dosage, can often uncover both underdosing and overdosing of the medications. Patients also may report taking narcotic medications, either obtained illegally or prescribed by other clinicians.

HERBAL MEDICATIONS

An increasing number of patients use herbal medications for prevention and treatment of migraine. The most common of these is the feverfew plant (*Tanacetum parthenium*), the active ingredient of which is parthenolide, which inhibits the action of both serotonin and prostaglandins. One study reported a 25-percent reduction in headache frequency, but this is the same reduction achieved by placebo treatment in other studies. Feverfew is typically consumed by either chewing the dry leaves or as a powdered extract. Its most common side effect is mouth ulcers, which occur most commonly in persons who chew the dry leaves.

NONMEDICINAL TREATMENTS

In addition to medications, many patients employ nonmedicinal techniques they have learned elsewhere or developed intuitively. These methods include neck massage, stress-reduction techniques, use of heat or cold, and adaptations of biofeedback techniques. Migraineurs and some tension-headache patients may develop patterns of behavior to minimize an attack, such as attempting to sleep in a darkened room using cold compresses or pillows and pads to maintain the least-painful body position. A surprising number of migraine sufferers self-induce vomiting to relieve nausea and reduce headache severity.

Clinician-Prescribed Treatments

A variety of strategies are available for treating headaches. They vary with the type of headache, patients' individual needs, and a variety of other considerations.

MIGRAINE HEADACHE

Effective management of migraine requires dual strategies. One strategy targets prevention of headaches through medications and avoidance of migraine-inducing stimuli. The other strategy provides relief from headaches when they occur.

Patients appreciate knowing about the different treatment strategies, and their full involvement in selecting a treatment is likely to foster confidence in the treatment. It also enhances the ability to change medication as is appropriate without invoking a sense of failure on the part of patient or clinician if treatment is not successful. This is important because the type and pattern of migraine attacks typically change over time, often making it necessary to alter therapies several times during a long-term relationship with a migraine patient.

In considering all migraine treatments, clinicians should keep in mind that the placebo effect in migraine treatment is of the order of 30 percent. This effect can be invoked and enhanced by clinicians who convey confidence in the management plan and take time to discover and address patients' uncertainties.

PREVENTIVE TREATMENTS   Prevention of migraine involves both nonpharmacologic and pharmacologic interventions. The choice depends on the frequency of headaches, a patient's willingness to comply with nonpharmacologic treatments, and the success of various preventive measures in a particular patient.

Nonpharmacologic Treatments   In some patients, specific foods (e.g., red wine, preserved meats, or chocolate), behaviors (e.g., sleeping late), or other stimuli (e.g., cigarette smoke, certain medications, fatigue, or menstruation) can precipitate a migraine attack. In theory, therefore, avoidance of these stimuli should decrease the frequency of migraine headaches. Theory, however, does not always translate into practice. It has been observed for at least 200 years that, for many patients, these factors are only important at certain times (i.e., when a migraine is "due"). Furthermore, potential headache stimuli are so ubiquitous that it may be unreasonable or impossible to expect patients to avoid them.

Most patients can identify precipitants of their headaches and be encouraged to take measures to minimize them to lower the chances of an attack. Strict or impractical avoidance regimens and punitive attitudes are not appropriate.

Pharmacologic Treatments Certain medications taken daily can reduce the frequency of migraine attacks by up to 65 percent. Research in this area, however, is complicated by the large placebo effect, need for individualized dosing of medications, subjectivity of migraine symptoms, and biased selection of patients for clinical trials. The medications commonly used for migraine prophylaxis are shown in Table 10-3.

Use of prophylaxis depends on balancing a number of issues, including the frequency of headaches, risk of side effects, compliance, cost, and reduction in migraine morbidity. Most ex-

perts consider prophylactic medication appropriate if migraine headaches occur more than twice per month. Preventive therapy may also be considered for patients whose migraines have a predictable onset (e.g., menstruation-associated migraine) and those who have infrequent headaches that are extraordinarily incapacitating. Regardless of the regimen selected, continuous prophylactic treatment for several months is usually necessary to assess any meaningful reduction in the pattern of migraine attacks.

Beta-Adrenergic Blocking Agents The best-studied medications for prevention of migraine are beta blockers that lack intrinsic sympathomimetic activity. In order of decreasing efficacy, these drugs are propranolol, nadolol, atenolol, timolol, and metoprolol. They are usually contraindicated in asthma, insulin-dependent diabetes, and heart failure. In addition, they may cause depression, fatigue, gastrointestinal upset, and neurologic symptoms, such as insomnia, memory changes, and disturbing dreams. Nadolol

Table 10-3

Medications for Prophylaxis of Migraine Headache

MEDICATION	DOSAGE	COMMON ADVERSE EFFECTS	COMMENTS
Propranolol	60–160 mg	Fatigue, depression, bradycardia, hypotension	Low cost
Atenolol	50–100 mg	Similar to propranolol, but fewer CNS effects	Greater cost
Amitriptyline	50–200 mg hs	Sedation, constipation, weight gain, dry mouth	Low cost; can be used in combination with propranolol
Verapamil	80–240 mg hs	Constipation	Low cost
Divalproex	250–1000 mg	Nausea, weight gain, sedation, hair loss, hepatic damage	Expensive
Naproxyn	325–550 mg	Gastrointestinal upset, hepatic/renal damage	May be used in short courses to prevent predictably recurring (e.g., menstrual) migraine

ABBREVIATIONS: CNS, central nervous system; hs, before bed.

and atenolol may have fewer neurologic effects because they are hydrophilic and, therefore, cross the blood-brain barrier less easily than the other agents.

The effective dose for each patient can be determined only by experience over several months of monitoring change in migraine activity, blood pressure, and side effects. It is surprising to note that patients who do not respond to one beta-blocking agent may do well with another.

Antidepressants The tricyclic antidepressant amitriptyline is widely used for migraine prophylaxis in doses of 50 to 200 mg/d, usually taken at night before sleep. Because of its anticholinergic effects, amitriptyline is not appropriate for patients with glaucoma, cardiac arrhythmias, or prostatism, and is a poor choice for elderly individuals. Published reports indicate widely varying effectiveness and recommended dosage. The effect on migraine is probably independent of its antidepressant properties.

There is surprisingly little research on the ability of other antidepressants, including tricyclics other than amitriptyline and selective serotonin reuptake inhibitors, to prevent migraine headaches. None of these other medications is approved for migraine prophylaxis by the U.S. Food and Drug Administration.

Other Drugs In spite of limited data, many other drugs have been used for migraine prophylaxis. Verapamil, a calcium channel blocking agent, may reduce the severity as well as the frequency of attacks in selected patients, but it is not universally effective. Divalproex sodium, an anticonvulsant drug containing a combination of valproic acid and sodium valproate, is effective in reducing headache frequency by about 40 percent, but it has several side effects, including tremor, alopecia, and rare occurrences of hepatotoxicity. Methysergide is effective for migraine prophylaxis but is not widely used because of the rare but serious side effects of retroperitoneal and endocardial fibrosis.

The NSAIDs, especially naproxyn, can be used for migraine prophylaxis. In predictable menstrual migraines, daily NSAID use starting 3 to 5 days before the expected onset of menses and continuing until the second day of flow can prevent or ameliorate headache symptoms.

SYMPTOMATIC TREATMENT OF ESTABLISHED MIGRAINE ATTACK   Nearly all migraine attacks ultimately resolve, even without treatment. Once a migraine headache develops, therefore, the goal of therapy is to minimize symptoms until the attack subsides. The most troublesome symptoms for patients are usually headache, nausea and vomiting, and exhaustion, and it is important that patients prioritize the symptoms for which treatment is most needed.

Treatments involve both nonpharmacologic and pharmacologic interventions. Nonpharmacologic interventions include biofeedback (usually with finger temperature), use of cold compresses, changing positions and activities, and sleep. Once patients seek care from a clinician, however, it is likely that medications will be required to diminish headache severity. For individual patients, the choice of medication depends on many factors, including type and severity of symptoms, vulnerability (if any) to side effects, available routes of administration (particularly the inability to use oral medications because of vomiting), side effects, cost, and how much value is placed on being able to "keep going" as opposed to "sleeping it off." The four main categories of medications for treating migraine headache include analgesics, antiemetics, ergotamines, and 5-HT-receptor agonists.

Analgesics and Antiemetics   When using analgesic and antiemetic medications, the lowest effective dose (Table 10-4) is the appropriate therapy. Combining analgesics with antiemetics, especially metoclopramide, is helpful because of synergy between the two types of medication. Rectal suppositories and injections are unpopular with patients but may be necessary if vomiting precludes ingestion of oral medication.

Table 10-4

Medications for Symptomatic Treatment of Migraine Headache

CATEGORY	MEDICATION AND DOSE
Analgesics	Aspirin, 350–650 mg q4h PO
	Acetaminophen, 500–1300 mg q4h PO
	Ibuprofen, 200–800 mg q4h PO
	Naproxyn, 275–550 mg bid PO
	Midrin* 2 caps × 1, then 1 q2h
	Ketorolac 30–60 mg IM
Antiemetics	Metoclopramide 5–10 mg PO or IM
	Promethazine 25 mg IM or PR
	Prochlorperazine 5–10 mg IM
Ergotamines	Ergotamine/caffeine (1–2 mg of ergotamine with 100 mg of caffeine) PO or PR
	Dihydroergotamine 1–4 mg IM, IV, or nasal spray
5-HT_1=receptor agonists	Sumatriptan 25–100 mg PO or 6 mg SC
	Zolmitriptan 2.5–5.0 mg PO

*Combination of isometheptane mucate (65 mg), dichloralphenazone (100 mg), and acetaminophen (325 mg).
NOTE: Medications are only one aspect of headache management. Patients should also consider life-style modifications, biofeedback, and relaxation techniques. Sleep may resolve many attacks without medication. If attack persists 3 days, consider prednisone 20–40 mg or hospital admission for hydration and intravenous ergotamine therapy.
ABBREVIATIONS: IM, intramuscularly; PO, orally; PR, per rectum; SC, subcutaneously; IV, intravenously; 5-HT, 5-hydroxytryptamine.

Treatment of migraine with narcotics, benzo-diazepines, barbiturates, and similar drugs should be discouraged. These drugs are frequently prescribed for migraine, however, either alone or in combinations with other analgesics (e.g., butalbital is combined with caffeine and acetaminophen in drugs such as Fiorinol and Fioricet). Use of these drugs risks "hangover" after an attack and raises concern about drug dependency in patients who have frequent migraine headaches. Furthermore, controlled trials have shown no advantage of these drugs over adequate dosages of the nonnarcotic analgesics or antiemetics shown in Table 10-4. With adequate analgesia, benzodiazepines and similar sedative drugs are rarely necessary because migraine attacks naturally end in sleep.

Ergotamines The ergotamines (ergot alkaloid derivatives) have a long tradition of use in migraine headache. Their action probably de-pends on direct effects on the neurotransmitter defects that causes migraine and also on their vasoconstrictive effect. Although effective and popular with many patients, their use is limited by nausea, vasoconstriction, bioavailability, and "rebound" headaches between doses when taken on more than 2 d/week or in dosages of over 10 mg/week. Practical considerations in prescribing include the need for awareness that other agents (mainly sedatives and atropine) are incorporated into the most popular formulations of oral and rectal ergotamines. In addition, ergotamines are sometimes unavailable to patients, since manufacturers have withdrawn several ergotamine-based medications from the commercial market.

Ergotamines may be given orally, sublingually, by injection, by nasal spray, or by rectal suppository (Table 10-4). They are most effective when taken early during a migraine attack, ideally during the aura or prodromal phase of the headache. Since ergotamines can cause considerable nausea, patients need to establish the lowest dose that is effective in terminating an early migraine headache but does not cause nausea. For many, this requires using fractions of standard doses, including suppositories (it is possible to create fractional doses of suppositories if they are first hardened in the refrigerator and then cut). Injectable ergotamines are useful in clinic or emergency room settings, where protocols usually include pretreatment with metoclopramide.

5-Hydroxytryptamine Receptor Agonists The effect of 5-HT-receptor agonists is based on the origin of migraine in the abnormal functioning of the serotonergic system. The prototype drug, sumatriptan, is available as a subcutaneous injection (6 mg) and oral tablets (25 and 50 mg). Subcutaneous injection is a somewhat more effective route of administration. Zolmitriptan is also available for use only by the oral route. Several other similar agents, including naratriptan, eletriptan, and rizatriptan, are expected to be available in the near future.

Effectiveness Sumatriptan can dramatically relieve migraine in some patients, even when taken during a well-established headache. It has become a popular treatment for migraine, advocated by many as the treatment of choice. However, early clinical studies and marketing may have overestimated its efficacy. A relatively recent, large double-blind study comparing sumatriptan to a combination of aspirin and metoclopramide found comparable symptom relief with both treatments, but higher cost and more side effects with sumatriptan.

Published trials of sumatriptan indicate that many patients (up to 40 percent) experience the return of headache after initial clearing, making repetitive administration necessary. This percentage may be lower in primary care practice, perhaps due to selection of more severe cases for the published drug studies. When headaches recur, pain returns up to 4 h after resolution of the initial symptoms. Discussion beforehand of the possibility of return of headache and instructions to take a second dose of sumatriptan, possibly with an antiemetic or analgesic agents, enables patients to be confident in managing their migraine.

Zolmitriptan, which is administered orally, has similar effects. A potential advantage of zolmitriptan is that its absorption is not affected by the presence of food in the stomach. About 40 percent of patients experience complete elimination of headache symptoms, and another 20 to 30 percent report substantial relief of headache within 4 h. As with sumatriptan, however, headache recurrence occurs, typically in about one-third of patients.

Contraindications and Side Effects Currently available 5-HT-receptor agonists should not be used in hypertensive or pregnant patients because of their vasoconstrictor effects. Similarly, caution is urged in older patients and those with cardiovascular risk factors because of the risk of coronary artery vasoconstriction. Concerns about vasoconstriction also make 5-HT receptor agonists inappropriate for patients who have recently used other vasoconstrictor drugs, including ergotamine and monoamine oxidase inhibitors.

Some patients experience an unpleasant acute autonomic reaction described as "like a panic attack," characterized by flushing, tingling, palpitations, "spaciness," and nausea, that occurs approximately 15 to 30 min after taking oral sumatriptan. These symptoms presumably represent a state of serotonergic excess. The symptoms do not last long and can often be prevented during future sumatriptan treatment by reducing the dose. If it is discussed beforehand, patients tolerate this effect and may even see it as a positive indication that the drug is working. Some patients report that the effect lessens after using sumatriptan over several months. There is too little experience with other 5-HT agonists to fully itemize their side effects, but they are likely to be similar to those of sumatriptan.

Other Treatments When patients do not respond to seemingly adequate treatment, clinicians should consider noncompliance as a possible cause. In addition, they should explore whether medications are being administered improperly or not being absorbed. If absorption is a concern because of vomiting, rectal suppositories or injectable medications (e.g., subcutaneous sumatriptan) can be considered. If compliance and absorption are not thought to be a problem, treatment with other medications, such as corticosteroids or intranasal lidocaine, can be considered.

Corticosteroids Corticosteroids may help terminate prolonged attacks. If steroids are necessary, however, the patient should be evaluated for dehydration and to confirm the diagnosis of migraine. Hospitalization for aggressive therapy with parenteral ergotamines, analgesic, antiemetics, or steroids may be appropriate in severe cases.

Intranasal Lidocaine Intranasal lidocaine is administered by dripping 0.5 mL of a 4% solution into the nose while the patient lies with the head hyperextended to 45° and rotated 30° to the side of the headache. When used in primary care settings, about half of patients will receive rapid relief, although return of headache, usually within an hour after treatment, occurs in about 40 percent of those who respond.

TENSION HEADACHE

Patients with tension headaches frequently ingest large quantities of analgesics but use these medications inappropriately. Thus, in designing an optimal treatment plan, it is important to establish what has already been tried and how it has been administered. In addition, clinicians should identify risk factors for medication side effects (particularly the risk of gastrointestinal bleeding from NSAIDs), and the presence and need for treatment of concomitant depression.

Management of tension headaches is a neglected research area, leaving clinicians unsupported by scientific evidence on which to base treatments. Based on experience and empirical evidence, however, a common treatment strategy for patients with chronic recurrent tension headaches includes both non-pharmacologic modalities and medications. Regardless of the treatment used, follow-up contact with patients by telephone or in the office is important for monitoring progress, encouraging compliance with treatment, and identifying the rare patient in whom the headache is caused by an intracranial pathologic condition.

NON-PHARMACOLOGIC TREATMENTS Daily vigorous exercise is frequently recommended to reduce the frequency of tension headaches. Typically, the type of exercise is determined by the patient's preferences. In addition, relaxation and stress-reduction techniques are frequently recommended both for prevention and treatment of tension headaches. These techniques include meditation, yoga, breathing exercises, isometric contraction-relaxation exercises of the neck muscles, and other modalities.

MEDICATIONS When headaches occur, patients can use a first-line analgesic, such as acetaminophen, aspirin, or other NSAIDs daily for 3 to 7 days. Doses are similar to those used for migraine headache (Table 10-4). In addition, patients should have a supplemental "rescue" medication available, usually another first-line analgesic medication, to take when pain recurs or persists despite use of their regular analgesic.

Evidence indicates that anti-migraine agents may be useful for tension headaches, serving as a backup to more conventional analgesic treatments. This recommendation is based on new discoveries suggesting that the pathophysiologic processes in tension headaches may be similar to those of migraine. Most clinicians, however, have not yet adopted a practice of treating classic tension headaches with ergotamines or 5-HT receptor agonists.

Antidepressants also have a place in the management of patients with chronic tension headaches, even in the absence of depression. Amitriptyline, nortriptyline, or doxepin in small doses, and more recently selective serotonin reuptake inhibitors, have been advocated as supplementary treatments for tension headaches. The choice of the individual agent is usually based on side-effect profile and other characteristics of the patient.

Patients with particularly severe or prolonged tension headaches were previously often treated with narcotic or benzodiazepine agents, in spite of the risks of dependence or rebound headaches. Most experts now consider these medications inappropriate.

CLUSTER HEADACHE

Since cluster headaches are rare, few large controlled studies are available to guide therapy. Management is based on the dual strategy of suppressing the cluster and providing symptom relief for any breakthrough headaches. Patients should also avoid alcohol and any other trigger substances, such as monosodium glutamate, during a cluster period.

SUPPRESSION   Suppression of the cluster can be achieved with steroids, verapamil, or lithium (Table 10-5). Assuming the patient has no contraindications, steroids can be started at the onset of a cluster of headaches. A typical dosing regimen is prednisone 20 to 40 mg/d for 3 to 5 days and then 10 mg/d for 10 days. Some prednisone regimens involve a longer period of treatment and tapering (Table 10-5). Prednisone may be used alone or in combination with verapamil (240 mg/d). Verapamil can then be continued until it is believed the cluster has completed its course. Lithium (300 to 900 mg/d) is an older therapy; while effective, it has many side effects. Methysergide and divalproex have also been recommended, but, as with lithium, side effects are

more frequent than with short courses of oral steroids.

PAIN RELIEF   Analgesic use for acute cluster headache is limited by the need for rapid onset of action, because any one headache within the cluster may resolve before an analgesic can take effect. Some patients can predict attacks with sufficient accuracy to take oral analgesics (e.g., NSAIDs) prior to the attack. In general, however, the rapid onset and relatively short duration of attacks require injected or inhaled medications. Inhaled oxygen (8 L/min by mask) is probably the treatment of choice. Intranasal lidocaine (4%) can be effective but is difficult to use in cluster headache patients, who are often agitated or restless. Patients or family members may also be comfortable using injections of ketorolac or sumatriptan. Ergotamines taken by suppository or sublingually are useful, but patients must be screened for contraindications. The older age and male predominance of cluster headaches means that many patients will have renal, hepatic, and cardiac (including hypertension) contraindications to ergotamine therapy.

SECONDARY AND MIXED HEADACHES

Secondary headaches require treatment of the underlying cause as well as appropriate analgesia to control pain. Treatment for mixed headaches should be directed at the headache type to which the patient's symptoms are most similar.

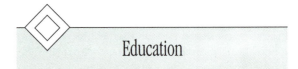

Education

Education plays an essential role in enabling patients to appropriately manage recurrent or chronic headaches with medical "coaching." Unfortunately, however, clinicians frequently de-

Table 10-5

Pharmacologic Treatment of Cluster Headache

	Dose	Common Side Effects	Comments
Suppression			
Prednisone	20–60 mg/d tapered over 2–4 weeks	GI upset, euphoria	Rebound when stopped
Verapamil	240–360 mg/d	GI upset	May be combined with prednisone
Lithium	300–900 mg/d	Diarrhea, nausea	Not in renal, cardiac disease
Divalproex	250–1000 mg	Nausea, weight gain, sedation, hair loss, hepatic damage	Not in hepatic disease
Acute Attacks			
100% oxygen	8 Liters/min for 10 min		Awkward to use
Lidocaine	4% intranasal		Awkward to use
Ketorolac	30–60 mg IM	GI upset or bleeding	Renal toxicity with prolonged use
Ergotamine	Suppository, sublingual	Vasoconstriction, nausea	Can use rectal or oral dose at onset of attacks
Sumatriptan	SC or oral	Not approved	Not in hypertension or angina

ABBREVIATIONS: GI, gastrointestinal; IM, intramuscularly; SC, subcutaneously.

liver educational information without first ascertaining the patient's beliefs, understandings, and fears. Headache patients and their families, along with coworkers and friends, may have fixed concepts of what causes headache, its most appropriate management, and its likely prognosis. Unless addressed, these preexisting concepts may interfere with even the best management plan.

Information must often be repeated and reinforced before patients incorporate it into their belief systems and daily routines. Printed materials and Internet sites can supplement education in appropriately motivated patients. Unfortunately, however, much commercially available educational material for patients is biased by personal perspectives, pharmaceutical company sponsorship, or other motivations; thus, this material must be carefully reviewed by clinicians before being given to patients.

Diagnosis and Causation

Patients should understand that headache is a symptom for which many diagnoses are possible. They should also understand that individual patients can have more than one type of headache, that headache types are not always clearly defined, and that neuroimaging is rarely essential because diagnosis is usually based on history alone. Recognizing that they can have more than one type of headache (e.g., a migraine patient who develops sinusitis) can relieve anxiety when headache symptoms change.

Many patients blame themselves for being vulnerable to headaches. Thus, it may be useful to explain that current evidence suggests that both tension and migraine headaches represent the effects of environmental or biological triggers on an underlying biochemical or neurologic vulnerability. A useful analogy is to compare headaches to diabetes or asthma, in which a predisposition to the condition is inherited, and symptoms can episodically worsen if there are inappropriate life-style behaviors or non-compliance with treatment.

Patients and others may also have beliefs about personality traits in headache sufferers. Many migraine patients never consult clinicians, suggesting that some migraineurs may be reluctant to disclose their condition to others for fear of being labeled as having a "migraine personality." In reality, there is no specific migraine personality but, rather, a wide variation in how migraine sufferers deal with and adjust to their headaches.

Prognosis

Although many textbooks and review articles state that tension and migraine headaches become less common with age, research to support this assertion is surprisingly sparse. Patients with both tension and migraine headaches should be counseled that they have a life-long vulnerability to headaches, but that the nature and frequency of attacks may change over time, as will the options available for management. Male patients can be told that they will probably have less frequent and less severe headaches as they age, but some may develop other headache syndromes. In women, menopause is reported to bring relief of migraine headaches, but there is minimal evidence to support this.

It may be appropriate to inform selected migraine patients that they have a slightly increased risk of stroke, epilepsy, and depression. However, migraine is also associated with lower rates of cardiovascular disease. These weak associations should not be over-emphasized and are only useful in encouraging patients to follow a healthy life-style.

Family Approach

Families vary enormously and unpredictably in their attitudes and behaviors regarding headaches. Most patients with migraine and tension headaches have relatives with the same conditions. Thus, expectations and coping behaviors may be conditioned by family experience and can range from using headaches to manipulate the family to stoical "no fuss" patterns of behavior.

When there is no family history of migraine, the first episode of migraine in a family member can be a frightening experience. This is particularly true when the patient is a teenager. In families with migraine history, the first headache can sometimes be anticipated because, it is interesting to note, the child who suffers most from motion sickness often turns out to be the migraineur.

Many migraine families struggle with helplessness and frustration because planned family events have to be deferred or canceled (many migraines occur with the relief of tension at weekends). In addition, families frequently experience anxiety because of concerns that the patient is not getting the best treatment, that there may be a more serious diagnosis than migraine, or that others in the family will develop the condition. In addition, the practical aspects of migraine (e.g., dark rooms, bans on cooking smells, arrangements for vomiting, and even explaining screams and crying to neighbors) are also stressful. Migraine families all have stories about embarrassing situations caused by the condition, and may enjoy the collection of such stories in a book by Sacks (see Bibliography).

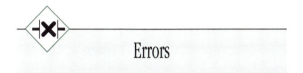

Errors

Primary care clinicians make three common errors in the treatment of headache: inappropriate overuse of narcotic analgesics, inappropriate underuse of nonnarcotic medications, and failure to develop a therapeutic clinician-patient relationship.

Inappropriate Overuse of Narcotic Analgesics

Perhaps the most common error in treating headaches is the inappropriate use of narcotic analgesics. This includes treating acute headaches with parenteral narcotics and giving patients oral or intranasal narcotics for home use.

Narcotic agents are rarely, if ever, indicated for treating headaches because other medications are more effective. Clinical trials involving migraine patients presenting to emergency rooms consistently demonstrate that adequate treatment with nonnarcotic agents (usually combined with antiemetics), antiemetics alone, or dihydroergotamine yield comparable or superior results to those obtained with narcotics and are associated with fewer side effects. For cluster headaches, administration of oxygen is a superior treatment, and headaches frequently resolve before narcotics would have time to achieve a therapeutic effect. Furthermore, because of the chronic and recurrent nature of most headache problems, narcotic use in headache can be complicated by abuse or dependence. For all of these reasons, narcotic use for treatment of headache should be discouraged.

Inappropriate Underuse of Nonnarcotic Treatments

First-line analgesics, such as acetaminophen, aspirin, and other NSAIDs, are frequently given in insufficient dosage or are not absorbed, leading to a perception that these medications are not sufficiently powerful for headache treatment. These analgesics should be administered in maximum anti-inflammatory doses. If patients have significant emesis, parenteral administration (e.g., intramuscular ketorolac) is preferred to ensure adequate absorption.

Similarly, nausea and vomiting are, for some patients, the most troublesome symptoms of an acute headache. Thus, antiemetic agents should be incorporated into the therapeutic regimen for many patients. In treating migraine, primary care clinicians frequently underuse appropriate alternative and second-line treatments, especially 5-HT agonists and ergotamine, and instead rely on narcotics when first-line therapies fail.

Problems in the Clinician-Patient Relationship

Many clinicians lack confidence in diagnosing and treating headaches, resulting in a lack of enthusiasm for treating headache patients. These feelings stem from the fact that patients with headaches often present with long-term chronic problems that do not resolve, the lack of objective symptoms, and a small but ever-present potential for missing an important diagnosis (i.e., intracranial pathology). In addition, patients with chronic recurrent headaches may be perceived as demonstrating "drug-seeking" behavior. Reference has already been made to the therapeutic power of patients' feeling that their concerns have been heard and the large placebo effect in headache treatment. These effects are easily lost if a clinician's lack of enthusiasm for headache management is transmitted to patients.

A related concern is that many clinicians focus too much attention on excluding the rare possibility of intracranial pathology, presumably because they are more comfortable with such a medical evaluation. While it is certainly important to provide patients with well-communicated assurances that no serious abnormalities are present, the therapeutic clinician-patient relationship will be lessened by concentration on ordering diagnostic tests instead of on selection of medications, adequate dosage, compliance, use of synergistic agents, and patients' expectations for treatment.

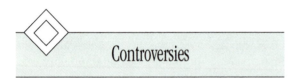

Controversies

Among controversial areas in headache management, several are pertinent to primary care practice.

Use of Diagnostic Imaging

Most studies on the role of diagnostic imaging (CT, MRI, positron emission tomography, etc.) come from tertiary care institutions and are not directly applicable to primary care practice because of the different frequency of structural neurologic abnormalities in primary care versus tertiary care patient populations. A recent review estimates the chances of detection of a "potentially treatable lesion" in patients with unspecified headache referred for radiologic investigation as between 0.4 and 2.4 percent, but the corresponding figures in primary care practice are unknown. While a National Institutes of Health consensus panel recommends that CT or MRI scans be obtained in patients with atypical headaches and neurologic signs or symptoms, the specific situations in which imaging is likely to be worthwhile have not been defined. The role of neuroimaging in primary care practice

and the role of positron emission tomography scans and other advanced imaging techniques for evaluating headaches in any practice setting remain unclear.

Use of Female Hormones (Contraception and Hormone Replacement Therapy)

Many reviews and texts offer the advice that oral contraceptives and post-menopausal hormone replacement therapy should not be used in women with migraine. This advice appears to be based on the perceived danger of exacerbating migraine attacks and/or contributing to the risk of stroke through the vasoconstrictive or thrombogenic actions of estrogen.

ORAL CONTRACEPTIVES

Although it is commonly stated that about half of women with migraine experience exacerbations when using oral contraceptives, this figure is based on studies with older, high-estrogen preparations. With current oral contraceptive formulations, the risk of exacerbating migraine may be as low as 5 percent, and some patients actually report improvement in migraine when cycles are regulated by oral contraceptives. Research data are not helpful for determining which patients will experience exacerbations of headache. Further investigations are needed to identify whether and which migraine patients are most appropriate candidates for oral contraceptive use.

For now, assuming there is no other risk factor for stroke or contraindication to oral contraception, the best evidence is that these medications can be prescribed to women with migraine. These women should be advised that hormone changes can influence migraine in unpredictable ways and that at least a 3-month trial is usually necessary to judge how they will react to oral contraception.

Patients who experience exacerbation of migraine but for whom oral contraception is the birth control method of choice can often be managed by continuing oral contraceptives and instituting more aggressive management of the headaches. Change of first-line therapy and/or addition of preventive therapy may be appropriate. Since attacks often occur around the time of breakthrough bleeding, use of NSAIDs or cyclical prolongation of estrogen levels using supplemental oral estrogen have been suggested.

POSTMENOPAUSAL HORMONE REPLACEMENT THERAPY

There is surprisingly little research evidence to support the long-held belief that headaches, especially migraine, disappear at menopause and are exacerbated by postmenopausal hormone replacement therapy (HRT). Many textbooks and other sources now state that women experience exacerbations of headaches around the time of menopause and can benefit from HRT. The HRT regimens with sustained estrogen levels are said to be most beneficial, while those with progestins and/or fluctuating estrogen levels are thought to negatively influence headache. Other observations are that synthetic estrogens are less strongly associated with headache than are naturally derived products and that addition of testosterone is also beneficial. While some of these statements and observations may be valid, primary care practice would benefit from research on the role of HRT for peri- and postmenopausal patients who have chronic headaches.

Emerging Concepts

Many new concepts in our understanding and management of headaches have already been mentioned, such as the notion that tension and migraine headache may have a common pathophysiologic basis. Research into the pathophysi-

ology and pharmacology of neurotransmitters and headache, especially migraine, is active and likely to provide important new understandings and new therapies in the future. The development of several additional 5-HT agonists is probably just the first step in developing new pharmacologic approaches to headache management. In addition to identifying new medications, research is likely to identify techniques to predict which patients will develop which headache syndromes and who will respond to which specific treatment strategies.

New neuroimaging techniques, including positron emission tomography (PET) scans, single photon emission computed tomography (SPECT), and others, will likely enhance our understanding of the pathophysiology of migraine, as well as offer new possibilities for diagnosis and classification of headache syndromes.

Bibliography

Akpek S, Arac M, Atilla S, et al: Cost-effectiveness of computed tomography in the evaluation of patients with headache. *Headache* 35:228, 1995.

Becker LA, Green LA, Beaufait D, et al: Use of CT scans for the investigation of headache: I. A report from ASPN. *J Fam Pract* 37:129, 1993.

Becker LA, Green LA, Beaufait D, et al: Detection of intracranial tumors, subarachnoid hemorrhages, and subdural hematomas in primary care patients: II. A report from ASPN. *J Fam Pract* 37:135, 1993.

Becker L, Iverson DC, Reed FM, et al: Patients with new headache in primary care: A report from ASPN. *J Fam Pract* 27:41, 1988.

Boureau F, Joubert JM, Lasserre V, et al: Double-blind comparison of an acetaminophen 400 mg–codeine 25 mg combination versus aspirin 1000 mg and placebo in acute migraine attack. *Cephalgia* 14:156, 1994.

Capobianco DJ, Cheshire WP, Campbell JK: An overview of the diagnosis and pharmacologic treatment of migraine. *Mayo Clin Proc* 71:1055, 1996.

Davis CP, Torre PR, Williams C, et al: Ketorolac versus meperidine plus promethazine treatment of migraine headache: evaluations by patients. *Am J Emerg Med* 13:146, 1995.

Frishberg BM: The utility of neuroimaging in the evaluation of headache in patients with normal neurologic examinations. *Neurology* 44:1191, 1994.

Harden RN, Gracely RH, Carter T, et al: The placebo effect in acute headache management: Ketorolac, meperidine, and saline in the emergency department. *Headache* 36:352, 1996.

Headache Classification Committee of the International Headache Society: Classification and diagnostic criteria for headache disorders, cranial neuralgias and facial pain. *Cephalgia* 8 8(suppl 7):1, 1988.

Linet MS, Celentano DD, Stewart WF: Headache characteristic associated with clinician consultation: A population-based study. *Am J Prev Med* 7:40, 1991.

Linet MS, Stewart WF, Celentano DD, et al: An epidemiologic study of headache among adolescents and young adults. *JAMA* 261:2211, 1989.

Maizels M, Scott B, Cohen W, et al: Intranasal lidocaine for treatment of migraine: A randomized, double-blind, controlled trial. *JAMA* 276:319, 1996.

Mitchell CS, Osborne RE, Grosskreutz SR: Computed tomography in the headache patient: Is routine evaluation really necessary? *Headache* 33:82, 1993.

Moore KL, Noble SL: Drug treatment of migraine: I. Acute therapy and drug-rebound headache. *Am Fam Phys* 56:2039, 1997.

Muller JL, Causon KA: Pharmaceutical considerations of common herbal medicine. *Am J Managed Care* 3:1753, 1997.

Noble SL, Moore KL: Drug treatment of migraine. II: Preventive therapy. *Am Fam Phys* 56:2279, 1997.

Robbins LD: *Management of Headache and Headache Medications.* New York, Springer-Verlag, 1994.

Sacks O: *Migraine.* Boston, Faber and Faber, 1991.

Scherl ER, Wilson JF: Comparison of dihydroergotamine with metoclopramide versus meperidine with promethazine in the treatment of acute migraine. *Headache* 35:256, 1995.

Schwartz BS, Stewart WF, Simon D, et al: Epidemiology of tension-type headache. *JAMA* 279:381, 1998.

Smith R: Chronic headaches in family practice. *J Am Board Fam Pract* 5:589, 1992.

Stewart WF, Lipton RB, Celentano DD, et al: Prevalence of migraine headache in the United States: Relation to age, income, race, and other sociodemographic factors. *JAMA* 267:64, 1992.

Tepper SL: Recent advances in antimigraine therapy: A clinical overview of zolmitriptan's efficacy and tolerability. *Postgrad Med* Special Report (Jan):20, 1998.

Tfelt-Hansen P, Henry P, Mulder LJ, et al: The effectiveness of combined oral lysine acetylsalicylate and metoclopramide compared with oral sumatriptan for migraine. *Lancet* 346:923, 1995.

Van Gijn J: Slip-ups in diagnosis of subarachnoid hemorrhage. *Lancet* 349:1492, 1997.

Weingarten S, Kleinman M, Elperin L, et al: The effectiveness of cerebral imaging in the diagnosis of chronic headache. *Arch Intern Med* 152:2457, 1992.

Welch KMA: Clinical Crossroads: A 27-year-old woman with migraine headaches. *JAMA* 278:322, 1997.

Woodwell DA: *National Ambulatory Care Survey: 1995 Summary. Vital and Health Statistics,* publication no. 286. Hyattsville, MD, National Center for Health Statistics, 1997.

Jay A. Swedberg

Chapter

11

Osteoarthritis

How Common Is Osteoarthritis?

Osteoarthritis is the most common form of arthritis seen in primary care practice, with a prevalence in the U.S. population of approximately 15 to 18 percent. The prevalence increases with age, with symptomatic osteoarthritis affecting 20 to 30 percent of individuals over 65 years of age. As the condition progresses in severity, patients may experience significant limitations of function, loss of independence, and diminished quality of life. In 2 to 3 percent of individuals with osteoarthritis, the condition results in long-term disability. Osteoarthritis is a major contributor to the use of health care services by older individuals, resulting in over 100,000 total hip arthroplasties and 120,000 total knee arthroplasties each year in the United States.

Principal Diagnoses

When older patients present to a primary care clinician with joint pain, four times out of five it is due to osteoarthritis. Pain that has been present for more than a few weeks in patients over age 55 is particularly suggestive of osteoarthritis.

Despite the prevalence of osteoarthritis, however, other causes of arthritis should always be considered for patients with joint pain. The most important of these are infectious arthritis (septic joint), crystal-induced arthritis (gout or pseudo-gout), and rheumatoid arthritis. Each of these common conditions is briefly discussed below. Additional causes of arthritis that are infrequently (but occasionally) seen in primary care practice include psoriatic arthritis, arthritis associated with connective tissue disorders other than rheumatoid arthritis (e.g., systemic lupus erythematosus), and infection-associated arthritis

(e.g., Lyme disease, Reiter's syndrome, Kawasaki's disease, viral hepatitis, non-specific viral infections, and others).

Osteoarthritis

Osteoarthritis is not a single disease with a single cause. Rather, a number of distinct but overlapping processes lead to the common clinical and pathologic manifestations of osteoarthritis. A recent national consensus conference developed the following definition of osteoarthritis: "Osteoarthritis is a group of overlapping distinct diseases which may have different etiologies but with similar biologic, morphologic, and clinical outcomes. The disease process not only affects the articular cartilage, but it involves the entire joint, including the subchondral bone, ligaments, capsule, synovial membranes, and periarticular muscles. Ultimately, the articular cartilage degenerates with fibrillation, fissures, ulceration, and full thickness loss of joint surface."

Osteoarthritis is often classified as primary (idiopathic) or secondary. Primary idiopathic osteoarthritis, the common arthritis seen in older individuals, does not have a clearly identifiable precipitating injury, condition, or event. It may be localized to one joint or a generalized process involving multiple joints. Secondary osteoarthritis is the result of an identifiable condition or injury that initiates degenerative osteoarthritic processes within a joint and surrounding structures. Thus, osteoarthritis may follow trauma to a joint or be associated with metabolic disorders (hemochromatosis, Wilson's disease, or alkaptonuria), endocrine disorders (acromegaly, hyperparathyroidism, or diabetes), crystal-induced arthritis (gout or pseudo-gout), or inflammatory arthropathy (rheumatoid or other connective tissue diseases).

EPIDEMIOLOGY

The prevalence of osteoarthritis progressively increases with age, and age is the strongest risk factor for development of osteoarthritis. Aging alone, however, does not cause osteoarthritis; thus, osteoarthritis is considered to be age related but not age dependent.

In addition to age, other risk factors for osteoarthritis include major joint trauma, repetitive stress or joint overload, obesity, genetic predisposition, and increased bone density. Osteoarthritis, in turn, is a risk factor for disability. The prevalence of disability is further increased when other chronic conditions (e.g., depression, heart disease, or lung disease) coexist with osteoarthritis, perhaps because these conditions interfere with an individual's ability to participate in rehabilitation or exercise programs.

PATHOGENESIS

The cause of osteoarthritis is not fully understood. As described later under "Controversies," various theories have been put forth to explain the development of osteoarthritis, but none fully clarifies the process.

The basic pathologic problem in osteoarthritis is that the normal equilibrium between synthesis and degradation of articular cartilage becomes unbalanced or poorly regulated. Current evidence suggests that the normal balance between synthesis and degradation of articular cartilage is maintained through cytokine-driven anabolic and catabolic processes. For example, interleukin-1 and tumor necrosis factor have been identified as cytokines that induce production of metalloproteinases (e.g., collagenase and stomelysin), which degrade macromolecules in the cartilage matrix. Other cytokines, such as insulin-like growth factor and transforming growth factor-β, inhibit metalloproteinase production, thereby limiting degradation of cartilage and promoting cartilage synthesis and repair. It is thought that if the catabolic processes mediated by the metalloproteinase-inducing factors predominate over reparative processes for an extended period of time, joint changes typical of osteoarthritis will develop.

Because cartilage, synovial membrane, and subchondral bone are closely interrelated, a change in one component of the joint invariably affects other components. Thus, damage to cartilage exposes underlying bone to abnormal stress, resulting in hypertrophy (increased density or sclerosis), cyst formation, and bone enlargement (osteophytes). The synovium responds to changes in subchondral bone and cartilage with mild inflammation.

Infectious Arthritis (Septic Joint)

When evaluating a patient with joint pain, it is essential to consider the possibility of septic arthritis, an acute bacterial infection within the joint space. If not diagnosed early, septic arthritis can rapidly damage a joint. It is essential to drain the joint (by serial arthrocentesis or surgical drainage) to reduce intra-articular pressure and the concentration of lytic enzymes found in pus. In addition, appropriate antibiotics must be administered.

Septic arthritis typically presents with rapid onset of joint pain, tenderness, and warmth, along with fever and/or chills. *Neisseria gonorrhea* is the most common cause of septic joint in many urban populations. The most common cause of non-gonococcal septic arthritis is *Staphylococcus aureus*, followed in frequency by group A and group B streptococcus. Non-gonococcal septic arthritis is more common in impaired hosts who have bacteremia (e.g., intravenous drug abusers with subacute bacterial endocarditis) or an abnormal joint (pre-existing rheumatoid arthritis, previous traumatic injury, or a prosthetic joint).

Crystal-Induced Arthritis

Crystal-induced arthritis is an acute or chronic joint inflammation caused by crystal deposition within the synovial cavity. Gout occurs with deposition of sodium urate (uric acid) crystals. Pseudo-gout occurs with deposition of calcium pyrophosphate dihydrate crystals. Crystal deposition leads to an acute inflammatory process associated with phagocytosis of crystals by polymorphonuclear leukocytes and release of chemotactic factors and other mediators of inflammation.

Gout

Gout, the most common crystal-induced arthritis, generally presents with a rapid onset of self-limited monoarthritis. In some patients, however, the condition is polyarticular. Gout typically involves the metatarsophalangeal joint of the great toe, another joint of the foot or ankle, or the knee. The prevalence of gout is about 1.5 percent in the general population, and its frequency increases with age. It most often occurs in men and postmenopausal women with hyperuricemia or a family history of gout. Hyperuricemia may be due to an idiopathic (probably genetic) increase in the synthesis or decrease in renal excretion of uric acid. Secondary causes of hyperuricemia include conditions with rapid turnover of cells (e.g., leukemia, chronic hemolytic anemia, psoriasis, sarcoidosis, and multiple myeloma) and medications that interfere with excretion of urate, such as thiazide diuretics, low-dose aspirin, or nicotinic acid.

Patients with gout usually have asymptomatic periods of months or years between acute attacks. During attacks, however, the affected joint is swollen, red, and warm, and the patient may be febrile. The diagnosis is made by identifying urate crystals in synovial fluid; in more advanced cases, the diagnosis can sometimes be made radiographically. Treatment for uncomplicated gout involves oral anti-inflammatory drugs, sometimes including colchicine. Anti-hyperuricemic medications will reduce the likelihood of recurrent attacks.

Pseudogout

Pseudogout, or calcium pyrophosphate deposition disease, also typically presents with acute joint inflammation, often associated with leukocytosis and fever. In some patients, however, pseudogout is manifest as a chronic polyarthritis. Calcium pyrophosphate crystals may be identified in joint fluid. More commonly, however, the diagnosis is made when the typical finding of calcified intra-articular cartilage (chondrocalcinosis) is seen on joint radiographs. Treatment most often involves non-steroidal anti-inflammatory drugs and, on occasion, intra-articular steroid injections.

Rheumatoid Arthritis

Rheumatoid arthritis is a chronic inflammatory disorder that affects joints as well as non-articular tissues. This disease often occurs in the third or fourth decade but may begin at any age, including the geriatric years. Usually, several joints are affected in a symmetrical pattern, most commonly the metacarpophalangeal and proximal interphalangeal joints of the hands and feet, the wrists, and the knees. The natural course varies, ranging from mild, slowly progressive disease to severe, rapidly progressive destructive arthritis.

Rheumatoid arthritis occurs in approximately 1 percent of the population, but it is three times more common in women than in men. Rheumatoid arthritis is often familial, thought to be due to a genetic predisposition. It also has been hypothesized that joint inflammation in rheumatoid arthritis is caused by an infectious organism, but at this time the cause remains unknown. It is possible that more than one cause can produce the clinical picture of adult rheumatoid arthritis.

Typical Presentation

Patients with osteoarthritis usually go to their primary care clinician because of recurrent aching joint pains that either interfere with activities or cause fear of disability. Often, patients have already found some relief from heat or non-prescription analgesics, but pain recurs and gradually may worsen. They suspect arthritis and are concerned that symptoms will progress and become crippling. If the patient's history and physical examination are consistent with osteoarthritis, then the probable diagnosis *is* osteoarthritis; no further laboratory tests or x-rays are necessary. The key history and examination findings associated with osteoarthritis are described below. If symptoms or examination findings are atypical (suggesting some other form of arthritis) or the patient remains unduly concerned, additional studies or tests may be warranted.

In contrast, patients usually see rheumatologists or orthopedists when they have advanced disease or disability and when treatments prescribed in primary care settings have not afforded sufficient relief of symptoms. Orthopedic surgeons frequently see patients being considered for surgical procedures such as insertion of prosthetic joints to relieve symptoms and disability of osteoarthritis.

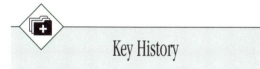

Key History

History is directed at determining whether a patient's symptoms are typical or atypical for osteoarthritis. Osteoarthritis causes slow-onset, deep, aching joint pains that remit and relapse. The pain is often aggravated by activity and relieved by rest. Patients often experience brief stiffness in the involved joints in the morning or after inactivity. This stiffness, however, lasts less than 30 min and is relieved by heat and movement of the joint. Stiffness that is body-wide or that lasts more than 30 min is atypical for osteoarthritis, and the presence of either should suggest the possibility of an inflammatory arthritis (i.e., rheumatoid arthritis or other collagen-vascular disorder).

Pain from osteoarthritis most often affects the hands, spine, knees, and hips. Pain in other locations would be unusual for osteoarthritis. Similarly, pain that is rapid in onset, throbbing, burning, or exquisitely tender would be unexpected in osteoarthritis. If such a history is elicited, diagnoses other than osteoarthritis should be considered. Systemic symptoms, such as fever, chills, rash, fatigue, and weight loss do not occur in osteoarthritis, and their presence should suggest inflammatory arthritis, infectious arthritis, or malignancy involving bone or joints.

Osteoarthritis of the spine causes back pain. In addition, neurologic symptoms, including sensory and/or motor problems in the arms or legs, may occur when osteoarthritic osteophytes cause stenosis of the spinal canal or impingement on nerve roots passing through neural foramina. Nerve root impingement in the cervical area is clinically manifested as radiculopathy in the upper extremities. Cervical spinal stenosis may also cause radiculopathies and/or myelopathic problems in the lower body, including bowel and bladder problems, lower extremity spasticity, and sensory abnormalities. Lumbar spinal stenosis is typically seen in older individuals. It causes pain radiating down the legs that is worse when walking upright and relieved by flexing forward or sitting.

Physical Examination

Physical examination is directed at determining whether the pain originates from a joint or whether it is referred pain or non-articular pain. Osteoarthritis pain (and the pain of any type of arthritis), by definition, originates from a joint. If the pain is joint-related, one must determine whether the findings are typical of osteoarthritis or of some other form of arthritis. In patients with symptoms of spinal osteoarthritis, the clinician must determine if there are neurologic abnormalities suggesting spinal stenosis, nerve root impingement, or a non-osteoarthritic back problem. Evaluation and treatment of patients with back pain are discussed in more detail in Chap. 12.

Does the Pain Originate in a Joint?

Pain originating in a joint typically occurs whether the joint undergoes passive or active movement. In contrast, non-articular pain occurs only (or is considerably worse) upon active movement. Thus, pain is likely to originate from within a joint if it occurs both when the examiner moves the joint and when the patient actively moves it. If the pain occurs only when the patient moves the joint but not when the clinician moves it passively, the pain is more likely to be non-articular.

Examples of non-articular pain that are often confused with osteoarthritis include the periarticular soft tissue inflammation seen in bursitis or tendinitis, and sciatica from lumbar disk disease that radiates into a patient's thigh and knee. Sciatic back pain often causes pain in the buttock or lateral thigh and is aggravated by bending, weight bearing, or raising the leg while holding it straight. Greater trochanteric bursitis produces tenderness over the lateral hip (i.e., in the trochanteric bursa) and is aggravated by lying on the affected side. Osteoarthritis of the hip causes limited and painful internal rotation while the hip is either flexed or extended; this does not occur with trochanteric bursitis.

Are Findings Typical of Osteoarthritis?

Typical osteoarthritic joints are enlarged, and there is mild joint-line tenderness to palpation. There may be limitation in range of motion, and crepitus or crackling with movement of the joint.

Effusions are unusual in osteoarthritis and should make the clinician suspect other diag-

noses. If effusion is detected, a diagnostic arthrocentesis should be performed to exclude crystal-induced, infectious, or rheumatoid arthritis.

Osteoarthritis most commonly involves the hands, knees, hips, and spine (cervical and lumbar). Osteoarthritis involving the hand has classic examination findings. The distal inter-phalangeal finger joints appear enlarged, an abnormality known as Heberden's nodes (Fig. 11-1). The proximal interphalangeal joints may sometimes be involved (Bouchard's nodes), as may be the first carpal-metacarpal joint of the thumb.

Involvement of the ankle, wrist, elbow, and shoulder are unusual unless there has been a history of significant past trauma to those joints. Pain in and about these joints, especially if unaccompanied by symptoms in joints commonly involved in osteoarthritis, should make the clinician suspect other forms of arthritis (e.g., pseudogout, gout, or rheumatoid arthritis) or

Figure 11-1

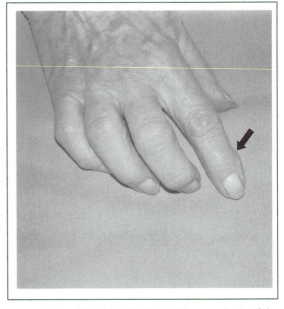

Osteoarthritis of the hand. Typical mild osteoarthritis of the hand, demonstrating classic widening of the distal interphalangeal joint (arrow), commonly referred to as a Heberden's node.

other disease processes (e.g., metastatic bone disease).

During the examination, it is useful to observe the patient's gait. The typical gait abnormality seen with severe osteoarthritis of the hips or knees is an antalgic gait (shortened length of stride on the affected side). Patients with severe osteoarthritis may also demonstrate a "giving way" when bearing weight on the affected side.

Ancillary Tests

If the history and examination findings are typical of osteoarthritis, a confident diagnosis can be made without need for laboratory or radiographic tests. Ancillary tests are necessary, however, when symptoms and examination findings do not fit the usual clinical pattern of osteoarthritis. In some cases, additional testing is needed to reassure patients that the diagnosis of osteoarthritis is correct.

Imaging Studies

PLAIN X-RAYS

Osteoarthritis joints demonstrate numerous radiographic findings (Figs. 11-2 and 11-3). These include (1) joint space narrowing, (2) osteophytes (calcified protrusions from bony surfaces), (3) sclerosis of subchondral bone, (4) subchondral cysts, and (5) osseous fragments within the joint space. Unfortunately, these radiographic findings do not correlate well with symptoms of osteoarthritis. Approximately 80 percent of individuals over 65 years of age will have typical findings of osteoarthritis on x-rays, but less than half of these persons will have significant symptoms of osteoarthritis.

X-rays of the affected joints are appropriate when the clinician is considering diagnoses

Figure 11-2

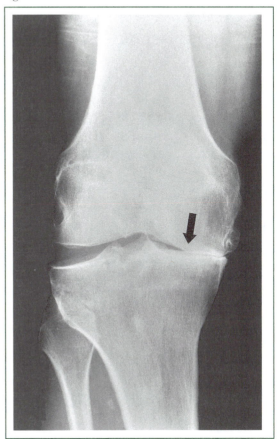

Osteoarthritis of the knee. Marked joint space narrowing is seen in the medial compartment of the knee joint (arrow). *(Photograph courtesy of James Heckman, M.D., University of Texas Health Science Center at San Antonio.)*

other than osteoarthritis. Such diagnoses include traumatic injuries, tumors, osteomyelitis, and so on. Radiographs may also show changes indicating other forms of arthritis (Fig. 11-4).

COMPUTED TOMOGRAPHY AND MAGNETIC RESONANCE IMAGING

Computed tomography and magnetic resonance imaging are almost never appropriate for routine evaluation of patients with suspected osteoar-

Figure 11-3

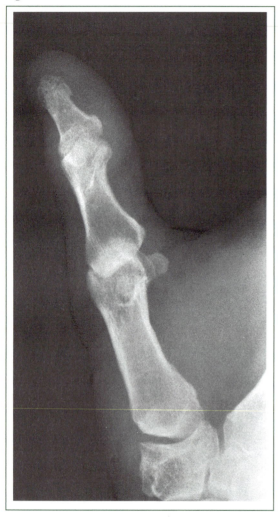

Osteoarthritis of the hand. Radiograph demonstrates bony enlargement at the interphalangeal joint (Heberden's node) and osteophyte formation at the first metacarpophalangeal joint. *(Photograph courtesy of James Heckman, M.D., University of Texas Health Science Center at San Antonio.)*

thritis. These imaging studies may, however, be useful in characterizing plain x-ray abnormalities found during evaluation of patients whose joint problems are not typical of osteoarthritis.

Figure 11-4

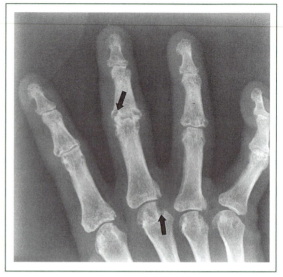

Rheumatoid arthritis. Destructive changes in bone adjacent to joints affected by rheumatoid arthritis appear as eroded, radiolucent areas, examples of which are marked with arrows.

NUCLEAR MEDICINE IMAGING

Results of nuclear medicine bone scans are usually abnormal for patients with osteoarthritis. However, they have poor specificity (i.e., results are positive in many conditions other than osteoarthritis). Therefore, they are not particularly helpful in the routine evaluation of osteoarthritis.

Diagnostic Joint Fluid Aspiration

Arthrocentesis and examination of synovial fluid should be performed if effusion is present. Knees are the most common joints in which effusions are found. Arthrocentesis can be performed with the knee extended or flexed. Figs. 11-5 and 11-6 provide information on how to perform arthrocentesis of the knee.

Synovial fluid obtained by arthrocentesis should undergo examinations including (1) cell count with differential count, (2) Gram's stain, (3) microbiologic cultures, and (4) polarized microscopic evaluation for crystals. In osteoar-

Figure 11-5

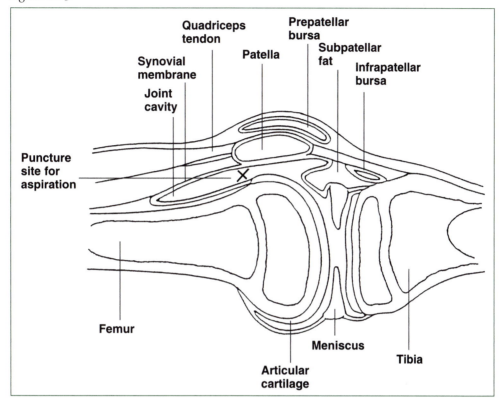

Anatomy of the knee and usual puncture site for performing arthrocentesis with the knee in an extended position. Position the patient comfortably in a supine position. Sterilely prep the area and use local anesthetic (Lidocaine 1% or 2% with epinephrine) to anesthetize the skin and synovium at the aspiration site. With the nonaspirating hand, apply pressure proximal to the patella and over the opposite side of the knee from the aspiration site. This will cause the synovium to bulge on the side of the knee (lateral or medial) to be aspirated. Direct a sterile 18-gauge needle parallel to the examination table into the bulging synovium going just inferior to the patella at the superior patellar pole. Note the appearance of synovial fluid (clear, cloudy, or bloody) and send for cell count, Grams stain cultures, and crystal analysis.

thritis the cell count shows less than 2000 white blood cells/μL (often less than 500 cells/μL), with no more than 15 to 25 percent polymorphonuclear leukocytes. On the other hand, synovial fluid in infectious (septic) arthritis often has 80,000 to 100,000 white blood cells/μL, with more than 90 percent polymorphonuclear leukocytes. In gout and pseudogout, joint fluid averages 20,000 white blood cells/μL, with ap-

proximately 60 percent polymorphonuclear leukocytes (Table 11-1).

Synovial fluid examination is also an important step in diagnosing crystal disease. Uric acid or calcium pyrophosphate crystals can be seen on polarized light microscopy in gout and pseudogout, respectively. When the physician diagnoses gout, blood uric acid levels do not substitute for joint crystal examination, because

Figure 11-6

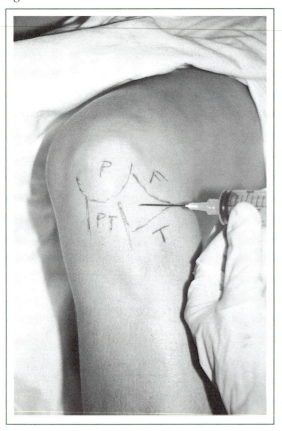

Arthrocentesis of the knee. Photograph demonstrates usual puncture site for performing arthrocentesis with the patient sitting and the knee flexed. The needle is inserted parallel to the floor. The outlines of anatomic landmarks are noted with the following abbreviations: F, femoral head; P, patella; T, tibial plateau; PT, patellar (quadriceps) tendon.

up to 20 percent of patients with gout have a normal uric acid level, and many patients with elevated uric acid levels never develop gout.

Blood Tests

There are no diagnostic blood tests for osteoarthritis. However, blood testing may be helpful in diagnosing or excluding other disease processes. For example, if arthritis is inflammatory and symmetrical in distribution, suggesting connective tissue disorders such as systemic lupus erythematosus or rheumatoid arthritis, it is appropriate to test for rheumatoid factor and/or antinuclear antibodies. If an inflammatory or infectious arthritis is suspected, obtaining a complete blood count and an erythrocyte sedimentation rate may be helpful, but joint fluid aspiration will provide more specific diagnostic information and should not be omitted.

Algorithm

The diagnostic algorithm shown in Fig. 11-7 emphasizes that, in the presence of typical history and examination findings, clinicians can make a presumptive diagnosis of osteoarthritis and initiate treatment. If history or physical examination findings are atypical, additional testing should be performed.

Table 11-1

Synovial Fluid Analysis in Common Arthridites

Fluid Sample	Leukocyte Count, per μL	Polymorphonuclear Leukocytes, %	Culture	Crystals
Normal fluid	<200	<25	Negative	Negative
Osteoarthritis	100–2,000	<25	Negative	Negative
Crystal disease	2,000–60,000	40–75	Negative	Positive
Rheumatoid arthritis	2,000–60,000	45–75	Negative	Negative
Septic joint	80,000–100,000	75–100	Positive	Negative

Figure 11-7

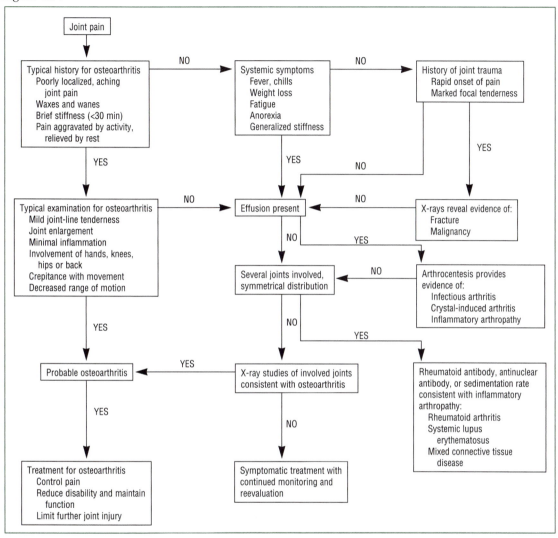

Algorithm for the differential diagnosis of osteoarthritis.

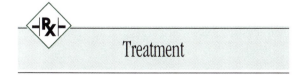

Treatment

Goals of Treatment

There are four primary goals in the treatment of osteoarthritis: (1) to control pain, (2) to reduce disability by improving function and maintaining independence, (3) to avoid or limit side effects and complications of therapy, and (4) to limit, if possible, further damage to the involved joints.

Successful treatment often requires stabilization of coexisting chronic diseases, such as coronary artery disease, chronic obstructive pulmonary disease, and depression, so that patients can participate fully in functional and physical therapies. Adequate social and psychological support is also necessary. The advantages, disadvantages, and costs of various medications and treatment interventions must be considered and discussed thoroughly with the patient before treatment is initiated (Tables 11-2 and 11-3).

Physical and Functional Therapy

EXERCISE

Patients should be encouraged to stay active and maintain a regular exercise regimen. Exercises are designed to maintain general condi-

Table 11-2

Nonpharmacologic Management of Osteoarthritis

EDUCATION
Education of patient and counseling to improve coping skills, management of stress, and understanding of the disease process Self-help information and resources

SOCIAL AND PSYCHOLOGICAL
Encouragement of social interaction (involvement in activities with family, friends, and community) Support groups Coordination of support services

EXERCISE
General conditioning with low-impact aerobic exercises, such as walking or aquatics Stretching and strengthening exercise for muscles around affected joints (isometric and/or isotonic exercises) Maintain range of motion and balance Treatment of coexisting diseases that might interfere with exercise ability

PHYSICAL MODALITIES
Application of heat: hydrotherapy, paraffin baths, short wave or microwave diathermy, ultrasound Applications of ice (cold) for spasm or to limit swelling Use of transcutaneous electrical nerve stimulation, especially for lumbar spine, hip, or knee involvement

JOINT PROTECTION
Reduction of body weight to ideal weight Modified use of affected joint and development of strategies for daily activities Tailoring of level and length of activity to degree of symptoms with rest periods at regular intervals Use of walking aids, such as canes and walkers Splints, orthotics, and appropriate shoes: wedges or shoe inserts to shift stress on the joint, cushioning of the soles to protect joints, nonslip soles to provide traction Use of assistive devices: grab bars, bath seats, mobile shower heads, dressing sticks, large tool grips and utensil handles

Table 11-3

Pharmacologic and Surgical Management of Osteoarthritis

PHARMACOLOGIC TREATMENTS
First-line treatments: nonnarcotic analgesics 　Acetaminophen (up to 4 g/d) 　Topical analgesic (methylsalicylate or cap- 　　saicin cream) Second-line treatments: anti-inflammatory 　NSAID agents, including nonacetylated sali- 　　cylates, for episodic pain uncontrolled by 　　nonnarcotic analgesics 　Intraarticular steroid injection (for intermit- 　　tent use, see text) Third-line treatments: narcotic analgesics (for 　short-term treatment of debilitating break- 　through pain) 　Codeine 　Tramadol 　Propoxyphene

SURGICAL TREATMENTS
Arthroscopic conservative débridement of car- 　tilage and joint space washout Joint replacement with total hip arthroscopy or 　total knee arthroplasty Joint osteotomy fusion

tioning, strengthen muscles around affected joints, and facilitate daily activities. Exercise should be individualized as much as possible to a patient's preferences and physical abilities. For most patients, simple walking can be effective. For others, especially those with severe osteoarthritis involving the back or knees, water aerobics or swimming may be preferable. In addition, specific exercises are recommended to stretch and strengthen muscles around affected joints.

Clinicians should titrate the level and duration of exercise to each patient's symptoms and activity tolerance, allowing adequate rest periods between exercise. Sometimes, several short exercise sessions are better tolerated than one longer period.

For patients who have difficulty with exercise because of osteoarthritis pain, several physical therapy modalities may be useful. Heat often relieves pain or stiffness and is beneficial prior to exercise. Cold application will reduce muscle pain associated with spasm and limit swelling after activity. Modalities such as ultrasound or transcutaneous electrical nerve stimulation may also be useful in reducing pain.

JOINT PROTECTION AND THERAPEUTIC AIDS

Exercise tolerance can be improved and joint function preserved with "joint protection." Joint protection involves reducing stress on affected joints with weight reduction, walking aids, and/or orthotic devices.

Reduction of body weight in overweight individuals reduces stress on weightbearing joints. Therefore, weight reduction is often recommended for osteoarthritis of the knees, hips, and low back (although there is no research evidence to support the contention that weight loss improves osteoarthritis). Regardless of its effect on arthritis, however, weight reduction may improve balance and thus decrease the risk of falls by patients whose mobility, agility, and balance are impaired by osteoarthritis. Use of walking aids, such as canes or walkers, can also decrease the risk of falls.

Footwear should be comfortable and sufficiently cushioned to decrease the stress of impact. However, research indicates that proprioception is better with bare feet or hard-soled shoes; thus, excessive cushioning is inappropriate, making shoe selection complicated for individuals at risk for falls. Regardless of sole hardness, shoes should have non-slip soles to promote traction. In addition, wedges or orthotics may be placed in shoes to shift stress from one portion of a joint to another and to improve joint alignment.

ASSISTIVE DEVICES
AND OCCUPATIONAL THERAPY

Assistive devices include grab bars next to toilet or bathtubs, benches in bathtubs and showers, mobile showerheads, elevated toilet seats, "dressing sticks" to aid in putting on clothes, and large-grip handles for tools and utensils. All of these devices can help maintain independent function and reduce the risk of injuries. Occupational therapists can assist patients in modifying the use of affected joints, developing strategies for independence in daily activities, and using aids and assistive devices.

Pharmaceutical Therapy

NONCONVENTIONAL TREATMENTS

Glucosamine, a constituent of normal articular cartilage, is available in the United States in health food stores as a "dietary supplement." Some glucosamine preparations also contain chrondroitin sulfate, a glycosaminoglycan thought to maintain joint viscosity and improve cartilage metabolism. In animals, glucosamine improves both mechanical and inflammatory arthritis. In humans, double-blind studies have found oral glucosamine to be more effective than placebo and similar in effect to ibuprofen for relieving osteoarthritis symptoms. No important side effects have been reported.

TOPICAL MEDICATION

In recent years, there has been interest in the use of topical agents to decrease pain from osteoarthritis. Sometimes, arthritic pain can be reduced with simple application of heat. The most effective topical analgesic medications are methylsalicylate or capsaicin. Methylsalicylate is widely used and available in non-prescription form. Capsaicin (usually administered as a 0.25-percent cream) reduces pain by depleting substance P, a neuropeptide pain transmitter, in peripheral sensory neurons. Because capsaicin requires several days to deplete substance P, it must be used regularly, rather than on an as-needed basis.

INTRA-ARTICULAR MEDICATIONS

STEROIDS   Injection of steroids into an osteoarthritic joint can provide considerable relief, typically lasting for 1 to 2 months or more. This form of treatment is most appropriate for individuals who have symptoms that predominate in just one or two joints. Steroid injections are performed using sterile technique, with a steroid solution typically mixed with either sterile saline solution or non-epinephrine-containing local anesthetics. Doses for intra-articular injections are provided in the package inserts for most steroid solutions.

Intra-articular steroid injection should be used infrequently, however, because repetitive exposure to steroids can weaken periarticular structures, such as tendons. For this reason, any one joint probably should receive no more than two or three injections per year. Systemic steroids are almost always inappropriate for the long-term treatment of osteoarthritis.

HYALURONIC ACID   In 1997, the U.S. Food and Drug Administration approved the use of cross-linked hyaluronan (hylan G-F20) for intra-articular treatment of osteoarthritis of the knee. Hyaluronan (hyaluronic acid) is a chemical that naturally occurs in synovial fluid and cartilage, and is thought to act as an intra-articular lubricant. It is believed that, in osteoarthritis, natural hyaluronan is abnormal in function and quantity.

After five intra-articular injections 1 week apart, a significant proportion of patients with osteoarthritis report improvement in their symptoms, with improvement lasting 4 to 6 months. Patients over 60 years of age with moderate symptoms and radiologic evidence of osteoarthritis are most likely to benefit. The degree of improvement is similar to that obtained with nonsteroidal anti-inflammatory drugs (NSAIDs) or intra-articular steroid injections.

ORAL MEDICATIONS

Nonsteroidal anti-inflammatory drugs, which have both anti-inflammatory and analgesic properties, are frequently used for treatment of osteoarthritis. However, several studies involving patients with knee arthritis have demonstrated that acetaminophen is equal or superior to NSAIDs for relieving osteoarthritis pain. This fact, combined with the risk of adverse gastrointestinal and renal effects from NSAIDs, makes it reasonable to initiate analgesic treatment with acetaminophen (up to 4 g/d), as needed to control symptoms.

When breakthrough pain occurs, a short course of NSAIDs may be considered. The analgesic dose of NSAIDs is less than the anti-inflammatory dose, so lower-than-usual doses may be effective, and larger doses may offer no advantage. Nonacetylated salicylates (choline magnesium trisalicylate or salsalate) appear to have less gastrointestinal and renal toxicity than other NSAIDs and thus may be preferable, especially in older individuals.

If regular treatment with NSAIDs is required to control pain, adjunctive treatment with misoprostol should be considered if the patient is over 65 or has a history of peptic ulcer disease. Misoprostol is a prostaglandin agonist that counters the decreased gastric blood flow that occurs because of the prostaglandin-inhibiting effect of NSAIDs on the gastric circulation. At a dose of 100 to 200 mg three to four times per day, misoprostol has been shown to reduce risk of gastrointestinal irritation and bleeding.

If pain continues to limit function or quality of life despite physical and pharmacologic treatments, short-term use of narcotic drugs, such as codeine, propoxyphene, or tramadol, may be appropriate for episodic breakthrough pain. Such medications have many potential side effects in older individuals, such as falling and confusion due to sedation, constipation due to decreased bowel motility, and urinary incontinence from interference with detrusor control. Thus, the use of narcotics to treat osteoarthritis should be discouraged and instituted only when essential.

Surgical Treatment

Surgery may be considered for patients with severe, debilitating osteoarthritis (Fig. 11-8) that

Figure 11-8

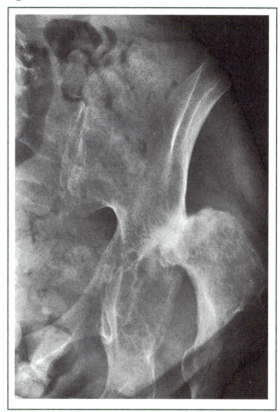

Osteoarthritis of the hip. This elderly patient had severe, debilitating, chronic hip pain. Because of the patient's advanced age, her clinician was reluctant to refer her for surgery, and she was treated instead with oral medications, physical therapy modalities, and even a narcotic infusion pump. Radiograph shows severe osteoarthritis in the left hip with sclerosis, degeneration of the acetabulum, and partial dislocation of the femoral head. Total hip arthroplasty was performed, and the patient is now ambulating without difficulty. *(Photograph courtesy of James Heckman, M.D., University of Texas Health Science Center at San Antonio.)*

has not been successfully treated with the measures outlined above. The most common surgical treatment is replacement of the osteoarthritic joint with a prosthetic joint. Joint replacement has been used with great success for osteoarthritis of the hip and knee and is appropriate for reasonably healthy individuals, including those of advanced age. As mechanical devices, artificial joints are subject to deterioration and have a limited functional half-life of about 10 to 15 years. Therefore, artificial joints may need replacement at a future time if inserted into younger individuals.

Other surgical procedures that can be considered in the treatment of osteoarthritis are arthroscopy and débridement of cartilage with washout of the joint space. Occasionally (especially in younger patients), lower-extremity wedge osteotomy is helpful to shift stress on weight-bearing joints to other parts of the cartilage. Joint fusion (arthrodesis) is effective in eliminating pain, but it also eliminates movement of the fused joint, thus further impairing function.

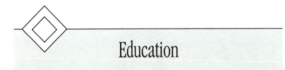

Education

It is essential that clinicians explain to patients the general difference between osteoarthritis and rheumatoid arthritis. Many patients (and their families) with osteoarthritis imagine developing joint deformities, such as they have seen in individuals with rheumatoid arthritis. They need to be reassured that osteoarthritis is a different condition with a different course, prognosis, and treatment.

However, patients and their families do need to understand the natural course of osteoarthritis so that they have appropriate expectations about what will occur over time. Clinicians should tell patients that osteoarthritis does not decrease life span. Rather, the condition typically progresses slowly, the course is variable, and constant pain and disability are by no means the norm. Joint pain may, however, become more constant or

lead to disability, but pain and limitation of activities can be minimized through treatment, which is aimed at maintaining activity and independent function. Patients should understand that current treatments do not retard or reverse the underlying process of the disease.

The importance of exercise in maintaining independent function and preventing disability should be emphasized. In addition, clinicians should explain that, although symptoms sometimes are aggravated by physical activity, activity does not cause the disease, nor does it cause the disease to progress. Furthermore, patients with moderate or severe osteoarthritis should be told about the availability of assistive devices, such as those mentioned above, which can reduce stress on joints to permit more activity with less pain.

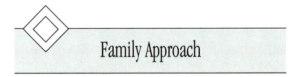

Family Approach

When an individual is diagnosed with arthritis, family members often assume that the individual should "take it easy" and reduce physical activity and work. They may try to do everything for the patient in an attempt to reduce pain and prevent worsening of arthritis. This approach, though well intentioned, often changes family dynamics so that the patient becomes dependent and isolated from activities with friends and family. To decrease the likelihood of this problem, clinicians should tell families to encourage patients to continue normal activities and maintain personal independence.

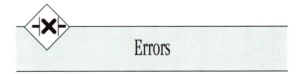

Errors

Clinicians make several errors in the diagnosis and treatment of osteoarthritis. The most common of these errors are misdiagnosing periarticular conditions as osteoarthritis, missing the diagnosis of infectious or crystal-induced arthritis, erroneously diagnosing connective tissue disorders, overusing NSAIDs, and failing to achieve adequate pain control.

Misdiagnosing Periarticular Conditions as Osteoarthritis

It is not uncommon for clinicians to erroneously attribute pain to joint diseases such as osteoarthritis when the pain is really caused by periarticular inflammation. This error occurs both when a periarticular condition is the sole cause of the pain and also when periarticular conditions accompany known osteoarthritis.

For example, anserine bursitis (inflammation at the site where the hip adductors insert on the medial side of the knee) can develop alone or coexist with osteoarthritis of the knee. It is often not recognized, and the symptoms are attributed to osteoarthritis. Greater trochanteric bursitis is often confused with osteoarthritis of the hip, even though the two can be distinguished by physical examination, as described earlier. Similarly, patients with shoulder arthritis may develop subacromial bursitis that is not recognized by their clinician. In comparison to osteoarthritis, pain due to bursitis does not respond as well to analgesics or NSAIDs but does respond to steroid injections.

Missing the Diagnosis of Septic Joint or Crystal-Induced Arthritis

A potentially serious error is to assume that a flare of joint pain is due to underlying osteoarthritis and thereby miss a diagnosis of septic arthritis. Arthritic diseases are not mutually exclusive, and patients with osteoarthritis may develop infectious arthritis. As a rule, an abrupt onset or worsening of joint pain in association with joint inflammation and/or effusion requires arthrocentesis to rule out joint infection.

Similarly, patients with osteoarthritis can develop gout or pseudogout. Synovial fluid obtained by arthrocentesis in a patient with worsening joint pain and effusion should be examined for crystals to exclude gout or pseudogout.

Erroneously Diagnosing Connective Tissue Disorders

In the process of evaluating patients with osteoarthritis, clinicians sometimes erroneously diagnose systemic connective tissue disorders on the basis of a falsely abnormal laboratory test result. In older individuals (the age group at risk for osteoarthritis), false-positive test results for rheumatoid factor and antinuclear antibodies are common, and the erythrocyte sedimentation rate may be elevated (up to 40 mm/h) even in persons with no apparent health problems. The result is that patients presenting with typical findings of osteoarthritis are sometimes incorrectly diagnosed with rheumatoid arthritis, systemic lupus erythematosus, or mixed connective tissue diseases simply because of a positive rheumatoid factor test result, a positive antinuclear antibody test result, or an elevated sedimentation rate. It is important to remember that diagnosis of these rheumatologic conditions requires a specific constellation of symptoms and signs and not solely an abnormal laboratory test result.

Overuse of NSAIDs

Adverse effects of NSAIDs are more common with age and with increasing doses and duration of therapy. The most important adverse effect is upper gastrointestinal bleeding. Gastric ulcers occur in 10 to 15 percent of chronic NSAID users, one-third of whom are asymptomatic. Renal insufficiency occurs in 10 to 15 percent of elderly persons treated with NSAIDs; the impairment of renal function is usually, but not always, reversible on discontinuing therapy. Other adverse NSAID effects include peripheral edema, hyperkalemia, and worsening control of blood pressure in hypertensive patients. Because of the potential adverse effects of chronic NSAID use, it is prudent to use shorter courses at the lowest effective dose for exacerbations of arthritic symptoms that are unrelieved by acetaminophen.

Inadequate Pain Control

The risk of inadequate pain control is that it may lead to a cascade of events that ultimately ends in disability. Persistent pain discourages use of the joint, which leads to loss of strength (deconditioning). Loss of strength results in decreased use of a joint, which leads to loss of range of motion (contractures), which further limit function and result in loss of independence. Thus, while it may not be necessary to totally eliminate osteoarthritic pain, clinicians should make every effort to control pain sufficiently to permit activity and use of the joint.

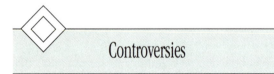

Controversies

Two current controversies about osteoarthritis are relevant to primary care practice. These issues include the cause of osteoarthritis and whether the progression of osteoarthritis can be slowed with currently available medications.

Cause of Osteoarthritis: Biomechanical or Metabolic?

Osteoarthritis has been referred to as degenerative joint disease, implying that joints simply deteriorate because of repetitive wear and tear that occurs with increasing age. Recent research,

however, has challenged this concept and suggests that osteoarthritis begins with changes in cartilage that are different than the changes associated with normal aging or wear and tear. For example, it has been found that, in comparison to cartilage in older persons without osteoarthritis, osteoarthritic cartilage has a higher water content, an increased ratio of chondroitin sulfate to keratin sulfate, and increased levels of degradative enzymes. As described earlier in this chapter, changes in osteoarthritic cartilage have been interpreted to reflect disruption of a dynamic process of cartilage biochemistry, and this disruption may precede development of clinical osteoarthritis. Furthermore, there are no convincing data indicating that the risk of osteoarthritis increases with normal use of joints or through regular exercise or low-impact sports, arguing against the concept of "wear-and-tear" arthritis.

On the other hand, major trauma to a joint clearly can result in osteoarthritis in that joint. For example, tri-malleolar ankle fractures, disruption of the anterior cruciate ligament of the knee, and meniscectomy of the knee are often followed by development of osteoarthritis in the affected joint. In addition, increased rates of osteoarthritis have been observed for persons in certain occupations (e.g., coal miners, shipyard laborers, and farmers), suggesting that repetitive joint stress can cause osteoarthritis. Thus, the cause of osteoarthritis is unclear, and further research is needed to clarify its pathogenesis.

Current Medications: Are They Symptomatic or Disease-Modifying Treatments?

Currently, osteoarthritis is treated symptomatically by alleviating pain with analgesics and maintaining function through physical modalities. There have been some claims that certain NSAIDs are chondroprotective, that is, they alter cartilage metabolism and slow or prevent the biochemical processes that result in cartilage destruction. These claims, however, are based solely on in vitro experiments. At this time, there is no convincing evidence that any of the NSAIDs provide protection or modify the disease process in humans with osteoarthritis.

There are some pharmaceutical agents, however, such as tetracycline (doxycycline) and tenidap (see below) that have demonstrated disease-modifying characteristics. They inhibit the action of metalloproteinases (i.e., collagenase, gelatinase, or stromelysin) that enzymatically break down cartilage matrix. Currently, the role of these drugs in treatment regimens for osteoarthritis is unclear.

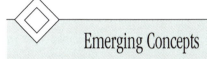

Emerging Concepts

Primary care clinicians should be aware of several developments likely to take place in the ability of clinicians to manage osteoarthritis. These innovations include development of markers to diagnose and predict progression of osteoarthritis, new treatments that halt or slow disease progression, and liquid polymers that serve as cartilage substitutes on osteoarthritic joint surfaces.

Markers for Diagnosing or Predicting Progression of Osteoarthritis

There is an ongoing search to find markers that will accurately diagnose osteoarthritis or predict its progression. X-rays have not been useful for this purpose because, as discussed earlier, radiographic findings do not correlate well with symptoms or progression of disease. Measurements of cartilage matrix-degradation products have also been evaluated, as have measurements of various cytokines that regulate the repair and

degradation process within articular cartilage. To date, measurements of these substances have shown some promise but are not sufficiently specific or sensitive to use them in clinical practice. It is likely that in the future reliable markers for the diagnosis and prognosis of osteoarthritis will become available for general use.

Treatments That Halt or Slow the Osteoarthritic Disease Process

A number of studies have found that tetracycline analogues, such as doxycycline, inhibit metalloproteinases, thereby reducing breakdown of cartilage. Similarly, because catabolic cytokines such as interleukin-1 and tumor necrosis factor-α induce production of metalloproteinases that cause proteolytic degradation of cartilage, inhibitors of these cytokines may halt or slow the progression of cartilage degradation. Anticytokine therapy with neutralizing monoclonal antibodies or soluble receptors that bind or block the activity of catabolic cytokines has been developed and used with some success in treatment of rheumatoid arthritis. These or similar anti-cytokine agents may ultimately be used to modify the disease process in osteoarthritis.

Tenidap sodium is another new chemical agent (an oxindole) that appears to modify the processes that cause osteoarthritis. Tenidap, like NSAIDs, inhibits cyclo-oxygenase and the production of prostaglandin. However, it is different from NSAIDs in its ability to inhibit production of anabolic cytokines, such as interleukin-1 and tumor necrosis factor-α. Although more research is needed, tenidap and similar medications may prove useful in the treatment of osteoarthritis.

Development of disease-modifying osteoarthritic drugs and anti-cytokine therapy is in its infancy, but these agents will be further developed and refined. The prospect of disease-modifying drugs for osteoarthritis gives hope that the disease process can be slowed or even reversed.

Intra-articular Treatments for Improving Cartilage Function

Research is progressing on liquid polymers that can be used to smooth the irregular surface of osteoarthritic cartilage. Polymers currently under investigation are injected into joints through an arthroscope and harden within minutes into a solid that is moldable for about 20 min. This moldable solid is shaped over damaged cartilage, where it subsequently hardens into a durable "cartilage substitute." Animal tests of these substances have been successful, and trials in humans are ongoing. If successful, these substances could result in major changes in the way osteoarthritis is managed.

Bibliography

Bellamy N: Changing perceptions of osteoarthritis; editorial. *MJA* 165:247, 1996.

Bellamy N, Bradley LA: Workshop on chronic pain, pain control, and patient outcomes in rheumatic arthritis and osteoarthritis: Conference summary. *Arthritis Rheum* 39:357, 1996.

Bjelle A: Age and aging in rheumatic disease, in Klipplel JH, Dieppe PA (eds): *Rheumatology.* Chicago, Mosby Yearbook, 1994, pp 15.1–15.6.

Blackburn WD: Management of osteoarthritis and rheumatoid arthritis: Prospects and possibilities. *Am J Med* 100:24S, 1996.

Brandt KD: Modification by oral doxycycline administration of articular cartilage breakdown in osteoarthritis. *J Rheumatol* 22(suppl 43):149, 1995.

Brandt KD: *Diagnosis and Nonsurgical Management of Osteoarthritis* Caddo, OK, Professional Communications, 1996, pp 15–23 and 183–186.

Brandt KD, Slemenda CW: Osteoarthritis: An epidemiology, pathology, and pathogenesis, in Schumacher HR Jr (ed): *Primer on the Rheumatic Disease,* 10th ed. Atlanta, The Arthritis Foundation, 1993, pp 184–187.

Firestein GS, Zvaifler NJ: Anticytokine therapy in rheumatoid arthritis. *New Engl J Med* 337:195, 1997.

Gabriel SE: Update on the epidemiology of the rheumatic disease. *Curr Opin Rheumatol* 8:96, 1996.

Glucosamine for osteoarthritis. *Med Lett* 39:91, 1997.

Greenwald RA: Treatment of destructive arthritic disorders with MMP inhibitors: Potential role of tetracyclines. *Ann N Y Acad Sci* 181, 1996.

Hall AP, Barry PE, Dawber TR, et al: Epidemiology of gout and hyperuricemia: A long-term population study. *Am J Med* 42:27, 1967.

Harris WH, Sledge OB: Total hip and total knee replacement. *New Engl J Med* 323:25, 1990.

Hochberg MC: Prognosis of osteoarthritis. *Ann Rheum Dis* 55:685, 1996.

Lane NE: Exercise: A cause of osteoarthritis. *J Rheumatol* 22(suppl):3, 1995.

Ling MS, Bathon JM: Osteoarthritis in older adults. *J Am Geriatr Soc* 46:216, 1998.

Pullar T: The pharmacokinetics of tenidap sodium: Introduction. *Br J Clin Pharmacol* 39:1S, 1995.

Ryan ME, Greenwald RA, Golub LM: Potential of tetracycline to modify cartilage breakdown in osteoarthritis. *Curr Opin Rheumatol* 8:238, 1996.

Stauffer RN: Correction of arthritic deformities of the hip, in: McCarty DJ, Koopman WJ (eds): *Arthritis and Allied Conditions,* 12th ed. Philadelphia, Lea & Febiger, 1993, pp 969–980.

Swedberg JA, Steinbauer JR: Osteoarthritis. *Am Fam Physician* 45:557, 1992.

Westacott CI, Sharif M: Cytokines in osteoarthritis: Mediators or markers of joint destruction? *Semin Arthritis Rheum* 25:254, 1996.

Appendix:
Resources for Patients

Lorig K, Fries JF: *The Arthritis Handbook: A Tested Self-Management Program for Coping with Your Arthritis.* 4th ed. New York, Addison-Wesley, 1995.

The Arthritis Foundation National Office, 1330 West Peachtree St., NW, Atlanta, GA, 30309.

Jeff Susman

Chapter

12

Back Pain

How Common Is Back Pain?

Almost everyone experiences low back problems at some time during their lives, and some degree of back pain affects up to 50 percent of adults each year. Fortunately, over 90 percent of these back-pain episodes have a self-limited course, resolving with minimal or no intervention. Nonetheless, from one-third to two-thirds of individuals with an episode of back pain have a recurrence within 1 year, and a significant percentage have chronic pain, disability, or both. In fact, low back problems are the most common causes of disability in working age adults. At any given time, up to 1 percent of the U.S. population is chronically disabled due to low back pain, and another 1 percent is temporarily disabled.

Overall, low back pain is the fifth most-common reason why patients see physicians, accounting for 2.8 percent of all office visits in the United States. It is the most common reason for visits to orthopedists and neurosurgeons, but the majority of individuals with low back pain are seen by primary care clinicians.

There were 15 million office visits in the United States for "mechanical" low-back pain in 1990. In almost 57 percent of these visits, the diagnosis was coded as nonspecific back pain. In 13 percent, the diagnosis was coded as back pain due to degenerative changes, and 11 percent were coded as herniated intervertebral disks. Surgical procedures related to low back pain are the third most-common operations performed in the United States.

Few interventions have been shown to change the natural history of pain and disability attributable to back pain. Thus, for most patients, clinicians must foster functional recovery by understanding patients' concepts of illness and providing appropriate education. In addition, a key challenge for primary care clinicians is to recognize, from among the majority of patients in whom back pain will resolve spontaneously, those few patients who require special management because of underlying surgical or medical problems or because of occupational or psychosocial issues.

Principal Diagnoses

The principal diagnoses to consider in persons with back pain vary with the patient's age. The most-practical age classification is the following three groups: working-aged adults, geriatric-aged adults, and children and adolescents.

Working-Aged Adults

NONSPECIFIC BACK PAIN

Acute low back problems in working-aged adults are usually defined as activity intolerance from back-related symptoms that have been present for 3 months or less. The vast majority of these individuals will have no specific identifiable cause for their back pain, and efforts to identify a specific pathophysiologic derangement are usually unsuccessful. Clinicians often use such terms as "back strain," "pulled muscle," "myofascial trigger points," or "sacroiliac syndrome" to describe the problem, or label the back pain as "degenerative," "facet syndrome," or "subluxation." However, there is no good evidence that any of these diagnostic terms are more accurate than simply labeling the problem nonspecific back pain. Furthermore, there is no evidence that using these various diagnostic terms affects treatment or influences outcome.

SPECIFIC BACK SYNDROMES

Less than 5 percent of patients will present with specific identifiable back pain syndromes. The most common of these is back pain with radiculopathy or associated with pain below the knee; such symptoms are highly suggestive of nerve-root compression due to a herniated lumbar intervertebral disk.

Spondylolysis and spondylolisthesis are other specific causes of back pain. Spondylolysis is a stress fracture or stress reaction of the isthmus of the pars interarticularis of the vertebra. Spondylolisthesis, which often follows spondylolysis, is slippage of one vertebra forward over another (Fig. 12-1). Reverse spondylolisthesis (i.e., backwards slippage) may also occur.

Cauda equina syndrome is a rare surgical emergency caused by impingement on the cauda equina by a herniated disk or other structural abnormalities. Cauda equina syndrome is characterized by saddle anesthesia, bowel or bladder incontinence, and muscle weakness.

SERIOUS SPINAL CAUSES OF BACK PAIN

In about one of 150 to 200 working-aged patients with low back pain, the pain is caused by a serious underlying disorder, such as malignancy, fracture, or systemic illness that involves the spine. The most common malignancies affecting the vertebral column are multiple myeloma and metastases from cancer of the breast, lung, prostate, colorectum, or kidney. Fractures can also cause low back pain, as can such systemic conditions as spinal infections (diskitis or osteomyelitis) and rheumatologic disorders (ankylosing spondylitis and rheumatoid arthritis).

SERIOUS NONSPINAL CAUSES OF BACK PAIN

It is important to realize that non-spinal conditions can also cause low back pain. While uncommonly confused with low back pain syndromes, some of these causes are serious, and

Figure 12-1

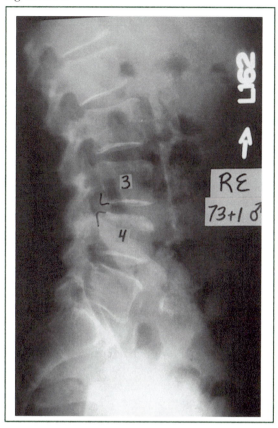

Spondylolisthesis. The vertebral body of L3 has moved forward in relation to the L4 vertebral body. (*Reproduced with permission from R Dee (ed): Principles of Orthopedic Practice, 2d ed. New York, McGraw-Hill, 1997.*)

clinicians should remain alert for possibility of these conditions, which are listed in Table 12-1.

PREGNANCY

Finally, back pain is common during pregnancy, affecting up to 90 percent of women. The prevalence of back pain during pregnancy increases with the age of the patient and is associated with later term, advanced parity, and previous back problems. Fortunately, most back pain in pregnancy is self-limited and of no clinical consequence. However, clinicians should be

Table 12-1

Selected Nonspinal Causes of Low Back Pain

Abdominal aortic aneurysm
Ectopic pregnancy
Pancreatitis
Perforated ulcer
Pyelonephritis
Pelvic tumor
Urolithiasis

alert for serious conditions that may mimic simple back pain in pregnant women, including appendicitis, pyelonephritis, ectopic pregnancy, and premature labor.

Geriatric-Aged Adults

As in younger adults, low back pain is common in older individuals. In younger adults, lumbar disk herniation and spondylolisthesis may be the underlying cause of back pain, but many cases of low back pain remain unexplained in older adults. Nonetheless, a careful exploration for underlying causes of persistent back pain is warranted because, in contrast to the situation in working-aged adults, back pain in older persons is more often associated with serious underlying disorders.

SERIOUS CAUSES OF BACK PAIN

Malignancy, including multiple myeloma and metastatic cancer, is more common in older individuals. Metabolic bone disorders, such as osteomalacia, osteoporosis, Paget's disease, and hyperparathyroidism, also occur more frequently. Vertebral compression fractures are much more common and may result from osteoporosis, osteomalacia, or trauma.

Another relatively common and important diagnosis to consider in older individuals is lum-

bar spinal stenosis. Symptoms occur by mechanical compression of nerve roots, due to narrowing of the lumbar spinal canal from osteophytic or other bone lesions. The structure of the lumbar spinal canal is such that it widens with flexion at the waist and narrows with upright posture. Thus, lumbar spinal stenosis often presents with pseudoclaudication (pain precipitated by walking or standing upright and relieved by sitting or leaning forward).

Children and Adolescents

In children and adolescents, non-specific low back pain is common, but most patients do not seek a clinician's attention. For youngsters who do present to a clinician, up to half have a specific or serious cause of their pain. Because children and adolescents have such a high incidence of identifiable and potentially serious causes of low back problems, clinicians must be more vigilant and quicker to use diagnostic tests to evaluate back pain in children.

Spondylolysis and spondylolisthesis are the most common specific causes of low back problems in children and adolescents; they occur most frequently at the fifth lumbar vertebra. Symptomatic spondylolysis and spondylolisthesis are more prevalent in boys and athletes, but they are also common occult radiographic abnormalities in asymptomatic individuals.

In adolescents, Scheuermann's disease (juvenile kyphosis) is a common cause of back pain. This diagnosis is made when x-rays reveal increased kyphosis and anterior wedging of at least three successive vertebrae. Typically, Scheuermann's disease causes pain in the upper back and neck, rather than in the lumbar area.

Other less common causes of low back pain in children and adolescents include malignancy, infection, scoliosis, and, less commonly, disk herniation and inflammatory rheumatologic conditions, such as ankylosing spondylitis.

Typical Presentation

Patents with low back pain typically present with back pain as the principal reason for an office visit. The most common complaints are pain in the lower lumbar or sacral area, with decreased mobility and activity intolerance. The back symptoms may be accompanied by pain in the buttock, in the thigh, or below the knee, often in a radicular pattern.

Many patients try nonprescription analgesics, bed rest, or activity modification or have visited another health provider (e.g., chiropractor) before or concurrently with visiting their primary care clinician. Indeed, managed-care plans encourage such self-care because low back pain is usually self-limited and nonprescription analgesics are as effective as more costly prescription medications.

As shown in Table 12-2, the causes of back pain among patients presenting to clinicians differ by specialty. The majority of patients with back pain in a primary care clinician's office have nonspecific back pain. Nonspecific back pain is somewhat less common in orthopedic practice and is relatively infrequent in the practices of neurosurgeons. While the diagnostic possibilities and management strategies remain the same regardless of specialty, the higher probability of nonspecific back problems in primary care practice makes it essential that primary care clinicians be alert for "red flags" that indicate the presence of more serious conditions, rather than evaluating all patients for the possibility of such conditions.

Finally, many patients seek care for chronic or recurrent low back problems, and complaints of chronic low back pain are common in primary care settings. In particular, primary care clinicians often see patients with long-term back problems that have not been successfully treated by other clinicians.

Key History

The goal of the history is to determine if (1) there is a serious underlying cause of low back pain, (2) the patient has radiculopathy, or (3) the patient is at high risk for protracted disability because of occupational or psychosocial factors. Examples of useful questions for the history are shown in Table 12-3.

Table 12-2

Diagnostic Mix of Low Back Pain by Physician Specialty

DIAGNOSIS	FAMILY PHYSICIAN, %	ORTHOPEDIC SURGEON, %	NEUROSURGEON, %
Nonspecific back pain	76	40	19
Herniated disk	3	20	46
Spinal stenosis	2	6	12
Degenerative disk disease	10	19	6
Other	9	15	17

SOURCE: Reproduced with permission from Deyo and Phillips.

Table 12-3

Suggested Questions for Patients with Low Back Problems

"Tell me about your low back problem."

"What symptoms are you having?"

"Have you experienced any weakness, numbness, or shooting pains?"

"Does the pain/numbness go anywhere?"

"Have you had any changes in your bowel or bladder habits?"

"How does your back problem affect your job/school/household performance?"

"How does your back problem affect what you do for fun?"

"How are things going in your life? Are there any problems at home or on the job?"

"Tell me what you know about back problems—have you experienced back pain before or do you have a friend or relative with back problems?"

"What concerns do you have about this problem?"

"What other tests do you expect?"

"What treatment do you expect?"

"What changes can you make at work/home/school to minimize your temporary discomfort?"

In addition, the history is important for developing rapport and a relationship with the patient that focuses on patient-centered care and functional rehabilitation. Many patients have underlying concerns, prior experiences with low back pain, or misconceptions about back pain. For example, patients may be concerned about developing disability, may fear they have cancer, or may expect x-rays or other inappropriate diagnostic or therapeutic interventions. The clinician should, therefore, use empathy, reflection of feelings, and legitimization of emotions to build partnership with patients so as to understand the meaning of illness to patients, its effect on their daily function, and their expectations for care.

Many clinicians do not enjoy interviewing patients with low back pain, especially if the patients are demanding, thought to be amplifying their pain, or suspected of malingering. The approach to such individuals should be similar to the approach described above, with added attention paid to the psychosocial and occupational aspects of illness. It is important that physicians face such patients with equanimity. Legitimizing the patient's concerns and discomfort is important. Working with the family, employer, other health providers, and state and federal agencies will often help ensure an appropriate approach to care.

Detecting Serious Underlying Causes of Back Pain

The history should seek symptoms associated with non-spinal or serious causes of low back pain, such as the conditions described above. Specific symptoms and their significance in predicting underlying causes of back pain are shown in Tables 12-4 and 12-5. For example, unremitting pain associated with constitutional symptoms such as weight loss suggests malignancy, a history of intravenous drug use suggests infection (osteomyelitis), and recent trauma indicates the possibility of fracture.

Detecting Radiculopathy

Radiculopathy can be caused by a herniated disk, spinal stenosis, abscess, tumor, osteophytes, or other structural abnormalities. Pain or numbness that extends below the knee (i.e., is not just localized to the posterior thigh) in a dermatomal distribution suggests radiculopathy. A potentially confusing mix of pain and numbness, associated with changes in bowel or bladder function, suggests cauda equina syndrome. The symptoms of spinal stenosis are described above.

Table 12-4

Historical Factors Associated with Serious Causes of Low Back Pain

SYMPTOM	DIAGNOSTIC SIGNIFICANCE
Current or prior neoplasm	Recurrent neoplasm
Corticosteroid use or immunosuppression	Infection, fracture
Intravenous drug use	Infection
Trauma (especially a significant fall or motor vehicle accident)	Fracture
Symptoms of infection (chills, fever)	Infection
Neurologic symptoms	Infection, neoplasm, herniated disk, cauda equina syndrome, spinal stenosis
Constitutional symptoms (weight loss, night sweats, anorexia)	Infection, neoplasm
Bowel or bladder dysfunction	Cauda equina syndrome
No relief with bed rest	Infection, neoplasm
Pain lasting more than 6–8 weeks	Infection, neoplasm

Detecting Risks for Protracted Pain or Disability

It is important to explore occupational and social issues that may indicate increased risk of chronicity or disability. Specifically, dissatisfaction with work and having previously received workers' compensation payments are important predictors of subsequent disability or chronic pain. Inconsistency in a patient's symptoms, overreaction, nonorganic complaints, or complaints with bizarre patterns (e.g., numbness below the waist on one side) suggest that a patient may be malingering and predict a lower likelihood of returning to work. Other factors that may increase the risk that pain will persist or that special psychosocial interventions might be needed are marital strife, stress, depression, and substance use.

Clinicians should ask about the functional effect of the back pain on the patient's daily activities, since this may have implications for recovery. For example, a truck driver who sits for long periods of time or a homemaker who must lift children may find it difficult to avoid these activities, despite the fact that they may aggravate back pain. Finally, although cigarette smoking does not cause back pain, low back problems are more common in smokers. Thus, interviewing a patient with back pain offers an opportunity to identify smokers and begin cessation counseling.

Physical Examination

The physical examination can usually be accomplished in 5 to 10 min. The purpose of the examination in primary care practice is to seek evidence of underlying causes of back pain or radiculopathy, either of which would suggest that the patient has something other than nonspecific back pain. The examination is not intended to determine a specific cause of nonspecific back pain, such as "degenerative changes," "sacroiliac syndrome," or "subluxations." In fact, use of such labels may tend to

Table 12-5

Accuracy of History for Detecting Serious Causes of Low Back Pain

MEDICAL HISTORY RED FLAGS	SENSITIVITY	SPECIFICITY
CANCER		
Age ≥50	0.77	0.71
Previous cancer history	0.31	0.98
Unexplained weight loss	0.15	0.94
Failure to improve with 1 month of therapy	0.31	0.90
Bed rest no relief	0.90	0.46
Duration of pain >1 month	0.50	0.81
SPINAL OSTEOMYELITIS		
Intravenous drug use, or urine or skin infection	0.40	NA
COMPRESSION FRACTURE		
Age ≥50	0.84	0.61
Age ≥70	0.22	0.96
Trauma	0.30	0.85
Corticosteroids use	0.06	0.995
HERNIATED INTERVERTEBRAL DISK		
Sciatica	0.95	0.88
SPINAL STENOSIS		
Pseudoclaudication	0.60	NA
Age ≥50	0.90	0.70
ANKYLOSING SPONDYLITIS		
Age at onset ≥40	1.00	0.07
Pain not relieved in supine position	0.80	0.49
Morning back stiffness	0.64	0.59
Duration of pain ≥3 months	0.17	0.54

ABBREVIATION: NA, not available.

SOURCE: Adapted from Bigos, Bowyer, Braen, et al.

"medicalize" back pain, rather than portraying it as an almost universal feature of life.

General Examination

A quick general screening examination should be performed to seek evidence of underlying causes of back pain. This examination should be targeted at whether the patient has fever or tachycardia (suggesting infection), abdominal or flank pain (suggesting the presence of conditions listed in Table 12-1), or a heart murmur (which, in an intravenous drug abuser, suggests septic emboli to the vertebral column). The examination should seek evidence of secondary causes of back pain, such as malignancy or rheumatologic conditions. The need for a more exhaustive physical examination will be suggested by the history and the initial screening examination.

Back Examination

Initially, the clinician should note the patient's general appearance and behavior. Specific attention should be paid to whether the patient appears to be in pain or has difficulty getting onto the examination table. In addition, the clinician should note whether there is obvious splinting, scoliosis, or kyphosis. Next, palpation of the vertebral column should be performed; localized spinal tenderness indicates the possibility of fracture, malignancy, or infection.

Most clinicians also test range of motion of the lumbar spine (flexion, extension, lateral bending, and rotation). Such functional testing is useful for documenting the degree of baseline impairment, against which treatment effects can be compared. It may also aid in selection of diagnostic tests or treatments by identifying patients with severe versus less-severe functional impairments.

TESTING FOR NERVE ROOT IMPINGEMENT

Several maneuvers can be used to evaluate for radiculopathy. The most common is straight-leg raising (SLR), which may be performed with the patient in a supine or sitting position (Fig. 12-2). A positive SLR test result requires the test to produce radicular pain below the knee, not just back discomfort. A positive crossed-SLR test result (i.e., radicular pain in the leg contralateral to the one being raised) is particularly suggestive of nerve root impingement. The sensitivity and specificity of common physical signs for detecting radiculopathy are outlined in Table 12-6.

Several variations of the SLR test can be used if there is concern that a patient is malingering. In the Hoover test, the clinician cups the patient's legs at the back of the foot and asks the patient to raise one leg. In the absence of severe bilateral muscle weakness, individuals who are truly trying to raise one leg will exert a downward counterforce in the opposite leg. Another testing maneuver is to perform the SLR test with the patient in a sitting position simply by straightening one leg at the knee. Patients who are malingering may not realize that the SLR test is being performed when they are in a sitting position, and this may reveal inconsistencies in their symptoms. Finally, pain drawings that map the location of pain, parasthesias, and neurologic symptoms may also be helpful in sorting out inconsistencies.

In considering the possibility of nerve root impingement, it is also useful to determine whether there is evidence of sensory and/or motor findings specific to a particular nerve root. Most nerve root impingement caused by lumbar disk disease involves nerve roots at the L3–L4 to L5–S1 levels.

SENSORY TESTING   Clinicians can easily test sensory nerve-root function by checking sensation of the foot (Fig. 12-3, on page 322). Impairment of tactile sensory function on the medial aspect of the foot implies impingement of the L3–L4 nerve root, impairment on the dorsum of the foot indicates L4–L5 nerve root impingement, and impairment of lateral foot sensation suggests impingement of the L5–S1 nerve root. Sensory innervation is somewhat variable, however, and impairment of sensation is not as accurate as motor testing in determining the level of nerve impingement.

MOTOR TESTING   Motor testing (Fig. 12-3) should include having patients walk on their heels and toes. Inability to heel-walk occurs with L4–L5 nerve root impingement, and inability to toe-walk suggests L5–S1 impingement. Having the patient squat checks for quadriceps strength (L3–L4 nerve root). In prolonged nerve impingement, atrophy of the innervated muscles may occur.

Additional testing of specific muscles includes dorsiflexion of the great toe (extensor hallucis longus, innervated by the L3–L4 nerve root), and

Figure 12-2

1. Ask the patient to lie as straight as possible
   on a table in the supine position.

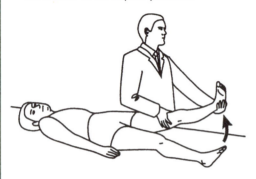

2. With one hand placed above the knee of
   the leg being examined, exert enough firm
   pressure to keep the knee fully extended.
   Ask the patient to relax.

3. With the other hand cupped under
   the heel, slowly raise the straight
   limb. Tell the patient, "If this bothers
   you, let me know, and I will stop."

4. Monitor for any movement of the pelvis
   before complaints are elicited. True sciatic
   tension should elicit compaints before the
   hamstrings are stretched enough to move
   the pelvis.

5. Estimate the degree of leg
   elevation that elicits complaint
   from the patient. Then
   determine the most distal
   area of discomfort: back, hip,
   thigh, knee, or below the knee.

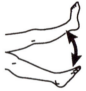

6. While holding the leg at the limit of straight
   leg raising, dorsiflex the ankle. Note whether
   this aggravates the pain. Internal rotation of
   the limb can also increase the tension on the
   sciatic nerve roots.

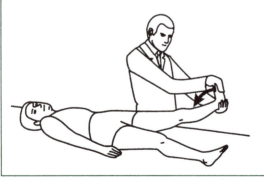

Instructions for the SLR test. *(From Bigos, Bowyer, Braen, et al.)*

Table 12-6
Accuracy of Physical Examination for Detecting Lumbar Disk Herniation*

TEST	SENSITIVITY	SPECIFICITY	COMMENTS
Ipsilateral SLR test	0.80	0.40	Positive result is leg pain at <60° of extension.
Crossed SLR test	0.25	0.90	Positive result is contralateral leg pain.
Ankle dorsiflexion weak	0.35	0.70	Usually signifies L4–L5 HNP
Ankle plantar flexion weak	0.06	0.95	—
Impaired ankle reflex	0.50	0.60	Usually signifies L5–S1 HNP; absent reflex increases specificity
Great toe extensor weak	0.50	0.70	Signifies HNP L5–S1 (60% of cases) or L4–L5 (30% of cases)
Sensory loss	0.50	0.50	Area of loss predicts HNP level poorly.
Patellar reflex	0.50	NA	For upper lumbar HNP only
Quadriceps weakness	<0.01	0.99	—

*Estimated accuracy of physical examination findings for lumbar disk herniation among patients with sciatica.
ABBREVIATIONS: HNP, herniated nucleus pulposis; SLR, straight-leg raising.
SOURCE: Adapted from Bigos, Bowyer, Braen, et al.

plantar flexion of the foot (flexor hallucis longus, innervated by L5–S1). Reflex testing should include the patellar (L3–L4) and ankle (L5–S1) reflexes. Finally, the Babinski reflex should be tested; its presence indicates the existence of an upper-motor neuron disorder.

Ancillary Tests

In the vast majority of patients, the history and physical examination alone provide sufficient information to establish a working diagnosis and either (1) initiate treatment for non-specific back pain or (2) perform further testing for nerve impingement or serious underlying causes of back pain. In the absence of red flags (i.e., findings on the history and physical examination suggesting serious underlying problems), however, the likelihood of such problems is extremely low.

Testing in Patients without Red Flags

For patients without red flags, even with evidence of radicular pain (but without a progressive neurologic deficit), further testing is almost never indicated in the first 1 to 3 months of symptoms. In fact, since the initial management of patients with non-specific back pain and of those with radiculopathy is the same (unless cauda equina syndrome or a progressive neurologic problem is present), imaging and further testing have little value in early management. While it is true that patients with radiculopathy may take longer to recover, initial management is not changed by results of additional tests.

Moreover, there is little evidence to suggest that imaging tests add more prognostic information to that which can be obtained with a good history and physical examination. Indeed, the history and physical examination are the basis for deciding whether the patient should ultimately have imaging tests performed.

Even plain x-rays of the back (i.e., lumbosacral spine films) have little value for patients

Figure 12-3

Nerve root	L4	L5	S1
Pain	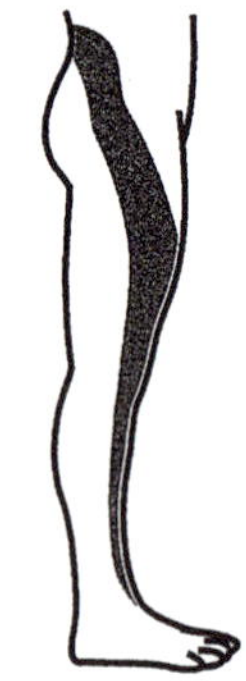	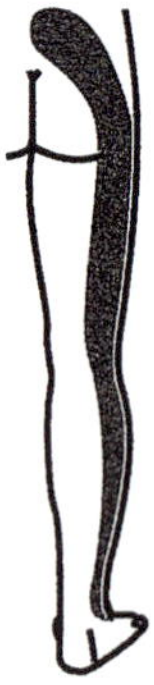	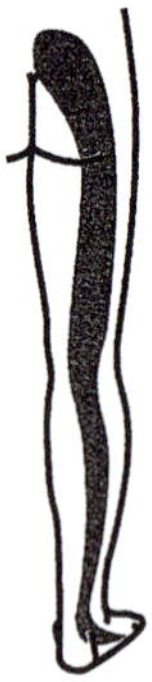
Numbness	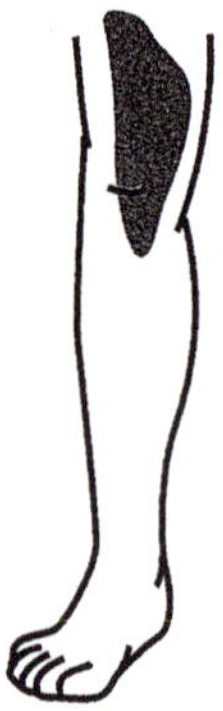	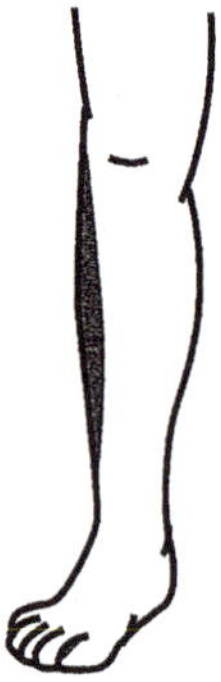	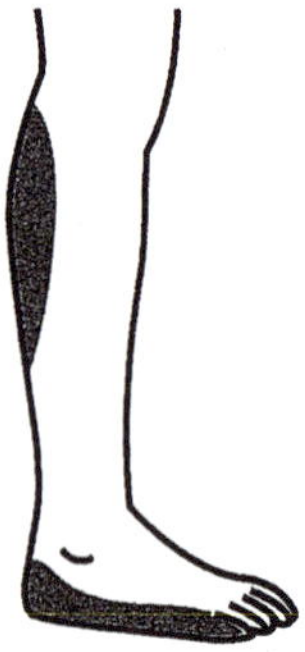
Motor weakness	Extension of quadriceps	Dorsiflexion of great toe and foot	Plantar flexion of great toe and foot
Screening examination	Squat and rise	Heel walking	Walking on toes
Reflexes	Knee jerk diminished	None reliable	Ankle jerk diminished

Testing for lumbar nerve-root compromise. *(From Bigos, Bowyer, Braen, et al.)*

in whom there is no suspicion of serious causes of back pain. X-rays (and other imaging modalities) frequently reveal incidental abnormalities that are unrelated to a patient's current symptoms. The rate of such false-positive results increases with the patient's age, and there is no good evidence that imaging is either specific or effective in altering the course of patients with uncomplicated low back pain.

Testing in Patients with Red Flags

In patients with red flags suggesting underlying malignancy, fractures, or infection (Tables 12-4 and 12-5), further testing should be directed at identifying or excluding the suspected cause. For example, magnetic resonance imaging (MRI) or computed tomographic (CT) scans might be used to diagnose a suspected fracture, malignancy, or herniated disk (Figs. 12-4 and 12-5). Electromyographic studies are used to confirm nerve root dysfunction. Bone scans can detect malignant, inflammatory, or infectious conditions.

Other common diagnostic tests can be useful in special situations, but they are of little value unless specific findings in the history and physical examination suggest that such tests might be helpful. For example, complete blood counts and determinations of erythrocyte sedimentation rates can provide evidence to support the possibility of infection, inflammation, or malignancy, but they are not ordered routinely because they are insensitive and nonspecific. Other biochemical tests (e.g., determination of serum calcium level, urinalysis, or determination of serum parathormone level) should only be ordered in individuals who have signs or symptoms suggesting that these tests might be helpful in diagnosis.

Special Considerations in Children and Older Adults

As noted previously, the prevalence of serious underlying abnormalities in children, adoles-

Figure 12-4

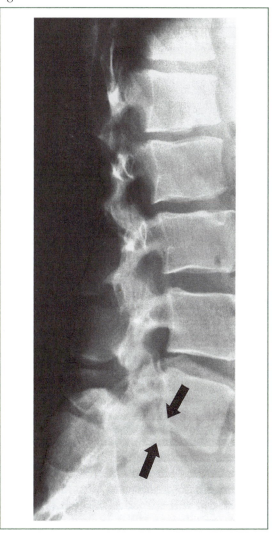

Plain x-ray of herniated lumbosacral disk. This patient has a herniated intervertebral disk at the L4–L5 level. The principal radiographic finding is narrowing of the L4–L5 interspace (arrows). *(Photograph courtesy of James Heckman, MD, Department of Orthopedics, University of Texas Health Science Center at San Antonio.)*

cents, and older adults with back pain is much higher than in working-aged adults. In adults over age 50, x-rays should be obtained more readily. Even in what appears to be non-specific back pain, plain x-rays may reveal evidence of

Figure 12-5

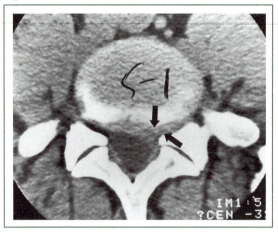

A CT scan of a herniated lumbosacral intervertebral disk. This scan is taken from the same patient whose x-ray is shown in Fig. 12-4. It shows a herniated nucleus pulposus (between the two arrows) that is impinging on the spinal canal. *(Photograph courtesy of James Heckman, MD, Department of Orthopedics, University of Texas Health Science Center at San Antonio.)*

spondylolysis, compression fractures, malignancies, and other abnormalities. Blood testing (e.g., for multiple myeloma or metabolic bone disorders) may be also important in elders who have persistent back pain. In children with suspected osteomyelitis or diskitis, radionuclide bone scans may be needed for diagnosis. The need for more specialized testing should be based on initial findings in the history and physical examination, and on the results of plain x-rays, blood tests, and bone scans.

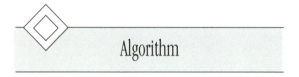

Algorithm

The U.S. Agency for Health Care Policy and Research (AHCPR) developed a series of algorithms for its clinical practice guidelines for the evaluation and management of acute low back pain. The five AHCPR back pain algorithms are shown in Figs. 12-6 to 12-10.

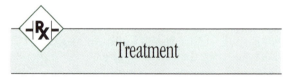

Treatment

After completing the history and physical examination, clinicians should be able to reliably decide whether a red flag or radiculopathy is present, and have a sense of the patient's underlying psychosocial situation. Because low back pain is a self-limited problem for the vast majority of patients, treatments should be used with caution, fully balancing the benefits, potential harm, and costs of therapy. In particular, treatment should seek, not just to diminish pain, but also to increase function. There is little evidence that outcome is influenced by the specific treatment chosen or by the type of clinician providing the treatment. However, some studies suggest that a practice style emphasizing self-care and depicting low back pain as a benign, self-limiting condition are associated with better outcomes, lower cost, and higher satisfaction on the part of the patient.

Treatment of Acute Low Back Pain

BED REST AND EXERCISE

One of the most important principles of treating low back pain is to keep patients active. A consensus is emerging that continuation of normal activities, as permitted by pain, provides recovery from back pain superior to that provided by bed rest or back exercises. For patients with typical low back pain whose pain prevents them from ambulating, bed rest should continue for no more than 2 days. Continuation of normal activities and return to work or school should be encouraged and should occur as early as possible. Specific exercise programs, the use of specialized machines, and structured back-pain

Figure 12-6

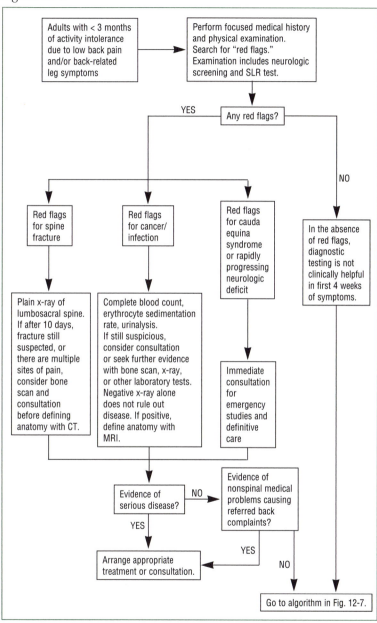

Algorithm for initial evaluation of acute low back problems. (*Adapted from Bigos, Bowyer, Braen, et al.*)

Figure 12-7

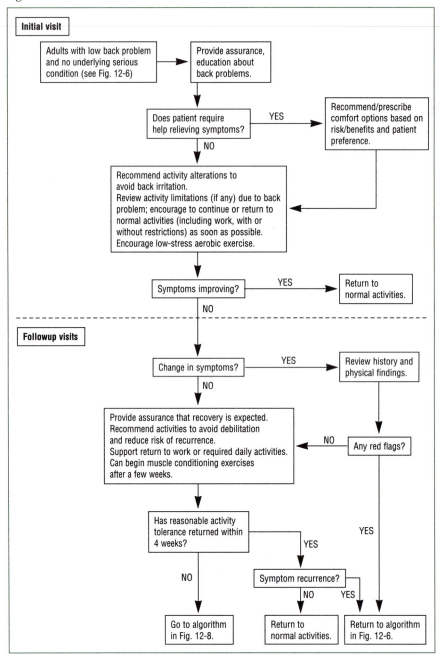

Algorithm for treatment of acute low back problems. (*Adapted from Bigos, Bowyer, Braen, et al.*)

Figure 12-8

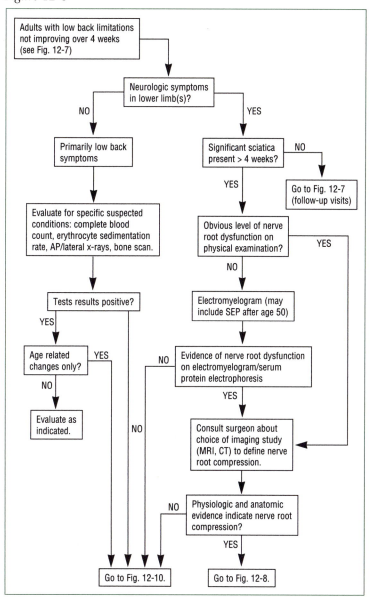

Algorithm for evaluating slow-to-recover back symptoms. *(Adapted from Bigos, Bowyer, Braen, et al.)*

Figure 12-9

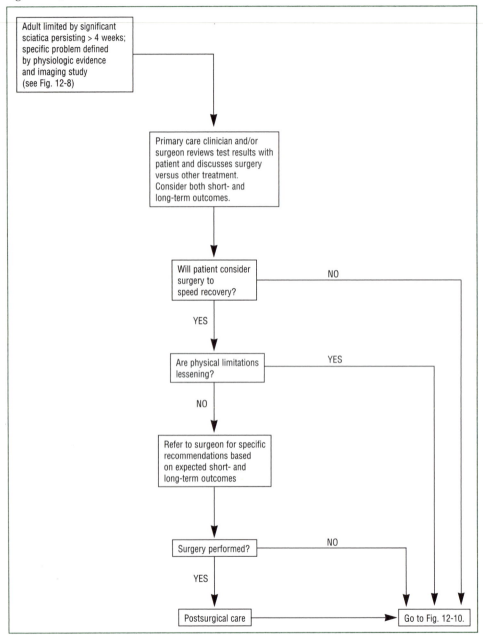

Algorithm for surgical consideration. (*Adapted from Bigos, Bowyer, Braen, et al.*)

Figure 12-10

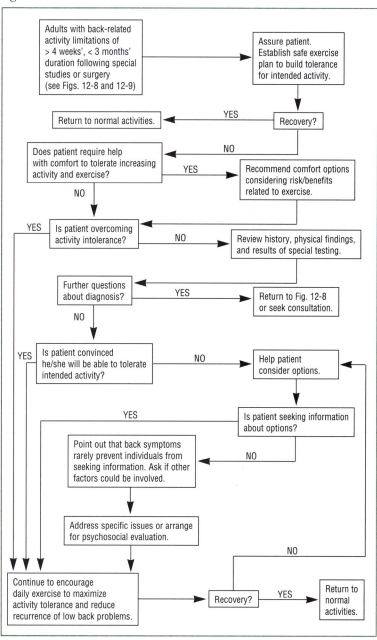

Algorithm for further management of low back problems. (*Adapted from Bigos, Bowyer, Braen, et al.*)

programs are costly and have not been shown to improve outcomes.

PHYSICAL AGENTS

There is little evidence to support the use of physical agents, such as application of heat or cold, in the treatment of low back pain. However, the use of cold or heat at home carries little risk and may offer some patients symptomatic relief. The only exception is for the elderly and for patients with impaired sensation, in whom there is a risk of burns or cold-induced cutaneous injury. Application of heat or cold may not be advisable in such individuals.

MEDICATIONS

There is considerable evidence that acetaminophen, aspirin, and other non-steroidal anti-inflammatory drugs (NSAIDs) are effective for treatment of low back pain. The margin of safety is reasonable, and these agents are relatively inexpensive. Thus, these agents are the medications of choice for analgesic treatment of low back pain. Standard dosing regimens are used, and continued as needed to facilitate ambulation and activity.

Medications classified as muscle relaxants (e.g., methocarbamol, chlorzoxazone, cyclobenzaprine, and carisoprodol) and benzodiazepines are often used for treatment of acute low back pain. Unfortunately, muscle relaxants cause drowsiness in up to 30 percent of patients, and sedation from benzodiazepines is almost universal. Therefore, these agents can impair or prevent patients from maintaining normal activity. Moreover, there is no clear evidence that these medications are effective in hastening recovery from low back pain. Thus, while they may relieve some degree of pain, muscle relaxants and benzodiazepines are not recommended for routine treatment of low back pain.

Antidepressants, corticosteroids, colchicine, and a host of other medications also are of unproven value in the treatment of low back pain and many carry risk of significant side effects. The use of opioid analgesics is controversial and is discussed later.

PHYSICAL THERAPY AND MANIPULATION

Despite widespread use, there are few data supporting the benefit of ultrasound, diathermy, and other modalities commonly used by physical therapists and others. The lack of data may reflect difficulty in demonstrating effectiveness of such treatments in a self-limited condition, methodological flaws in studies, or true lack of efficacy. Regardless of the reason, these methods of treatment are probably not appropriate for routine treatment of low back pain.

On the other hand, spinal manipulation, commonly performed by chiropractors and osteopathic physicians, is clearly effective for treatment of low back pain. Although many clinicians perceive manipulation as a controversial therapy, the bulk of evidence supports the effectiveness of manipulation for patients with and without radiculopathy. Spinal manipulation has a low incidence of complications (e.g., cauda equina syndrome occurs in about 1 case per million manipulations). However, although manipulation is effective and safe, the financial costs associated with manipulation may be higher than those of other treatments, probably reflecting the fact that manipulation usually involves a greater number of visits to the clinician. Limiting the number of manipulations per week and limiting the total duration of therapy to 2 to 4 weeks may be a reasonable way to control the cost of manipulation therapy.

SURGERY

Surgery is recommended for patients with serious underlying causes of low back problems (e.g., tumors) and in those with radiculopathy unresponsive to a 4- to 6-week trial of conservative treatment, as outlined above. Even with a herniated intervertebral disk, it is generally accepted that surgery is appropriate only for the abovementioned indications and then only if (1) examination reveals evidence of nerve-root compromise with significant disability or pain, and (2) an imaging test corroborates the presence of a herniated disk. Because surgery for herniated disks has not been conclusively shown to have better long-term outcomes than conservative management, most patients with sciatic radiculopathy can safely pursue conservative measures beyond 6 weeks, provided that there is no evidence of cauda equina syndrome or progressive weakness. Urgent surgery is indicated for individuals with cauda equina syndrome or progressive weakness.

When surgery is performed for properly selected patients with herniated disk, it is often effective. Standard diskectomy is the traditional procedure for herniated lumbar discs. However, microdiskectomy has similar outcomes and may have fewer complications. Injection of chymopapain is an acceptable alternative approach to open surgical procedures, but it is less efficacious and occasionally has adverse outcomes, including allergic reactions, diskitis, thrombophlebitis, pulmonary embolism, and transverse myelitis. Percutaneous diskectomy and other newer surgical approaches await further evidence of effectiveness. Spinal fusion is rarely indicated.

Surgery for spinal stenosis is often appropriate, even for individuals of advanced age. However, careful selection of patients and a frank discussion of the benefits and risks of surgery are important.

Unproven Interventions

A variety of non-surgical interventions, many of which have been commonly used, are of unproven benefit. For example, the use of traction, shoe insoles or shoe lifts (in patients without significant leg length discrepancy), acupuncture, transcutaneous electrical nerve stimulation (TENS), and biofeedback have never been shown to benefit patients with acute low back pain. The use of corsets, back belts, and braces is controversial because of concern that these external support devices may result in deconditioning of the patient's own musculature, and firm evidence of benefit is not available.

Evidence also indicates that local injections of anesthetics or corticosteroids are ineffective. Some studies, however, support the use of epidural corticosteroid injections, but the evidence for this is controversial and widely contested. It may be reasonable to try epidural steroid injections as a possibly effective nonsurgical treatment before proceeding to surgery for a herniated disk.

Treatment of Chronic Low Back Problems

The treatment of chronic low back pain, particularly when tied to disability, is a difficult problem. A detailed discussion of chronic pain management is beyond the scope of this chapter, but early identification of individuals with low back pain who are at risk for chronic disability may lead to better outcomes if clinicians can introduce appropriate therapies early in the course of treatment. These therapies include early resumption of activity, treatment of underlying psychosocial and occupational issues, exercise programs geared to increasing general physical activity, work-hardening (progressive reintroduction of work activities), education of the patient, and functionally-oriented programs that target improvement of activity tolerance.

A variety of psychosocial and behavioral interventions, such as cognitive-behavioral therapy and contingency management, may also be effective for alleviating or reducing pain in patients with chronic low back problems. Cognitive-behavioral therapy and contingency management programs are psychological interventions that address patients' perceptions and reactions to common tasks, restructure unproductive thought patterns, and create new, more positive behaviors.

Treatments such as traction, TENS, and analgesics are probably less effective than the more "holistic" approaches outlined above, since the latter emphasize functional improvement and coping strategies. Multidisciplinary pain or rehabilitation programs may offer benefits to individuals with chronic back pain unresponsive to the abovementioned treatments.

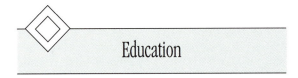

Education

Education of patients is widely felt to be important both for patients at risk for back problems and for those who already have acute or chronic back pain. Several educational interventions are discussed here.

Education for Prevention of Back Pain

There is limited evidence that low back pain can be prevented. Some research suggests that recurrent episodes of low back pain may be prevented by regular physical exercise (not necessarily specific back exercise, but physical fitness exercise in general). The benefits of other interventions to prevent low back pain, including group educational programs, work-site programs, and mechanical supports, remain controversial, and there is some evidence to suggest they are not effective. While ergonomic principles should govern patients' work and home environments, including tasks such as sitting, lifting, or bending, there is little definitive evidence demonstrating that characteristics of chairs, beds, or work equipment have beneficial effects on outcomes.

Education for Treatment of Back Pain

Education is a key part of the treatment of low back pain. It involves educating patients about the cause and universality of back pain, negotiating a plan of treatment that includes early return to activity, and motivating patients to follow the predetermined plan. The AHCPR patient guide, *Understanding Acute Low Back Problems*, is a useful pamphlet for emphasizing key educa-

tional messages for patients. It may be obtained from the AHCPR (phone number 1-800-358-9295, Internet site www.ahcpr.gov). Key educational messages for patients are summarized in Table 12-7. Organized educational programs, such as "back schools," have been widely used in occupational settings, but recent large-scale studies show no evidence that they are beneficial.

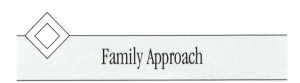

Family Approach

As in most of primary care practice, recognition of underlying psychosocial issues and capitalizing on family dynamics are important in caring for patients with low back pain. In fact, studies suggest that family and psychosocial problems may have more negative influence on developing or resolving chronic disability than do traditional biomedical factors.

For patients with subacute and chronic low back pain, involvement of the family can be important to functional recovery. A supportive family member may help encourage the patients to enter a rehabilitation program. Furthermore, family members may provide important information about substance use, psychiatric conditions, or family dysfunction, which, if addressed, may increase the likelihood of successful treatment.

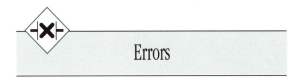

Errors

There are wide variations in how clinicians evaluate and treat low back problems. Evidence suggests that these variations may contribute to errors in care. The three most common errors are (1) inappropriate use of imaging modalities, (2) use of ineffective treatments, and (3) not spend-

Table 12-7

Key Educational Messages for Patients
with Acute Low Back Pain

> Over 90% of patients recover within 4–8
> weeks of presentation.
>
> While we have traditionally talked about back
> strains, subluxations, slipped disks, and
> other diagnostic labels, no clear classifica-
> tion predicts outcome—probably because
> the prognosis is so good anyway.
>
> Blood tests, x-rays, and other diagnostic inter-
> ventions are seldom necessary.
>
> You should maintain routine, nonstrenuous
> activities.
>
> Treatment is as close as your medicine chest:
> acetaminophen, aspirin, or ibuprofen are as
> effective as any other analgesic when taken
> appropriately.
>
> Other effective treatments include NSAIDs,
> manipulation, and mild, unsupervised exer-
> cise.
>
> Physical modalities (e.g., ice) may bring com-
> fort, but their effectiveness is uncertain.
> They are safe, however.
>
> Ineffective, unproven, and potentially harmful
> interventions include bed rest, traction, mus-
> cle relaxants, and a host of other medica-
> tions and procedures.
>
> Radiculopathy may require longer to subside;
> surgery is an option in patients with func-
> tional compromise who fail to respond to
> conservative measures.

ing enough time conducting a thorough history
and physical examination and educating the
patient. These common errors are relatively easy
to avoid when faced with patients who have
acute low back pain.

Inappropriate Use of Imaging Tests

As noted earlier, in working-aged adults with no
red flags, there are few indications for imaging
tests with patients who have otherwise uncomplicated acute low back pain unless symptoms
persist for more than a month (or more than 3
months if significant improvement or resolution
is occurring). Nonetheless, clinicians commonly
obtain imaging studies without these indications,
leading to unnecessary costs and radiation exposure.

On the other hand, clinicians sometimes fail
to obtain imaging studies with patients for whom
such testing is indicated. Probably the most common situations involve children with back pain
or apparently healthy-appearing older individuals with seemingly mild back pain who may, in
fact, have myeloma, metastatic cancer, Paget's
disease, or other potentially treatable conditions.
In both children and older persons, the rate of
important pathologic conditions is usually sufficient to warrant imaging studies in the initial
evaluation of back pain.

Use of Ineffective Treatments

As already discussed, there is no evidence that
many of the conventional treatments for back
pain are effective. Despite this lack of evidence,
many clinicians prescribe these treatments, some
of which have substantial cost implications for
patients and the health care system.

Perhaps the most treatment common error is
prescribing bed rest and limitations on activity,
because patients improve more rapidly when
they remain active and return to normal activities as quickly as possible. Similarly, clinicians
frequently prescribe drugs with limited proven
efficacy and potential harm, such as muscle
relaxants, while failing to prescribe clearly effective medications, such as NSAIDs. Finally,
clinicians sometimes encourage patients to participate in unproven and expensive rehabilitation programs for which no benefit has been
demonstrated. Participation in such programs
should be carefully considered and undertaken
cautiously, with structured, functional goals in
mind.

Spending Inadequate Time with Patients

Because job dissatisfaction, social and family stress, and psychological dysfunction all increase the likelihood of developing chronic back problems, the quality of the clinician-patient relationship is important to successful management of back pain. The realities of day-to-day practice, however, are such that clinicians often cannot spend sufficient time with patients to develop a high-quality relationship or to deal with the various psychosocial issues that contribute to poor outcomes. However, primary care clinicians are uniquely situated to offer patients, patients' families, and patients' employers a realistic assessment of the situation without losing the ability to work effectively with patients. A few extra minutes with a patient who has back pain can help establish an atmosphere of empathy, thereby facilitating education about the favorable natural history of back pain, the frequent lack of need for diagnostic tests, and the ineffectiveness of many common treatments.

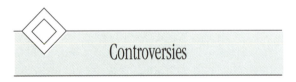

Controversies

The use of muscle relaxants and opioid analgesics for treating low back pain is particularly controversial. The role and effectiveness of many other unproven therapies are uncertain. There is also controversy about the effectiveness and timing of various surgical and anesthetic interventions.

Muscle Relaxants

A meta-analysis conducted by the AHCPR Low Back Problems Guideline Panel methodologists suggested a small beneficial effect of muscle relaxants on relief of pain and other back symptoms. However, the analysis also found potential risks from these medications, such as sedation that decreases activity levels. In addition, some muscle relaxants have potent anticholinergic properties, making them generally unsuitable for use in older patients. Despite this, many clinicians regularly prescribe muscle relaxants for patients with back problems. Further research is needed to clarify the role of these medications in treating back pain.

Opioids

For treating acute low back pain, NSAIDs are generally preferred because they have similar or greater effectiveness than opioids and other analgesic medications. In addition, opioids have the potential to cause sedation and, therefore, decrease early return to activity. With patients predisposed to substance abuse problems or at risk for developing chronic pain, opioids also have the potential for abuse. Nonetheless, many clinicians argue that short-term use of opioids carries little risk of addiction or dependence, and they are effective for pain relief. The general consensus, however, is that, because acute low back pain typically occurs in self-limited episodes and NSAIDs are at least as effective as opioids, NSAIDs should generally be the first-line analgesic therapy for acute back pain.

For chronic back pain, opioid analgesic therapy is considerably more controversial. Opioids are effective for pain relief, but there are many potential pitfalls and unanswered questions about using opioids for treatment. If opioids are given for chronic recalcitrant back pain, they are likely to be continued as long-term or life-long therapy, creating a potential for addiction and misuse, and no beneficial effects have been demonstrated with such therapy.

Thus, other treatment modalities, including non-pharmacologic interventions and management by a multidisciplinary pain clinic, are often preferred. If used for chronic back pain, opioid therapy should have clear objectives and anticipated functional outcomes. Patients should be evaluated at intervals to assess progress toward those objectives and outcomes, and opioids should be discontinued if objectives are not met. In addition, patients should be fully informed of the potential risks of narcotic therapy for a chronic back pain syndrome.

Unproven Therapies

As discussed earlier, the effectiveness of a wide variety of commonly used treatments has never been demonstrated. These treatments include various physical therapy modalities, exercises, braces and supports, and back pain education programs. Despite lack of demonstrated benefit, many clinicians are convinced of the advantage of using these treatments and continue to prescribe them. While rarely harmful, the cost of these interventions is substantial. Clarification of the benefit and role of these controversial treatments is needed.

Other Controversies

Many controversies exist among orthopedists, neurosurgeons, and other referral specialists about the management of low back pain. Key unresolved issues include the roles of epidural steroid injections and facet-joint injections, the timing of surgery relative to pharmacologic and nonpharmacologic interventions, and the best procedures to perform when invasive interventions are needed.

In particular, the AHCPR back pain guideline stimulated considerable controversy with its recommendation against early imaging studies and early surgical interventions for patients with radiculopathic syndromes. Many surgical specialists felt that the guideline recommendations were too conservative, despite lack of evidence to support earlier interventions. However, recent studies suggest that, rather than being conservative, the AHCPR recommendations may actually be overly interventional. When they are applied in primary care practice, many unnecessary x-rays are obtained, leading to a needless increase in

costs. Additional research is needed to demonstrate potential benefits, if any, from early radiographic or surgical interventions.

Emerging Concepts

Perhaps the most important new trend in the approach to back pain is to view the problem as an expected part of life, rather than as an illness. Management now focuses on early return to normal activity, delay in surgical interventions, and non-use of the many common treatments that have no proven benefit. Research, in turn, is focusing on determining which of these treatments, if any, are beneficial. It is likely that continued development of managed care and cost-containment pressures will further emphasize the need to use only treatments with established benefits.

Another important area of future emphasis will be refining the ability to determine which patients with acute low back pain are at risk of developing chronic back problems or disabilities, and in which patients the acute episode will resolve uneventfully. The recent realization that psychosocial factors appear more strongly associated with chronicity and disability than medical factors will provide a rational basis for developing such predictive models. The ability to accurately identify patients at risk for chronicity and disability can alter the way in which primary care clinicians approach patients with low back pain.

Bibliography

Assendelft WJJ, Bouter LM, Knipschild PG: Complications of spinal manipulation. *J Fam Pract* 42:475, 1996.

Bigos SJ, et al: A longitudinal, prospective study of industrial back injury reporting. *Clin Orthop Relat Res* 279:21, 1992.

Bigos SJ, Battie MC, Spengler DM, et al: A prospective study of work perceptions and psychosocial factors affecting the report of back injury. *Spine* 16:3, 1991.

Bigos SJ, Bowyer O, Braen G, et al: *Acute Low Back Problems in Adults: Clinical Practice Guideline Number 14*, AHCPR publication no 95-642. Rockville, MD, U.S. Department of Health and Human Services, Public Health Service, Agency for Health Care Policy and Research, 1994.

Boos N, Lander PH: Clinical efficacy of imaging modalities in the diagnosis of low-back pain disorders. *Eur Spine J* 5:2, 1996.

Borenstein DG, Burton JR: Lumbar spine disease in the elderly. *J Am Geriatr Soc* 41:167, 1993.

Brown RL, Fleming MF, Patterson JJ: Chronic opioid analgesic therapy for chronic low back pain. *J Am Board Fam Pract* 9:191, 1996.

Carey TS, Garrett J: The North Carolina Back Pain Project: Patterns of ordering diagnostic tests for patients with acute low back pain. *Ann Intern Med* 125:807, 1996.

Carey TS, Garrett J, Jackman A, et al: The outcomes and costs of care for acute low back pain among patients seen by primary care practitioners, chiropractors, and orthopedic surgeons. *New Engl J Med* 333:913, 1995.

Daltroy LH, Iversen MD, Larson MG, et al: A controlled trial of an educational program to prevent low back injuries. *New Engl J Med* 337:322, 1997.

Deyo RA, Phillips WR: Low back pain: A primary care challenge. *Spine* 21:2826, 1996.

Deyo RA, Rainville J, Kent DL: What can the history and physical examination tell us about low back pain? *JAMA* 268:760, 1992.

Frymoyer JW: Predicting disability from low back pain. *Clin Orthop Relat Res* 279:101, 1992.

Hadler NM: Workers with disabling back pain. *New Engl J Med* 337:341, 1997.

Hartigan C, Miller L, Liewehr SC: Rehabilitation of acute and subacute low back and neck pain in the work-injured patient. *Orthop Clin North Am* 27:841, 1996.

Hollingworth P: Back pain in children. *Br J Rheum* 35:1022, 1996.

Indahl A, Velund L, Reikeraas O: Good prognosis for low back pain when left untampered. *Spine* 20:473, 1995.

Jensen MC, Brant-Zawadzki MN, Obuchowski N, et al: Magnetic resonance imaging of the lumbar spine in people without back pain. *New Engl J Med* 331:69, 1994.

Karas BE, Conrad KM: Back injury prevention interventions in the workplace. *Am Assoc Occup Health Nurs J* 44:189, 1996.

Katz JN, Dalgas M, Stucki G, et al: Degenerative lumbar spinal stenosis. *Arthritis Rheum* 38:1236, 1995.

Kummel BM: Nonorganic signs of significance in low back pain. *Spine* 21:1077, 1996.

Lechner DE: Work hardening and work conditioning interventions: Do they affect disability? *Phys Ther* 74:471, 1994.

Malmivaara A, Hakkinen U, Aro T, et al: The treatment of acute low back pain: Bed rest, exercises, or ordinary activity? *New Engl J Med* 332:351, 1995.

Payne WK, Ogilvie JW: Back pain in children and adolescents. *Pediatr Clin North Am* 43:899, 1996.

Rungee JL: Low back pain during pregnancy. *Orthopedics* 16:1339, 1993.

Shekelle P, Markovich M, Louie R: An epidemiologic study of episodes of back pain care. *Spine* 20:1668, 1995.

Simmonds MJ, Kumar S, Lechelt E: Psychosocial factors in disabling low back pain: Causes or consequences? *Disabil Rehabil* 18:161, 1996.

Spaccarelli KC: Lumbar and cauda epidural corticosteroid injections. *Mayo Clin Proc* 71:169, 1996.

Suarez-Almazor ME, Belseck E, Russel AS, et al: Use of lumbar radiographs for the early diagnosis of low back pain: Proposed guidelines would increase utilization. *JAMA* 227:1782, 1997.

U.S. Preventive Services Task Force: *Guide to Clinical Preventive Services*, 2nd ed. Baltimore, Williams & Wilkins, 1996.

Weber H: The natural history of disc herniation and the influence of intervention. *Spine* 19:2234, 1994.

James L. Moeller
Douglas B. McKeag

Chapter

13

Sprains and Strains

How Common Are Sprains and Strains?

Various epidemiologic studies have shown that sprains and strains are the most common injuries to the musculoskeletal system. They account for 30 to 60 percent of the musculoskeletal problems seen in clinical practice and are among the top 20 reasons why patients seek treatment from primary care clinicians. Sprains and strains are usually acute injuries.

In both primary care and orthopedic practice, the most common sprains and strains are to joints of the lower extremity, most often the ankles and knees. Other common strains and sprains involve the thigh, wrist, and shoulder. This chapter reviews the diagnosis and management of the most common sprain or strain in each of these areas.

Sprains

Sprains are injuries to ligaments. Ligaments attach bone to bone (e.g., the anterior cruciate ligament of the knee runs between the femur and tibia). Injury to ligaments can be fairly minor (e.g., a mild stretch) or major (e.g., complete rupture of a ligament). Grading systems have been developed to quantitate the severity of sprains based on the amount of ligamentous disruption. The grade is determined clinically by stressing the ligament with a passive range of motion test to observe (1) the ligament's excursion relative to the contralateral side, (2) the quality of the ligament's "end point" (i.e., how effectively the ligament stops the joint's excursion), and (3) the intensity of pain (Table 13-1). Higher-grade injuries typically take longer to heal, and the return to full activity usually takes longer than with lower-grade injuries.

Strains

Strains are injuries to muscles or musculotendinous tissue. They usually occur during specific traumatic events, which distinguishes them from overuse injuries, in which repetitive micro-stress causes injury to tissue. Strains can also be graded, based on whether a musculo-tendinous unit has been stretched, partially torn, or completely torn. The assessment of grade depends on retention of strength, intensity of pain, and whether there is a visible defect in the musculo-

Table 13-1

Grades of Ligamentous Injuries (Sprains)

GRADE	COMMON TERM	DEGREE OF INJURY	EXCURSION	END POINT	PAIN INTENSITY
I	Mild	Overstretch of ligament fibers but no tearing of fibers	Same as uninjured side	Firm	+
II	Moderate	Partial tear (i.e., tear of some fibers)	Increased in comparison to uninjured side	Present	+ +
III	Severe	Complete tear	Increased in comparison to uninjured side	Soft or absent	±

tendinous unit (Table 13-2). As with sprains, recovery from higher-grade strains takes longer than that from lower-grade strains.

ANKLE SPRAINS

The ankle is the most common site of sprains and strains. Approximately 12 percent of musculoskeletal injuries encountered in acute-care settings involve the ankle, and ankle injuries make up a large portion of sports-related injuries. The majority of ankle injuries (up to 85 percent) are sprains, and most of these sprains are due to inversion of the joint, leading to injury of lateral ligamentous structures of the ankle. Sprains of the medial and tibiofibular ligamentous structures also occur, but they are less common in comparison to lateral ankle sprains.

Typical Presentation

Patients with a lateral ankle sprain typically complain of pain on the outside of the ankle after an inversion injury ("I rolled my ankle over"). A thorough history will often reveal some degree of foot plantar flexion as well. Many patients will have applied ice to the injured area, while others may have used heat, and some will have taken nonsteroidal anti-inflammatory drugs (NSAIDs) prior to seeking care for their injury.

Office-based primary care clinicians are often the first to provide care for these injuries, but sometimes patients are first treated in an emergency room and then present to office-based clinicians for follow-up care. In the latter situation, they may already be wearing a splint or brace, using crutches, and may or may not have x-rays in hand.

Key History

Along with the main complaint of lateral ankle pain, patients also commonly complain of swelling and bruising, primarily over the lateral aspect of the ankle. They may or may not be able to bear weight on the injured ankle, and, if they can walk, they typically walk with a limp. A precise description of the mechanism of injury, if the patient can recall the injury, can be helpful

Table 13-2

Grades of Muscle and Musculotendinous Injuries (Sprains)

GRADE	COMMON TERM	DEGREE OF INJURY	STRENGTH	VISIBLE DEFECT OR BULGE WITH MUSCLE CONTRACTION	PAIN INTENSITY
I	Mild	Stretch of muscle fibers, no tearing	Full, but testing causes discomfort	No	+
II	Moderate	Partial tear	Decreased compared to uninjured side	Possible	+ +
III	Severe	Complete tear	Significantly decreased compared to uninjured side	Possible	+ + +

in identifying the injured structure. In addition, six other questions that have importance for diagnosis and treatment are listed in Table 13-3.

Physical Examination

Physical examination should be performed systematically, and the uninjured side should always be examined and compared to the injured side.

Inspection

The first step is inspection of the patient's gait and of the ankle itself. While the patient attempts to walk, the clinician observes the gait, looking for evidence of a limp or inability to bear weight. Patients with lateral ankle sprains limp favoring the injured side. Then, after removal of the patient's shoes and socks from both feet, the ankles are inspected for swelling and ecchymosis. General ankle swelling is usually present on the injured side and is often more prominent laterally. Ecchymosis is a variable finding, ranging from extensive to absent, depending on the severity of and the time elapsed since the injury.

Palpation

The next step is gentle palpation, with the area of expected maximal tenderness palpated last. The most commonly injured and most tender structures in ankle inversion injuries are the anterior talofibular and calcaneofibular ligaments (Fig. 13-1). Other ankle structures that should be palpated include the posterior talofibular ligament, anterior tibiofibular ligament, deltoid ligament complex, navicular tubercle, posterior portion of the medial and lateral malleoli, and the tibialis anterior, peroneal, and Achilles tendons.

Ankle inversion with or without plantar flexion may also injure other structures. The most common are the proximal fibula and base of the

Table 13-3
Useful Questions for Patients with Lateral Ankle Injuries

QUESTION	SIGNIFICANCE
"Did you hear or feel a snap or pop at the time of the injury?"	Yes response indicates possible fracture, ruptured ligament, or ruptured tendon.
"What types of activities does this injury keep you from doing?"	Response indicates functional severity of injury.
"Does the ankle feel numb or weak, or is it just painful?"	Numbness suggests injury to common peroneal nerve, which can occur from ankle inversion.
"Have you ever injured this ankle, or the other ankle, previously?"	Ligamentous instability, if detected, may be the result of an old injury.
"Are you experiencing any problems in other places such as the knee, leg, or foot?"	Ankle inversion can also cause fractures of the proximal fibula and/or base of fifth metatarsal.
"What have you done to treat this injury on your own?"	Response is useful in prescribing treatment.

Figure 13-1

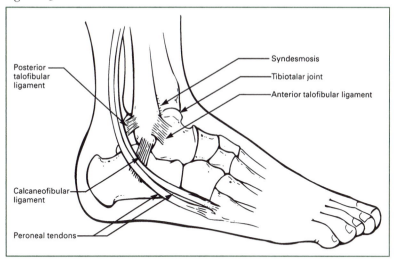

Ligamentous structures of the ankle. The ligaments most often sprained in ankle inversion injuries are the anterior talofibular ligament and the calcaneofibular ligament. (*From AM McBryde and DL Morrow. Reproduced with permission of © The McGraw-Hill Companies, Inc.*)

fifth metatarsal, and palpation should also include these areas. In fact, when examining an injured ankle, it is advisable to also briefly examine the knee and foot.

Assessing Neurovascular Integrity

An assessment of neurovascular integrity should always be performed when evaluating an injured ankle. Specifically, the dorsalis pedis and posterior tibial pulses should be palpated and compared to pulses on the uninjured side. Nerve function should be briefly tested by determining the patient's ability to sense a light touch.

Assessing Ligamentous Stability

The final step in the physical examination is assessment of ligamentous stability. Lateral ankle ligaments are evaluated by the anterior drawer test and talar tilt test. However, some patients may not tolerate these tests due to pain from the injury. In addition, it is important to remember that all patients have some degree of "native laxity" in their joints, and this laxity varies from person to person. This is why comparison to the opposite ankle is imperative. Finally, prior injury may alter findings on these stress tests.

ANTERIOR DRAWER TEST

Anterior drawer testing assesses stability of the anterior talofibular ligament, which is usually the first ligament injured during an inversion stress to the ankle. The test is performed by stabilizing the distal portion of the leg with one hand while the other hand attempts to move the talus anteriorly (Fig. 13-2). Placing the patient's foot in a slight degree of plantar flexion adds to the specificity of this test. Increased excursion compared to the opposite side constitutes a positive test result (i.e., injury to the anterior talofibular ligament).

Figure 13-2

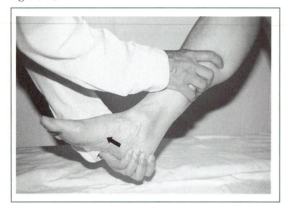

Anterior drawer test for ligamentous stability of the ankle. The anterior drawer test assesses stability of the anterior talofibular ligament. The test is performed by stabilizing the distal portion of the leg with one hand while the other hand attempts to move the talus anteriorly, in the direction shown by the arrow.

TALAR TILT TEST

The talar tilt test assesses integrity of the calcaneofibular ligament. This test is performed by stabilizing the distal leg with one hand while using the other hand to apply inversion stress to the ankle (Fig. 13-3). Increased excursion compared to the opposite side constitutes a positive test result. Since this test often causes substantial pain, it is usually performed at the end of the examination.

Ancillary Tests

Many clinicians routinely obtain plain x-rays of patients with ankle injuries. However, the appropriateness of obtaining routine ankle x-rays has been called into question by development of the "Ottawa clinical decision rules," which selectively identify patients for whom x-rays are required. Implementation of the Ottawa rules

Figure 13-3

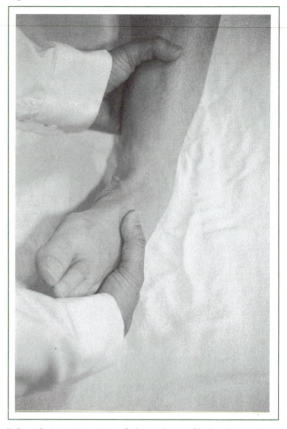

Talar tilt test. Integrity of the calcaneofibular ligament is assessed by stabilizing the distal leg with one hand while the other hand applies inversion stress to the ankle.

has been shown to decrease the use of x-rays for ankle and foot injuries, lower cost, and lessen the time patients spend having ankle injuries evaluated with no loss of sensitivity for detecting fractures.

According to the Ottawa rules, x-rays of the ankle are only required in cases of blunt ankle trauma if there is pain in the malleolar area plus (1) tenderness along the posterior aspect or tip of the lateral malleolus, (2) tenderness along the posterior edge or tip of the medial malleolus, or (3) inability to bear weight. In addition, patients over 55 years of age should generally have ankle x-rays because of the higher likelihood of occult fractures in older patients. However, in the absence of any of these findings, patients can be assumed not to have a fracture, and treatment for ankle sprain can be instituted. While the Ottawa rules were developed for patients over the age of 18 in emergency department settings, recent studies indicate they are also valid for children. They have not been validated, however, in office settings.

Treatment

Treatment of Acute Injury

Treatment of sprains initially involves protection, rest, ice, compression, and elevation (PRICE). For ankle sprains, protection may include splinting. Rest can be achieved with immobilization boots, inflatable plastic splints, or other in-shoe splint devices, and crutches may also be required if patients are unable to bear weight. If crutches are necessary, their use should be limited and discontinued as quickly as pain permits. Ice is typically applied in 20-min sessions, four to six times per day immediately following the injury, and then the frequency is decreased as swelling abates. Compression can be achieved with the use of an elastic wrap, and elevation (to above the level of the heart) should occur as much as possible until swelling is resolved.

Pain control can be achieved with acetaminophen or NSAIDs. Optimal timing of NSAID administration, however, is controversial. Some experts suggest that NSAIDs not be administered for 24 to 48 h after the injury because of concern that earlier use of these platelet-inhibiting medications might increase bleeding into the injured area. On the other hand, there is evidence that early administration of NSAIDs may speed healing. Thus, at this time, the preferred schedule for NSAID use is uncertain.

Rehabilitation

TIMING

In the past, many experts recommended that use of the ankle not occur until after 7 to 10 days of immobilization. In mild to moderate lateral ankle sprains, however, active rehabilitation can often be started within 24 to 72 h of injury. In fact, Eiff and colleagues demonstrated that patients with first-time lateral ankle sprains tend to return to activity earlier and with less discomfort when treated with early mobilization. Compared to patients initially treated with 10 days of immobilization, there is no increase in late residual symptoms or ankle instability when mobilization begins early following mild to moderate sprains.

REHABILITATION PROGRAM

Most patients do well with a simple, home-based rehabilitation program. Typical home programs include range-of-motion exercises, strengthening exercises, and restoration of proprioception, followed by resumption of normal activity and measures to prevent future ankle sprains.

RANGE OF MOTION   Ankle motion is improved by range-of-motion exercises, such as "foot alphabet" exercises. These exercises are conducted by having patients imagine that their great toe is a pencil and then having them write the alphabet in the air with their toe.

STRENGTHENING EXERCISES   When motion has been restored, patients may begin strengthening exercises by moving the ankle, against resistance, through its various motions. Elastic tubing, physical therapy bands, towels, or an old bicycle-tire tube can be used to provide resistance. It is important, however, not to limit strengthening only to the ankle. Rather, the muscles of the lower leg, particularly those that provide secondary support to the lateral ankle (i.e., the peroneal muscles) should also be involved in strength training.

PROPRIOCEPTION Restoration of proprioception is the next goal. This portion of the rehabilitation is often the most difficult. Balance boards are used in formal rehabilitation programs, but other, simpler methods can be used in a home program. For example, having a patient balance on one foot (the foot of the injured extremity) is simple and effective. Another technique is to have patients control a tennis ball on the floor with their foot without looking at the foot.

RESUMING NORMAL ACTIVITIES Before resuming full activity, patients should go through a graded increase in functional activity to assure that their ankle can perform normally and without discomfort. This is particularly important for patients who will be resuming vigorous, sports-related movements of the injured ankle. Return to activity follows the principle of "start low, go slow." The process typically begins with straight-ahead jogging and slowly graduates to straight-ahead running. Next, patients can add gentle turns to the jogging or running routine and then advance to zig-zags and sharp cutting maneuvers. Eventually, patients should be able to return to full activities.

The entire routine of increasing activity may require a very short time, perhaps as little as 1 week, for patients with mild ankle injuries. For others, resumption of normal activities may take weeks or months, depending on the severity of the injury, treatment success, rehabilitation efforts, and compliance on the part of the patient.

PREVENTING FUTURE INJURIES After patients have successfully completed rehabilitation and returned to full activities, the goal is to prevent recurrent ankle sprains. Maintenance of ankle motion, strength, and proprioception are important for preventing future injuries.

For individuals participating in sports, external stabilization using tape, ankle stirrups, or other types of ankle support is often helpful.

Ankle taping has been shown to restrict range of motion of the ankle and reduces the incidence of ankle sprains. However, the supportive benefit of taping is typically lost within 10 to 20 min. Other, probably more effective devices include lace-up stabilizers and semi-rigid (stirrup) orthoses. In contrast, high-top athletic shoes have not been consistently shown to be of benefit in reducing ankle sprains.

KNEE SPRAINS

Knee injuries are common in active individuals and very common in sports. Most of the knee problems evaluated by primary care clinicians are overuse injuries (e.g., patellofemoral dysfunction, patellar tendinitis, and quadriceps tendinitis). The purpose of this chapter, however, is to review common sprains and strains. Sprains of the knee can involve any of the four major ligaments that provide stability to the knee: the medial collateral, lateral collateral, anterior cruciate, and posterior cruciate ligaments.

This discussion focuses on sprains of the medial collateral ligament (MCL), the most common ligamentous injury of the knee. It is also an injury that usually requires no surgical intervention and therefore can often be managed by primary care clinicians. The MCL connects the medial aspect of the distal femur to the medial aspect of the proximal tibia and provides restraint against valgus forces applied to the knee, which, if excessive, can injure the MCL.

Typical Presentation

Typically, patients will describe a blow to the lateral knee, causing the knee to "buckle," with pain present since the time of injury. Sometimes, however, patients will not remember the mechanism or occurrence of an injury. Some swelling may be present, and the patient may have difficulty walking, changing directions while walking, or performing normal daily activities because of knee pain.

As with ankle injuries, patients will often have used rest, ice, and non-prescription medications before seeking medical attention. Some will have been seen in an emergency room before presenting to a clinician's office.

Key History

The precise mechanism of injury should be sought, since mechanisms other than a direct valgus stress suggest other or concomitant injuries. For example, valgus stress with a twisting component suggests injury to the medial meniscus, and a posterior blow suggests injury to the anterior cruciate ligament. Other important questions for the history are shown in Table 13-4.

Physical Examination

A systematic approach to the knee examination is important, and it is imperative for the examiner to differentiate between a guarded versus a relaxed examination. An examination performed when a patient is in pain and guarding can elicit inaccurate results.

Inspection

The patient's gait should initially be evaluated for ability to bear weight. General observation for gross deformities, swelling, and ecchymosis should then be performed.

Palpation

Gentle palpation is the next step of the examination. Palpation should include an assessment of the active and passive range of motion of the knee, and of the integrity of neurovascular function below the knee.

Table 13-4

Useful Questions for Patients with Knee Injuries

QUESTION	SIGNIFICANCE
"Were you able to bear weight immediately after the injury?"	No response indicates higher likelihood of fracture or ligamentous injury.
"Did you hear or feel a snap or pop at the time of the injury?"	Yes response indicates possible fracture, patellar dislocation, or anterior cruciate ligament tear.
"How long did it take for swelling to develop?"	Rapid swelling often indicates anterior cruciate ligament tear.
"Have you noticed any feelings of knee instability since the injury?"	If yes, higher likelihood exists of anterior or posterior cruciate ligament injury.
"Has your knee 'locked up' since the injury?"	Yes response suggests possible meniscus injury or bone/cartilage fragment within joint.
"Have you ever injured this knee before?"	Yes response suggests that ligamentous instability, if detected, may be the result of an old injury.

Tenderness to palpation may be isolated or more severe at the injury site, thereby facilitating identification of the injured structure. Sites that should be palpated are the quadriceps tendon, patella, patellar tendon, tibial tubercle, medial joint line, lateral joint line, medial and lateral collateral ligaments, hamstring tendons, fibular head, and popliteal fossa. Patients with an acute MCL sprain often have tenderness over the medial joint line and MCL, particularly where the ligament attaches to the femur. Marked tenderness in other areas suggests other injuries.

The next step in palpation is to determine whether a joint effusion is present. Effusions in the setting of an acute knee injury are usually due to hemarthrosis and suggest a fracture or a ligamentous tear.

Finally, palpation should include maneuvers to detect injuries in other structures of the knee. Patellar tests, including patellar motion (both passive and with quadriceps activation) and patellar apprehension and compression tests, should be performed to exclude patellar injury.

Assessing Ligamentous Stability

The next step in examining the knee is to assess the integrity of the ligaments. Valgus and varus stress tests are performed to evaluate the medial and lateral collateral ligaments, respectively (Fig. 13-4). These tests should be performed with the patient's knee in full extension and repeated again with the knees in 25 to 30° of flexion. While Fig. 13-4 depicts stress testing with x-ray images, stress testing in clinical practice is commonly performed without radiographs. Partial knee flexion enables the posterior joint capsule to relax, allowing isolation of the collateral ligament. Increased laxity noted with the knee in full extension indicates capsular injury in addition to collateral ligament injury. In cases of mild (grade I) MCL sprain, no laxity may be noted and the end point of any motion induced by the stress is usually firm. In severe (grade III) sprains, the laxity is significant and the end point is soft or nonexistent.

Because multiple ligamentous knee injuries may coexist, the stability of other ligaments should also be assessed. To test the anterior cruciate ligament, Lachman's test is considered the most sensitive and specific clinical test (Fig. 13-5). The anterior drawer test is commonly used to evaluate the anterior cruciate ligament, but it is less reliable than Lachman's test. Posterior drawer testing evaluates the integrity of the posterior cruciate ligament.

Tests of meniscal integrity, particularly the McMurray test, complete the general physical examination of the knee. In cases of isolated MCL sprain, the results of these tests should all be negative.

Ancillary Tests

The most important ancillary tests for evaluating knee injuries are plain x-rays of the knee, computerized tomography (CT) scans, and magnetic resonance imaging (MRI). In special situations, such as when knee pain and effusion are thought to be due to infection or crystal-induced arthritis, joint fluid analysis is important.

Plain X-rays

The most commonly ordered test to evaluate knee injury is the plain x-ray. The need for x-rays is often obvious, and they can reveal a great deal of information, including the presence or absence of fractures and loose bodies or degenerative changes within the joint.

Despite the importance of x-rays, they are not required in all cases, even when trauma is the cause of injury. Decision rules for the use of x-rays in acute knee injuries have been developed and validated by the same group in Ottawa that developed decision rules for obtaining x-rays in ankle injuries.

Figure 13-4

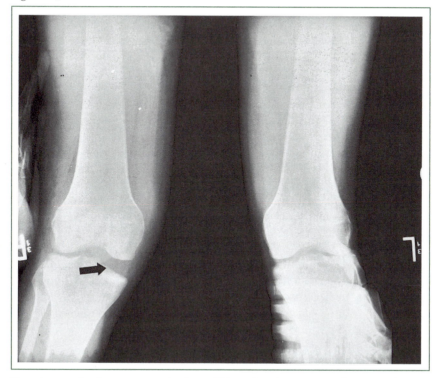

X-ray image of valgus stress to the knee. This patient has a ruptured MCL in the right knee. Application of valgus stress demonstrates widening of the medial joint space (arrow). *(Courtesy of James Heckman, M.D., University of Texas Health Science Center at San Antonio.)*

According to the Ottawa knee rules, x-rays are needed for acute knee injuries only if one or more of five factors is present: (1) age 55 years or older, (2) tenderness at the head of the fibula, (3) isolated tenderness of the patella (i.e., no tenderness anywhere but the patella), (4) inability to flex to 90°, or (5) inability to bear weight both immediately after the injury and for four steps when evaluated by a clinician (i.e., unable to transfer weight twice onto each lower limb regardless of limping). The Ottawa guidelines for knee x-rays were developed for adults and do not apply to individuals under 18. They are not applicable to persons who present with chronic knee problems.

Computed Tomography and Magnetic Resonance Imaging

Computed tomography scans are useful when fracture is strongly suspected but no fracture is seen on plain x-rays. Magnetic resonance imaging scans are highly sensitive and reasonably specific for evaluating soft tissue injuries in the knee, particularly meniscal and ligamentous injuries, including MCL injury. However, MRI should be used to confirm clinical diagnoses or suspicions, not to search for occult ligamentous injuries. In cases of isolated MCL sprains, MRI scans are often unnecessary, but they may be useful if an additional pathologic condition is

Figure 13-5

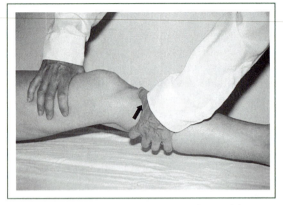

Lachman's test. Lachman's test assesses stability of the anterior cruciate ligament of the knee. While the knee is positioned in 10 to 15° of flexion, the examiner attempts to pull the tibia forward relative to the femur, while stabilizing the femur with the other hand. Any forward movement of the tibia relative to that in the contralateral knee indicates anterior cruciate ligament injury.

suspected based on the clinical examination. The results of MRI can help primary care clinicians make decisions regarding treatment and referral, and can help orthopedists make decisions regarding possible surgical interventions.

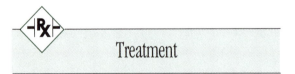

Treatment

Non-operative management is the treatment of choice for isolated MCL injuries, even in cases of complete tears. Furthermore, early functional rehabilitation of these injuries should be instituted for optimal results. Depending on their level of experience managing MCL injuries, primary care clinicians may wish to seek assistance from an orthopedist or physical therapist in developing and executing a treatment and rehabilitation plan.

Treatment of Acute Injury

The mainstay of early management of isolated MCL sprains of any degree is PRICE. Protection following acute injury can be provided with knee-immobilization splints, but complete immobilization should be avoided, regardless of the degree of injury. The benefits of knee bracing and knee sleeves have not been clearly established in grade I and II injuries. In grade III injuries, laterally hinged functional knee braces are helpful. Use of these protection devices is usually continued into the rehabilitation phase of treatment.

Although pain may preclude weight bearing immediately after the injury, weight bearing is allowed, as tolerated, in all cases of MCL sprain. However, crutches and avoidance of weight bearing may be needed in grade III injuries. Pain control can often be achieved with NSAIDs, but narcotic pain medications may also be needed. Icing and elevation should be provided in the acute post-injury period.

Rehabilitation

Early functional rehabilitation includes active range-of-motion exercises and quadriceps strengthening started as soon as possible after the injury. Quadriceps strengthening usually begins with unweighted straight-leg raises. Physical therapy modalities such as cold whirlpool and electrical muscle stimulation can be useful.

Once the patient is able to fully bear weight, closed kinetic-chain exercises, such as bicycling and mini-squats, can be added. Progressive resistive exercises (e.g., weighted straight-leg raises using exercise machines) are begun when the patient is able to flex the knee to 90°. When full range of motion is present, a running program can be started.

Patients may return to full activity once they demonstrate complete motion, minimal discomfort, ability to successfully complete functional testing, and quadriceps strength of at least 90 percent of that of the uninjured leg. Continued use of knee sleeves or braces after completion of the rehabilitation program is at the discretion of the patient and treating clinician.

THIGH MUSCLE STRAINS

Tears of the quadriceps and hamstring muscles are extremely common. These strains may be partial or complete, and usually occur at the musculotendinous junction.

Muscle strains typically occur during eccentric muscle activity: forced lengthening of a muscle while it is contracting. An example of eccentric quadriceps injury occurs when soccer players trying to kick the ball have their leg simultaneously struck from the front. An eccentric hamstring injury typically occurs during running when, while the hamstring is pulling the tibia backwards, the leg is struck from behind and pushed forward.

Typical Presentation

Patients will often complain of a "pulled muscle" in the thigh, although they may or may not recall the specific injury. Discomfort is usually present when the patient tries to use the injured muscle, particularly against resistance. Although patients usually can tolerate normal daily activities, vigorous activities are more difficult to perform.

Key History

The primary issue to address in the history is whether the problem is due to a muscle strain or simply a muscle contusion. Ascertaining the specific mechanism of injury can help differentiate these two entities. Contusions are generally due to direct blunt trauma to a muscle, whereas strains, as noted above, are caused by stretching of contracted muscles. Distinguishing strains from contusions is important because the initial therapy may differ, and rehabilitation will progress more slowly for patients with a thigh strain.

Physical Examination

Quadriceps Strains

Palpation of a strained quadriceps muscle reveals fairly superficial tenderness, typically over the rectus femoris. Tenderness may be exacerbated by resisted activation of the quadriceps and by passive stretching of the rectus femoris.

A palpable defect may be noted with contraction of the strained quadriceps muscle, representing the site of torn muscle fibers, particularly in an acute grade II or grade III strain. Swelling and hematoma formation may obscure the defect, but contraction of the quadriceps may cause a noticeable bulge in the thigh.

Hamstring Strains

In hamstring strains, swelling and ecchymosis may be present over the muscles, and palpation causes tenderness at the site of injury. Resisted hamstring contraction is often also uncomfortable for the patient, as is passive stretching. A palpable defect in the muscle may be detected early, but, as with quadriceps injuries, this defect may subsequently be obscured by swelling. Nonetheless, contraction of the hamstring musculature may still reveal a bulge.

Avulsion of the hamstring from its bony origin on the ischium sometimes occurs. This injury should be suspected when the patient has a palpable defect extending proximally from the retracted muscle belly to the ischium.

Ancillary Tests

X-rays are rarely helpful in cases of quadriceps and hamstring strains. The only exception is with children, in whom bony epiphyseal avulsions can occur in association with muscle strains. X-rays should be obtained of children with thigh muscle strains if bony tenderness is present.

Generally, CT and MRI are not needed to assist in making diagnostic or treatment decisions for patients with quadriceps or hamstring strains. Some studies have indicated, however, that CT scanning may aid in choosing between non-surgical and surgical interventions, and that MRI may be helpful in predicting recovery following hamstring injuries. Thus, CT and MRI scans may be appropriate with severe injuries or when surgical interventions are being considered.

Treatment

Treatment for quadriceps and hamstring strains begins with PRICE and also includes pain control with acetaminophen or NSAIDs and crutches if needed. This early phase of treatment, referred to as the "acute phase," is aimed at reducing swelling, inflammation, and pain.

The goal of the next "subacute phase" is to regain normal gait and normal motion, but there is no consensus on optimal treatment following this phase. The most common approach is to undertake a program of gentle stretching along with muscle strengthening.

Once recovery has advanced to the point where the patient has a normal gait and mobility, more vigorous strengthening efforts and functional exercises can begin. Return to full activity is allowed when strength is estimated to be within about 90 percent of that of the uninjured side and function is pain free.

Indications for Surgical Repair

Surgical intervention generally is not needed. In fact, even large quadriceps tears with significant palpable defects seldom require surgical repair. However, when avulsion of the hamstring complex at or near the proximal bone-tendon junction occurs, surgical reconstruction is generally advisable to avoid chronic pain and functional deficits. As noted above, CT or MRI scans can be useful for confirming the presence of bone avulsions when such injuries are suspected.

WRIST SPRAINS

The anatomy of the wrist is complex, consisting of eight carpal bones aligned in two transverse rows, multiple ligaments, and a rich vascular supply. Wrist injuries can involve fractures and/or sprains of any of these structures. This section focuses on the common wrist sprain seen in primary care practice—sprain of the scapholunate articulation—along with comments about scaphoid (navicular) fracture, which is a commonly overlooked injury that may mimic a wrist sprain.

Scapholunate sprains involve injury to the three ligamentous structures that connect the scaphoid and lunate bones (Fig. 13-6). These ligaments are the interosseous scapholunate ligament, the dorsal scapholunate ligament, and the volar radioscapholunate ligament. The importance of scapholunate sprains lies not only in their frequency, but also in the fact that they are

Figure 13-6

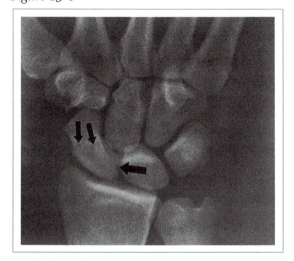

Scaphoid bone fracture. This patient was initially suspected of having a sprain of the scapholunate ligament, which connects and stabilizes the scapholunate articulation (large arrow). In reality, however, there is a fracture of the scaphoid bone (small arrows), which is somewhat difficult to see. *(Courtesy of James Heckman, M.D., University of Texas Health Science Center at San Antonio.)*

sometimes difficult to detect, diagnosis is often delayed or missed, and symptoms may really be due to scaphoid bone fracture.

Consideration of scaphoid bone fracture is an important aspect of evaluating wrist injuries. Fractures of the scaphoid make up 70 percent of all carpal bone injuries, but these fractures are often missed because x-rays immediately after the injury often appear normal, even when a scaphoid fracture is present. The frequency with which this occurs is sufficiently large that missed scaphoid fractures are among the top ten reasons for malpractice actions against family physicians.

Typical Presentation

Patients with wrist sprains typically present with pain, decreased motion, and swelling. As with other acute injuries, patients may have tried a number of treatments at home, such as ice, heat, elastic wraps, and nonprescription NSAIDs, prior to presenting to a clinician's office.

Many wrist injuries seen by primary care clinicians are mild in nature and involve no obvious fracture or dissociation. These cases may be diagnosed simply as wrist sprain and treated with rest, ice, NSAIDs, and immobilization in a cock-up style wrist splint. In most cases, treatment is successful, but some patients either fail to improve or have difficulty returning to normal activities. It is only then that a more significant injury is discovered.

Key History

The mechanism of the injury is important. Typically, patients with scapholunate sprains report having fallen on an outstretched hand with the wrist in a hyperextended position. Other wrist derangements should be suspected if patients report a different mechanism of injury.

Several additional questions are also helpful. For example, it is useful to know whether the patient is left- or right-handed, and whether the injury is interfering with specific activities, since injuries to the dominant hand pose functional limitations during immobilization and also in the future if recovery is not complete. Patients should be questioned about the precise location of pain and any radiation of the pain, since the responses may suggest others injuries (e.g., fractures, nerve injuries, etc). Similarly, patients should be asked whether they are experiencing any numbness or tingling in the wrist, hand, or fingers (and, if so, which fingers), since the responses provide clues to possible nerve impingement. Finally, information about past wrist injury can be helpful in interpreting abnormalities and comparisons with the non-injured wrist.

Physical Examination

Physical examination begins with observation, looking for generalized or localized swelling in the wrist. Range of motion in all planes (palmar flexion, dorsiflexion, ulnar deviation, radial deviation, supination, and pronation) should be tested actively and passively. All facets of the examination should be compared to the uninjured side.

Palpation

The entire wrist should be palpated, as well as the distal forearm and hand, to determine the area of maximal tenderness. Because a variety of bone fractures can be present in what appears to be an otherwise uncomplicated wrist sprain, it is important to palpate bony structures, including each carpal bone, the ulnar and radial styloid processes, and the anatomical "snuffbox." The anatomical snuffbox lies between the extensor pollicis longus and abductor pollicis tendons (Fig. 13-7), and tenderness in this area indicates a scaphoid bone fracture until proven otherwise.

Assessing Ligamentous Stability

The Watson test is used to assess stability of the scapholunate ligaments. To perform the test, the examiner stabilizes the scaphoid by placing his or her thumb over the volar pole of the scaphoid bone while the wrist is held in ulnar deviation. As the hand is brought into radial deviation, pain is produced as the force is transmitted through the uninjured scaphoid bone to the scapholunate ligaments. In the absence of suspected navicular fracture, a positive Watson test result is taken as evidence that a scapholunate sprain is present.

Assessing Neurovascular Integrity

While an assessment of neurovascular integrity should be performed with all sprains and strains,

Figure 13-7

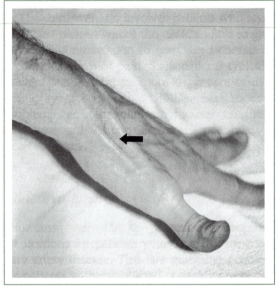

The anatomical "snuff box." The hollow between the extensor pollicis longus and abductor pollicis tendons is known as the anatomical snuff box (arrow). It overlies the scaphoid (navicular) bone.

this assessment is particularly important with wrist injuries. The radial and ulnar pulses should be palpated, and, when necessary, the Allen test can be used to confirm circulatory integrity. General sensation is best tested by two-point discrimination in each dermatomal region. Strength testing can be performed manually or with the help of a dynamometer.

Tinel's and Phalen's tests can be used if carpal nerve impingement is suspected. Tinel's test is performed by gently striking the flexor retinaculum on the volar surface of the wrist with a reflex hammer; if carpal tunnel impingement is present, patients will experience a shooting pain in the distribution of the median nerve. Phalen's test involves having the patient fully flex at the wrist and maintain this position for at least 1 min. This wrist position will compress structures within the carpal tunnel and cause symptoms if carpal tunnel impingement is present. These symptoms include numbness, tingling, or shooting pain in the distribution of the median nerve.

Ancillary Tests

Plain x-rays should be obtained in most cases of acute wrist trauma and should always include anterior-posterior, lateral, and oblique views. These standard views are sufficient for diagnosis and formulating a treatment plan in most cases, but special views may be appropriate if specific injuries are suspected (Table 13-5).

As noted above, results of initial x-rays are often negative with scaphoid fractures. If a scaphoid fracture is suspected based on snuff-box tenderness, treatment for a scaphoid fracture should be instituted. If there is need for a more prompt or definitive diagnosis, bone scanning can help rule out scaphoid (and other) fractures if performed more than 48 h after the injury. A CT scan and MRI scan can also be helpful in diagnosing scaphoid and other carpal bone fractures, but the cost of these studies makes them impractical for routine use.

Treatment

Because the scaphoid bone receives its blood supply via a single, retrograde intraosseous vessel, avascular necrosis of the distal bone fragment can occur if the bone is not properly immobilized (Fig. 13-8), and sometimes even if it is properly immobilized. Therefore, if snuff-box tenderness is present, scaphoid fracture should be suspected even if x-ray results are negative, and the patient's wrist should be immobilized in a short-arm thumb spica cast. Reevaluation (repeat x-rays) should occur in 2 weeks; if a fracture is present, it will be visible on the repeat x-ray. If no fracture is seen at the time of reevaluation, the cast can be removed.

If scaphoid fracture is not suspected, scapholunate sprain is the more likely diagnosis. This diagnosis is corroborated by a positive Watson test

Figure 13-8

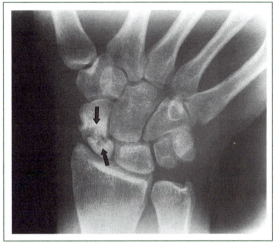

Scaphoid fracture. The arrows on this x-ray identify a fracture with non-union of the scaphoid bone accompanied by avascular necrosis of the distal bone fragment. *(Courtesy of James Heckman, M.D., University of Texas Health Science Center at San Antonio.)*

result (described above). If it is concluded that no true ligamentous dissociation has occurred, based on normal findings of special x-ray views (Table 13-5), and the injury is less than 3 weeks old, cast immobilization can be a successful treatment. The wrist is immobilized in a position of full supination, mild dorsiflexion, and ulnar deviation. However, if scapholunate dissociation has occurred and scapholunate instability is present by x-ray, treatment options include closed reduction with immobilization, percutaneous pinning, or open reduction with internal fixation.

Chronic scapholunate injuries, usually defined as injuries of greater than 3 months' duration, pose a complex and difficult management challenge. Several surgical options are available, and orthopedic consultation should be considered.

SHOULDER SPRAINS

The differential diagnosis of acute shoulder injuries includes dislocation, acute rotator cuff tear,

Table 13-5

Special Radiographic Views for Evaluating Wrist Injuries

SUSPECTED INJURY	RADIOGRAPHIC VIEW
Scapholunate widening (sprain)	Anterior-posterior clenched fist or supination
Suspected scaphoid (navicular) fracture	Ulnar deviation
Wrist instability	Lateral flexion and extension, anterior-posterior ulnar and radial deviation
Tear of ulnar-side triangular fibrocartilage complex	Wrist arthrograms or MRI
Perforations of the scapholunate ligament	Wrist arthrograms or MRI

proximal biceps tendon rupture, fractures, acromioclavicular injury, and a variety of other conditions. Many of these injuries (e.g., capsular joint injury, rotator cuff tendon injuries, and biceps tendon injury) are often called sprains even though no ligamentous structures are involved. The most common true ligamentous injury in the shoulder area, and the topic of discussion in this chapter, is acromioclavicular (AC) joint sprain.

Typical Presentation

Patients with AC sprain commonly present after receiving a blow to the superior surface of the shoulder, such as occurs when skiers fall on their shoulder. Depending on degree of pain and limited function, presentation to a clinician may occur soon after an injury or be delayed until several days later.

Key History

As with other injuries, history is important when trying to establish a diagnosis when patients present with shoulder injuries. Of particular impor-

tance is the mechanism of injury, which can involve direct or indirect trauma to the shoulder.

Any significant trauma causing elevation, depression, retraction, or anterior/posterior movement of the shoulder will transmit force to the axial skeleton. This force is transmitted via the clavicular complex anteriorly and through the periscapular muscles posteriorly. Because the clavicular complex is the more rigid of the two, failure along this complex is more common than injury to the periscapular muscles.

Whereas direct blows to the clavicle, such as those occurring in contact or stick sports, often result in clavicle fracture, blows that direct a downward force at the superior aspect of the acromion lead to an AC sprain. An AC sprain can thus occur when a patient falls and strikes the top of the shoulder on the ground. It also commonly occurs in contact sports during player-to-player, player–to–playing surface, or player-to-wall contact.

In addition to eliciting information about mechanism of injury, the history should cover other factors that might influence diagnosis or management. These factors are listed on Table 13-6.

Finally, the history should focus, not only on the musculoskeletal system, but also on the range of potentially serious non-musculoskeletal conditions that can present as shoulder pain. Of these, cardiac ischemia is of most concern because it is an acute life-threatening illness in which misdiagnosis can have fatal conse-

Table 13-6

Useful Questions for Patients with Shoulder Injuries

QUESTION	SIGNIFICANCE
"Where is the majority of the pain located?"	Response helps localize the site of injury.
"Does the pain radiate?"	Yes response may suggest cardiac disorder or neurologic injury.
"Are you experiencing any numbness, tingling, or weakness?"	Yes response suggests neurologic injury.
"Do you have any associated neck pain?"	Yes response suggests cervical radiculopathy.
"Does the shoulder feel like it came out of joint?"	Yes response suggests possible glenohumeral dislocation.
"Have you injured this shoulder before?"	Yes response indicates previous ligamentous instability; may warrant surgical intervention
"How does this injury interfere with your normal daily activities?"	Response indicates functional impairment associated with the injury.

quences. Thus, adults with shoulder pain, especially left shoulder pain, should always be questioned about cardiac risk factors and symptoms of acute heart disease, particularly when there is no clear history of trauma. Other important nonmusculoskeletal causes of shoulder pain include diaphragmatic irritation from hepatic or gallbladder disease, and intrathoracic neoplastic disease, such as a Pancoast tumor.

Physical Examination

Patients with AC sprain usually present with their shoulder in a guarded position, keeping the arm internally rotated and adducted, and supporting the injured side with the uninjured arm.

Inspection

The first step is to compare the injured and uninjured shoulders. In cases of acute AC sprain, swelling and deformity (a bump) over the AC joint are often readily visible. In addition to seeking evidence of AC joint injury, the clinician should look for signs of other injuries, such as obvious deformity of the clavicle (suggesting fracture) or deformity of the biceps muscle ("Popeye sign") that may indicate biceps tendon rupture.

Palpation

The second step in the examination is to test range of motion of the shoulder and the neck, simultaneously palpating the shoulder and scapula. Normally, movement of the humerus should account for about the first two-thirds of shoulder abduction, while scapulothoracic motion accounts for the final one-third of abduction. An AC joint injury is accompanied by reduction in scapulothoracic movement.

Palpation should then proceed to test for tenderness in specific locations. The usual routine for palpation is to begin at the sternoclavicular joint, progressing distally along the length of the clavicle to the AC joint and subacromial area. The biceps tendon in the bicipital groove, the anterior glenohumeral joint, and the coracoid process are palpated next. Finally, the clinician should palpate the muscles of the shoulder and neck. Pain over the AC joint is compatible with a diagnosis of AC joint sprain, but pain over any of these other anatomic sites should alert the examiner to the possibility of other injuries.

Neuromuscular Testing

Because the brachial plexus lies in close proximity to the shoulder, testing for neuromuscular defects is important in shoulder injuries. Neuromuscular examination begins with sensory testing throughout the upper extremity. Strength testing of the trapezius, deltoid, rotator cuff (supraspinatus, infraspinatus, subscapularis, and teres minor), biceps, and triceps should be performed and compared to the opposite side. While testing strength, it is important to pay attention to whether the patient experiences pain with muscle movement, since pain may indicate injury in the painful muscle. Testing of deep tendon reflexes, with comparison to the uninjured side, completes the neurologic evaluation.

Special Tests

There are many special tests used to determine integrity of the shoulder joint. Some of these tests are listed in Table 13-7 and discussed below.

CROSSOVER TEST

The crossover test is a test for AC joint injury. It is performed by having the patient place the hand of the injured side on the shoulder of the uninjured side, and then asking the patient to keep the arm parallel to the ground as the examiner applies a slight downward force to the elbow (Fig. 13-9). Pain at the AC joint constitutes a positive test result, indicative of AC joint injury. Since patients with a fractured clavicle also experience pain with crossover testing, it is important to carefully localize the site of pain and to obtain x-rays to exclude clavicle fracture if necessary.

APPREHENSION TEST

The apprehension test is useful for detecting an unstable (dislocatable) glenohumeral joint. It is performed by placing the patient's arm in an abducted and externally rotated position. Patients whose shoulders can be dislocated will experience pain, but, more important, they will resist any further motion and will probably have a noticeable look of alarm on their face. Pain without true apprehension is a negative test result. A positive test result suggests that the injury is a shoulder dislocation and not an AC joint problem.

SPEED'S AND YERGASON'S TESTS

These tests detect abnormalities in the biceps tendon. Speed's test is performed by having the patient extend the elbow and flex the shoulder to approximately 90°. While in this position, the patient resists downward force applied to the arm. Pain in the area of the bicipital groove constitutes a positive test result for a biceps tendon problem rather than an AC joint sprain. Yerga-

Table 13-7

Special Tests of the Shoulder

TEST	ANATOMIC STRUCTURE TESTED	DIAGNOSIS WITH POSITIVE RESULT
Crossover	AC joint	AC sprain
Apprehension	Anterior joint capsule	Anterior instability
Speed's	Biceps tendon (proximal)	Biceps tendinitis
Yergason's	Biceps tendon (distal)	Biceps tendon injury
Drop arm	Rotator cuff	Rotator cuff tear

Figure 13-9

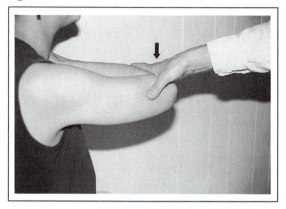

The crossover test. The patient places the hand of the injured shoulder onto the shoulder of the uninjured side, keeping the arm parallel to the ground. The examiner applies downward force to the elbow (arrow). In the absence of clavicle fracture, pain at the AC joint indicates AC joint injury.

son's sign is elicited by having the patient supinate the forearm against resistance while the elbow is flexed. Weakness and/or pain indicate a pathologic condition of the biceps.

DROP-ARM TEST

The drop-arm maneuver is used to detect rotator cuff injury. It is performed by having patients fully abduct the arm and then slowly and smoothly lower the arm to their side. If there is a tear in the rotator cuff (especially the supraspinatus muscle), the arm will typically drop abruptly to the side from about 90° of abduction. If the patient is able to hold the arm in abduction, a gentle tap on the forearm may cause the arm to drop.

Ancillary Tests

When AC injuries of the shoulder are suspected clinically, plain x-rays should be obtained (Fig. 13-10). Plain x-rays will not only detect the extent of the AC injury but also exclude the possibility of distal clavicle fractures. The x-rays should include anterior-posterior and axillary views of the AC joint, along with images of the uninjured side for comparison. If standard x-rays do not show disruption of the AC joint but AC injury is still suspected, anterior-posterior stress views may be obtained by applying downward weighting to the patient's arm (e.g., having the patient hold a sandbag or pail of water). Other studies, such as CT or MRI scans, are not generally required unless there is suspicion of soft tissue interposition between the disrupted aspects of the AC joint.

Treatment

Treatment of AC sprains is based upon the severity of the injury (Table 13-8). Types I and II injuries are treated conservatively with ice, rest, NSAIDs, a sling for comfort, and early range-of-motion. Rotator cuff and scapulothoracic strengthening can begin when pain permits. It may take 2 to 3 weeks for patients to be able to return to full activity after type I or II injuries. For athletes who wish to participate in contact activity during their rehabilitation, a doughnut-shaped pad over the AC joint can be helpful. For football players, "spider pads" (foam pads that fit under the regular shoulder pads), may provide significant relief and allow the player to participate in competition.

Proper initial treatment of type III injuries is controversial. Rockwood and colleagues reported that type III injuries can be treated conservatively initially with a 90 to 100 percent rate of satisfactory outcomes. Conservative treatment of type III AC joint injuries is similar to that for types I and II injuries.

Use of special braces to stabilize the AC joint, such as the Kenny-Howard sling, was common in the past but is infrequent today. The reason these devices are no longer used is that they pull

Figure 13-10

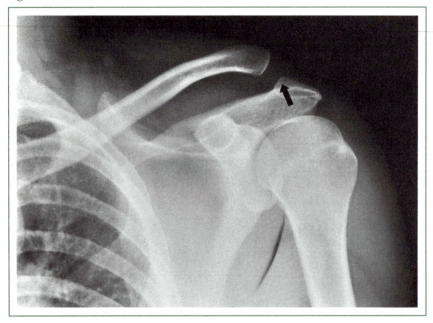

Grade III AC joint separation. The distal clavicle is displaced above the acromion (arrow). *(Courtesy of James Heckman, M.D., University of Texas Health Science Center at San Antonio.)*

the arm superiorly, reducing the space between the acromion and the clavicle; this position results in complications including skin breakdown, recurrence of deformity, and neurologic problems. Recovery from type III injuries managed conservatively may take up to 3 months.

Patients who fail conservative therapy for type III AC injuries should be referred to an orthope-

Table 13-8

Classification of AC Joint Injuries

Type	Description	Treatment
I	AC ligament sprain, joint and ligaments intact	Conservative
II	AC ligament disrupted, coracoclavicular ligament sprained, slight AC separation noted on x-ray	Conservative
III	AC and coracoclavicular ligaments disrupted, distal clavicle displaced above the acromion	Conservative*
IV	Complete AC dislocation, clavicle displaced posteriorly into the trapezius muscle	Orthopedic referral
V	Gross disparity between distal clavicle and acromion, with displacement of one to three times that of contralateral side	Orthopedic referral
VI	Clavicle displaced inferior to the acromion or coracoid process (rare)	Orthopedic referral

*Consider orthopedic referral if skin over AC joint is compromised.

dic surgeon. In addition, persons with type III injuries who perform overhead activities in their occupation should be considered for surgery initially, as should any patient whose injury compromises the integrity of the skin overlying the joint. Types IV, V, and VI injuries all require surgical consultation at the time of initial diagnosis.

Bibliography

Bach BR, VanFleet TA, Novak PJ: Acromioclavicular injuries. *Physician Sportsmed* 20:87, 1992.

Backx FJG, Beijer HJM, Bol E, et al: Injuries in high-risk persons and high-risk sports: A longitudinal study of 1818 school children. *Am J Sports Med* 19:124, 1991.

Barrett JR, Tanji JL, Drake C, et al: High- versus low-top shoes for the prevention of ankle sprains in basketball players: A prospective randomized study. *Am J Sports Med* 21:582, 1993.

Best TM, Garrett WE Jr: Hamstring strains: Expediting return to play. *Physician Sportsmed* 24:37, 1996.

DuPont M, Beliveau P, Theriault G: The efficacy of antiinflammatory medication in the treatment of the acutely sprained ankle. *Am J Sports Med* 15:41, 1987.

Eiff MP, Smith AT, Smith GE: Early mobilization versus immobilization in the treatment of lateral ankle sprains. *Am J Sports Med* 22:83, 1994.

Fumich RM, Ellison AE, Guerin GJ: The measured effect of taping on combined foot and ankle motion before and after exercise. *Am J Sports Med* 9:165, 1981.

Hutchinson MR, Ahuja GS: Diagnosing and treating clavicle injuries. *Physician Sportsmed* 24:26, 1996.

Hutton KS, Julin MJ: Shoulder injuries, in Mellion MB, Walsh WM, Shelton GL (eds): *The Team Physician's Handbook*, 2d ed. Philadelphia, Hanley & Belfus, 1997, p 438–460.

Keading CC, Sanko WA, Fischer RA: Quadriceps strains and contusions: Decisions that promote rapid recovery. *Physician Sportsmed* 23:59, 1995.

McBryde AM, Morrow DL: Pitfalls of early mobilization for patients with ankle sprains. *Your Patient and fitness* 12(1)29: 1997.

McCue FC, Bruce JF: The wrist, in DeLee JC, Drez D (eds): *Orthopaedic Sports Medicine*, Philadelphia, Saunders, 1994, pp 913–923.

McGrew C, Lillegard W, McKeag D, et al: Profile of patient care in a primary care sports medicine fellowship. *Clin J Sport Med* 2:126, 1992.

Meislin RJ: Managing collateral ligament tears of the knee. *Physician Sportsmed* 24:67, 1996.

Moeller JL, Lamb MM: Anterior cruciate ligament injuries in female athletes: Why are women more susceptible? *Physician Sportsmed* 25:31, 1997.

Pomeranz SJ, Heidt RS Jr: MR imaging in the prognostication of hamstring injury: Work in progress. *Radiology* 189:897, 1993.

Reider B, Sathy MR, Talkington J, et al: Treatment of isolated medial collateral ligament injuries in athletes with early functional rehabilitation: A five-year follow-up study. *Am J Sports Med* 22:470, 1993.

Rettig AC: Wrist injuries: Avoiding diagnostic pitfalls. *Physician Sportsmed* 22:33, 1994.

Rifat SF, McKeag DB: Practical methods of preventing ankle injuries. *Am Fam Phys* 53:2491, 1996.

Rockwood CA Jr, Williams GR, Young DC: Injuries to the acromioclavicular joint, in Rockwood CA Jr, Green DP, Bucholz RW (eds): *Fractures in Adults*, 3d ed. Philadelphia, Lippincott, 1991, pp 1181–1239.

Rovere GD, Clarke TJ, Yates CS, et al: Retrospective comparison of taping and ankle stabilizers in preventing ankle injuries. *Am J Sports Med* 16:498, 1988.

Rubin A, Sallis R: Evaluation and diagnosis of ankle injuries. *Am Fam Phys* 54:1609, 1996.

Sloan JP, Hain R, Pownall R: Benefits of early anti-inflammatory medication following acute ankle injury. *Injury* 20:81, 1989.

Speer KP, Lohnes J, Garrett WE Jr: Radiographic imaging of muscle strain injury. *Am J Sports Med* 21:89, 1993.

Stiell IG, McKnight RD, Greenberg GH, et al: Implementation of the Ottawa ankle rules. *JAMA* 271:827, 1994.

Stiell IG, Wells GA, Hoag RH, et al: Implementation of the Ottawa knee rule for the use of radiography in acute knee injuries. *JAMA* 278:2075, 1997.

Surve I, Schwellnus MP, Noakes T, et al: A fivefold reduction in the incidence of recurrent ankle sprains in soccer players using the sport-stirrup orthosis. *Am J Sports Med* 22:601, 1994.

Yergason RM: Rupture of biceps. *J Bone Joint Surg* 13:160, 1931.

Michael S. Klinkman

Chapter
14

Chest Pain

How Common Is Chest Pain?

Chest pain is a common complaint in primary care practice. Each year, approximately 2 percent of all ambulatory visits to clinicians in the United States are for a chief complaint of chest pain. These statistics put chest pain on the list of the ten most common problems seen in primary care. The situation is similar in Europe, where data from the Dutch Transition Project show that each year chest pain is the initial reason for encounter in 56 of every 1000 adults who visit primary care clinicians.

Chest pain is not limited to a specific age group, but it occurs more commonly in adults than children. Incidence is highest in adults over 65 years old, with a secondary peak in males between 45 and 65 years of age.

The major importance of chest pain lies in the fact that it is a key symptom of several life-threatening conditions that must be recognized and treated promptly (Table 14-1). Of perhaps equal importance, however, is that most chest pain in primary care practice is not caused by the life-threatening conditions. Thus, the need to distinguish urgent from non-urgent chest pain is critically important and may be the single most difficult decision-making task in primary care practice.

When evaluating patients with chest pain, clinicians must weigh the relative probabilities of potential causes of the pain, determine when intervention is necessary or urgent, and choose from almost limitless diagnostic and therapeutic strategies. This must all be achieved while responding to the distress felt by patients who are concerned about the presence of life-threatening heart disease. The diagnostic difficulty is made even more challenging by the fact that

Table 14-1

Principal Life-Threatening Causes of Acute Chest Pain

ORGAN SYSTEM	CONDITION
Cardiac	Acute or unstable angina pectoris
	Myocardial infarction
	Dissecting aortic aneurysm
	Acute pericardial tamponade
Pulmonary	Pulmonary embolism
	Tension pneumothorax

chest pain often represents a complex interplay of physiology, pathology, and psychosocial factors, making it a quintessential primary care problem.

Principal Diagnoses

Chest pain can be caused by almost any condition affecting the thorax or abdomen, as well as by mental health conditions, such as anxiety or panic disorder. Two studies conducted in networks of primary care practices have documented the diagnoses given to patients with chest pain (Table 14-2). The studies emphasize the wide variety of conditions to which chest pain can be ascribed. One study, by researchers in the national Ambulatory Sentinel Practice Network (ASPN), reported diagnoses established after a first visit for chest pain. The other study, by investigators in the Michigan Research Network (MIRNET), reported final diagnosis for patients with chest pain after as many visits as were needed to establish a diagnosis. Table 14-3 displays MIRNET data demonstrating the most common causes of chest pain identified after a full evaluation. These data show that more than

Table 14-2

Most Common Diagnoses for Chest Pain in Primary Care Practice

		FREQUENCY	
ORGAN SYSTEM	SPECIFIC DIAGNOSIS	MIRNET, %*	ASPN, %†
Musculoskeletal	Muscular chest wall pain	20.4	20.9
	Costochondritis	13.1	7.8
	Rib fracture	<1.0	
Cardiac	Unstable angina/myocardial infarction	1.5	2.9
	Angina pectoris	10.3	31.6
	Mitral valve prolapse syndrome	1.3	
	Cardiac arrhythmias	<1.0	
	Pericarditis	0.0	
Gastrointestinal	Unspecified gastrointestinal problem		13.8
	GERD	13.4	
	Peptic ulcer disease	0.8	
	Esophageal spasm	3.8	
	Cholecystitis	<1.0	
Psychological	Anxiety disorder or stress	7.5	7.5
Pulmonary	Bronchitis	1.3	
	Pleurisy, pleurodynia	1.3	4.3
	Pneumonia	<1.0	
Neurologic	Herpes zoster ("shingles")	<1.0	
	Radiculopathy	<1.0	
Other/unknown	"Atypical" chest pain	12.6	11.3

NOTE: Blank space indicates that the diagnosis was not reported in the study.
*Frequency of specific diagnoses reached at end of chest pain episode
†Frequency of specific diagnoses reached after initial visit for chest pain

Table 14-3

Frequencies of Diagnoses, by Age and Gender, in the MIRNET Chest Pain Study

GENDER	AGE GROUP	NO.	MOST COMMON DIAGNOSES	FREQUENCY, %
Men	18–24	11	1. Gastroesophageal reflux	46
			2. Muscular chest wall pain	18
	25–44	81	1. Gastroesophageal reflux	26
			2. Muscular chest wall pain	25
			3. Costochondritis	12
	45–64	62	1. Angina/unstable angina/myocardial infarction	23
			2. Muscular chest wall pain	21
			3. "Atypical" chest pain	16
	65 and over	27	1. Muscular chest wall pain	26
			2. "Atypical" chest pain or coronary artery disease	22
Women	18–24	15	1. Costochondritis	40
			2. Anxiety/stress	27
	25–44	97	1. Muscular chest wall pain	21
			2. Costochondritis	19
			3. "Atypical" chest pain	12
			4. Gastroesophageal reflux	11
	45–64	63	1. Angina/unstable angina/myocardial infarction	18
			2. "Atypical" chest pain	16
			3. Muscular chest wall pain	13
	65 and over	39	1. Angina/unstable angina/myocardial infarction	31
			2. Muscular chest wall pain	15
			3. "Atypical" chest pain or costochondritis	13

85 percent of chest pain in primary care practice is *not* due to heart conditions.

Most literature on the subject of "chest pain" deals with life-threatening causes, often in emergency room settings where the probability of acute coronary artery disease or unstable cardiac ischemia is relatively high. As noted, however, it is non-emergent chest pain that most commonly faces primary care clinicians in office settings, where the frequency of musculoskeletal, gastrointestinal, and psychological causes of chest pain exceed that of urgent chest pain conditions. Thus, in addition to discussing the differential diagnosis of chest pain to facilitate identification of urgent situations, this chapter discusses the approach to the problem of non-urgent chest pain in office practice.

Musculoskeletal Conditions

In both the ASPN and MIRNET chest pain studies, musculoskeletal conditions were common causes of chest pain. In fact, in the MIRNET study, musculoskeletal problems were common sources of chest pain in adults of all ages. Several types of musculoskeletal conditions have been associated with chest pain; of these, muscular chest pain and costochondritis are the most common. Rib fractures are also occasionally seen in office practice.

MUSCULAR CHEST PAIN

Muscular chest pain, also known as chest wall muscle pain or pectoralis strain, most commonly occurs in active young men or women. It is the cause of chest pain in between 20 and 33 percent of primary care patients and is the most frequent diagnosis for both men and women between ages 25 and 65.

The pain is probably the result of overuse of chest wall muscles and a resulting strain (partial tear) within a muscle body or at its insertion site. The strain may cause well-localized pain that occurs upon movement of the affected muscle, or it can result in generalized pain and tightness that mimics angina pectoris. History suggesting musculoskeletal chest pain includes pain with movement, sharp pain of recent onset associated with minor trauma or repeated use of arms or shoulders, or pain radiating to the shoulder, back, or arm. The characteristic physical examination finding is tenderness to palpation of the chest wall muscles. In many cases, palpation of the affected muscle reproduces the chest pain experienced by the patient. When this occurs, the diagnosis is clear and no additional testing is necessary.

COSTOCHONDRITIS

Also known as Tietze's syndrome, costochondritis is most often seen in young women, particularly African-American women. In both the MIRNET and ASPN studies, costochondritis was most often diagnosed in women under 65 and in men between 25 and 44 years of age, but the condition also occurs in the geriatric age group.

The chest pain of costochondritis is thought to be due to inflammation of the costochondral articulation of the upper rib cage, most often at the third or fourth left costochondral junction. Suggestive history includes pain with use of chest wall muscles. In addition, the pain may occur at rest or with deep inspiration, and there usually is no history of recent trauma or muscular exertion. If the patient has tried them, nonprescription anti-inflammatory agents have often provided relief. The characteristic physical examination finding is tenderness to palpation over a costochondral junction. Laboratory studies are not helpful in establishing this diagnosis.

RIB FRACTURES

Rib fractures are a less common cause of musculoskeletal chest pain than either muscle strain or costochondritis, accounting for only about 1 percent of cases. Rib fractures usually follow chest trauma, and they cause sharp pain at the site of the trauma, exacerbated by deep inspiration, movement, or anything that causes movement of the injured rib or ribs. Rib fractures can also occur without trauma in patients with abnormal bone strength or structure (pathologic fracture), such as patients with osteopenia or malignancy.

Cardiac Conditions

The two most common cardiac conditions that cause chest pain in primary care practice are ischemic heart disease and mitral valve prolapse. Other, less common conditions include cardiac arrhythmias and pericarditis. Cardiac ischemia is perhaps the most serious causes of chest pain encountered in office practice and, because of its potentially life-threatening nature, ischemic heart disease is the focus of most investigations undertaken to diagnose chest pain.

The medical literature provides many clinical algorithms designed to diagnose or exclude acute cardiac ischemia in emergency room settings. Unfortunately, this diagnostic process has been carried over into office-based practice despite significant differences in the epidemiology of chest pain in the two settings. For example, cardiac conditions accounted for less than 15 percent of chest pain episodes in the MIRNET study, with a diagnosis of unstable coronary artery disease (myocardial infarction or unstable angina) in only 1.5 percent of episodes. In the older patient population captured in the ASPN study, myocardial infarction was diagnosed in only 3 percent of cases. In contrast, studies of chest pain in emergency room settings describe the need to admit 15 to 25 percent or more of patients with chest pain to the hospital for probable ischemic heart disease.

Thus, while cardiac disease is potentially serious, the low relative presence of serious heart disease in primary care practice makes it unnecessary to "rule out" cardiac disease definitively in every patient with chest pain. Careful attention to the patient's history and the characteristics of the pain will often enable the clinician to diagnose noncardiac conditions and to identify those who do require further consideration of cardiac disease.

CARDIAC ISCHEMIA DUE TO ATHEROSCLEROTIC HEART DISEASE

Cardiac ischemia is most commonly seen in middle-aged to elderly men and in postmenopausal women. However, it can occur in younger individuals, including men in their thirties and, occasionally, men in their twenties.

The classic history is that of angina pectoris, caused by atherosclerotic coronary artery disease. The symptoms of angina include diffuse substernal chest tightness or discomfort that occurs with physical exertion and sometimes emotional stress, often associated with radiation to the jaw, left arm, or back. It is sometimes accompanied by dyspnea, nausea, diaphoresis, and/or sudden fatigue. During episodes, patients may have hypertension or hypotension, a palpably displaced point of maximal cardiac impulse, systolic murmur of mitral insufficiency, transient third or fourth heart sound (S_3 or S_4), or other signs of congestive heart failure.

The pain of angina pectoris is not affected by respiration, nor is it relieved by antacids or changing body position, and it is not reproduced by chest wall palpation. Angina pectoris is usually relieved by rest or sublingual nitroglycerin, and between episodes there are no characteristic physical examination findings.

UNSTABLE ISCHEMIA　If angina is suspected as the cause of chest pain, the clinician's most important immediate task is to determine whether the patient has stable or unstable angina. Unstable angina is a medical emergency and has been defined as angina with any of the following characteristics: (1) symptoms at rest, especially if longer than 20 min; (2) new onset of angina; and/or (3) a recent change in severity of angina. Unstable angina is associated with a significantly higher risk of myocardial infarction and sudden death than is stable angina, and it is sometimes difficult to distinguish unstable angina from acute infarction on clinical grounds alone. A variety of ancillary tests, described later, can aid in clarifying the nature of angina-like chest pain.

Current clinical practice guidelines call for intensive in-hospital management of patients with unstable ischemic heart disease. In practical terms, if the patient has no previous diagnosis of angina, or if there is an increase in frequency, intensity, or other change from an established pattern of anginal episodes, the diagnosis is probably unstable angina or infarction, and in-hospital management is indicated. Patients with suspected unstable angina or infarction should be transported to a hospital by paramedic ambulance equipped with cardiac monitoring and resuscitation equipment.

STABLE ISCHEMIA　Angina not meeting the characteristics of unstable angina is often referred to as "chronic stable angina." Chronic stable angina typically involves ischemic pain that develops with exertion, is relatively reproducible after the same amount of exertion, and is relieved by rest or nitroglycerin. Because symptoms are not always classic, stable angina can be easily confused with other chest pain syndromes. The diagnosis is often confirmed with exercise treadmill testing. Treatments include anti-anginal medications and/or various coronary revascularization procedures.

CARDIAC ISCHEMIA DUE TO CORONARY ARTERY VASOSPASM (VASOSPASTIC ANGINA PECTORIS)

Vasospastic angina, also known as atypical, variant, or Prinzmetal's angina, is characterized by symptoms similar to those of classic angina pectoris but that occur at rest rather than with exertion, and for which the underlying patho-physiology is coronary artery vasospasm instead of atherosclerotic lesions. Vasospastic angina has been associated with cardiac arrhythmias and sudden cardiac death.

Vasospastic angina is believed to affect young to middle-aged women more frequently than men, but the true prevalence is unknown. It can occur as an isolated condition or concomitantly with angina from atherosclerotic coronary artery disease. Vasospastic angina is far less common than classic angina, and no specific diagnoses of vasospastic angina were reported in either the ASPN or MIRNET chest pain studies (although undiagnosed cases may have been included in the "atypical chest pain" or "other" categories of these studies).

Patients with vasospastic angina experience diffuse substernal chest tightness or discomfort while at rest, sometimes radiating to the jaw, left arm, or back, occasionally accompanied by dyspnea, nausea, diaphoresis, or sudden fatigue. The pain is not associated with exertion, inspiration, or expiration and is not relieved by antacids or position changes. Between episodes there are usually no specific physical examination findings. The most helpful ancillary tests include the electrocardiogram (ECG), which will show ST segment elevation during pain, and cardiac catheterization with ergonovine challenge testing to induce coronary artery vasospasm.

Mitral Valve Prolapse Syndrome

This condition is most often diagnosed in young to middle-aged women, although it can be detected in men and in older individuals, and it occurs more frequently in persons with connective tissue disorders, such as Marfan's syndrome. Mitral valve prolapse has a prevalence of 1.5 to 6 percent in the general population, and it was diagnosed in 1.5 percent of patients in the MIRNET study.

Patients with chest pain due to mitral valve prolapse report substernal chest discomfort of variable duration. It can be sharp or dull, and it may be accompanied by palpitations. The symptoms are often worse with physical exertion or emotional stress. The pathophysiologic basis of the chest pain associated with mitral valve prolapse in unclear; some experts attribute the pain to ischemia of the papillary muscles.

The characteristic physical examination finding is a mid-systolic click followed by a systolic murmur on cardiac auscultation; however, the "click-murmur" is often variable in intensity and may not be easily heard. Two-dimensional echocardiographic studies will reveal the characteristic bowing of the mitral valve leaflet that confirms this diagnosis (Fig. 14-1).

Cardiac Arrhythmias

Cardiac arrhythmias can exacerbate existing angina by decreasing coronary artery perfusion. This situation can occur, for example, from decreased diastolic filling time in tachyarrhythmias or diminished cardiac output from loss of atrial contraction in atrial fibrillation. In addition, tachyarrhythmias (particularly supraventricular tachycardia) have also been associated with chest pain in persons without coronary artery disease. The physiologic basis of chest pain in the absence of coronary artery disease is not known.

Based on MIRNET data, about 1 percent of chest pain episodes in primary care practice can be attributed to a cardiac rhythm disturbance. The chest pain associated with arrhythmias is typically of variable quality and intensity, and may be accompanied by dyspnea. If patients present for care while symptoms are occurring, an ECG may confirm the presence of a potentially causative arrhythmia. If a rhythm disorder is detected, however, it should not be considered the cause of chest pain before cardiac ischemia has been excluded.

Pericarditis

Pericarditis is a relatively uncommon (less than 1 percent) cause of chest pain in primary

Figure 14-1

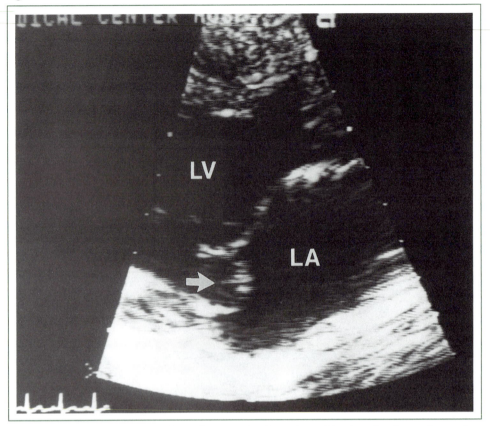

Mitral valve prolapse. A parasternal two-dimensional echocardiographic view showing prolapse of a redundant posterior mitral leaflet toward the left atrium during systole. LV, = left ventricle; LA, = left atrium. *(Reproduced with permission from RW Alexander et al: The Heart. New York, McGraw-Hill, 1998.)*

care practice. When it occurs, it is typically due to one of several disorders ranging from infection to malignancy to a variety of inflammatory conditions. The pain of pericarditis is typically sharp, localized to the left side of the chest, and made worse by lying down, coughing, or deep breathing. A pericardial "friction rub" (a scratchy, high-pitched sound heard at varying levels of intensity throughout the cardiac cycle) on cardiac auscultation strongly supports the diagnosis. The ECG may show characteristic abnormalities (decreased voltage and widespread ST-segment changes), but the diagnosis is usually made by an echocardiographic study. Laboratory studies are aimed at diagnosis of the underlying condition causing pericarditis.

Gastrointestinal Condition

Gastrointestinal conditions are a common cause of chest pain in primary care practice, accounting for between 15 and 20 percent of cases. The two most important conditions are gastroesophageal reflux disease (GERD) and esophageal spasm. Although GERD is more common, esophageal spasm commands considerable attention due to the similarity of its symptoms to those of angina pectoris. Efforts are now being made to improve techniques for diagnosing esophageal spasm, to minimize unnecessary invasive cardiac imaging in those with angina-like chest pain due to esophageal spasm. In addition to GERD and esophageal spasm, other common gastrointestinal causes of chest pain include peptic ulcer disease and gallbladder disorders.

GASTROESOPHAGEAL REFLUX DISEASE

Also known as reflux esophagitis, GERD affects persons of all ages and both sexes. Based on MIRNET data, it is the most common cause of chest pain in men under the age of 45. Chest pain associated with GERD is thought to be the result of the erosive effect of unbuffered gastric acid on the mucosal lining of the distal esophagus. Due to the imprecise localization of pain originating in the upper gastrointestinal tract, the pain of GERD may be felt in the back, in the epigastrium, in the flank, or deep in the chest, and patients may experience anything between a mild discomfort and a sharp stabbing pain. As described in Chap. 15, the most helpful studies for establishing the diagnosis of GERD are esophagogastroduodenoscopy and esophageal pH measurements.

ESOPHAGEAL SPASM

Esophageal spasm typically occurs in the distal esophagus and may be caused by a variety of conditions. The most common is GERD, in which reflux of gastric acid into the distal esophagus induces spasm of the esophageal smooth muscle. Spasm can also have its origin in the esophagus, such as from a primary esophageal motility disorder or from stimulation of esophageal smooth muscle by sympathetic nervous system activity.

Since there are no firm criteria or classic clinical signs on which to base the diagnosis, esophageal spasm is often not considered as a diagnostic possibility until after coronary artery disease has been ruled out. The clinical presentation can be similar to that of coronary artery disease, with squeezing substernal chest pain or pressure or sharp substernal pain. However, in contrast to angina pectoris, the pain of esophageal spasm occurs at rest, is worse when recumbent, is often relieved by antacids or eructation, and at times can be localized by the patient with one finger. The pain can last from moments to hours and can be associated with dysphagia. There are no characteristic physical examination findings.

Laboratory studies are often necessary to establish the diagnosis. The most useful tests are the barium swallow test, which can provide a visual image of spasm, and esophageal manometric studies, which can detect pressure changes associated with abnormal esophageal contractions.

In the setting of acute pain thought to be due to GERD or esophageal spasm, administration of an oral "GI cocktail," described later, can serve as a confirmatory diagnostic study as well as a therapeutic maneuver. Nonetheless, the diagnosis is difficult, and most clinicians have a high level of uncertainty when making a presumptive diagnosis of esophageal spasm.

PEPTIC ULCER DISEASE

Peptic ulcer disease, discussed in more detail in Chap. 15, generally causes pain of a constant nature, often waking patients from sleep. The pain of peptic ulcer disease may be localized to the epigastrium, radiate from the epigastrium to the back, or be localized to the back. However, peptic ulcer disease may cause chest pain and be confused with ischemic heart disease.

GALLBLADDER DISEASE

Gallbladder disease is an infrequent cause of chest pain, but pain from gallstones can be referred to the lower chest as well as the shoulder.

Postprandial chest discomfort, especially if associated with radiation to the back or abdomen and accompanied by nausea, is suggestive of gallbladder disease.

Anxiety Disorders

Anxiety disorders are common causes of chest pain in primary care practice. In fact, anxiety was diagnosed as the cause of 6 to 7 percent of chest pain episodes in both the ASPN and MIR-NET studies, as well as in other studies involving general internal medicine patients. It is also common for patients with chest pain to become anxious about the possibility that the pain is of cardiac origin, sometimes making it difficult to determine whether chest pain is causing anxiety or anxiety is causing chest pain.

NONSPECIFIC ANXIETY OR "STRESS"

Chest pain caused by anxiety or emotional stress most commonly occurs in healthy young men or women, but it can occur at any age. Characteristic symptoms include chest tightness associated with dyspnea, difficulty in taking a deep breath, or hyperventilation. These symptoms are often associated with other stress-related complaints (e.g., headache or nausea) or the presence of significant situational stress. Chest pain episodes may last from hours to days. On physical examination, patients often exhibit distress out of proportion to objective findings.

The diagnosis is often relatively clear in young, otherwise healthy individuals but may be difficult to determine in patients at risk for cardiac disease or with known cardiac ischemia. Failure to diagnose ischemia can have serious adverse consequences, but subjecting patients with anxiety to invasive cardiac studies also carries risk. Laboratory studies are usually not helpful in reaching a diagnosis. In some cases, brief mental health screening instruments may assist in establishing the diagnosis.

PANIC DISORDER

Panic disorder is common among primary care patients with unexplained chest pain. In emergency room settings, up to half of patients with unexplained chest pain have panic disorder. Chest pain with panic disorder has also been associated with mitral valve prolapse, but the basis for this association is unclear.

Patients suffering from panic attacks often present with sudden episodes of chest tightness accompanied by autonomic symptoms including dyspnea, a smothering sensation, dizziness, palpitations, trembling, sweating, nausea, parasthesias, hot flashes, depersonalization, or fear of dying or of "going crazy." Rapid respiratory rate and tachycardia are usually present. Between episodes, physical examination is nonspecific, but sometimes patients will be overtly anxious during the examination. The diagnosis and management of panic disorder are described in Chap. 9.

Pulmonary Conditions

Pulmonary problems are a relatively infrequent cause of chest pain in primary care, accounting for less than 5 percent of diagnoses in all published studies. The most common pulmonary conditions associated with chest pain in primary care practice are pleurodynia, acute bronchitis, and pneumonia.

PLEURODYNIA

Pleurodynia (pleurisy), caused by inflammation of pleura, often accompanies viral or bacterial respiratory infections. It may also occur in collagen vascular disorders. Pleurodynia is diagnosed in 2 to 4 percent of patients with chest pain in primary care practice. History suggesting pleurodynia includes acute onset of sharp pain associated with breathing or movement, sometimes accompanied by systemic symptoms of infection. Physical examination may reveal a pleural friction rub. A chest x-ray should be obtained to exclude pneumonia, pleural effusion, or other intrathoracic processes. Laboratory studies, such as a serum rheumatoid factor test, an antinuclear antibody (ANA) test, and determination of the erythrocyte sedimentation rate, may be useful to exclude pleuritis caused by an underlying rheumatologic or connective tissue disease.

ACUTE BRONCHITIS

Bronchitis occurs in all age and gender groups and is more common in smokers. Published studies indicate that it accounts for about 2 percent of cases of chest pain in primary care practice. Acute bronchitis is discussed in more detail in Chap. 7, but when it causes chest pain, patients usually complain of a dull chest ache, often accompanied by a painful, productive cough. Lung examination may reveal upper airway congestion, bronchi, or diffuse wheezing on pulmonary auscultation. Laboratory studies are not necessary unless a chest x-ray is needed to exclude pneumonia.

PNEUMONIA

Pneumonia is an uncommon cause of chest pain in primary care practice. It was diagnosed in less than 1 percent of patients in the MIRNET study. Pneumonia is also discussed in Chap. 7.

Neurologic Conditions

Conditions such as herpes zoster ("shingles") or cervical or thoracic radiculopathies can cause chest pain. However, they account for less than 1 percent of cases.

Nonspecific or Atypical Chest Pain

Nonspecific or atypical chest pain is pain for which no cause can be identified. Depending on the population of patients being studied, the percentage of chest pain patients who receive a diagnosis of nonspecific or atypical chest pain can vary from 10 to 80 percent. In the MIRNET and ASPN studies, 11 to 13 percent of patients had non-specific pain.

Most reports of nonspecific chest pain describe relatively young patients with vaguely defined pain occurring without a specific pattern. Pain is often described as "squeezing" and is not well localized. Patients are usually alarmed by these symptoms, attribute them to cardiac disease, and seek reassurance. Unfortunately, reassurance often cannot be provided until completion of an evaluation for cardiac disease. It is likely that many of these episodes represent psychological problems that do not receive specific diagnosis, often due to their undifferentiated, "subsyndromal" nature or the reluctance of clinicians and/or patients to accept a potentially stigmatizing psychological diagnosis on the basis of a physical symptom.

Life-Threatening Causes of Chest Pain

There are six life-threatening causes of chest pain that must be considered in every patient with chest pain (Table 14-1). Two of these conditions, unstable angina and myocardial infarction, have already been discussed. The other conditions are dissecting aortic aneurysm, pulmonary embolism, tension pneumothorax, and pericardial tamponade. Acute pericardial tamponade, however, is virtually never seen in office-based practice and will not be discussed.

DISSECTING AORTIC ANEURYSM

Dissecting aortic aneurysm may occasionally present to office-based clinicians. While it is an extremely rare cause of chest pain in office practice, it must be recognized at once and patients transported immediately to a hospital equipped for diagnosis of and emergency intrathoracic surgery for the condition. The pain of dissecting aneurysm is usually described as sharp and tearing, and is unrelated to breathing. Patients are almost always hemodynamically unstable at presentation.

PULMONARY EMBOLISM

Pulmonary embolism most often occurs in older individuals who have risk factors for thromboembolic disease (e.g., smoking, venous occlusive disease, prolonged immobility, or hypercoagulable states). The pain associated with pulmonary embolism is thought to be caused by ischemia in the affected lung parenchyma, and the pain can be sharp, squeezing, or dull. The pain may worsen with inspiration or be constant, and it may be severe or very mild.

Pulmonary embolism has been called the "great imitator" because of its protean clinical manifestations. Thus, the diagnosis is frequently overlooked and often not detected until autopsy. Diagnosis depends on maintaining a high degree of suspicion with patients with atypical chest pain, especially in the presence of risk factors. The diagnosis is suggested by noninvasive studies such as radionuclide ventilation-perfusion lung scanning, which characteristically shows a ventilation-perfusion mismatch. If necessary, the diagnosis can be confirmed by pulmonary angiography. Treatment requires anticoagulation and supportive pulmonary care. In the past, treatment almost always involved in-hospital anticoagulation with intravenous heparin, but recent studies suggest that outpatient treatment with subcutaneous low-molecular-weight heparin is safe and effective for hemodynamically stable patients.

TENSION PNEUMOTHORAX

Tension pneumothorax most commonly occurs following chest trauma or diagnostic thoracentesis. However, occasionally patients will present to office-based clinicians with tension pneumothorax without an antecedent history of trauma or thoracentesis. These individuals typically have either a spontaneous pneumothorax or chronic obstructive pulmonary disease with air trapping, in which case pneumothorax occurs when a pulmonary "bleb" ruptures. Diagnosis is suggested by physical examination (deviated trachea and asymmetric breath sounds) and confirmed by chest x-ray. Emergency needle aspiration in the second intercostal space to decompress the pneumothorax can be lifesaving, but definitive treatment involves placement of a thoracostomy tube.

Typical Presentation

Chest pain is almost always a patient's primary reason for visiting a clinician, rather than an incidental complaint. In primary care office practice, patients with chest pain typically present with one of three clinical scenarios.

In the "gradual" scenario, pain is mild, intermittent, and difficult to describe or localize, and has not affected functional status. Patients have usually tried to self-treat with medications (antacids or histamine antagonists such as cimetidine or ranitidine), dietary changes, or rest. They present to a clinician because self-treatment has not worked.

In the "acute" scenario, pain has begun recently and abruptly without obvious cause and has limited the patient's activities. These patients are usually concerned about the possibility of serious cardiac disease. Depending on the severity of pain, they seek care within one or a few days after symptoms begin.

In the third scenario, which might be labeled the "worry" scenario, pain is usually mild and without observable pattern, and has not limited function. However, patients are nonetheless concerned about the possibility of cardiac disease and often present with a request for cardiac testing.

These scenarios are very different from those seen in emergency room and subspecialty settings. The typical emergency room presentation of chest pain is that of acute onset of chest discomfort, often accompanied by dyspnea, nausea, diaphoresis, or feeling ill, and not resolving with rest or self-care over minutes to hours. This emergent chest pain has a relatively high probability of representing acute cardiac ischemia, and the major task of emergency room clinicians is to determine whether a life-threatening condition is sufficiently likely to warrant hospital admission or referral, and then turn the patient's care over to the admitting clinician.

Subspecialists usually deal with yet other clinical scenarios. Patients seen by subspecialists have often passed through the filter of emergency room or primary care assessment, and either have a known problem that is difficult to manage or chest pain that is difficult to diagnose. Consequently, patients referred to a cardiologist have a higher probability of having cardiac disease than unselected primary care patients, patients referred to gastroenterologists have a higher prior probability of having gastroesophageal conditions, and so on. In some ways, the diagnostic task of subspecialists is to confirm that a disease in "their" organ system is causing the chest pain and then institute appropriate evaluation and treatment.

Primary care clinicians, who must evaluate unselected patients, face the most complex diagnostic task. They must first determine whether an acute, life-threatening condition is present. If such a condition is not present, they must then pursue multiple diagnostic possibilities of intermediate likelihood that may not be mutually exclusive (e.g., GERD and anxiety may coexist and have a clinical presentation that resembles acute cardiac ischemia).

Key History

The chest pain history should contain at least the following five elements: (1) predisposing factors,

(2) characteristics of the onset of pain, (3) duration of pain episodes, (4) characteristics of the pain itself, and (5) factors that provide relief from pain. The pattern of responses regarding these elements can direct the clinician to the organ system most likely causing the patient's chest pain: cardiac, gastrointestinal, or musculoskeletal, as shown in Table 14-4. If the pattern of responses does not suggest any of these organ systems, the clinician should consider other causes of chest pain, such as pulmonary disease and/or anxiety disorder, and ask questions pertinent to these conditions.

Physical Examination

A complete physical examination is usually not necessary. In many cases, a "most likely diagnosis" will emerge after the key history elements have been reviewed, and a directed, organ system–focused physical examination can be performed to support or confirm that diagnosis. If the diagnosis remains uncertain after the history is taken, a general physical examination focusing on the systems most closely associated with chest pain (cardiac, pulmonary, musculoskeletal, and gastrointestinal) is warranted. Physical examination findings suggesting each of the common organ systems involved in chest pain are shown in Table 14-4. In addition, key physical examination findings associated with specific chest pain diagnoses have already been described.

However, many of the more serious conditions causing chest pain may have no characteristic physical findings. In addition, many abnormal physical findings are nonspecific and cannot be used to make a diagnosis in the absence of other clinical evidence. Of most importance is the fact that there are no physical examination findings that can confirm or exclude acute cardiac ischemia or pulmonary embolism, the most common life-threatening causes of chest pain.

Table 14-4

History and Physical Examination Findings for Discerning the Cause of Chest Pain

	DIAGNOSTIC CATEGORY		
FINDINGS	**CARDIAC**	**GASTROINTESTINAL**	**MUSCULOSKELETAL**
History			
Predisposing risk factors	Male gender Smoking Hypertension Hyperlipidemia Family history of myocardial infarction	Smoking Alcohol use	Physically active New activity Overuse Repeated activity
Onset	At consistent level of exertion or under emotional stress	After meals and/or on empty stomach	With or after activity
Duration	Minutes	Minutes to hours	Hours to days
Character	Pressure or "tightness"	Pressure or "gnawing" pain	Sharp, localized, movement-related
Relieved by	Rest Sublingual nitrates	Food Antacids Histamine blockers	Rest Analgesics NSAIDs
Physical examination			
Supportive finding(s)	During anginal episodes may have S_3 gallop, arrhythmia, or murmur	Epigastric tenderness	Pain on palpation

Ancillary Tests

In general, ancillary diagnostic tests should be used to confirm or support a specific diagnosis for patients whose history and physical examination suggest an intermediate or high probability of having a particular condition. This section focuses on the indications for and characteristics of several of the diagnostic tests most often used to evaluate patients with chest pain.

In most cases, ancillary tests should not be used to rule out a specific condition in patients with a low probability of having that condition. This is especially true for patients with chest pain, since cardiac studies such as exercise stress tests performed on patients with a low probability of cardiac ischemia yield more false-positive than true-positive results and lead to potentially risky follow-up studies and unnecessary treatments.

Cardiac Tests

A variety of noninvasive tests are available for evaluating the possibility that chest pain is of cardiac origin. These tests include resting ECG, stress ECG, and noninvasive cardiac imaging studies. The ability to effectively interpret many of these tests in primary care practice is limited because the published predictive values for these tests have been derived in relatively high-risk populations, usually in cardiology practices or in-hospital settings. The predictive values of these tests in unselected primary care populations are unknown. Invasive cardiac imaging (e.g., coronary angiography) should be reserved for clinical situations in which the diagnosis is not clear after noninvasive studies are completed or when ischemia is confirmed and surgical therapy is being considered.

ELECTROCARDIOGRAM

A resting ECG is by far the most frequently performed test for evaluating patients with chest pain. If obtained during an episode of acute coronary ischemia, the ECG may demonstrate ST-segment elevation or depression, and ST-seg-

ment elevation is often seen with acute infarction (Fig. 14-2).

However, ECG is also one of the most inappropriately used tests. While an ECG is obtained in the initial evaluation of more than half of chest pain patients in office-based primary care settings, the test has surprisingly little diagnostic value. If the patient is not in pain at the time of the visit, the ECG will probably demonstrate no evidence of ischemia. Similarly, if a patient has pre-existing heart disease (e.g., prior myocardial infarction or left bundle branch block), it may not be possible to identify acute ischemia from an ECG even if ischemia is present. In fact, in some studies, up to 50 percent of individuals have a normal ECG in early phases of acute myocardial infarction. Thus, if history suggests acute ischemia, clinicians should not be inappropriately reassured by a "negative" ECG result.

Figure 14-2

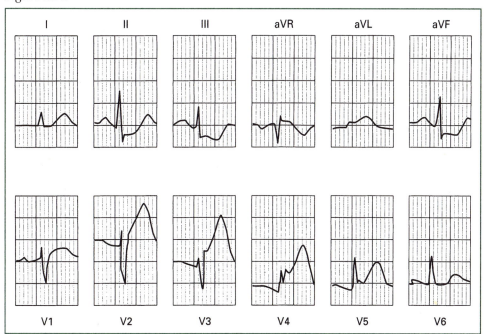

Myocardial infarction. The ECG shows an extensive acute anterior wall myocardial infarction with ST-segment elevation in the anterior leads (V_1–V_5 and aV_L), along with reciprocal ST-segment depression in the inferior leads (II, III, and aV_F). *(Reproduced with permission from RW Alexander et al: The Heart. New York, McGraw-Hill, 1998.)*

However, the ECG is useful for chest pain evaluation in two situations. The first is excluding acute cardiac ischemia in patients with low or intermediate probability of having coronary artery disease, such as persons with atypical chest pain or typical angina without cardiac risk factors. If an ECG is completely normal in such individuals and it is obtained while pain is present, the likelihood of acute coronary ischemia is extremely low. The second situation in which an ECG is helpful in evaluating chest pain is when the resting ECG reveals evidence of preexisting cardiac disease (e.g., prior myocardial infarction or left ventricular hypertrophy), since such a finding raises the likelihood that the current chest pain is of cardiac origin.

EXERCISE STRESS TESTING

In patients with chest pain who are not acutely ill and do not have symptoms suggestive of unstable ischemia, additional testing is sometimes needed to determine whether the chest pain has a cardiac source. The exercise stress test, which measures ECG response to exercise-induced tachycardia, can be used for this purpose. For individuals who cannot exercise adequately, tachycardia can be induced with arbutamine or dobutamine. A "positive" exercise test result (tachycardia-induced ST-segment depression of at least 1 mm in ECG leads corresponding to the inferior, anterior, or lateral regions of the myocardium) suggests the presence of myocardial ischemia. Unfortunately, exercise stress testing has poor positive predictive value in persons at low risk for coronary artery disease, such as premenopausal women, leading to high rates of false-positive test results in such individuals.

Several methods have been developed to more accurately score stress tests based on exercise level, extent of ST depression, and presence of angina. As a diagnostic test, however, exercise testing is probably most useful for corroborating a clinical suspicion of angina before referring

patients for further or invasive cardiac evaluation. Patients suspected of having acute, unstable ischemia should not be evaluated with stress testing but, rather, as noted above, should be admitted to a hospital for evaluation and treatment.

BLOOD TESTS

Serum levels of creatine kinase, an enzyme released from necrotic muscle cells, is the standard test used to detect myocardial infarction. Measurement of the myocardium-specific MB isoenzyme of creatine kinase enhances accuracy of the test. In addition, creatine kinase MB measurement permits detection of minor myocardial injury that may occur in some patients with unstable angina and no clinically apparent infarction. However, creatine kinase MB levels do not increase until hours after myocardial necrosis begins, and they remain normal in most patients who have unstable ischemia without infarction. Thus, creatine kinase levels cannot be used to determine with certainty whether acute chest pain has a cardiac origin. Suspicion of acute coronary ischemia, even if the creatine kinase levels are normal, should prompt hospital admission or referral to an emergency room–based chest pain evaluation unit for further evaluation.

Serum levels of lactate dehydrogenase, another cardiac enzyme, also increase following myocardial necrosis. However, since levels rise later (48 to 72 h after necrosis begins) than do creatine kinase levels, lactate dehydrogenase levels can only be used to diagnose infarctions that occurred days before a patient presents for care. New blood tests for detecting myocardial necrosis are discussed below under "Controversies and Emerging Concepts."

OTHER TESTS

Several other tests can be used to aid in determining whether chest pain is of cardiac origin.

These include both noninvasive and invasive imaging tests. The MIRNET study revealed that these tests are rarely ordered by primary care clinicians. In fact, such tests were performed in less than 3 percent of chest pain episodes. Rather, these imaging tests are usually performed in conjunction with or after referral to a cardiologist of patients with a high probability of cardiac ischemia.

RADIONUCLIDE-ENHANCED EXERCISE TESTING Myocardial perfusion imaging with thallium 201 or technetium 99m sestamibi, at rest and during exercise, offers increased accuracy for detecting myocardial ischemia. For example, one published estimate of the sensitivity and specificity of routine exercise stress testing in referral settings was 70 and 84 percent, respectively, while the addition of radionuclide-enhanced perfusion imaging increased both the sensitivity and specificity to approximately 90 percent. These imaging tests are also useful diagnostic techniques for patients who have preexisting ECG abnormalities that make it difficult to measure ST-segment changes on routine exercise ECG testing.

Myocardial perfusion imaging can also be used for patients who cannot exercise. In such cases, ischemia can be diagnosed by detecting thallium- or sestamibi-enhanced myocardial perfusion defects after injection of vasodilating drugs such as dipyridamole or adenosine.

STRESS ECHOCARDIOGRAPHY Echocardiography performed during exercise may detect ischemia-induced defects in cardiac wall motion. These wall-motion defects may be due to exercise-related ischemia or to preexisting myocardial infarction.

CARDIAC CATHETERIZATION Diagnostic cardiac catheterization is most useful in three general situations. The first is for detection of vasospastic angina, as described earlier. The second is when cardiac ischemia is strongly suspected on clinical history, but noninvasive tests, such as those outlined above, fail to diagnose or exclude ischemia with sufficient certainty. The third situation is evaluation of coronary artery anatomy in patients being considered for invasive therapeutic procedures, such as bypass surgery, angioplasty, or placement of a coronary artery stent.

Gastrointestinal Tests

Diagnostic strategies for evaluating patients with dyspeptic syndromes, including endoscopy, barium contrast radiography, *Helicobacter pylori* tests, and esophageal pH monitoring, are described in Chap. 15. Although they are not reviewed here, the same tests are useful in determining whether a patient's chest pain can be attributed to gastroesophageal disorders.

In addition, several tests not described in Chap. 15 can be used to identify gastrointestinal causes of chest pain. These tests include the "GI cocktail," the Bernstein test, and esophageal manometry.

"GI COCKTAIL"

In the setting of acute pain thought to be due to reflux esophagitis or esophageal spasm, administration of an oral "GI cocktail" can serve as both a confirmatory diagnostic study and a therapeutic maneuver. The precise proportion of ingredients varies among institutions, but nearly all contain some combination of viscous xylocaine and a liquid antacid as active ingredients. Relief of symptoms within several minutes of ingestion lends strong support to the diagnosis of esophageal reflux or spasm.

BERNSTEIN TEST

The Bernstein test involves the infusion of 0.1 *N* hydrochloric acid into the esophagus (with infusion of saline solution as control). It is a provocative maneuver that can reproduce esophageal pain and establish a causal relationship between acid in the esophagus and a patient's symptoms. Several published studies show the Bernstein procedure to have an overall sensitivity of roughly 80 percent and a specificity of 86 percent in outpatients referred to gastroenterologists. The test cannot determine the severity of symptoms or the magnitude of reflux, nor have test performance characteristics been defined in primary care patient populations.

ESOPHAGEAL MANOMETRY

Esophageal manometry can detect abnormal esophageal contractions, increased resting esophageal pressure, and dysfunction of the lower esophageal sphincter (LES), all of which are manometric correlates of GERD or esophageal spasm. While the sensitivity of decreased LES pressure as an indicator of GERD is quite low (57 percent), the combination of decreased LES pressure and the presence of abnormal contractions is more highly associated with severe GERD.

Psychological Tests

Several brief mental health screening instruments have been validated for use in primary care settings, most oriented toward determining whether patients meet diagnostic criteria for major depressive or generalized anxiety disorders. These instruments may occasionally be useful with patients with unexplained chest pain, and they are discussed in Chaps. 8 and 9.

Other Tests

Few other tests are useful in the routine evaluation of chest pain. Chest x-ray may confirm or exclude pneumonia or pneumothorax when these diagnoses are suspected, but it is not indicated in all cases of chest pain. Blood tests, such as serum chemistries and complete blood counts, are not useful in the absence of a specific indication for the test.

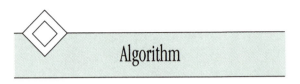

Algorithm

As noted, diagnosis of chest pain in office-based practice can be a complex task because of the variety of conditions that cause chest pain and the many tests that can be used to evaluate it. The diagnostic process can be simplified, however, by following the several steps described here (Fig. 14-3).

Perform Severity and Acuity Assessment

When patients present to a primary care office for acute onset of severe pain or pain associated with diaphoresis or difficulty breathing, they should be considered to have one of the urgent causes of pain outlined in Table 14-1, unless there is evidence to the contrary. Because of its prevalence, evaluation should initially focus on the possibility of severe, acute, or unstable cardiopulmonary disease, as outlined above. If one of these conditions is present, the patient should be stabilized while plans are set in motion to transport the patient to a facility with staff and equipment capable of dealing with serious cardiopulmonary emergencies.

Use Probabilities to Focus Attention on the Most Likely Diagnostic Possibilities

If there is no initial evidence of a cardiopulmonary emergency, the next step is to focus on the most likely diagnoses for the patient's age and gender group. A crude estimate of these

Figure 14-3

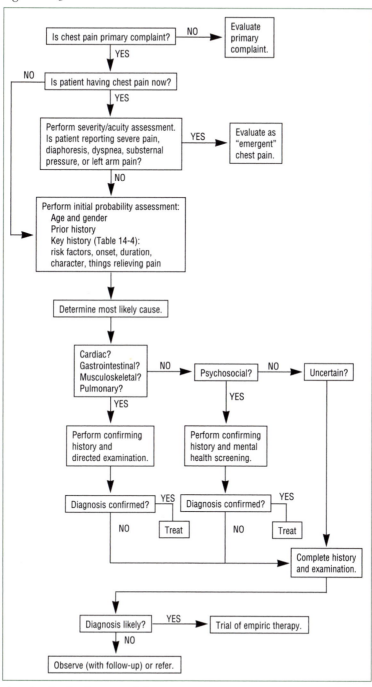

Algorithm for the diagnosis of chest pain.

probabilities is shown in Table 14-3. Probabilities can then be adjusted upward or downward based on key clinical findings and, to some extent, the clinician's experience.

Perform a Directed History, Physical Examination, and Laboratory Assessment

A complete history and physical examination are rarely necessary. In many cases, a brief history and/or examination can strongly suggest a specific cause of chest pain. For example, patients with reproducible pain on palpation of the costochondral junction have costochondritis, and there is little need for further examination or laboratory studies. At the other extreme, however, a thorough diagnostic evaluation, including multiple ancillary tests, may fail to identify a cause of chest pain for some patients.

Use Follow-Up Visits When Diagnosis Is Uncertain

If the diagnosis is unclear, and assuming there is no continued suspicion of serious cardiopulmonary disease, time can be used as both a diagnostic and a therapeutic agent in primary care settings. By following a patient over time, clinical clues to the diagnosis may appear, or pain may resolve spontaneously.

Consider Empiric Therapy

When a specific diagnosis is likely but not yet confirmed, clinicians may consider a trial of empiric therapy based on the tentative diagnosis. If therapy is successful, confirmation of the diagnosis through laboratory studies or ancillary testing may no longer be necessary. In fact, this is the strategy now recommended by the American College of Gastroenterology for managing patients with suspected GERD; if symp-

toms are compatible with GERD and patients respond to therapy, no further diagnostic tests are needed.

Treatment

It is far beyond the scope of this chapter to provide detailed recommendations regarding treatment of the dozens of conditions that might cause chest pain. In addition, detailed protocols for treating any of these conditions rapidly become outdated, especially for conditions on which research is progressing rapidly (e.g., management of acute coronary artery disease or GERD).

Consequently, rather than providing detailed treatment recommendations, this section focuses on the principles of treatment for several of the most common conditions causing chest pain in primary care practice, including costochondritis and muscular chest wall pain, angina pectoris, and esophageal spasm. Treatments of other common causes of chest pain, such as GERD, peptic ulcer disease, and anxiety (including panic) disorders, are reviewed in other chapters of this book.

Costochondritis and Chest Wall Pain

Standard therapy for costochondritis and muscular chest wall pain is both simple and effective, and can be based on the specific clinical circumstances. For acute chest wall pain that is improving by the time of the encounter, short-term treatment with ice, heat, or topical or oral analgesic or anti-inflammatory medications is all that is needed. If the pain is related to overuse injury, this treatment, accompanied by education of the patient about overuse syndromes, may prevent recurrences.

If the problem is chronic or not improving, a more intensive approach to treatment is needed. For muscular chest wall pain, therapy may include full-dose oral anti-inflammatory medications (aspirin or nonsteroidal anti-inflammatory drugs), physical therapy regimens prescribed by the primary care clinician or a physical therapist, and education of the patient designed to minimize future overuse or injury. For costochondritis, treatment with topical or oral anti-inflammatory agents is effective, with length and intensity of treatment dictated by the duration and severity of symptoms. For both costochondritis and muscular pain, trigger-point injections, using a combination of local anesthetic and corticosteroid, can sometimes afford substantial relief. However, caution must be taken to avoid penetrating the chest wall, since pneumothorax has been reported following trigger-point injections. When performing trigger-point injections, the needle should be inserted approximately parallel, not perpendicular, to the chest wall.

It is also important to discuss with patients the often intermittent and long-term nature of chest wall symptoms, in order to prevent concern if the problem persists. If possible, long-term use of analgesics or anti-inflammatory medications should be avoided because of potential gastro-erosive, hepatic, and renal side effects.

Angina Pectoris

Therapy for angina is aimed at preventing (and treating) episodes ischemia, preventing myocardial ischemia and infarction, treating other medical conditions that may complicate or aggravate ischemia, and maintaining function and overall well-being.

PREVENTING AND TREATING ISCHEMIA

Both medical and invasive therapies are used to prevent and treat ischemia. Medical therapy involves several classes of drugs, the most widely used of which are nitrates, beta blockers, and calcium channel blockers. Invasive treatments include coronary artery bypass surgery and cardiac catheterization procedures, such as angioplasty and placement of coronary artery stents.

NITRATES Nitrates are smooth muscle relaxants that cause vasodilation (primarily venous), thereby reducing left ventricular filling pressure (preload). To a lesser degree, they also reduce systemic blood pressure (after-load). Reductions in pre-load and after-load reduce cardiac work and myocardial oxygen demand. There is evidence that nitrates may also reduce coronary vasospasm.

For acute anginal episodes, nitrates can be administered by sublingual tablets or sprays. For chronic ischemia, nitrates are usually given orally by tablet or transdermally via paste or patch. The major side effects attributed to nitrates are headache, decreased exercise tolerance, and postural hypotension. Use of long-acting nitrate preparations, including transdermal patches, may cause nitrate tolerance and decreased effectiveness, leading to the recommendation that nitrates not be used on a round-the-clock basis.

BETA BLOCKERS Beta-adrenergic blocking agents reduce myocardial contractility, blood pressure, and heart rate, all of which tend to reduce myocardial oxygen demand. These agents have documented effectiveness in preventing death after acute myocardial infarction, and there is growing evidence that they can reduce the likelihood of first infarction in patients with angina. Beta blockers are often used in combination with nitrates to manage angina.

Beta blockers vary as to half-life, lipid solubility, cardioselectivity, and intrinsic sympathomimetic activity (which can minimize the drug's effect on heart rate and contractility). The choice of a specific drug can be guided by these characteristics in specific patients. Side effects common to this class of drugs include fatigue and decreased exercise tolerance, depression, and sexual dysfunction. Because beta blockers slow conduction through the atrioventricular node, they generally should not be used in patients with underlying cardiac conduction system abnormalities.

CALCIUM CHANNEL BLOCKERS Calcium channel blockers block calcium ion transport through the cell membrane in smooth muscle, which results in coronary artery vasodilation and reduced myocardial contractility, in theory, reducing myocardial oxygen demand and increasing oxygen supply. However, there is no evidence that these drugs increase survival rates among patients with angina, and recent studies have shown higher mortality rates in patients treated with short-acting calcium channel blockers. Therefore, as described later, the use of calcium channel blockers as antianginal therapy has become controversial. Long-acting calcium channel blockers, however, have not been associated with decreased survival rates, and they are still considered a first-line treatment for vasospastic angina.

The most common side effects of calcium channel blockers are fatigue and decreased exercise tolerance, postural hypotension, and peripheral edema. The incidence of these side effects varies for individual drugs. Like beta blockers, calcium channel blockers slow atrio-ventricular nodal conduction, and some decrease cardiac contractility. Thus, these drugs generally should not be used for patients with underlying cardiac conduction system abnormalities and should be used with caution for patients who have impaired ventricular function.

INVASIVE THERAPY Percutaneous transluminal angioplasty and coronary artery bypass grafting of stenotic coronary arteries are the principal invasive treatments for preventing ischemia. Coronary artery bypass grafting has been shown to improve survival rates of patients with proximal high-grade stenosis of the left main coronary artery and patients with high-grade three-vessel stenosis with impaired left ventricular function. It is not yet clear whether percutaneous transluminal angioplasty will also provide long-term survival benefits or simply offer an alternative way of managing symptoms without altering long-term prognosis.

PREVENTING MYOCARDIAL INFARCTION

Two agents (beta blockers and aspirin) have been proven effective in preventing myocardial infarction in patients with coronary artery disease. As mentioned above, beta blockers have been proven effective in secondary prevention trials. Aspirin has also been shown to be effective in primary prevention, although the ideal dose is not certain. Recommendations range from 80 to 325 mg/d, and some regimens involve alternate-day dosing. No other antiplatelet agents have demonstrated effectiveness for prevention of myocardial infarction. At present, all patients with known coronary artery disease should receive beta blockers and aspirin unless specific contraindications exist.

TREATING OTHER MEDICAL CONDITIONS

Congestive heart failure, cardiac arrhythmias (particularly atrial fibrillation), and hypertension can contribute to increased myocardial oxygen demand and/or reduced myocardial oxygen availability. Management and control of these conditions is, therefore, essential for preventing further ischemia. Similarly, because diabetes, hyperlipidemia, cigarette smoking, and lack of physical activity have all been associated with coronary artery disease, treatment of and counseling about these conditions are considered important components of coronary artery disease management.

MAINTAINING FUNCTION

As with other chronic diseases, a primary goal of treatment is to help patients maintain function and quality of life. This goal can be achieved with management of angina and associated conditions, cardiac rehabilitation programs, and education of the patient. When clinicians emphasize functional status and quality of life, they send a message to patients that it is the person with the disease, not the disease process itself, that is of primary importance.

Esophageal Spasm

Several effective therapies are available for symptomatic treatment or prevention of esophageal spasm. These treatments include both non-pharmacologic and pharmacologic modalities.

NONPHARMACOLOGIC THERAPY

Some patients note a relationship between esophageal spasm and emotional stress or intake of certain foods. Therefore, many clinicians recommend relaxation therapy and/or diet modification to reduce symptoms of esophageal spasm. However, the benefit of eliminating such environmental triggers has not been formally investigated. Similarly, education of the patient centered on explaining the pathophysiology of spasm is often used to reduce patients' anxiety about the condition, but the benefit of such education for esophageal spasm has also not been studied.

PHARMACOLOGIC THERAPY

The principal medications used to treat episodes of esophageal spasm are nitrates and calcium channel blockers. Some patients require prophylactic therapy, rather than treatment of symptomatic episodes. Such individuals include those with frequent or severe esophageal spasm and those failing pharmacologic treatment of spasm episodes. Nitrates and calcium channel blockers are both effective prophylactic agents, with calcium channel blockers preferred because they cause fewer side effects when used on a daily basis. Promotility drugs may also be effec-

tive prophylactic agents. Nitrates can be used to treat acute episodes.

NITRATES   In addition to their beneficial effect on angina pectoris, the smooth-muscle-relaxing property of nitrates is effective for relieving esophageal spasm. Sublingual (tablet or spray) nitrates usually relieve spasm gradually within several minutes. Before using nitrates to treat esophageal spasm, however, clinicians *must* carefully establish that esophageal spasm is the correct diagnosis and that the patient's symptoms are not due to coronary artery disease, because anginal episodes from undiagnosed coronary artery disease also respond to this treatment. Masking coronary artery disease in this way may have serious, even fatal, consequences for patients.

CALCIUM CHANNEL BLOCKERS   Sublingual or oral calcium channel blockers, particularly verapamil, may also relieve esophageal spasm. As with nitrates, calcium channel blockers can mask symptoms of coronary ischemia. Therefore, the diagnosis of esophageal spasm must be confirmed and coronary artery disease excluded before embarking on a course of therapy with calcium channel blockers.

PROMOTILITY AGENTS   Promotility agents, such as cisapride, enhance smooth muscle motility. They can markedly improve esophageal spasm in some patients while exacerbating it in others. These agents can be tried with patients who require therapy but fail to respond to calcium channel blockers and/or nitrates.

OTHER TREATMENTS   Esophageal spasm in patients with GERD may be triggered by acid reflux into the esophagus. Effective treatment of GERD may, therefore, resolve symptoms of esophageal spasm. In fact, esophageal spasm in some patients is caused by "occult" reflux (i.e., reflux without overt reflux symptoms). Thus, empiric treatment with antireflux agents may eliminate and prevent spasm in some patients.

Rapid-acting benzodiazepines, such as alprazolam, can also relieve esophageal spasm. However, they do not act as quickly as nitrates and are not recommended for long-term or frequent use because chronic treatment can result in tachyphylaxis and drug dependence.

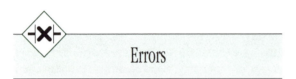

Errors

Several errors are common in the diagnosis and management of chest pain in primary care practice. These include errors of misdiagnosis, undertreatment, overly extensive evaluations, and failure to deal with patients' emotional response to chest pain.

Misdiagnosis

Failure to diagnose acute coronary ischemia is perhaps one of the most serious errors a clinician can make in caring for patients with chest pain. In fact, this error is one of the major causes of malpractice allegations against primary care clinicians. There are three common scenarios in which misdiagnosis occurs.

The first scenario involves patients whose chest pain is recognized as being due to ischemic heart disease but for which appropriate treatment is not instituted. For example, a patient with new or worsening angina symptoms may be given a prescription for anti-anginal medications, when appropriate management would have been hospital admission.

The second scenario involves patients with typical angina symptoms in whom the clinician excludes the possibility of coronary artery disease on the basis of a normal resting ECG. As noted earlier, ECG often fails to demonstrate

diagnostic abnormalities, even in patients with overt ischemia or an evolving infarction.

The third scenario involves patients with atypical chest pain in whom the clinician fails to give sufficient consideration to coronary ischemia as a possible cause of pain. Such patients typically present with symptoms more suggestive of dyspeptic syndromes (e.g., GERD) or pulmonary problems, and the clinician focuses on these diagnoses without considering the possibility of heart disease.

Undertreatment

Clinicians often fail to prescribe appropriate medications for patients with or at risk for coronary artery disease. This is a particular problem for patients with established coronary artery disease manifested by a previous myocardial infarction, for whom beta blockers and aspirin are recommended to prevent future coronary events. Several studies have demonstrated that primary care clinicians, both internists and family physicians, fail to prescribe these medications for many at-risk patients.

Similarly, studies have demonstrated that women with coronary artery disease, as a group, are treated less aggressively than are men who have the same clinical presentation. This tendency toward undertreatment may be one reason why women have poorer outcomes from acute coronary events than do men.

Overly Extensive Evaluations

It is appropriate that many clinicians fear that they will fail to recognize and treat an acute cardiac condition for patients who complain of chest pain. While this is a rational concern, it also leads to the most common error that clinicians make in evaluating chest pain: overusing cardiac studies in an attempt to achieve certainty by definitively excluding cardiac disease in all cases. Given the epidemiology of chest pain in primary care practice (Table 14-3), the probability of heart disease causing chest pain in certain age and gender groups is quite low. In the absence of a typical cardiac presentation, overemphasis on excluding heart disease in such patients is a wasteful use of health care resources. Furthermore, as discussed earlier, when cardiac testing is applied to individuals at low risk of heart disease, abnormal test results are frequently false-positive results. Follow-up of these abnormal test results can lead to further testing that is unnecessary, and potentially invasive and risky.

Failure to Deal with Patients' Emotional Responses

Fear and uncertainty drive the actions of many patients and clinicians during an episode of chest pain. Failure to recognize and address these issues explicitly can have adverse consequences. Patients with chest pain worry that they have a life-threatening disease, and when clinicians diagnose a minor or non-life-threatening condition, they must adequately reassure patients about the cause of symptoms and certainty of the diagnosis. Clinicians who fail to do so leave patients with unanswered questions, leading to emotional suffering for patients, as well as unnecessary use of health services as patients continue to seek answers from other clinicians.

This error can be avoided through effective clinician-patient communication. Clinicians who elicit patients' fears about the possible causes of chest pain can more effectively address them. This will permit the clinician to defer cardiac evaluation of patients with a low probability of unstable cardiac disease, while explaining to patients the reasons for doing so. The use of follow-up appointments for further evaluation can be an effective strategy for facilitating communication.

Controversies and Emerging Concepts

Role of Calcium-Channel-Blocking Medications

As mentioned earlier, a major current controversy in treating anginal chest pain relates to the use of short-acting calcium-channel-blocking drugs. Meta-analyses and case-control studies have indicated an association between these medications and a higher risk of myocardial infarction. Because of these studies, many experts now recommend against use of short-acting calcium channel blockers for treatment of angina and hypertension. However, there is also concern that some studies demonstrating the relationship between calcium blockers and infarction may have been biased by financial relationships between investigators and pharmaceutical firms that manufacture calcium-channel-blocking medications. Additional controversy has arisen because of recent research linking use of calcium channel blockers to cognitive impairment. Because of the minimal short-term side-effect profile of these drugs, which makes them an otherwise excellent choice for treatment, it will be important for future research to resolve controversies about the safety of calcium channel blockers.

New Tests for Detection of Myocardial Infarction

A variety of new blood tests have been developed for early detection of myocardial infarction. In comparison to creatine kinase and its MB isoenzyme, these new tests are more sensitive and produce a positive result earlier in the course of an acute ischemic event.

Blood tests for the cardiac contractile proteins, troponin I and troponin T, are most likely to see widespread clinical use. Compared with total creatine kinase and other proteins, such as myoglobin, troponin I and troponin T are highly sensitive and specific for myocardial necrosis. In addition, elevated levels of these proteins appear in the serum within just a few hours of the onset of ischemic symptoms. Furthermore, troponin I and troponin T are excellent predictors of adverse outcomes from acute ischemic events, making them useful for identifying patients at highest risk for complications. Recent development of a rapid (20-min) bedside test for measuring troponin levels offers the possibility of early decision making in evaluation of patients with suspected ischemic chest pain in chest pain evaluation units.

Chest Pain Evaluation Units

The availability of modalities, such as bedside troponin tests, to permit early and accurate identification of patients whose chest pain is due to acute coronary artery ischemia and infarction has led to the developments of outpatient chest pain evaluation units. These chest pain units, usually associated with a hospital-based emergency room, have access to a variety of diagnostic testing capabilities, including blood testing, ECG, cardiac monitoring, echocardiography, chest radiography, and sometimes treadmill testing, nuclear medicine cardiac perfusion scanning, and computer-based diagnostic algorithms. Most studies thus far have shown that, when patients with suspected ischemia are evaluated in these chest pain units, fewer patients are admitted to the hospital unnecessarily or sent home inappropriately, and costs and time spent in evaluation are reduced. Given the current expense of treating the 5 million patients who seek care in U.S. emergency rooms each year because of chest pain, the diagnostic accuracy and reduced cost of chest pain evaluation units is likely to result in increased use of this approach to evaluating chest pain.

Noninvasive Detection of Coronary Artery Disease

Several new imaging techniques are being studied to detect coronary artery disease and measure its severity. These include ultra-fast computerized tomography (which measures coronary artery calcification) and transesophageal color-flow Doppler imaging (which measures coronary artery blood flow). Other techniques, such as positron emission tomography and single-photon emission computerized tomographic scanning, are also under investigation; these techniques can be combined with exercise or dipyridamole administration to generate a functional image of coronary artery perfusion. Finally, expired gas analysis during exercise is likely to be useful in distinguishing whether a patient's symptoms are related to cardiac or pulmonary conditions.

Bibliography

Barret-Conner EL, Cohn BA, Wingard DL, et al: Why is diabetes mellitus a stronger risk factor for fatal ischemic heart disease in women than in men? *JAMA* 265:627, 1991.

Braunwald E, Mark DB, Jones RH, et al: *Unstable Angina: Diagnosis and Management*, Clinical Practice Guideline no 10, AHCPR publication no 94-0602. Rockville, MD, Agency for Health Care Policy and Research and the National Heart Lung and Blood Institute, Public Health Service, U.S. Department of Health and Human Services, 1994.

Conwell CF, Lyell R, Rodney WM: Prevalence of *Helicobacter pylori* in family practice patients with refractory dyspepsia: A comparison of tests available in the office. *J Fam Pract* 41:245, 1995.

Eagle KA: Medical decision making in patients with chest pain. *New Engl J Med* 324:1282, 1991.

Fleet RP, Dupuis G, Marchand A, et al: Panic disorder in the emergency department chest pain patients: Prevalence, comorbidity, suicidal ideation, and physical recognition. *Am J Med* 101:371, 1996.

Furberg CD, Psaty BM, Meyer JV: Nifedipine: Dose-related increase in mortality in patients with coronary heart disease. *Circulation* 92:1326, 1995.

Glassman PA, Kravitz RL, Petersen LP, et al: Differences in clinical decision making between internists and cardiologists. *Arch Intern Med* 157:506, 1997.

Gottlieb SS, McCarter RJ, Vogel RA: Effect of beta-blockade on mortality among high-risk and low-risk patients after myocardial infarction. *New Engl J Med* 339:489, 1998.

Hamm CW, Goldmann BU, Heeschen C, et al: Emergency room triage of patients with acute chest pain by means of rapid testing for cardiac troponin T or troponin I. *New Engl J Med* 337:1648, 1997.

Hull RDE, Raskob G, Carter CJ, et al: Pulmonary embolism in outpatients with pleuritic chest pain. *Arch Intern Med* 148:838, 1988.

Katerndahl DA, Realini JP: Where do panic attack sufferers seek care? *J Fam Pract* 40:237, 1995.

Kennedy RL, Harrison RF, Burton AM, et al: An artificial neural network system for diagnosis of acute myocardial infarction (AMI) in the accident and emergency department: Evaluation and comparisons with serum myoglobin measurements. *Comput Methods Prog Biomed* 52:93, 1997.

Klinkman MS, Stevens D, Gorenflo DW: Episodes of care for chest pain: A preliminary report from MIRNET. *J Fam Pract* 38:345, 1994.

Malacrida R, Genomi M, Maggioni AP: A comparison of the early outcome of acute myocardial infarction in women and men. *New Engl J Med* 338:8, 1998.

Mikhail MG, Smith FA, Gray M, et al: Cost effectiveness of mandatory stress testing in chest pain center patients. *Ann Emerg Med* 29:88, 1997.

Pryor DB, Shaw L, Harrel F: Estimating the likelihood of severe coronary artery disease. *Am J Med* 90:553, 1991.

Roberts RR, Zalenski RJ, Mensah EK, et al: Costs of an emergency department-based accelerated diagnostic protocol vs hospitalization in patients with chest pain: A randomized controlled trial. *JAMA* 278:1670, 1997.

Rosser W, Henderson R, Wood M, et al: An exploratory report of chest pain in primary care. *J Am Board Fam Pract* 278:1670, 1990.

Sox HC: Decision-making: A comparison of referral practice and primary care. *J Fam Pract* 42:155, 1996.

Sox HC, Hickam DH, Marton KI, et al: Using the patient's history to estimate the probability of coronary artery disease: a comparison of primary care and referral practices. *Am J Med* 89:7, 1990.

Stelflox HT, O'Rourke K, Detsky AS: Conflict of interest in the debate over calcium-channel antagonists. *N Engl J Med* 338:101, 1998.

Svaavrsrdsdottir AE, Jonasson MR, Gudmundsson GH, et al: Chest pain in family practice. *Can Fam Physician* 42:1122, 1996.

Tatum JL, Jesse RL, Kontos MC, et al: Comprehensive strategy for the evaluation and triage of the chest pain patient. *Ann Emerg Med* 29:116, 1997.

Thijs JC, van Sweet AA, Thijs WJ, et al: Diagnostic tests for *Helicobacter pylori*: A prospective evaluation of their accuracy, without selecting a single test as the gold standard. *Am J Gastroenterol* 91:2125, 1996.

Alan M. Adelman

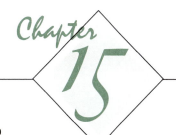

Abdominal Pain: Dyspepsia

Medications If H. pylori *Infection Is Absent*	Inappropriate Treatment of H. *pylori* Infection
DUODENAL ULCER	**Controversies**
GASTRIC ULCER	Empirical Treatment
GASTRITIS	Treatment Based on H. *pylori* Testing
Medications If H. pylori *Infection Is Present*	Routine Endoscopy before Treatment
	Resolving the Controversy
Education	**Emerging Concepts**
Errors	Diagnosis and Management of Dyspeptic
Errors in Diagnosis	Syndromes
Inappropriate Use of Antisecretory Medications	Adenocarcinoma of the Esophagus

How Common Is Abdominal Pain?

The complaint of abdominal pain encompasses a wide variety of clinical presentations and diagnoses, ranging from mild gastrointestinal infections to such life-threatening conditions as peritonitis and bowel obstruction. Thus, it can be challenging to identify the cause of abdominal pain, especially in primary care practice, because the various conditions that cause abdominal pain do not always present with classic findings. With so many conditions resulting in abdominal pain, a review of all possible causes of abdominal pain, or even all causes seen in primary care practice, would require an entire textbook. This chapter focuses on one of the most common abdominal pain syndromes seen in primary care practice: dyspepsia.

Prevalence

According to the National Ambulatory Medical Care Survey, abdominal pain, classified as stomach ache, cramps, or spasms, is one of the top ten reasons why patients in the United States make office visits to physicians. The majority of these visits are to primary care clinicians.

Virtually all individuals experience abdominal pain at some time in their lives, and between 14 and 27 percent report having had abdominal pain within the last 6 to 12 months. Of those who report abdominal pain, 20 to 38 percent seek medical care for their pain, with women more likely to seek care than men.

It is not surprising to note that individuals who have severe or frequent pain are more likely to seek medical attention than others, averaging between 1 and 3 visits to a clinician for each episode of abdominal pain. Despite the fact only the more severe cases come to medical attention, almost 90 percent of patients who are evaluated by a clinician for abdominal pain will be pain-free within 2 to 3 weeks of the evaluation, even without any specific treatment. Only about 10 percent of patients seen in primary care practice for abdominal pain are referred to specialty clinicians for further evaluation. Fewer than 10 percent are admitted to a hospital.

Heartburn, the most common symptom of dyspepsia, is extraordinarily common. Over 6 million individuals in the United States experience heartburn every day, and nearly half of all adults in the United States have heartburn at least monthly. The problem is so common that 18 million Americans take antacids to relieve heartburn more than twice per week.

Principal Diagnoses

Many conditions can cause abdominal pain, and the likelihood of encountering various conditions in primary care practice is different than that in other settings, such as emergency departments and surgical practices. The most common diagnoses for abdominal pain in outpatient primary care settings are listed in Table 15-1. The diversity of diagnoses is impressive and includes gastrointestinal problems as well as conditions unrelated to the gastrointestinal tract. The most important diagnoses to consider in relation to upper abdominal pain from dyspeptic disorders are discussed here.

Nonspecific Abdominal Pain

The single most common diagnosis of patients with abdominal pain is "nonspecific abdominal pain" (also referred to as "abdominal pain of unknown etiology"). Nonspecific abdominal pain is defined as a pain or discomfort anywhere in the abdomen for which a specific cause cannot be determined. This condition is generally self-limited and is particularly common in children, in whom the vast majority of cases of abdominal pain has no identifiable cause. In contrast, when elderly individuals experience abdominal pain, they are more likely to seek medical care for the pain and more likely to have an identifiable, and often serious, organic condition causing the pain.

Table 15-1

Final Diagnoses for the Presenting Symptom of Abdominal Pain in Primary Care Settings

DIAGNOIS	A FAMILY PRACTICE IN THE UNITED STATES %	A FAMILY PRACTICE IN THE UNITED STATES %	A GENERAL PRACTICE IN THE NETHERLANDS %
Adominal pain, nonspecific	50.4	20.6	63.1
Nonulcer dyspepsia			7.7
Acute gastroenteritis	9.2	6.3	1.5
Urinary tract infection	6.7		0.2
Irritable bowel syndrome	5.8	6.9	14.8
Pelvic inflammatory disease	3.8		
Gastroesophageal reflux	2.3	6.9	0.7
Diverticulosis	2.2		1.3
Diarrhea, cause undetermined	1.6		
Cholelithiasis	1.6	3.2	0.3
Tumor, benign	1.4		0.9
Duodenal ulcer	1.4	3.7	1.8
Urolithiasis	1.3		0.4
Appendicitis	1.1		0.1
Ulcerative colitis	0.9		1.2
Muscular strain	0.9		
Gastritis		9.0	
Malignancy, gastrointestinal			1.0
Other	9.5		

SOURCE: From Adelman et al (a family practice in the United States), Klinkman (a family practice in the United States), and Muris et al (a general practice in the Netherlands).

Dyspeptic Conditions

Dyspepsia describes a constellation of symptoms consisting predominantly of upper abdominal or epigastric pain or discomfort. Heartburn—the feeling of acid in the stomach—is also common. Other symptoms of dyspepsia include bloating, nausea, vomiting, hiccuping, and/or belching.

About one-quarter of individuals with dyspepsia consult a clinician. After evaluation by a clinician, the five diagnoses accounting for 80 to 90 percent of dyspepsia are nonulcer dyspepsia, gastroesophageal reflux disease (GERD), duodenal ulcer, gastritis, and gastric ulcer.

NONULCER DYSPEPSIA

The most common cause of dyspeptic symptoms is "nonulcer dyspepsia," or dyspepsia for which no specific cause can be identified. Thus, as with the general category of abdominal pain, the most common diagnostic outcome for patients with dyspepsia is to identify no specific cause for the symptoms.

The cause of nonulcer dyspepsia is unknown, but some experts believe it may represent a gastrointestinal motility disorder. Patients with nonulcer dyspepsia have normal levels of gastric acid secretion, and the prevalence of *Helicobacter pylori* infection, the apparent cause of peptic ulcers, is no greater in persons with nonulcer dyspepsia than in the general population. In addition, treatment of *H. pylori* infection does not predictably lead to resolution of nonulcer dyspepsia.

The incidence of nonulcer dyspepsia decreases with advancing age. Thus, when young adults complain of dyspeptic symptoms, the likelihood that no specific pathologic condition will be discovered (i.e., the diagnosis will be nonulcer dyspepsia) is relatively high. With increasing age, however, especially after age 50, the diagnosis of specific conditions, such as gastritis, gastric cancer, peptic ulcer disease, or GERD, becomes more common.

GASTROESOPHAGEAL REFLUX DISEASE

The next most common cause of dyspeptic symptoms in primary care practice is GERD. This condition involves reflux of stomach contents into the esophagus, which can cause injury to the esophagus [Fig. 15-1 (Plate 8)]. Most symptoms of GERD are caused by reflux of acid, but pepsin, bile salts, and pancreatic enzymes may also contribute to symptoms and esophageal injury.

The principal pathophysiologic process that permits reflux to occur is weakness or incompetence of the lower esophageal sphincter. However, other processes also contribute to reflux, including abnormal esophageal motility, diminished resistance of the esophageal mucosa to refluxed gastric contents, and delayed postprandial emptying of the stomach.

Figure 15-1 (Plate 8)

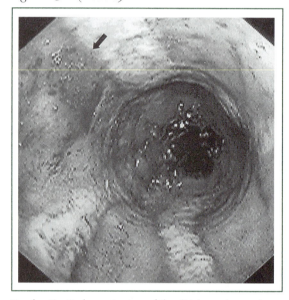

Esophagitis. Endoscopic view of the distal esophagus showing inflammation of the esophageal mucosa. The arrow indicates the most-inflamed area. *(Courtesy of Gregory Gambla, D.O., Milton Hershey Medical Centers, Penn State Geisinger Health System.)*

Simple heartburn is the most common manifestation of GERD. However, gastric contents can damage esophageal mucosa, causing esophagitis, including erosive esophagitis [Fig. 15-2 (Plate 9)]. Esophageal mucosa that is chronically exposed to gastric contents can also develop strictures. In addition, between 10 and 20 percent of patients who seek care for GERD will develop Barrett's esophagus (metaplasia of normal squamous esophageal epithelium into columnar epithelium). Barrett's esophagus is of concern because the metaplastic epithelium can undergo further transformation to adenocarcinoma. Finally, in some patients, refluxed gastric contents can enter their airway, resulting in laryngitis, chronic cough, asthma-like wheezing, aspiration pneumonia, or chest pain.

DUODENAL ULCER

Duodenal ulcers are typically small (less than 1 cm) ulcerations of the proximal duodenal mucosa [Fig. 15-3 (Plate 10)]. They occur at one time or another in about 10 percent of the U.S. population. Duodenal ulcers are thought to result from the action of gastric acid and digestive enzymes on a duodenal mucosa that is inadequately protected by mucus, bicarbonate, and prostaglandins. However, the gram-negative bacteria H. pylori also plays a critical role, since the organism is present in nearly all individuals who develop duodenal ulcers. In addition, eradication of H. pylori with antibiotic therapy markedly reduces the risk of ulcer recurrence.

Duodenal ulcers are more common in persons who smoke cigarettes and in individuals with chronic renal failure, alcoholic liver disease, and hyperparathyroidism. Persons with blood type O are also at increased risk, possibly

Figure 15-2 (Plate 9)

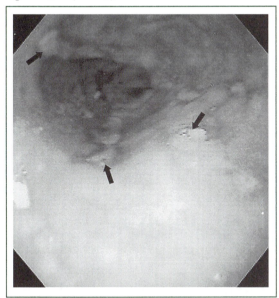

Esophagitis with ulcerations. Endoscopic view of the distal esophagus demonstrating erythema and multiple erosions and ulcerations (examples marked with arrows). *(Courtesy of Gregory Gambla, D.O., Milton Hershey Medical Centers, Penn State Geisinger Health System.)*

Figure 15-3 (Plate 10)

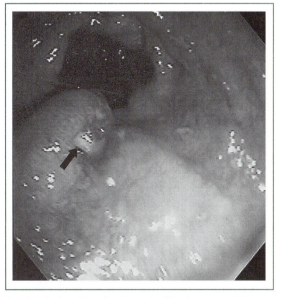

Duodenal ulcer. The ulcer is marked by the arrow. *(Courtesy of Gregory Gambla, D.O., Milton Hershey Medical Centers, Penn State Geisinger Health System.)*

because the O antigen facilitates binding of *H. pylori* to duodenal mucosa.

Aside from the discomfort of dyspeptic symptoms, the major risk of duodenal ulcers is bleeding. Bleeding can be abrupt and of large volume, resulting in upper gastrointestinal hemorrhage. It can also be occult and manifested as chronic iron-deficiency anemia. Duodenal inflammation and edema associated with the ulcer can cause gastric outlet obstruction. Less commonly, duodenal ulcers can perforate the duodenal wall, spilling gastrointestinal contents into the peritoneal cavity or penetrating adjacent structures, such as the pancreas.

Gastric Ulcer

Gastric ulcers are typically deep ulcerations through the mucosa of the stomach, often surrounded by areas of gastritis. They can be caused by ingestion of nonsteroidal anti-inflammatory drugs (NSAIDs), but they also occur in the absence of NSAID use. Gastric acid and pepsin are both involved in the pathogenesis of gastric ulcers, but, as with duodenal ulcers, there is also strong evidence that *H. pylori* infection is of primary importance in gastric ulcers. In fact, *H. pylori* is present in the stomach of virtually all individuals who develop gastric ulcers, and, even in the 20 to 25 percent of gastric ulcers caused by NSAIDs, *H. pylori* is still thought to play an etiologic role in many individuals. The mechanism by which *H. pylori* causes gastric ulcers is not certain, but the organism secretes a variety of factors that may damage gastric mucosa and gastric mucus.

Gastric ulcers may be benign or malignant. Benign gastric ulcers are typically small and occur in the antrum of the stomach. They are almost always accompanied by antral gastritis due to *H. pylori* infection. Ulcers in the gastric fundus, on the other hand, and larger ulcers are more likely to be malignant. Endoscopic studies and biopsy are required to determine whether a gastric ulcer is benign or malignant. Barium contrast radiological studies are unreliable, since they

may be falsely negative in the presence of malignant gastric ulcers.

Gastric ulcers may also cause serious acute complications, including hemorrhage, gastric outlet obstruction, and perforation of the stomach either into the abdominal cavity or posteriorly into the pancreas. It should be noted that duodenal ulcers are simultaneously present in about 10 percent of patients with benign gastric antral ulcers.

Gastritis

Gastritis (inflammation of the gastric mucosa) can result from a variety of causes, and it may be acute or chronic. In primary care practice, the most common causes of acute gastritis are *H. pylori* infection and NSAID ingestion. Acute gastritis may be mild and asymptomatic [Fig. 15-4 (Plate 11)], or it may cause dyspeptic symptoms or gastrointestinal bleeding [Fig. 15-5 (Plate 12)].

Figure 15-4 (Plate 11)

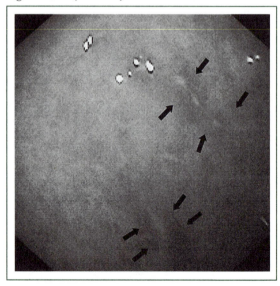

Gastritis. This patient has mild gastritis, manifested as areas of erythema on the gastric mucosa (arrows). *(Courtesy of Gregory Gambla, D.O., Milton Hershey Medical Centers, Penn State Geisinger Health System.)*

Figure 15-5 (Plate 12)

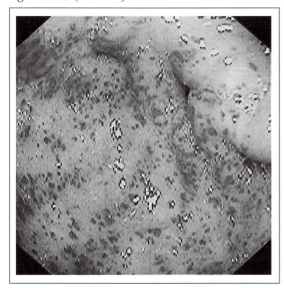

Gastritis. This patient has marked gastritis, with areas of intense erythema and numerous small mucosal hemorrhages. *(Courtesy of Gregory Gambla, D.O., Milton Hershey Medical Centers, Penn State Geisinger Health System.)*

The common form of chronic gastritis in primary care practice is related to *H. pylori* infection. In younger patients, the *H. pylori*-related inflammation is typically in the gastric antrum (antral gastritis), whereas in older individuals, the entire stomach may be affected. Over time, the gastric mucosa involved in *H. pylori* gastritis may become atrophic, which increases the risk of gastric adenocarcinoma; however, the mechanism by which *H. pylori* infection causes gastric cancer is not understood. It may be that the infection renders gastric mucosa more susceptible to dietary or environmental carcinogens, or it may be simply that the chronic inflammation leads to cell proliferation and subsequent development of cancer. It is interesting to note that chronic *H. pylori* gastritis is also associated with an increased risk of gastric lymphoma.

Another, relatively uncommon, cause of gastritis is autoimmune gastritis. In this condition, antibodies develop against gastric parietal cells and intrinsic factor, resulting in malabsorption of vitamin B_{12} and subsequent pernicious anemia. There are also many other causes of gastritis that are almost never seen in primary care practice. These disorders include sarcoidosis; Crohn's disease; and parasitic, mycobacterial, and fungal infections of the stomach.

Other Diagnoses to Consider

In addition to the common dyspepsia syndromes described above and the common causes of abdominal pain listed in Table 15-1, there are also several serious or life-threatening conditions that should be considered with any patient who presents with abdominal pain. A discussion of these conditions is beyond the scope of this chapter, but a few of the more common conditions are listed in Table 15-2.

Finally, ischemia of the inferior myocardium sometimes presents with symptoms indistinguishable from dyspepsia, including heartburn, nausea, vomiting, belching, and/or hiccups. Typical angina, with chest pressure and arm discomfort, may or may not also be present. Thus, in any patient with dyspeptic symptoms, especially those with risk factors for cardiac disease, myocardial ischemia should be considered as a diagnostic possibility, as described in Chap. 14.

Typical Presentation

There is no typical presentation for individuals with abdominal pain; about two-thirds of patients present with pain below the umbilicus and one-third with pain above the umbilicus. Dyspeptic syndromes, by definition, present with pain above the umbilicus. However, in primary care practice, patients' symptoms often do not fit classic patterns described in textbooks. This can make diagnosis difficult. The infre-

Table 15-2

Serious or Life-Threatening Causes of Nontraumatic Abdominal Pain

CAUSE OF PAIN (EXAMPLES)	KEY HISTORY	KEY EXAMINATION
Bowel obstruction (due to adhesions, volvulus, duodenal edema, tumor)	Bloating, abdominal distention, persistent emesis, vomiting fecal material	Tympanitic abdomen, abnormal bowel sounds (rushes, tinkles), distention, succussion splash
Cancer (colon, pancreatic)	Weight loss, anorexia, fatigue	Jaundice, abdominal mass, rectal bleeding, anemia
Abdominal aortic aneurysm	Ripping or tearing pain, pain radiating or boring to the back, history of hypertension	Loss of femoral pulses, pulsatile abdominal mass, hypotension
Bowel perforation (duodenal ulcer, diverticulitis)	Pain, fever	Absent bowel sounds, abdominal muscle rigidity
Bowel infarction (mesenteric ischemia)	History of atrial fibrillation, myocardial infarction, or atherosclerosis	Absent bowel sounds, rectal bleeding, septic appearance
Acute gastrointestinal bleeding	Dizziness, weakness, hematemesis, melena, hematochezia	Guiac-positive emesis or stool, tachycardia, hypotension
Pelvic organ disease (ectopic pregnancy, pelvic inflammatory disease, ovarian cyst)	Menstrual history, vaginal discharge or bleeding	Pelvic examination

quency of classic patterns in primary care practice occurs for two main reasons.

First, patients often present to primary care clinicians early in the course of their disease. It is only with time that patients display the classic presentations of a particular condition. This lack of classic symptoms is most well known for appendicitis, which may present initially with periumbilical pain rather than the right lower quadrant pain that develops later. Similarly, dyspeptic syndromes, such as duodenal ulcer, may initially present with nonspecific complaints, such as nausea or lack of appetite, and only later will the possibility of an ulcer become apparent.

The second reason that classic presentations are uncommon in primary care is that most patients simply do not have the classic conditions described in textbooks. Rather, they have undifferentiated symptoms that are not easily labeled. As shown in Table 15-1, approximately 50 percent of patients in primary care settings have nonspecific diagnoses and never are diagnosed with an identifiable cause for their pain.

Key History

The history of patients with abdominal pain can be both helpful and confusing because serious diagnoses occur infrequently and many conditions have the same or overlapping symptoms.

The combination of low prevalence of serious disease and overlapping symptoms makes the positive predictive value of most symptoms quite low.

For example, duodenal ulcer and non-ulcer dyspepsia both can present with pain relieved by food or antacids. However, duodenal ulcer is fairly uncommon, whereas nonulcer dyspepsia is extremely common. The low frequency of duodenal ulcer means that, even if a patient presents with the "classic" ulcer symptom of pain relieved by food or antacids, the positive predictive value of these symptoms for duodenal ulcer is actually very low. Furthermore, the presence of these symptoms is not a good discriminator between ulcers and nonulcer dyspepsia. In such situations, in which the prevalence of serious disease is low, the challenge in taking a history is to distinguish those few patients with potentially serious problems from the majority who have no specific treatable problem or diagnosis.

Thus, the basic plan in taking a history from a patient with dyspepsia and/or abdominal pain is to first search for symptoms indicative of serious or life-threatening conditions. In addition, the patient should be asked about use of NSAIDs. Then, the clinician should seek symptom clusters that suggest or exclude one of the specific dyspepsia syndromes described above. If none are detected, the patient probably has nonulcer dyspepsia or a nonspecific abdominal pain syndrome.

Symptoms Indicative of Serious Conditions

The first step in taking a history from patients with upper abdominal pain is to seek clues to the presence of serious or life-threatening disease, such as gastric-outlet obstruction, bowel perforation, gastrointestinal bleeding, cholecystitis, and cancer. Important clues to these diagnoses include severe pain or vomiting, weight loss, melena, hematochezia, hematemesis, and orthostatic dizziness. Table 15-2 shows key his-

tory items for a number of serious conditions that may be encountered in primary care. As mentioned above, the conditions in Table 15-2 are uncommon in everyday office practice, but clinicians should briefly consider them for any patient with abdominal pain.

Myocardial ischemia, on the other hand, is somewhat more common in primary care practice. Therefore, clinicians must always consider the possibility of ischemia or infarction with patients who have dyspeptic symptoms. The likelihood of a cardiac cause of dyspepsia is higher in older patients, particularly those with risk factors for atherosclerosis, recent onset of symptoms, or other symptoms associated with heart disease. If ischemia is considered a possible cause for a patient's symptoms, the patient should be evaluated with resting and stress electrocardiographic studies if the symptoms are chronic and hospital admission to exclude acute infarction or unstable angina if the symptoms are acute.

Non-steroidal Anti-inflammatory Drugs

Patients with dyspeptic symptoms should always be asked about use of NSAIDs, since these medications are the second most common cause of peptic ulceration after *H. pylori* infection. NSAIDs are also a common cause of gastrointestinal bleeding, especially in older individuals.

Dyspeptic Symptoms

Assuming that the patient's history does not suggest any of the serious conditions discussed above, and the patient is not taking NSAIDs, the next step is to focus on symptoms of dyspepsia. Differentiating the symptoms of nonulcer dyspepsia from the specific dyspeptic syndromes (duodenal ulcer, gastric ulcer, gastritis, and GERD) can be difficult, since there is a poor correlation between symptoms and endoscopic findings. In addition, in primary care practice the classic history items, such as the relationship of pain to food, the timing of pain, and the severity of pain, are all poorly predictive of the patient's actual diagnosis.

SINGLE SYMPTOMS

Single symptoms of patients with dyspepsia are poor predictors of the final diagnosis, with one exception. The exception is in GERD, in which the presence of heartburn with a sensation of reflux into the esophagus or mouth (pyrosis) is highly suggestive of GERD. Other,

less common, but relatively typical symptoms of GERD include dysphagia (manifested as food boluses getting stuck in the esophagus) and/or chronic cough not explained by a respiratory tract problem.

SYMPTOM CLUSTERS

Experienced clinicians tend to rely on patterns and clusters of symptoms for clues to the diagnosis, rather than seeking any one specific symptom. Table 15-3 summarizes the operating

Table 15-3

Operating Characteristics of Symptom Clusters in Dyspepsia

	SYMPTOM CLUSTERS	DISEASE	SENSITIVITY	SPECIFICITY	LR+	LR−	PV+	PV−
1.	Food or milk aggravates pain, mild pain, no night pain, no vomiting or weight loss, age under 40	Nonulcer dyspepsia	57	94	9.5	0.46	90	67
2.	Pain relieved by antacids, age above 40, previous ulcer disease, male gender, symptoms provoked by berries, night pain relieved by antacids or food	Organic dyspepsia	84	51	1.7	0.31	41	88
3.	Previous peptic ulcer, pain relieved with antacids, age above 40, smoking, pain relieved by food	Peptic ulcer	90	55	2.0	0.18	27	93
4.	Pain radiating to the back	Cholelithiasis	83	74	3.1	0.23	36	96
5.	Vomiting, smoking, previous peptic ulcer or hiatal hernia, higher age, male gender	Organic dyspepsia	97	30	1.4	0.10	34	97
6.	Nocturnal pain, pain before meals or when hungry, absence of nausea, higher age, male gender	Peptic ulcer	51	83	3.0	0.59	49	84

ABBREVIATIONS: LR+, likelihood ratio that the disease is present if the symptom cluster is present, compared to if the symptom cluster were absent; LR−, likelihood ratio that the disease is absent if the symptom cluster is absent, compared to if the symptom cluster were present; PV+, positive predictive value for the disease if a symptom cluster is present; PV−, negative predictive value of a symptom cluster.
SOURCE: Adapted and reprinted by permission of Appleton & Lange, Inc., from Muris JWM, Starmans R, Pop P, et al: Discriminant value of symptoms in patients with dyspepsia. *The Journal of Family Practice* 38(2):139–143, 1994.

characteristics of various symptom clusters in patients with dyspepsia.

SYMPTOMS SUGGESTING NON-ULCER DYSPEPSIA The first symptom cluster in Table 15-3 (food or milk aggravates pain, mild pain, no night pain, no vomiting, no weight loss, and age under 40) is highly suggestive of nonulcer dyspepsia. If this symptom cluster is present, there is a 90-percent chance that the patient has nonulcer dyspepsia, and it is almost 10 times more likely that the patient has nonulcer dyspepsia than not. Thus, the presence of this symptom cluster is useful in diagnosing nonulcer dyspepsia.

SYMPTOMS SUGGESTING AN ORGANIC CAUSE OF DYSPEPSIA The presence of nocturnal pain and older age are common to all the clusters associated with organic (i.e., other than non-specific) causes of dyspepsia. In addition, clusters 4 and 6 in Table 15-3 are moderately useful in diagnosing cholelithiasis and peptic ulcer, respectively.

SYMPTOMS EXCLUDING AN ORGANIC CAUSE OF DYSPEPSIA The absence of cluster 3 in Table 15-3 is useful for excluding peptic ulcer disease, and the absence of cluster 5 tends to exclude all organic causes of dyspepsia. Lack of previous peptic disease and younger age are common to all the clusters that tend to exclude organic dyspepsia.

SYMPTOMS SUGGESTING RISK FOR CHRONIC PAIN Certain symptoms may not be useful for diagnosis but have prognostic value for identifying patients at risk of chronic abdominal pain. Muris and associates found that several symptoms and symptom clusters in individuals with non-organic abdominal pain tend to predict that abdominal pain will persist for longer than 1 year. These symptoms included the combination of abdominal pain, flatulence, and bowel irregularities; pain described by the patient as sharp, burning, and intense; and/or pain that, at the time of the initial consultation, was long-lasting or recurrent. Women and patients with depression were also more likely to have persistent abdominal pain.

Physical Examination

In general, physical examination is usually not helpful in the diagnosis of abdominal pain in primary care practice. While classic signs of peritonitis, appendicitis, cholecystitis, or other serious conditions may sometimes be present and have classic examination findings, the more common situation in office practice is that the examination reveals few physical findings, most of which are nonspecific.

Nonetheless, an important purpose of the physical examination is to detect serious conditions, if they are present, and to seek findings suggestive of the specific dyspeptic syndromes. The absence of specific or classic signs, however, does not rule out any particular condition.

Detecting Serious Conditions

As with the history, initial attention during the physical examination should be focused on detecting signs of serious or systemic conditions. These signs include findings such as fever, significant weight loss, jaundice, abdominal rigidity, orthostatic hypotension, and blood in the stool. In addition, the examination should include the lungs and, in women, a pelvic examination if gynecological conditions are a possibility. Table 15-2 shows key examination findings for some of the serious conditions that can present with abdominal pain.

Identifying Dyspeptic Conditions

Most patients with dyspepsia have no examination findings or minimal epigastric tenderness. If present, however, findings that suggest complications of dyspeptic syndromes (i.e., perforated ulcer or bleeding from ulcers, gastritis, or GERD-related esophagitis) include orthostatic hypotension; blood in the stool; and peritoneal signs, such as abdominal rigidity, distention, or absent bowel sounds.

Ancillary Tests

As with the history and physical, ancillary tests for patients with dyspepsia are used to detect serious conditions or complications and to diagnose and guide management of dyspeptic syndromes. There are no tests that should always be ordered in evaluating patients with abdominal pain, since such an approach to testing seldom leads to diagnoses not already suspected by the clinician. Instead, imaging and laboratory testing should be guided by findings of the history and physical examination.

Blood Tests, Stool Tests, Urine Tests, and Plain X-Rays

For patients with abdominal pain, only a small percentage of routine abdominal x-rays will detect serious abnormalities, such as free air or an obstructive pattern, and, usually, serious conditions are already suspected in most of these patients. Similarly, routine blood, stool, and urine testing are rarely helpful unless there is reason to think the tests results might be abnormal.

The only exception to routine testing is at the extremes of age. In infants and elderly individuals with abdominal pain, there is a higher rate of serious abnormalities, including surgical emergencies, than in older children, adolescents, and working-aged adults. Infants and the elderly frequently have atypical presentations and may not be able to communicate their symptoms to clin-

icians. Thus, while testing in infants and geriatric-aged individuals should still be guided by the history and physical examination, clinicians should regularly consider obtaining complete blood counts, radiographic imaging, urinalyses, chemistry panels, and stool testing for blood for patients in these age groups who have abdominal pain. A similar approach is needed for immunocompromised patients, in whom symptoms and presentations are also frequently atypical and may represent serious disease.

Specific Tests for Dyspeptic Syndromes

Testing of patients with dyspepsia is designed to answer two questions. The first is to determine the underlying cause of a patient's dyspeptic symptoms. That is, does the patient have an ulcer, gastritis, or GERD? The second question, if an ulcer or gastritis is present, is whether the patient has *H. pylori* infection.

DETERMINING THE CAUSE OF SYMPTOMS

The tests most commonly used for diagnosing the cause of dyspepsia are endoscopic esophagogastroduodenoscopy and barium-contrast upper gastrointestinal (UGI) radiography. Esophageal pH monitoring is a useful adjunctive test for diagnosing GERD.

ENDOSCOPY For most patients who require examination of the UGI tract, endoscopy is the preferred test. Endoscopy can reliably diagnose gastritis and is more sensitive and specific than radiographic imaging for diagnosing ulcers and GERD. In fact, endoscopy is considered the "gold standard" for diagnosing ulcers, gastritis, and esophageal injury from GERD. Second, the ability to obtain biopsies during endoscopic procedures permits identification of *H. pylori* infection.

The American College of Physicians has published recommendations for when endoscopy should be performed. While written before the role of *H. pylori* in dyspeptic disorders was understood, the recommendations are still clinically applicable. They suggest endoscopy be performed if (1) there is no response to medical therapy after 7 to 10 days of medical treatment, (2) symptoms persist after 6 to 8 weeks of medical therapy, (3) signs of ulcer complications develop, (4) signs of systemic illness are present, or (5) symptoms recur after treatment. As discussed later, some experts now recommend that endoscopy be performed at the beginning of the evaluation of dyspepsia. Endoscopy is also recommended in patients with a long-standing history of untreated GERD, because such patients may have Barrett's metaplasia.

UPPER GASTROINTESTINAL RADIOGRAPHY Upper gastrointestinal x-rays are considerably less costly than endoscopy (the 1996 Medicare reimbursement for physician and hospital costs of UGI radiographic studies was $100.35, while the cost of endoscopic studies was $412), and they can diagnose peptic ulcer, gastric ulcer, and GERD. Unfortunately, the false-negative rates are substantial. For peptic ulcers, the false-negative rate of UGI studies exceeds 18 percent, and it is much higher for GERD. In addition, UGI examinations are falsely positive for ulcers in up to one-third of examinations. For these reasons, UGI x-rays are not usually considered the test of choice for evaluating dyspeptic symptoms.

The UGI series still has a role in diagnosis, however. In particular, UGI x-rays can be useful as an initial diagnostic test for patients with isolated dysphagia and for patients for whom the sedation required for endoscopy would be excessively risky.

ESOPHAGEAL pH MONITORING AND MANOMETRY Esophageal pH monitoring is useful for selected patients suspected of having GERD in whom endoscopy reveals no evidence of the condition. The procedure is performed by placing a probe through the nares into the distal esophagus to monitor esophageal pH. A fall in pH to less than 4 occurs when gastric contents reflux into the

esophagus. Esophageal manometric studies can also be performed to measure the contractility of the lower esophageal sphincter, which is impaired in GERD. However, manometric studies are not routine in the evaluation of patients with dyspepsia or GERD.

DETECTING *H. PYLORI*

Testing for *H. pylori* infection is indicated for patients with gastric or duodenal ulcers or gastritis, since each of these conditions is highly associated with *H. pylori* infection, and treatment of infection markedly reduces the chance of recurrence. Methods of detection include blood testing, breath analyses, and several tests that can be performed in conjunction with endoscopy.

BLOOD TESTS Qualitative tests for anti–*H. pylori* antibodies in serum are widely available The serum tests are reasonably accurate (sensitivity 93 percent, specificity 90 percent, positive likelihood ratio 9, and negative likelihood ratio 0.08). However, not all individuals who test positive have ulcers or gastritis, and the test cannot be used to distinguish active from previously treated infection because serologic test results remain positive even after treatment.

A quantitative enzyme-linked immunosorbent assay (ELISA) can also be used. Although less widely available, it is even more accurate than a qualitative serologic analysis (sensitivity 95 percent, specificity 95 percent, positive likelihood ratio 19, and negative likelihood ratio 0.05). More important, it can be used to document resolution of infection because ELISA titers decrease after successful treatment of *H. pylori* infection. In addition to its use as a diagnostic test, repeat ELISA measurements can be performed following therapy (usually at 1, 3, and 6 months after treatment) to document eradication of the organism.

BREATH ANALYSIS The urea breath test is based on the fact that *H. pylori* is a urea-splitting organism. The test involves ingesting a gelatin-coated capsule that contains carbon-14-labeled urea. If *H. pylori* is present in a patient's stomach, the urea is split and releases radio-labeled CO_2, which can be detected in the patient's exhaled breath. The test is sensitive (96 percent) and specific (98 percent), and has positive and negative likelihood ratios of 48 and 0.04, respectively. Breath analysis can be used for initial diagnosis of infection and to test for eradication of *H. pylori* after treatment.

ENDOSCOPIC TESTS   If endoscopic testing is performed, several methods can be used to detect *H. pylori* infection in biopsy specimens. The "gold standard" method is to culture the biopsy tissue specimen for *H. pylori*. In clinical practice, however, culture is used primarily when there is concern about antibiotic resistance.

Currently, the fastest and most frequently used method is the rapid urease test, also known as the *Campylobacter*-like organism (CLO) test, which tests the specimen of mucosa for bacterial urease. The CLO test detects the change in pH that occurs as a result of urease activity by changing the color of a phenol-red indicator. The CLO test has a sensitivity of about 95 percent and near-perfect specificity.

Histologic examination of the tissue specimen for the *H. pylori* organism can also be used. Special stains may be needed, however, and studies report variable sensitivity compared to culture, ranging from less than 90 percent to as high as 99 percent.

Finally, polymerase chain reaction testing of the biopsy specimen has almost perfect sensitivity and specificity compared to culture. It is likely to be the test of choice in the future.

to approach diagnosis. The algorithm in Fig. 15-6 shows one diagnostic approach that can be used to evaluate patients with new symptoms of dyspepsia in a primary care setting. Note that this algorithm does not apply to patients with chronic or recurrent dyspepsia, in whom it is often appropriate to perform endoscopy at the onset of the evaluation.

For the individual with new-onset dyspepsia, the first step is to determine whether the patient is taking a NSAID. If so, the NSAID should be discontinued. If dyspepsia persists after stopping the NSAID, the clinician should undertake further investigation. This evaluation should include endoscopic study as an initial test if the patient has symptoms or signs suggesting malignancy or if the patient is older than 50. It also should include appropriate ancillary tests if there is suspicion of a malignancy or other systemic illness.

Assuming that the patient is not taking NSAIDs and has no findings suggesting malignancy or systemic disorder, the next step is to seek specific symptoms of GERD or the symptom clusters typical of non-ulcer dyspepsia (see Table 15-3). If either is present, the patient should be treated accordingly. If symptoms persist despite treatment, endoscopy should be performed.

If there are no symptoms typical of GERD or non-ulcer dyspepsia, a test for *H. pylori* is ordered. A negative test result suggests that neither peptic ulcer nor antral gastritis is present, and the patient can be treated for non-ulcer dyspepsia. If the *H. pylori* test result is positive, endoscopy should be performed to detect and confirm the presence of *H. pylori*-associated conditions, such as duodenal ulcer, gastric ulcer, gastritis, or gastric cancer.

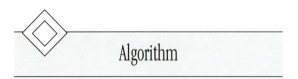

Algorithm

As discussed later, the ideal method of evaluating dyspepsia is controversial, and many different recommendations have been made for how

Treatment

Before seeking care from a clinician, many patients unsuccessfully self-treat with nonpre-

Figure 15-6

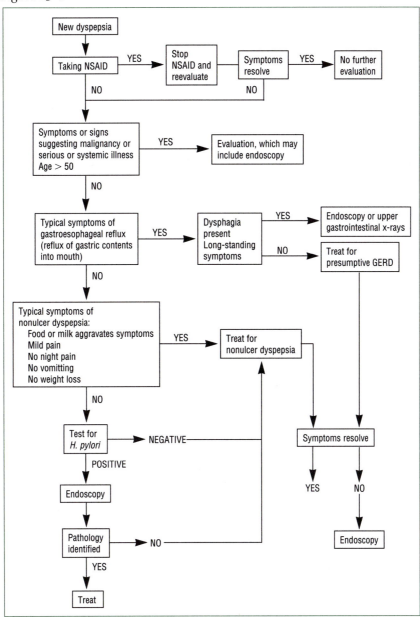

Algorithm for the diagnosis of new-onset dyspepsia in a primary care setting.

scription medications. The most commonly used medications are antacids and antisecretory histamine-2 (H-2) receptor antagonists, such as cimetidine, ranitidine, or famotidine. Because non-prescription H-2 blockers and antacids are frequently taken in lower than the recommended prescription dose, clinicians should ascertain the dose being used before concluding that the patient's self-administered nonprescription treatment was truly unsuccessful.

In addition, some patients try nontraditional self-treatments, including herbal remedies. One of the more widely used herbal remedies for dyspepsia is ginger, the underground stem of the *Zingiber officinale* plant. Several studies have shown some benefit from this treatment, and there are no reported side effects.

When symptoms are related to use of NSAIDs, these drugs should be stopped if at all possible. If patients have gastric or duodenal ulcers from NSAID use, antisecretory medications such as H_2 blockers or proton-pump inhibitors, described below, can hasten healing of the ulcers. Proton-pump inhibitors are the most effective treatment for NSAID-induced ulcers.

Nonspecific Abdominal Pain and Nonulcer Dyspepsia

Many treatments have been used for both nonspecific abdominal pain and for nonulcer dyspepsia, but no formal studies have evaluated the effectiveness of these treatments. For abdominal pain of unknown etiology, many clinicians prescribe a fixed-dose "antispasmodic" drug combination (marketed as Donnatal) containing phenobarbital, hyoscyamine, atropine, and scopolamine. Others prescribe dicyclomine, an anticholinergic agent marketed as Bentyl, or similar agents. None of these treatments has been conclusively demonstrated to benefit patients with nonspecific abdominal pain. They carry the risk of anticholinergic side effects, and, in the case of those containing barbiturates, there is potential for dependence and addiction. Acetaminophen and a heating pad applied to the abdomen are preferable to anticholinergic and barbiturate medications for most patients.

Likewise, for nonulcer dyspepsia, no treatment has been shown to be consistently effective. Antacids and antisecretory agents (H_2 blocking agents) are often prescribed (Table 15-4), but there is no convincing evidence that they alter the course of nonulcer dyspepsia. Similarly, as mentioned earlier, *H. pylori* infection is not

Table 15-4

Standard Medication Doses for Treatment of Dyspeptic Syndromes

MEDICATION	DOSE
H_2 BLOCKERS (ANTISECRETORY)	
Cimetidine (Tagamet)	400 mg bid
Famotidine (Pepcid)	20 mg bid
Nizatidine (Axid)	150 mg bid
Ranitidine (Zantac)	150 mg bid
PROTON-PUMP INHIBITORS	
Omeprazole (Prilosec)	20 mg qd
Lansoprazole (Prevacid)	15 mg qd
PROTECTIVE COATING AGENT	
Sucralfate (Carafate)	1 g qid
ANTACIDS (ALUMINUM HYDROXIDE/MAGNESIUM HYDROXIDE/SIMETHICONE)	
Liquids	30 mL qid or prn
Tablets	2 tablets qid
PROKINETIC AGENTS (FOR GERD)	
Cisapride (Propulsid)	10 mg qid
Metoclopramide (Reglan)	10 mg qid

NOTE: Some medications require dosing adjustments for patients with renal or hepatic disease. Consult complete prescribing information before administering to patients.

thought to play a role in non-ulcer dyspepsia, and treating the infection, if present, does not consistently improve symptoms. Thus, antibiotic treatment of *H. pylori* for patients with nonulcer dyspepsia is not considered appropriate therapy. Overall, despite the prevalence of nonulcer dyspepsia, clinical research provides clinicians with little guidance about how to approach treatment of the condition.

Gastroesophageal Reflux Disease

Treatment of GERD involves life-style modifications, medications, and, in some cases, surgery.

In addition, an important part of managing GERD is surveillance for Barrett's metaplasia and esophageal adenocarcinoma.

LIFE-STYLE MODIFICATIONS

Life-style modifications for GERD are aimed at decreasing exposure to substances that cause relaxation of the lower esophageal sphincter and avoiding physical and/or mechanical factors that predispose to reflux or esophageal irritation. Substances that decrease lower esophageal pressure include alcohol, caffeine, chocolate, and fatty foods. Physical and mechanical interventions include avoiding the supine position for several hours after eating, elevating the head of the bed during sleep, and avoiding large meals (which distend the stomach and predispose to reflux). Substances that directly irritate the esophageal mucosa include citrus, coffee, and spicy or tomato-based foods.

These life-style modifications are inexpensive and safe, but there is limited information about their benefit. The only study that has examined long-term effectiveness of these treatments in primary care practice evaluated life-style modifications in combination with intermittent antacid therapy, rather than life-style modifications alone. Forty percent of patients in this study experienced relief of symptoms.

MEDICATIONS

Medications for treating GERD include antisecretory agents (H_2 blockers and proton-pump inhibitors) and prokinetic agents. Treatment, including presumptive treatment based on symptoms, typically begins with an H_2 blocker and/or a prokinetic drug. Proton-pump inhibitors are generally used when GERD is accompanied by erosive esophagitis and for patients with GERD that has not responded to H_2 blockers.

H_2 RECEPTOR ANTAGONISTS The H_2 blockers include cimetidine, famotidine, nizatidine, and ranitidine. All of the H_2 blockers inhibit about two-thirds of total daily gastric acid secretion, and they are more effective at decreasing nighttime acid production than postprandial acid secretion. None of the H_2 blockers has been shown to be superior to any of the others, although cimetidine interacts with the metabolism of many drugs, making it less desirable for some patients. The usual doses of H_2 blockers are shown in Table 15-4.

PROKINETICS Prokinetic drugs can be used as initial therapy, but they are more commonly used as adjuncts to H_2 blockers. Prokinetic drugs enhance esophageal peristalsis and gastric emptying, and they improve function of the lower esophageal sphincter. Prokinetic drugs include metoclopramide (a dopamine antagonist) and cisapride (a serotonin agonist that enhances release of acetylcholine from the esophageal myenteric plexus). Metoclopramide's extrapyramidal side effects limit its use, especially as a long-term therapy or for older patients, but cisapride appears to be safe. For best effect, however, cisapride must be taken four times per day, which is inconvenient for most patients. The usual doses of the prokinetic drugs are shown in Table 15-4.

PROTON-PUMP INHIBITORS The proton-pump inhibitors, which include omeprazole and lansoprazole, block the proton pump in gastric parietal cells that is responsible for acid secretion. Their effect on gastric acid secretion is far superior to that of H_2 blockers, decreasing acid production by over 90 percent. These drugs are the treatment of choice for patients with endoscopically documented erosive esophagitis. Resolution of esophagitis occurs in 80 to 90 percent of patients after 6 to 8 weeks of treatment. Proton-pump inhibitors are also indicated for documented GERD that has not responded to H_2 blocker treatment. In addition, patients who relapse after successful treatment with H_2 blockers may be candidates for therapy with proton-pump inhibitors. Finally, some patients will require long-term treatment with a proton-pump inhibitor to prevent relapse of GERD symptoms or esophagitis.

SURGERY

Antireflux surgery can be considered for patients whose condition is refractory to medical treatment, who develop recurrent esophagitis, or who develop complications of esophagitis, such as stricture or hemorrhage. Open surgical procedures for GERD have been available for years, but complication rates are relatively high and outcomes not optimal. In recent years, however, laparoscopic surgical techniques have been used with success. The most common procedure is fundoplication, in which the gastric fundus is wrapped around the lower esophagus, increasing lower esophageal sphincter pressure. Success rates exceed 90 percent.

SURVEILLANCE FOR BARRETT'S METAPLASIA

About 10 percent of patients with GERD develop Barrett's metaplasia, and these individuals have a risk of esophageal cancer up to 300 times higher than that of the general population. Thus, patients with esophagitis should be monitored for development of metaplasia and cancer. The ideal interval for monitoring is uncertain, but typical recommendations are that patients who have esophagitis without Barrett's changes should undergo an endoscopic examination every 2 to 3 years, while those with Barrett's metaplasia should be monitored endoscopically every 6 to 12 months.

Gastritis, Duodenal Ulcers, and Gastric Ulcers

GENERAL CONSIDERATIONS

Patients with gastritis and peptic ulcers, including both duodenal and gastric ulcers, should avoid NSAIDs and alcohol (which irritate gastric and duodenal mucosa), discontinue or minimize nicotine and caffeine (both of which stimulate acid secretion), and avoid foods that aggravate symptoms. However, there is no evidence that any specific diets, such as "bland" diets or diets free of spices, are effective in relieving symptoms. Similarly, there is no evidence that "coating" the stomach with milk or cream is beneficial. In fact, milk and cream may actually be harmful because they stimulate gastric acid secretion; they also contribute to hyperlipidemia and atherosclerotic vascular disease.

For treatment of uncomplicated gastritis, duodenal ulcers, and gastric ulcers, the critical factor is the presence or absence of *H. pylori*. If *H. pylori is* absent, then acid-reduction therapy with anti-secretory drugs is indicated (Table 15-4). If *H. pylori* is present, antibiotics are prescribed, usually in combination with acid-reduction therapy (Table 15-5).

MEDICATIONS IF *H. PYLORI* INFECTION IS ABSENT

DUODENAL ULCER　For duodenal ulcers in the absence of *H. pylori* infection, treatment with H_2 blocking agents or proton-pump inhibitors is indicated. The H_2 blocking agents are typically used as the first-choice treatment, but proton-pump inhibitors can also be used. Sucralfate, a complex salt of sucrose and aluminum that binds to ulcer craters, is also an acceptable first-line treatment. With sucralfate bound to the ulcer crater, the ulcer is protected from gastric acid, pepsins, and bile acid. Combination therapy (i.e., H_2 blockers plus proton-pump inhibitors, or H_2 blockers plus antacids, etc.) has not been shown to be more effective than a single agent. Antacids are not appropriate for primary therapy for duodenal ulcer. Instead, they are used for breakthrough symptoms that occur while taking standard acid-reduction medications.

GASTRIC ULCER　For gastric ulcers in the absence of *H. pylori* infection, proton-pump inhibitors are the medications of choice because gastric ulcers heal faster with proton-pump inhibitors than

Table 15-5

Several Drug Regimens for Eradication of *Helicobacter pylori* Infection

REGIMEN	DOSE	EFFECTIVENESS, %	COST
MOC		87–90	$200
Metronidazole*	500 mg bid × 14 days		
Omeprazole	20 mg bid × 14 days		
Clarithromycin	250 mg bid × 14 days		
Helidac†		77–90	$45
Bismuth subsalicylate	2 tablets qid × 14 days		
Metronidazole	250 mg qid × 14 days		
Tetracycline	500 mg × 14 days		
O + C		64–90	$350
Omeprazole‡	40 mg/d × 14 days‡		
Clarithromycin	500 mg tid × 14 days		
BMTO		75–95	$100
Bismuth	2 tablets qid × 10 days		
Metronidazole	250 mg qid × 10 days		
Tetracycline	500 mg qid × 10 days		
Omeprazole	20 mg bid × 10 days		
Tritec + clarithromycin		73–84	$200
Ranitidine/bismuth§	400 mg bid × 14 days		
Clarithromycin	500 mg tid × 14 days		

*Substitute amoxicillin (1g bid) for metronidazole if metronidazole resistance is suspected.
†Helidac is nearly identical to classic "triple therapy."
‡Continue omeprazole (20 mg d) for 2 additional weeks if active ulcer is present.
§Continue ranitidine/bismuth (400 mg bid) for 2 additional weeks if active ulcer is present.

with H_2 blockers. Benign gastric ulcers should heal within 2 to 3 months of beginning therapy. Failure to heal within that time interval suggests the possibility of malignancy and is an indication for endoscopy and biopsy.

GASTRITIS Gastritis in the absence of *H. pylori* infection is not often encountered in primary care practice. As discussed earlier, it is usually due to autoimmune processes, such as pernicious anemia. Patients with non–*H. pylori* typically have gastric mucosal atrophy and decreased acid secretion. Thus, acid-reduction therapy is not indicated. Treatments are directed at the underlying cause of the gastritis.

MEDICATIONS IF *H. PYLORI* INFECTION IS PRESENT

If *H. pylori* infection is detected, eradicating infection is the single most important intervention. While acid-reduction therapies are also used, they are of secondary importance. Failure to effectively treat and eliminate the infection is the major cause of recurrent ulcers and gastritis.

Several antibiotic regimens are effective for eradicating *H. pylori* infection, some of which combine antibiotics with acid-reduction therapy (Table 15-5). If the chosen antibiotic regimen does not include acid-reduction therapy, it may be added as an adjunctive treatment, using the recommendations outlined above.

The most successful and widely used antibiotic regimen is the "triple-therapy" combination of bismuth subsalicylate, metronidazole, and either amoxicillin or tetracycline. When combined with omeprazole, this regimen is effective at eradicating infection and healing ulcers in up to 90 percent of patients. However, the triple-therapy regimen is somewhat cumbersome, in that patients must take pills four times per day and side effects may occur, including constipation, discoloration of the tongue and stool, and antibiotic-induced colitis. Therefore, alternative regimens are being used with increased frequency. For example, the combination of clarithromycin and omeprazole, while considerably more expensive than triple therapy, is nearly as effective and much easier to administer (Table 15-5). In practice, the choice of treatment regimen is frequently determined by the drugs available on the formulary of the health care organization in which a clinician practices.

The National Institutes of Health consensus conference recommended antibiotic therapy only for patients with documented ulcers or gastritis and confirmed evidence of *H. pylori* infection. This recommendation stems from concerns about the developing problem of antibiotic-resistant *H. pylori*. Resistance is a particular problem with metronidazole but may occur with all antibiotic regimens.

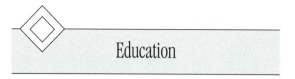

Education

The U.S. public has substantial misconceptions about the causes of dyspeptic syndromes. For example, most people believe that ulcers are caused by emotional stress and have no awareness that ulcers and gastritis are associated with an infection.

Thus, patients with peptic ulcers and gastritis should be provided with information about the cause of their condition and the lack of effect of dietary changes. Those with GERD should receive instruction regarding life-style interventions that may improve symptoms. Individuals with GERD and esophagitis should know about the importance of periodic surveillance for Barrett's metaplasia and cancer.

In the many patients for whom no specific diagnosis for abdominal pain is identified, clinicians should provide reassurance and emphasize that most abdominal pain resolves spontaneously. This is important because patients who seek medical attention for dyspepsia often are concerned about having cancer or heart disease. When possible, therefore, clinicians should explain the cause of symptoms to patients. If uncertainty about the diagnosis exists, the uncertainty should also be explained.

Finally, it is important to inform patients about the need to seek medical attention if changes in symptoms indicate development of complications. Examples of such symptoms include increasing pain, hematemesis, melena, or orthostatic dizziness. Patients with GERD should seek attention for symptoms of dysphagia, as this symptom may represent stricture or malignancy.

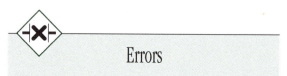

Errors

A variety of errors occur in the diagnosis and treatment of dyspeptic abdominal pain. The three most common errors are failure to consider important alternative diagnoses, inappropriate use of acid-reduction therapy, and inappropriate treatment of *H. pylori* infection.

Errors in Diagnosis

The most common serious error in diagnosis of dyspeptic symptoms is failure to consider and/or properly evaluate the possibility that symptoms are caused by myocardial ischemia. As noted earlier, inferior-wall myocardial ischemia frequently causes nausea, heartburn, and other symptoms typically associated with dyspeptic disorders. Failure to diagnose myocardial infarction is one of the ten most common causes of malpractice allegations against family physicians in the United States, and mistaking myocardial ischemia for dyspeptic symptoms is one of the common scenarios in which this failure occurs. Exclusion of a cardiac cause for dyspeptic symptoms should always take precedence over treatment of dyspepsia. If the diagnosis is uncertain, or if ischemia cannot be reliably excluded during an office encounter, clinicians should consider treadmill or other diagnostic testing, or hospital admission for cardiac monitoring and exclusion of ischemia and/or infarction.

Another error is disregarding signs or symptoms that indicate diagnoses other than the common dyspeptic syndromes. These missed diagnoses include the various conditions listed in Table 15-2. This error sometimes occurs because clinicians put too much weight on individual symptoms, signs, or laboratory tests; this can be avoided by knowing the operating characteristics of patients' symptoms (Table 15-3), signs, and test results. Errors in diagnosis also occur when clinicians fail to perform a systematic history and physical examination. For example, many clinicians do not routinely perform pelvic examinations, creating the risk of overlooking such nongastrointestinal conditions as pelvic inflammatory disease, ovarian torsion, or ectopic pregnancy. In addition, failure to perform a rectal examination for detection of fecal blood is a potentially serious error in evaluating patients with dyspepsia, because management can be substantially different in the presence of bleeding from gastritis, ulcers, or esophagitis.

A third diagnostic error is not being cognizant of the atypical presentation of abdominal pain and dyspepsia in elderly or immunocompromised individuals. As discussed earlier, such individuals warrant more-intensive investigation because they frequently lack the expected signs and symptoms of serious intra-abdominal problems.

Inappropriate Use of Antisecretory Medications

While empirical treatment with anti-secretory medications is acceptable, some clinicians prescribe these medications in inappropriate situations. For example, empirical antisecretory therapy is not appropriate for patients whose symptoms persist despite treatment, who have symptoms of dysphagia in association with reflux symptoms, or who have blood in their stool. Such individuals should undergo diagnostic tests (usually endoscopy) to accurately determine the cause of their symptoms.

Similarly, acid-reduction is not appropriate as sole treatment for ulcers or gastritis if *H. pylori* infection is present. Many clinicians make the error of prescribing H_2 blockers or proton-pump inhibitors without testing for *H. pylori*, perhaps because such tests are not readily available in the clinician's office. Failure to detect and treat *H. pylori* infection, however, markedly increases the rate of recurrence for ulcers and gastritis. Acid-reduction therapy should be considered an adjunct to antibiotic treatment of *H. pylori*–related ulcers and gastritis, not as principal treatment.

Inappropriate Treatment of H. pylori Infection

In addition to not detecting and treating *H. pylori*, some clinicians make the error of treating *H. pylori* infection without confirmation that such infection is present. In fact, some clinicians prescribe antibiotics for patients with non-specific dyspeptic symptoms, without confirming that the patient has gastritis or an ulcer. As discussed above, current recommendations are that antibiotic therapy is not appropriate for nonulcer dyspepsia and should be reserved for patients with documented ulcers or gastritis.

Controversies

The principal controversy in diagnosis and management of dyspeptic disorders currently surrounds the issue of how much diagnostic testing is necessary before treatment can be prescribed. That is, is it necessary to establish definitive diagnoses before beginning treatment, or is empirical treatment acceptable and appropriate? Because of the large number of individuals affected by these dyspetic conditions, this controversy has substantial cost implications for society. At least seven specific approaches to diagnosis and management have been proposed, but they all fall into three basic strategies: empirical treatment, treatment based on *H. pylori* testing, and routine endoscopic studies before treatment.

Empirical Treatment

The first strategy involves empirical treatment. In this approach, patients are treated presumptively with antisecretory agents, antibiotics, or both, based on symptoms indicative of gastritis or ulcers. The potential drawback of empirical antisecretory treatment is that malignant gastric ulcers will not be detected, nor will the presence of GERD-associated erosive esophagitis or Barrett's metaplasia. The drawback of empirical antibiotic treatment is an increase in antibiotic-resistant *H. pylori*.

Treatment Based on H. pylori Testing

A second strategy is to perform serological or breath analysis tests for *H. pylori* for patients who have symptoms suggesting ulcers or gastritis. Individuals who test positive are treated with antibiotics, while those who test negative are treated empirically with anti-secretory agents. This strategy is attractive because it eliminates the need for and cost of endoscopy. However, it will result in treatment of many persons who do not have demonstrable organic disease, because no diagnosis is established.

Routine Endoscopy before Treatment

The third strategy is to perform endoscopy to make a definitive diagnosis in all patients with dyspepsia. If gastritis or ulcers are detected, testing for *H. pylori* is performed at the time of endoscopy. The cost of routine endoscopy would appear to make this approach expensive, but, as noted below, a controlled trial of various approaches to dyspepsia found it was more cost-effective to perform endoscopy early in the diagnostic evaluation. In addition, this strategy corresponds to the National Institutes of Health consensus recommendations calling for a definitive diagnosis of ulcers or gastritis, as well as a positive test for *H. pylori*, before treating with antibiotics.

Resolving the Controversy

Over the past few years, several investigators have performed decision analyses to determine which of these or other strategies leads to the best outcomes at the lowest cost. Unfortunately, there were differences between the specific strategies examined, and each analysis reached different conclusions. Ebell and associates examined seven strategies and identified two that were most cost-effective: empirical *H. pylori* treatment and use of serologic tests to identify and treat patients with *H. pylori* infection. Ofman and associates examined patients who tested positive on serologic tests for *H. pylori* and found that the most cost-effective approach was to treat the infection without documenting an ulcer. Silverstein and associates compared initial endoscopy and empirical therapy, with or without initial testing for *H. pylori*, and found that no strategy showed a clear advantage. Finally, the analysis of Fendrick and associates advocated initial empirical treatment of ulcers and *H. pylori* infection.

There is only one randomized clinical trial to support any specific strategy. Bytzer and associates compared initial endoscopy before treatment to empirical treatment with anti-secretory agents. The investigators found that it was more cost-effective to perform prompt endoscopy. Individuals whose dyspepsia was managed in this fashion required less medication, lost fewer days from work, and used fewer health services than those treated empirically. A major limitation of this study, however, is that identification and treatment of *H. pylori* infection was not addressed.

Thus, while some evidence suggests that performing endoscopy before treatment may be the preferred approach to diagnosis and management of dyspeptic complaints, the ideal strategy has not yet been defined. With wider availability of quantitative serologic and breath analysis tests for *H. pylori*, current approaches to dyspeptic syndromes are likely to undergo continued revision.

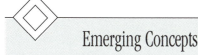

Emerging Concepts

Over the next few years, several emerging concepts may change the approach to dyspeptic abdominal pain syndromes. These include (1) development of new information on diagnosis and management of dyspeptic syndromes and (2) the possible relationship between acid-reduction therapy and adenocarcinoma of the esophagus.

Diagnosis and Management of Dyspeptic Syndromes

As the influence of evidence-based medicine continues to grow, more information about the predictive values of symptoms, signs, and laboratory tests will emerge, permitting more accurate and rational diagnoses and treatment of dyspeptic disorders. Furthermore, controversies in the evaluation and management of dyspepsia, as outlined above, are likely to be clarified. The possible development of office-based tests (e.g., breath analyses) for detecting *H. pylori* will further modify and facilitate the evaluation process.

Adenocarcinoma of the Esophagus

The incidence of adenocarcinoma among white men in the United States has increased substantially since 1970. Although it is controversial, some authors have proposed that the increase may be related to increased use of H_2 blockers for treatment of GERD. The rationale for this hypothesis is that, when used to treat GERD, anti-secretory agents only diminish acid production. While diminished acid production can eliminate the acid-related symptoms of reflux, anti-secretory agents do not prevent reflux of pepsin and other gastric contents into the esophagus. Thus, patients' symptoms are relieved by anti-secretory drugs, while reflux of pepsin and/or other gastric contents may continue to injure the esophagus and cause Barrett's metaplasia and adenocarcinoma. This concern has led some authorities to advocate increased use of laparoscopic fundoplication for treatment of GERD, as fundoplication decreases reflux of all gastric contents. However, some studies have demonstrated reversal of Barrett's metaplasia with proton-pump inhibitor therapy, suggesting that acid-reduction therapy is unrelated to the increased incidence of esophageal cancer. More research is needed to clarify these concerns.

Bibliography

Adelman A: Abdominal pain in the primary care setting. *J Fam Pract* 25:27, 1987.

Adelman A, Koch H: New visits for abdominal pain: The NAMCS experience. *Fam Med* 23:122, 1991.

Adelman A, Metcalf L: Abdominal pain in a university family practice setting. *J Fam Pract* 16:1107, 1983.

Adelman AM, Revicki DA, Magaziner J, et al: Abdominal Pain in an HMO. *Fam Med* 27:321, 1995.

Boyle JT: Recurrent abdominal pain: An update. *Pediatr Rev* 18:310, 1997.

Bytzer P, Hansen JO, deMuckadell OB: Empirical H_2 blocker therapy or prompt endoscopy in management of dyspepsia. *Lancet* 343:811,1994.

Chang L: Gastroesophageal reflux disease: Pathophysiology, clinical symptoms, and diagnosis. *J Managed Care* 3(suppl):S6, 1997.

Chow WH, Finkle WD, McLaughlin JK, et al: The relation of gastroesophageal reflux disease and its treatment of adenocarcinoma of the esophagus and gastric cardia. *JAMA* 274:474, 1995.

Ebell MH, Warbasse L, Brenner C: Evaluation of the dyspeptic patient: A cost-utility study. *J Fam Pract* 44:545, 1997.

Fendrick AM, Chernew ME, Hirth RA, et al: Alternative management strategies for patients with suspected peptic ulcer disease. *Ann Intern Med* 123:260, 1995.

Foodborne and Diarrheal Disease Branch, Division of Bacterial and Mycotic Diseases, National Center for Infectious Diseases: Knowledge about causes of peptic ulcer disease: United States, March–April 1997. *MMWR* 46:985, 1997.

Fraser AG, Ali MR, McCullough S, et al: Diagnostic tests for *Helicobacter pylori*: Can they help select patients for endoscopy? *N Z Med J* 109:95, 1996.

Health and Public Policy Committee, American College of Physicians: Endoscopy in the evaluation of dyspepsia. *Ann Intern Med* 102:266, 1985.

Johnsen R, Bernersen B, Straume B, et al; Prevalences of endoscopic and histological findings in subjects with and without dyspepsia. *BMJ* 302:749, 1991.

Jones RH, Lydeard SE, Hobbs FDR, et al: Dyspepsia in England and Scotland. *Gut* 31:401, 1990.

Klinkman MS: Episodes of care for abdominal pain in a primary care practice. *Arch Fam Med* 5:279, 1996.

Kuster E, Rose E, Toledo-Pimentel V, et al: Predictive factors of the long-term outcome in gastrooesophageal reflux disease: Six-year follow-up of 107 patients. *Gut* 35:8, 1994.

Lukens TW, Emerman C, Effron D: The natural history and clinical findings in undifferentiated abdominal pain. *Ann Emerg Med* 22:690, 1993.

Mendall MA, Jazrawi RP, Marrero JM, et al: Serology for *Helicobacter pylori* compared with symptom questionnaires in screening before direct access endoscopy. *Gut* 36:330, 1995.

Muller JL, Clauson KA: Pharmaceutical considerations in common herbal medicine. *Am J Managed Care* 3:1753, 1997.

Muris JWM, Starmans R, Fijten GH, et al: One-year prognosis of abdominal complaints in general practice: A prospective study of patients in whom no organic cause is found. *Br J Gen Pract* 46:715, 1996.

Muris JWM, Starmans R, Pop P, et al: Discriminant value of symptoms in patients with dyspepsia. *J Fam Pract* 38:139, 1994.

NIH Consensus Conference: *Helicobacter pylori* in peptic ulcer disease: NIH Consensus Development Panel on *Helicobacter pylori* in Peptic Ulcer Disease. *JAMA* 272:65, 1994.

Ofman JJ, Etchason J, Fullerton S, et al: Management strategies for *Helicobacter pylori*–seropositive patients with dyspepsia: Clinical and economic consequences. *Ann Intern Med* 126:280, 1997.

Sampliner RE:. Effect of up to 3 years of high-dose lansoprazole on Barrett's esophagus. *Am J Gastroenterol* 89:1844, 1994.

Silverstein MD, Petterson T, Talley NJ: Initial endoscopy or empirical therapy with or without testing for *Helicobacter pylori* for dyspepsia: A decision analysis. *Gastroenterology* 110:72, 1996.

Soll AH, for the Practice Parameters Committee of the American College of Gastroenterology: Medical treatment of peptic ulcer disease: Practice guidelines. *JAMA* 275:622, 1996.

Talley NJ: Nonulcer dyspepsia: Current approaches to diagnosis and management. *Am Fam Phys* 47:1407, 1993.

Yeomans ND, Tulassay ZT, Racz I, et al: A comparison of omeprazole with ranitidine for ulcers associated with nonsteroidal antiinflammatory drugs. *New Engl J Med* 338:719, 1998.

Wang HH, Hsieh CC, Antoniolo DA: Rising incidence rate of esophageal adenocarcinoma and use of pharmaceutical agents that relax the lower esophageal sphincter. *Cancer Causes Control* 5: 573, 1994.

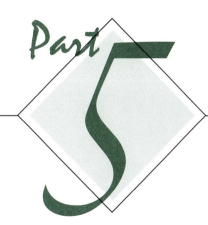

Part 5

Some Other
Common Problems

Patricia E. Boiko
Susan Boiko
with contributions from
Ron Singler and Michael W. Piepkorn

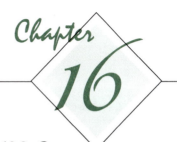

Chapter

16

Dermatitis-Eczema

How Common Is Dermatitis-Eczema?

Eczema, from the Greek "to boil over," is the most common skin disorder treated by primary care clinicians. Eczema is actually a group of skin conditions that have common symptoms, signs, and histologic characteristics. They share the sensation of itching and dryness, the clinical appearance of redness and scaling, and the histologic appearance that the epidermis is "boiling" because of intercellular edema (spongiosis). Clinically, eczematous skin conditions range from mild and transient to chronic and disabling.

Primary care clinicians are trained to evaluate and treat skin diseases. However, among individual practitioners there is considerable variability in the ability to diagnose skin disorders. In this chapter, written descriptions of eczema and its imitators are supplemented by photographic images, an algorithm, and tables to help clinicians make a diagnosis, choose therapy, order additional tests if needed, and make specialty referrals when appropriate.

"Rash" is among the top five symptoms for which patients state they seek care from primary care clinicians. In large health maintenance organizations, the diagnostic cluster of dermatitis-eczema is in the top 15 diagnoses seen in primary care practice. The Group Health Cooperative of Puget Sound in Seattle, Washington, reports that each year diagnoses of dermatitis-eczema account for over 14,000 visits and more than 1 million dollars in health care costs.

The most common form of eczema, atopic dermatitis, affects 10 to 15 percent of the population at some point during their lifetimes. It is particularly common in children, and primary care clinicians diagnose eczema in one-third of all children between 1 and 4 years old.

Principal Diagnoses

Many skin conditions fall under the diagnostic rubric of eczema or dermatitis-eczema, but five are particularly common in primary care practice: (1) atopic dermatitis, (2) allergic contact dermatitis, (3) irritant contact dermatitis, (4) seborrheic dermatitis, and (5) nummular eczema.

Atopic Dermatitis

DEFINITION

Atopic dermatitis is a genetically determined skin disorder characterized by superficial scaling, erythema, papules, and vesiculation whose expression is modulated by the environment. One system used to define the diagnosis of atopic dermatitis involves sets of major and minor criteria. To diagnose atopic dermatitis, an individual must have at least four of five major features plus three or more of ten minor features. Questions that can be useful in detecting the major and minor features of atopic dermatitis are shown in Table 16-1.

The specific, or major, features are pruritus, onset during infancy [Fig. 16-1 (Plate 13)] or childhood [Fig. 16-2 (Plate 14)], a typical appearance and distribution, a chronic or chronically relapsing course, and a personal or family history of atopy (asthma, allergic rhinoconjunctivitis, or atopic dermatitis). Onset in adulthood suggests a diagnosis other than atopic dermatitis.

The 10 less-specific, or minor, features include xerosis (dry skin), ichthyosis vulgaris (rough scaling of the skin, usually of the feet), palmar hyperlinearity (deep linear grooves that are perpendicular to the long axis of the thenar or hypothenar eminence of the palm), keratosis pilaris (dry, itchy bumps on the upper arms), and perifollicular accentuation (prominence of the rash around hair follicles, commonly seen in darker-skinned individuals). Other minor features include involvement of the hands and feet, lips (cheilitis), and/or nipples and an increased susceptibility to cutaneous infections. An additional minor feature is an immediate type 1 skin test response to intradermally injected allergen.

A second scheme for defining the diagnosis of atopic dermatitis is based on identification of 17 signs and symptoms that occur more frequently in individuals with atopic dermatitis than in those without the condition. In this diagnostic scheme, the presence of at least 14 of the signs or symptoms is diagnostic of atopic dermatitis (Table 16-2).

For about 30 percent of individuals, atopic dermatitis first occurs on the hands, and 70 percent have hand involvement at some time during their lives. Other characteristic signs and symptoms of atopic dermatitis include excessive dandruff (or cradle cap in infants) and cracked or crusting skin around the ears. Eye findings include dark circles under the eyes ("allergic shiners"), absence of the lateral third of the eyebrows (Hertoghe's sign), and lower eyelids that appear to have two folds (Dennie-Morgan fold).

EPIDEMIOLOGY

Atopic dermatitis occurs in most countries of the world. It is interesting to note that individuals who are genetically susceptible to atopic dermatitis who live in rural areas may have no skin problems until they move to an urban area. The reason for this is not fully understood, but air pollutants such as sulfur dioxide and nitrogen oxide increase IgE synthesis and are associated with increased incidence of atopic dermatitis. Further indications that atopic dermatitis is more prevalent in urban or industrialized areas come from Japan, where, prior to 1988, severe atopic dermatitis was most prevalent among infants and children, with no predominance among urban dwellers. In recent years, however, 83 percent of patients with severe atopic dermatitis (i.e., requiring hospital admission) were between 13 and 30 years old and were typically from urban and/or industrialized areas.

An additional epidemiologic risk for atopic dermatitis is cigarette smoking. Maternal smoking during pregnancy and lactation is associated with a 2.3 times greater risk of eczematous skin conditions in the offspring.

The natural history of atopic dermatitis is highly variable. Over the course of 15 to 20 years, atopic dermatitis will resolve in about 40 percent of affected individuals. In others, it may

Table 16-1

Sample Questionnaire for Diagnosis of Atopic Dermatitis

To diagnose atopic dermatitis, a person must answer yes or respond as indicated by the explanation in italics, to 4 of the specific (major) features plus 3 of the less specific (minor) features.

MAJOR FEATURES (REQUIRES 4 OR MORE)

1. ONSET DURING CHILDHOOD

   Were you between 2 months and 12 years old when the rash first began?

   COMMENT: Atopic dermatitis usually begins in infancy and 85 percent of cases are manifest by age 5. If the rash began in adulthood consider scabies, contact dermatitis, cutaneous lymphoma, or other diagnosis.

2. PRURITUS

   Does your skin and/or rash itch?

   COMMENT: Pruritus is virtually always present in atopic dermatitis. In fact, atopic dermatitis is often referred to as "the itch that rashes."

3. TYPICAL DISTRIBUTION

   Where was your rash and itching mostly located when you were a child? Where was it when you were an adolescent?

   COMMENT: During childhood, atopic dermatitis occurs most commonly on facial and extensor surfaces. Infants below age 2 may have a rash on the cheeks that is dry, red, and scaly. During adolescence, the rash most commonly occurs on flexural surfaces (i.e., antecubital or popliteal) and demonstrates lichenification and linearity.

4. CHRONIC OR CHRONICALLY RELAPSING

   Does your rash and itching go away and come back, or just gets a little better but is always present?

   COMMENT: Atopic dermatitis is, by definition, a chronic or chronically-relapsing condition. Finding that a patient has received numerous treatments with topical steroids or oral antipruritics establishes chronicity.

5. PERSONAL OR FAMILY HISTORY OF ATOPY

   Do you, or does anyone in your family, have a similar rash, or eczema, asthma, or allergies that affect the nose and eyes?

   COMMENT: 31 percent of individuals with atopic dermatitis have a personal history of allergic rhinitis or asthma, 62 percent have a family history of respiratory allergies, and only 21 percent have no such personal or family history. 50 percent of persons with atopic dermatitis will ultimately develop allergic rhinitis or asthma. A medical record that documents prescriptions for asthma or allergy medications can establish this criteria in the absence of a specific atopic diagnosis.

MINOR FEATURES (REQUIRES 3 OR MORE)

1. XEROSIS

   Is your skin dry?

   COMMENT: Dry skin is often present since birth.

Table 16-1

Continued

2. ICTHYOSIS VULGARIS

Do you, or does anyone in your family, have heels that are so dry and cracked that they rip thin socks or hose?

COMMENT: Feet with thick, rough scaling may be a sign of ichthyosis vulgaris which is sometimes associated with atopic dermatitis.

3. PALMAR HYPERLINEARITTY

Do you have deep grooves or folds on your palms? Can I see them?

COMMENT: Hyperlinearity of the palms is seen as deep linear grooves crossing perpendicular to the long axis of the thenar or hypothenar eminence.

4. KERATOSIS PILARIS

Do you have bumps on your upper arms (cheeks in children) that get dry and itchy?

COMMENT: Keratosis pilaris is present in one-third to half of persons with atopic dermatitis.

5. PERIFOLLICULAR ACCENTUATION

Is the rash more prominent around the hair or pores of your skin?

COMMENT: Perifollicular accentuation is most easily seen in individuals with darker skin.

6. INVOLVEMENT OF HANDS OR FEET

Do you have a rash on your hands and/or feet?

COMMENT: While not highly specific for atopic dermatitis, involvement of the hands and/or feet is common. In about 30 percent of patients, atopic dermatitis begins on the hands and 70 percent have hand dermatitis at some time in their life.

7. CHEILITIS

Do your lips chap easily?

COMMENT: Upper lip cheilitis is common in atopic dermatitis.

8. NIPPLE ECZEMA

Do you have a rash on your nipples?

COMMENT: Nipple eczema is uncommon, but is a relatively specific indicator of atopic dermatitis if it is present.

9. INCREASED SUSCEPTIBILITY TO CUTANEOUS INFECTION

Are there any problems now, or have you had problems in the past, with skin redness or crusting that looked infected?

COMMENT: There is an increased susceptibility to cutaneous infections (especially S. Aureus, *molluscum contagiosum, varicella and herpes simplex viruses)*

10. TYPE I IMMEDIATE HYPERSENSITIVITY

Have you ever had allergy tests that showed you were allergic to something?

COMMENT: Typically, immediate type I hypersensitivity is seen following intradermal skin testing. Hypersensitivity may also be manifest as increased serum IgE levels, or a positive RAST or prick test to a specific antigen.

SOURCE: Adapted with permission from JM Haniflin: *Pediatr Clin North Am* 38:763, 1991.

Figure 16-1 (Plate 13)

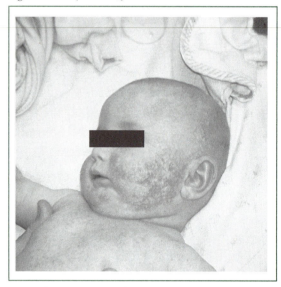

Atopic dermatitis in an infant. Note the typical facial distribution of redness and scaling. *(Courtesy of Peggy R. Cyr.)*

Figure 16-2 (Plate 14)

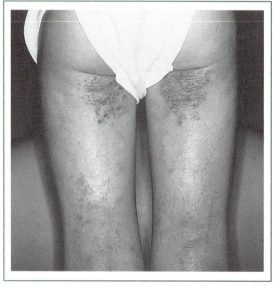

Atopic dermatitis in a child. Note the typical distribution of dermatitis in flexural surfaces of the extremities. *(Photograph by Susan Boiko.)*

spontaneously clear after childhood and then recur later in the individual's life as hand, neck, genital, or facial dermatitis. Children with severe disease and/or with a history of food allergy have a higher chance of persistent disease.

PATHOPHYSIOLOGY

The precise pathophysiology of atopic dermatitis is still under investigation. It is likely that atopic dermatitis is multifactorial, due to an interaction between genetic, sensory, immunologic, mechanical, and psychological factors.

GENETICS   It seems clear that genetics are involved in the pathogenesis of atopic dermatitis, since there is a definite familial tendency to develop this condition. However, genetics do not completely explain the cause of atopic dermatitis, since there is 86-percent, but not 100-percent, concordance between identical twins.

SENSORY AND IMMUNOLOGIC FACTORS   Sensory and immunologic properties of the skin are important in the pathophysiology of pruritus that occurs in atopic dermatitis. The skin of patients with atopic dermatitis has a lower than normal itch threshold for mechanical and chemical stimuli. In experimental situations, wool fiber stimulation causes patients to scratch their atopic skin, which introduces antigens from the skin surface into the epidermis. Langerhans cells in the epidermis [Fig. 16-3 (Plate 15)], which are immunocytes whose dendrites spread throughout the epidermal keratinocytes, find and trap these antigens and present them to the immune system. The skin subsequently thickens in response to chronic inflammation caused by the scratching.

IgE Antibodies   Large amounts of IgE antibodies are produced in response to antigen exposure. Allergen-specific IgE in the skin causes mast cell activation, which results in release of histamine, leukotrienes, cytokines, and other mediators. The mediators induce further itching, leading to further scratching (the "itch-scratch cycle"),

Table 16-2

Seventeen Symptoms and Signs for a Specific Diagnosis of Atopic Dermatitis

SYMPTOMS	SIGNS
Seasonal variation	Xerosis (dry skin)
Worsening with stress	Serum IgE >80 kU/l
Itch in uninvolved skin when perspiring	Hand eczema (can also be by history)
Personal history of allergic rhinitis	Facial pallor or erythema
Family history of allergic rhinitis	Lichenified eczematous knuckle dermatitis
Irritation from textiles (especially wool)	Keratosis pilaris
Family history of atopic dermatitis	Nipple eczema
Personal history of asthma	Nummular eczematous patches
Food intolerance	

NOTE: Presence of 14 or more symptoms or signs is specific for the diagnosis of atopic dermatitis.
SOURCE: Adapted with permission from B Svensson, B Edman, DH Moller: *Acta Derm Venereol Suppl (Stockh)* 114:33, 1985.

Figure 16-3 (Plate 15)

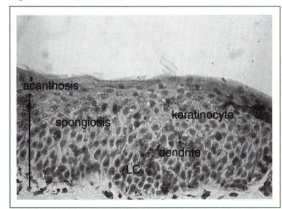

Microscopic appearance of atopic dermatitis. The dendrites of Langerhans cells (brown stain) spread between epidermal keratinocytes, trap antigens, and present them to the immune system. Inflammation leads to acanthosis (thickening of the spinous epidermal layer from the normal three to four cells thick to eight to nine cells thick) and spongiosis (clear spaces around the cells). Immunoperoxidase stain, S100, at 400×. *(Courtesy of Michael W Piepkorn.)*

which in turn leads to further immunologic activation of keratinocytes. This excessive immune activation is thought to occur because of decreased suppressor T-cell function.

T-cell Dysfunction   Saurat and others provided evidence in support of a T-cell–mediated basis for atopic dermatitis by demonstrating clearing of flexural dermatitis in patients with a T-cell immunodeficiency disease [Wiskott-Aldrich syndrome; Fig. 16-4 (Plate 16)] following successful engraftment of non-atopic T-cell–producing bone marrow. Further evidence of T-cell involve-

Figure 16-4 (Plate 16)

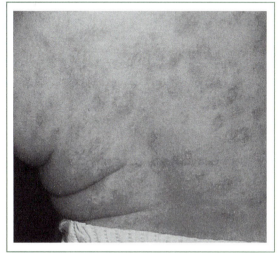

In the T-cell immunodeficiency disease (Wiskott-Aldrich syndrome), an atopic dermatitis-like rash typically occurs as eczematous patches, often with petechiae, in the flexural folds. *(Photograph by Susan Boiko.)*

ment comes from several reports that most patients with atopic dermatitis have a decreased proportion of circulating CD3+ T-cells and CD8+ suppressor T-cells. In contrast, persons with other skin conditions, such as contact dermatitis and psoriasis, do not have a reduction of circulating/suppressor T-cells. Also, patients who have outgrown atopic dermatitis have a normal proportion of circulating CD8+ cells.

Food Allergy Another immunologic aspect of atopic dermatitis involves allergens in food, especially eggs, cow's milk, wheat, fish, and soy. Studies indicate that, in about 28 percent of atopic dermatitis patients, the condition is exacerbated by food allergy. The problem may have its genesis early in life, since a birth cohort study of 1265 children found a 3-times higher risk of recurrent or chronic eczema in infants exposed to 4 or more solid foods before the age of 4 months. Several other studies have demonstrated development of pruritic rash in a typical atopic dermatitis distribution after ingesting food allergens. The rash generally arises abruptly and persists for one-half to 2 h.

Inhaled Allergens In addition to ingestion of allergens in food, inhalants can also serve as allergens that cause atopic skin problems. After the age of 2, inhalant allergy, especially to dust mites, is an important precipitant of atopic dermatitis.

MECHANICAL AND PSYCHOLOGICAL FACTORS Mechanical and psychological factors also contribute to atopic dermatitis. Mechanical factors include dry skin (xerosis) and psychological stress. Dry skin, which commonly occurs in centrally dry air–heated homes and buildings, has a water content of less than 10 percent, compared to 15 percent in normal skin. The stratum corneum in dry skin becomes hard and brittle, thereby impairing the skin's barrier functions and permitting external agents to penetrate the skin, which leads to itching. For unclear reasons, itching due to various processes, and the rash of atopic dermatitis, get worse under psychological stress.

Allergic Contact Dermatitis

DEFINITION

Allergic contact dermatitis is a localized pruritic, vesiculated, weeping, and sometimes swollen rash that occurs because of re-contact with an allergen on skin already sensitized to that antigen [Fig. 16-5 (Plate 17)]. A person can develop allergic contact dermatitis from over 2800 known environmental antigens, including agents to which they have been exposed for many years without problems.

Common household products that can cause allergic contact dermatitis include cleaning chemicals, nickel (in jewelry, wrist-watch bands, and clothing snaps) [Fig. 16-6 (Plate 18)], plants, animals, cosmetics, perfumes, rubber, epoxy glues, and fabrics. A classic example of allergic contact dermatitis is poison ivy.

EPIDEMIOLOGY

The epidemiology of allergic contact dermatitis depends on the nature, frequency, and pat-

Figure 16-5 (Plate 17)

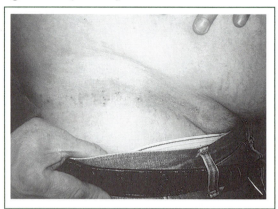

Allergic contact dermatitis. This 42-year-old man had a 2-week history of pruritic rash in a belt-like distribution. There is a localized pruritic, maculopapular rash on skin probably sensitized to latex contained in the elastic of his underwear. Perspiration may have increased contact sensitivity to elastic. *(Courtesy of Peggy R. Cyr.)*

Figure 16-6 (Plate 18)

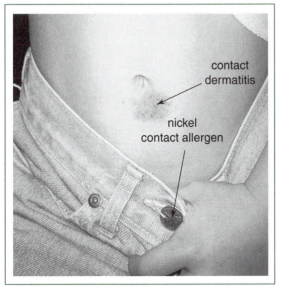

contact
dermatitis

nickel
contact allergen

Allergic contact dermatitis. This 6-year-old girl has dermatitis on the abdomen, caused by contact with a nickel-containing pants snap. *(Courtesy of Peggy R. Cyr.)*

terns of exposure to allergens. Allergic contact dermatitis is most important in relation to the workplace. It is estimated to account for 7 percent of all occupationally related illnesses and costs $250 million annually in lost worker productivity, medical care, and disability payments.

PATHOPHYSIOLOGY

The development of allergic contact dermatitis occurs in stages. In the first stage, the skin becomes sensitized to an allergen (hapten). The process of sensitization takes 14 to 21 days from the time of exposure. During this interval, epidermal Langerhans cells bind the hapten and present it to CD4+ T-cells (T-helper cells). For many allergens, sensitization is the result of repeated exposures, rather than a one-time event. Since haptens can more easily penetrate the skin's protective stratum corneum layer when skin integrity is broken down, sensitization is more likely to occur in patients with atopic or

other dermatitis and in areas with increased heat, occlusion, friction, or sweating.

The second stage of allergic contact dermatitis involves antigen reexposure, which can occur days or even years after initial exposure. With reexposure, memory T-cells aggregate at the sites of allergen contact and initiate an inflammatory process. As with initial sensitization, antigen reexposure may be more effective at initiating an inflammatory response if skin integrity is impaired.

Irritant Contact Dermatitis

DEFINITION

Irritant contact dermatitis has a clinical appearance similar to that of allergic contact dermatitis, but it is caused by the direct chemical action of an irritant, rather than an allergic response. It presents as a stinging, burning rash with erythematous patches and papules confined to the areas of exposure [Fig. 16-7 (Plate 19)].

Figure 16-7 (Plate 19)

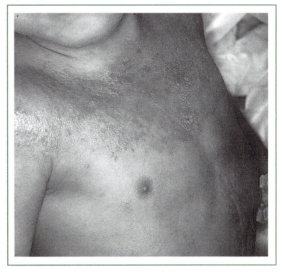

Irritant contact dermatitis. This child has severe developmental delay and drools onto his chest. Note the erythematous patches confined to the area of direct contact with chemical action of saliva. *(Photograph by Susan Boiko.)*

In contrast to allergic contact dermatitis, irritants can cause dermatitis the first time a person comes in contact with them. There are over 85,000 known irritants. Some of the most common are soaps, solvents, paint, abrasives, cleansers, cosmetics, skin lubricants, antiseptic creams, and topical corticosteroids. The dermatitis these agents cause ranges in severity from mild erythema to severe chemical burns.

EPIDEMIOLOGY

Irritant contact dermatitis accounts for 80 percent of all occupational skin disease. There is a large variation in whether individuals develop dermatitis from a given irritant.

PATHOPHYSIOLOGY

Irritants damage the skin directly. The severity of damage depends on both an individual's skin condition and the concentration, duration, and type of irritant. Some substances irritate the epidermis by stripping protective skin lipids from the stratum corneum. Others, because of their physical properties and pH, may cause specific types of skin lesions. For example, ulceration can be caused by a strong acids or alkalis, salts, solvents, or gases. Arsenic, glass fibers, oils, tars, asphalt, and halogenated compounds can cause folliculitis or acneiform lesions. Ultraviolet and infrared radiation, aluminum chloride, and tapes and dressings can cause a "prickly heat" (miliaria) type of dermatitis.

Seborrheic Dermatitis

DEFINITION

Seborrheic dermatitis is an erythematous scaling rash that typically affects the scalp, eyebrows, eyelids, and the nasolabial and retroauricular folds. The condition can exhibit a spectrum of illness ranging from mild dandruff in normal individuals to extensive skin lesions in immunocompromised patients.

EPIDEMIOLOGY

Seborrheic dermatitis affects 2 to 5 percent of the U.S. population. There are two age peaks in normal immunocompetent individuals. One peak occurs in early infancy [Fig. 16-8 (Plate 20)], and the second occurs in adulthood during the fourth to seventh decades of life. Seborrheic dermatitis is more common in immunocompromised individuals; it occurs in between 38 and 50 percent of HIV-infected patients. The frequency of seborrheic dermatitis is also increased in neurologic conditions such as Parkinson's disease, cerebrovascular disease, epilepsy, facial nerve palsy, and syringomyelia.

PATHOPHYSIOLOGY

The precise cause of seborrheic dermatitis is not known. Hormonal, neurologic, infectious, and nutritional mechanisms have been implicated. It is known that seborrheic dermatitis is associated with increased sebum production, and therefore it occurs most commonly on areas that have higher activity and concentration of sebaceous follicles (i.e., face and trunk). Sebaceous glands in these areas are enlarged, and their lipid and triglyceride secretions are

Figure 16-8 (Plate 20)

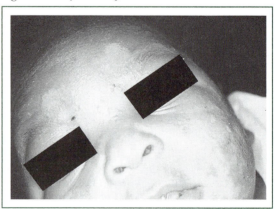

Seborrheic dermatitis in an infant. Note the classic scaling and erythematous rash on the infant's scalp, eyebrows, and eyelids. *(Photograph by Susan Boiko.)*

increased in comparison to other parts of the body.

There is some evidence that an infection with *Pityrosporum ovale*, the lipophilic yeast that causes tinea versicolor, may have some role in seborrheic dermatitis. *Pityrosporum ovale* is more abundant in infants and HIV-infected patients with seborrheic dermatitis. *Pityrosporum ovale* is theorized to activate the alternate complement pathway and cause an inflammatory response when it combines with sebum.

The reason why seborrheic dermatitis is more common in patients with neurologic disorders is unclear. We do know that, in patients with syringomyelia or hemiplegia, sebum production is increased in paralyzed areas of the body. However, this does not explain the frequency of seborrheic dermatitis in other neurologic conditions.

Nummular Eczema

DEFINITION

Nummular eczema has a characteristic morphology that helps to distinguish it from other eczematous eruptions. Initially, nummular eczema presents with tiny papules and vesicles and then assumes the characteristic clinical appearance of coin-shaped plaques. Typically, nummular eczema is seen on the legs, but it can also appear on the upper extremities and trunk [Fig. 16-9 (Plate 21)].

EPIDEMIOLOGY

Nummular eczema occurs more often in men than in women. It peaks at ages 55 to 65. In women, an additional peak occurs between 15 and 25 years of age.

PATHOPHYSIOLOGY

The pathophysiology of nummular eczema is not understood. Xerosis, infectious agents, and varicose veins have all been associated with

Figure 16-9 (Plate 21)

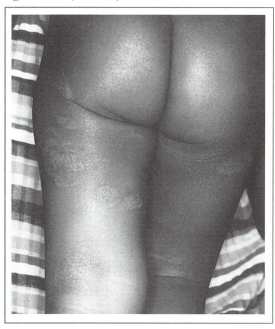

Nummular eczema. Note the characteristic coin-shaped plaques on the legs. *(Photograph by Susan Boiko.)*

nummular eczema, but their role in its pathogenesis is unclear.

Other Diagnoses to Consider

In primary care practice, most patients with eczematous dermatitis have one of the five conditions described above. However, the differential diagnosis of eczema also involves a variety of other conditions, as described below and outlined in Table 16-3.

The differential diagnosis for common, non–life-threatening causes of eczema includes scabies, fungal and yeast infections, and psoriasis. Rare and/or serious disorders may also present with an eczematous rash. These conditions include cutaneous lymphomas, hypothyroidism, severe nutritional deficiencies, systemic lupus erythematosus (SLE), invasive *Staphylococcus aureus* infection (hyper-IgE syndrome), and immunodeficiency syndromes.

Table 16-3

Eczema Differential Diagnosis Conditions and Comparative Features

DIAGNOSIS	APPEARANCE	DISTINGUISHING FEATURES	LABORATORY DIAGNOSIS
Scabies	Linear papulovesicular rash and burrows; occasional bullae	Severe pruritus (especially at night); distribution over the finger webs, axillary, and genital regions	Mineal oil preparation positive for scabies mite
Crusted scabies	Thick white scale overlying erythematous plaque or patch	Occurs in immuno-compromised adults; severe pruritis; no improvement with topicals or single scabies treatment	Scales teem with the scabies mite
Tinea corporis	Erythematous patches and plaques with peripheral scale, crusts, vesicles and pustules	May spontaneously resolve or worsen with topical steroid treatment	KOH test positive for hyphae, fungal culture positive
Psoriasis	Thick white scale overlying erythematous plaque or patch	Auspitz sign, "oil spots" on nails, silvery scale that looks like the mineral mica	Not applicable
Hypothyroidism		Systemic signs of thyroid disease, loss of lateral eyebrows, pretibial myxedema	Low T4, high TSH
Systemic lupus erythematosus	Malar prominence	Symmetric polyarthralgias, lack of scratching, photoinduced or -aggravated	Positive SLE serology, skin biopsy positive with immunofluo-rescent stain
Hyper-IgE syndrome	Unremitting, severe atopic dermatitis	Begins in infancy, recurrent systemic infections, intertriginous, retroauricular and hairline areas involved	IgE > 2000 IU/mL
Immunodeficiency diseases	Severe unremitting eczema in ill-appearing infant	Triad of erythroderma, diarrhea, and failure to thrive	Abnormal complement and immunoglobulins

ABBREVIATIONS: KOH, potassium hydroxide; T$_4$, thyroxine; TSH, thyroid-stimulating hormone; SLE, systemic lupus erythematosus.

COMMON NON–LIFE-THREATENING DISORDERS ASSOCIATED WITH ECZEMATOUS DERMATITIS

SCABIES Scabies is a linear papulovesicular and occasionally bullous rash that typically occurs in axillary and genital regions and on the hands and feet. Scabies is a mite infection caused by *Sarcoptes scabiei*. Acquisition of the mite requires skin-to-skin contact with someone who is infected. Following initial infection, symptoms of rash and itching may not occur for a month or more. Symptoms may be mild, and the initial infection may provide partial immunity against re-infection. However, if re-infection occurs, it can cause an inflammatory eczematous skin eruption in as little as 24 h, accompanied by elevated IgE levels, with rash and intense pruritus.

DERMATOPHYTE AND YEAST INFECTIONS Fungus and yeast invade the epidermis superficially and produce scaly, erythematous, or discoid lesions in areas of the body that promote growth of the infecting organism. These characteristic areas include the scalp (tinea capitis), extremities (tinea pedis), and trunk [tinea corporis; Fig. 16-10 (Plate 22)]. Tinea capitis (scalp ringworm) is caused by a variety of dermatophytes. In the U.S., *Trichophyton tonsurans* is the most common cause. In other areas of the world, tinea capitis is caused by *Microsporum canis*, a highly contagious dermatophyte. Dermatophytes can cause a primary skin infection or predispose to secondary bacterial infection in the involved skin. Yeast infections with Candida species occur mostly in skin fold areas and the groin, with characteristic satellite papules and pustules outside the margin of the main rash.

PSORIASIS Psoriasis is a chronic T-cell–mediated disease characterized by rapid turnover and build-up of epidermal cells. The disease appears clinically as symmetrical erythematous, silvery, scaled papules and plaques. Psoriasis affects about 2 percent of the U.S. population, with an estimated 150,000 new cases diagnosed annually. Psoriasis is responsible for about 3 million

Figure 16-10 (Plate 22)

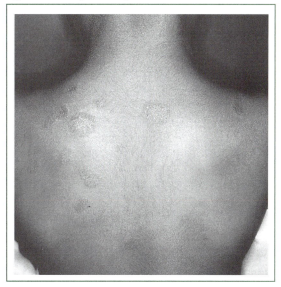

Tinea corporis on the back. This fungal infection invades the epidermis to the level of keratin and produces scaly, erythematous, discoid lesions that resemble the lesions of nummular eczema. *(Photograph by Susan Boiko.)*

outpatient visits to practitioners each year and results in more repeat office visits than any other skin disease.

Characteristic physical findings of psoriasis are distribution of lesions on extensor surfaces of the extremities, pitting of the fingernails, development of psoriatic lesions in previously traumatized skin (Koebner's phenomenon), and punctate bleeding points when the scale is removed (Auspitz's sign).

RARE OR SERIOUS DISORDERS ASSOCIATED WITH ECZEMATOUS DERMATITIS

ERYTHRODERMA Erythroderma (exfoliative erythroderma) is a medical emergency caused by over 30 different diseases, including T-cell lymphoma and severe flares of atopic dermatitis or psoriasis. The skin becomes acutely inflamed, with extreme capillary dilation that can lead to high-output cardiac failure. The skin appears lobster red and is hot to touch, but the body core is hypothermic because of heat loss from dilated skin capillaries. Exfoliation occurs as epidermal scales literally "fall off" the patient.

CUTANEOUS T-CELL LYMPHOMA Cutaneous T-cell lymphoma (CTCL) is difficult to diagnose in its early stages, and the diagnosis typically is made an average of 6 years after onset of the rash. Early on, the rash may appear as single or multiple erythematous, scaly macules. Months to years after this early rash, a second stage occurs with development of sharply demarcated, scaly elevated red to violaceous plaques (mycosis fungoides). These plaques may coalesce to form larger plaques with annular, arcuate, or serpiginous borders, or they may completely regress. Biopsy specimens obtained during these first two stages may not show a pattern specific for CTCL.

The disease may progress to brown or purplish red dermal nodules (tumors). The nodules often (but not exclusively) occur on the face, body folds, and, in women, the inframammary area. The tumor stage can progress further, or exfoliative erythroderma can occur. Through much of the process, CTCL may resemble atopic dermatitis, with diffuse erythema and scaling. Unlike atopic dermatitis, however, there are symmetrical islands of uninvolved skin.

HYPOTHYROIDISM The syndrome of hypothyroidism can include an eczematous skin rash. The low thyroid hormone level leads to accumulation of hyaluronic acid in the skin, which results in the typical boggy, non-pitting edema (myxedema) of hypothyroidism. In pituitary hypothyroidism, however, the epidermis becomes thin, and a generalized eczematous rash may develop. The hypothyroidism rash is distinguished from eczema by the fact that it is more generalized, and the patient has signs, symptoms, and laboratory findings of thyroid dysfunction.

NUTRITIONAL DEFICIENCIES Deficiencies of vitamins A, B, C, and K, and a variety of malab-sorption syndromes can present with an eczematous rash. This usually occurs in association with advanced small bowel diseases, such as sprue and celiac disease. Patients receiving parenteral nutrition may develop eczematous skin symptoms if the formula is deficient in vitamins or essential fatty acids.

SYSTEMIC LUPUS ERYTHEMATOSUS Systemic lupus erythematosus is an autoimmune collagen vascular disease that may involve multiple organs, including the kidneys, blood, nervous system, serosal surfaces, and skin. It is most common in young adult women. When the skin is involved, typically there is a butterfly-shaped malar rash that can look like facial seborrheic dermatitis. However, the absence of pruritus, scaly-red plaques, and axillary involvement tends to exclude the diagnosis of seborrheic dermatitis.

STAPHYLOCOCCAL INFECTION (HYPER-IgE SYNDROME) Skin infections with *S. aureus* are common in routine atopic dermatitis, occurring at some point in over 90 percent of patients. Although recurrent staphylococcal pustulosis can be a significant problem in atopic dermatitis, it can usually be treated with anti-staphylococcal medications. However, systemic and deep skin infections beginning in infancy, combined with high elevations of serum IgE, should raise suspicion of hyper-IgE syndrome.

IMMUNODEFICIENCY SYNDROMES The clinical presentation of several rare immunodeficiency syndromes may include dermatitis. These include Leiner's disease, Wiskott-Aldrich syndrome, and Langerhans cell histiocytosis (histiocytosis X). Leiner's disease is one name for a group of complement defects characterized by generalized seborrheic dermatitis, diarrhea, and failure to thrive. Wiskott-Aldrich syndrome is a disorder of males that consists of flexural dermatitis, multiple deep infections, purpura, and immunodeficiency problems. Langerhans cell histiocytosis can masquerade as seborrheic dermatitis, with papular, erythematous, and sometimes purpuric lesions associated with greasy scale [Figs. 16-11 (Plate 23) and 16-12 (Plate 24)].

Typical Presentation

Most eczematous skin lesions encountered in primary care practice are seen early in the course of the skin problem and are usually without complications. In contrast, dermatologists see a greater percentage of patients with advanced, chronic, or recalcitrant eczema.

Atopic Dermatitis

Atopic dermatitis frequently has its first presentation in infancy or childhood. Children may

Figure 16-11 (Plate 23)

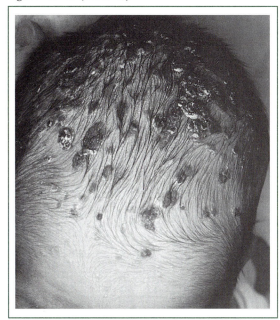

Langerhans cell histiocytosis. This dermatologic condition can appear as "cradle cap" (seborrheic dermatitis) with hemorrhage. Compare it with true seborrheic dermatitis in Fig. 16-12. *(Photograph by Susan Boiko.)*

Figure 16-12 (Plate 24)

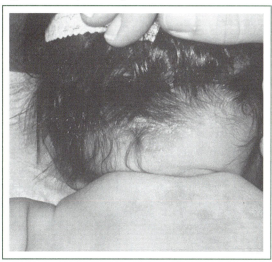

Seborrheic dermatitis. Compare with Langerhans cell histiocytosis in Fig. 16-11. *(Courtesy of Peggy R. Cyr.)*

have a persistent or recurrent dry, red, and scaly rash, with a history of dry skin since birth. The face is the common location for atopic dermatitis in infants and small children [Fig. 16-13 (Plate 25)]. In older children and adolescents, atopic dermatitis often involves the flexural folds of the extremities [Fig. 16-2 (Plate 14)].

Allergic Contact Dermatitis

Patients with allergic contact dermatitis most commonly complain of sudden onset of itching, blistering, and weeping of the skin. The rash is often accompanied by edema and may seem to spread. The offending allergen may or may not have been identified by the patient, but it may be possible to elicit a history of increased pressure, friction, sun exposure, heat, and/or sweating in the area of the rash.

Irritant Contact Dermatitis

In irritant contact dermatitis, patients complain of a stinging, burning rash in the area of expo-

Figure 16-13 (Plate 25)

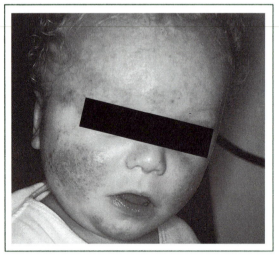

Atopic dermatitis. Atopic dermatitis in young children has its typical location on the face. Note the characteristic dry, scaling lesions. *(Photograph by Susan Boiko.)*

sure to the irritant. As with allergic contact dermatitis, patients may or may not recall exposure to an offending irritant.

Seborrheic Dermatitis

The most common presentation of seborrheic dermatitis is scaling of the scalp, most commonly manifested as "cradle cap" in infants and "dandruff" in children or adults. Adults with more marked seborrhea may also frequently complain of scaling and waxy lesions in the eyebrows, beard, anterior chest, and sometimes the groin.

Nummular Eczema

Nummular eczema is an often-indolent condition that may or may not cause significant symptoms. It is most commonly seen in older individuals with chronic dry skin who complain of new, chronic, or recurrent, skin lesions on the legs.

Key History

Most key items for the medical history have already been discussed. The items listed in Tables 16-1, 16-2, 16-4, and 16-5 are useful for detecting key characteristics of the various types of eczematous rashes and their effect on a patient's daily activities.

Physical Examination

In addition to seeking the general characteristics of the five common forms of eczema, and noting characteristics suggestive of other eczematous

Table 16-4

Assessment of Exacerbating Factors and Past Treatment for Atopic Dermatitis

Goal: To delineate factors that can be modified to improve eczema treatment

What makes your rash get better?

What treatments have you used in the past that consistently work for your skin?

What makes your rash get worse?

What skin products, foods, drugs, or other thing consistently make your skin worse?

Does a shower or bath make your eczema better or worse?

If worse: How often do you shower or bathe?

Do you use soap? If yes, what type of soap do you use?

After bathing do you use anything on your skin?

If yes: How long after bathing do you use it and what do you use?

Please list all products that you put on your skin.

Table 16-5

Assessment of Eczema Severity and Effect on Daily Life

Goal: To measure the effect of eczema in a person's daily life by open-ended questions that can lead to a dialogue and qualitative assessment of the psychological and physical difficulties

  How do you feel about having eczema?

  How does your eczema affect your daily life?

  How does your eczema affect your emotional behavior?

  How does eczema affect relationships with your family and friends, or meeting new people?

  How does your eczema affect your sleep and ability to rest?

  How does your eczema affect your work?

  How does your eczema affect your fun, recreation, and hobbies?

Figure 16-14 (Plate 26)

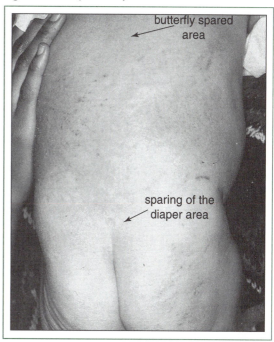

Atopic dermatitis. In atopic dermatitis, there is often relative sparing of skin in the moist diaper area and also relative sparing of skin in areas where the patient is unable to reach and scratch, such as the upper back. *(Photograph by Susan Boiko.)*

skin conditions (Table 16-3), several key findings on physical examination can serve as clues to differentiating the various types of eczema.

Atopic Dermatitis

In infants, lesions are typically on the face and trunk, with sparing of the moist diaper area. In older individuals, lesions frequently occur on the flexural folds of the extremities. An important finding in atopic dermatitis is that there are fewer lesions where patients cannot easily reach to scratch the skin, such as on the back [Fig. 16-14 (Plate 26)].

Other important physical findings in atopic dermatitis are erythematous papules and/or excoriations, which, in older children and adults, develop lichenification (epidermal thickening)—a hallmark of atopic dermatitis—due to persistent scratching and rubbing. Lichenified skin may develop hypopigmentation or hyperpigmentation that may persist for 10 years or more.

Sometimes, lichenification can be so marked that it is difficult to distinguish lichenification of atopic dermatitis from scales of psoriasis [Fig. 16-15 (Plate 27)]. The distinction can be particularly difficult if the psoriatic plaques are red and itchy instead of white and shiny. However, the distribution of the two conditions often permits a distinction to be made. Atopic dermatitis in adolescents and adults appears on the flexor surfaces of the extremities, while in psoriasis the lesions are most often found on the scalp and the extensor surfaces of the knees and elbows. Examination for the fingernails can also be helpful because, in psoriasis, nail pitting occurs. In atopic dermatitis, no pitting is seen, although patients may have dried blood or keratin debris under the nails from scratching.

Figure 16-15 (Plate 27)

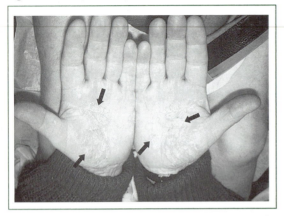

Atopic dermatitis on the hands. In atopic dermatitis, the lichenified skin lesions (margins indicated by arrows) may appear similar to the plaques of psoriasis. *(Courtesy of Peggy R. Cyr.)*

Contact Dermatitis

The initial distribution of allergic or irritant contact dermatitis is an important clue to its cause. Rash on uncovered skin suggests airborne allergens or ultraviolet light as the offending agent. In contrast, when the rash occurs in clothed areas, a textile-related substance is more likely to be the cause. Dermatitis on the face or neck may be related to cosmetics or fragrances, either alone or in combination with ultraviolet light. A rash in the shape of linear stripes suggests a plant-induced dermatitis, such as from poison ivy leaves rubbing on the skin. A rash at the umbilicus or in the belt line suggests a nickel-containing trouser clasp or latex elastic as the allergen.

Seborrheic Dermatitis

Classic seborrheic dermatitis has already been described. Tinea capitis, however, can mimic seborrheic dermatitis of the scalp. Examination findings in tinea capitis include a rash with an advancing edge, central clearing, and peripheral scale beyond the scalp line. When seborrheic dermatitis occurs in the groin, it may resemble or be superinfected with candida or dermatophytes. Important findings for distinguishing these conditions are that lesions due to dermatophytes are usually asymmetrical, while groin lesions from seborrheic dermatitis are usually accompanied by seborrheic dermatitis elsewhere, such as the scalp, eyebrows, or chest.

Nummular Eczema

Individual patches of nummular eczema are pruritic and have uniform scaling. In contrast, superficial fungal infections appear as annular lesions with circumferential papules and pustules and central clearing.

Ancillary Tests

The history and physical examination are often sufficient to make the diagnosis of eczema and to identify it as atopic, allergic contact, irritant contact, seborrheic, or nummular. In addition, atypical history and physical examination findings often provide clues that the differential diagnosis should be expanded to include some of the conditions described earlier that may mimic routine causes of eczema. Several ancillary procedures and tests can help in distinguishing and identifying the various types of eczema and excluding other conditions.

Photographs

One of the most useful procedures in evaluating an eczematous rash is to take photographs. Primary care providers have found it useful to take photographs with a small 35-mm camera with automatic focus and flash, using 100 ISO-speed

Plate 8 *(Figure 15-1)*
Esophagitis. Endoscopic view of the distal esophagus showing inflammation of the esophageal mucosa. The arrow indicates the most-inflamed area.
(Courtesy of Gregory Gambla, D.O., Milton Hershey Medical Centers, Penn State Geisinger Health System.)

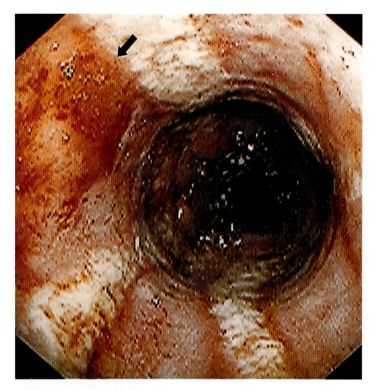

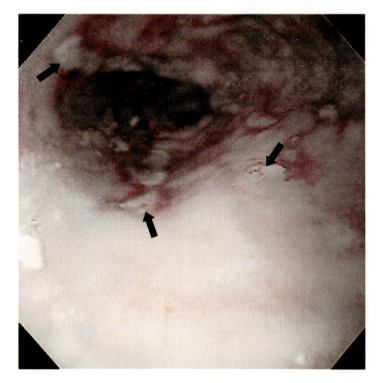

Plate 9 *(Figure 15-2)*
Esophagitis with ulcerations. Endoscopic view of the distal esophagus demonstrating erythema and multiple erosions and ulcerations (examples marked with arrows).
(Courtesy of Gregory Gambla, D.O., Milton Hershey Medical Centers, Penn State Geisinger Health System.)

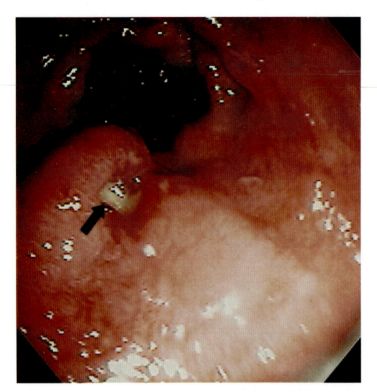

Plate 10 *(Figure 15-3)*
Duodenal ulcer. The ulcer is marked by the arrow.
(Courtesy of Gregory Gambla, D.O., Milton Hershey Medical Centers, Penn State Geisinger Health System.)

Plate 11 *(Figure 15-4)*
Gastritis. This patient has mild gastritis, manifested as areas of erythema on the gastric mucosa (arrows).
(Courtesy of Gregory Gambla, D.O., Milton Hershey Medical Centers, Penn State Geisinger Health System.)

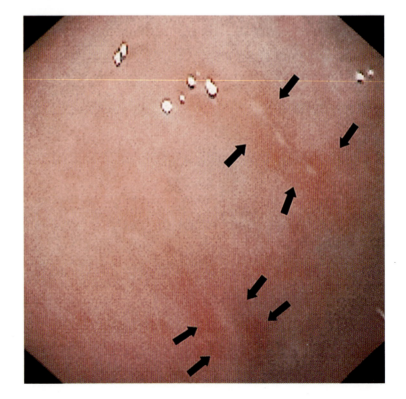

Plate 12 *(Figure 15-5)*
Gastritis. This patient has
marked gastritis, with areas
of intense erythema and
numerous small mucosal
hemorrhages.
*(Courtesy of Gregory Gambla,
D.O., Milton Hershey Medical
Centers, Penn State Geisinger
Health System.)*

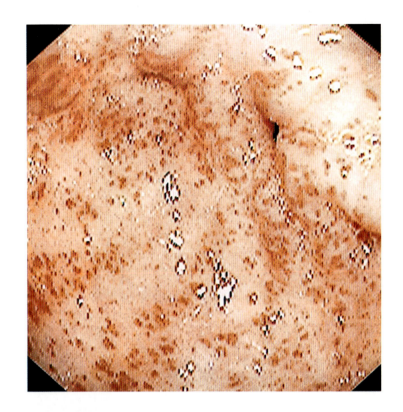

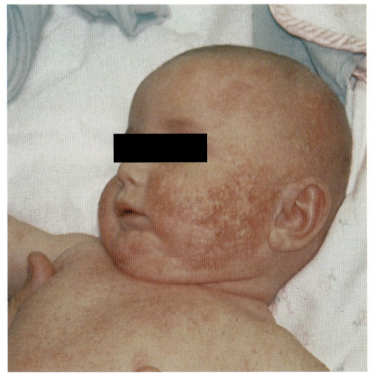

Plate 13 *(Figure 16-1)*
Atopic dermatitis in an infant.
Note the typical facial distribu-
tion of redness and scaling.
(Courtesy of Peggy R. Cyr.)

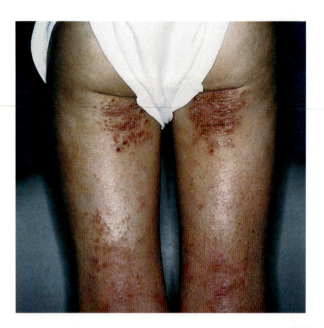

Plate 14 *(Figure 16-2)*
Atopic dermatitis in a child. Note the typical distribution of dermatitis in flexural surfaces of the extremities.
(Photograph by Susan Boiko.)

Plate 15 *(Figure 16-3)*
Microscopic appearance of atopic dermatitis. The dendrites of Langerhans cells (brown stain) spread between epidermal keratinocytes, trap antigens, and present them to the immune system. Inflammation leads to acanthosis (thickening of the spinous epidermal layer from the normal three to four cells thick to eight to nine cells thick) and spongiosis (clear spaces around the cells). Immunoperoxidase stain, S100, at 400X.
(Courtesy of Michael W. Piepkorn.)

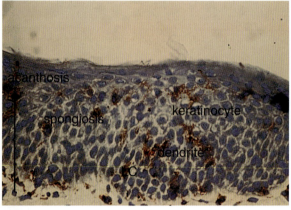

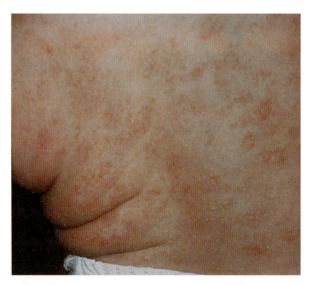

Plate 16 *(Figure 16-4)*
In the T-cell immunodeficiency disease (Wiskott-Aldrich syndrome), an atopic dermatitis-like rash typically occurs as eczematous patches, often with petichiae, in the flexural folds.
(Photograph by Susan Boiko.)

Plate 17 *(Figure 16-5)*
Allergic contact dermatitis. This 42-year-old man had a 2-week history of pruritic rash in a belt-like distribution. There is a localized pruritic, maculopapular rash on skin probably sensitized to latex contained in the elastic of his underwear. Perspiration may have increased contact sensitivity to elastic.
(Courtesy of Peggy R. Cyr.)

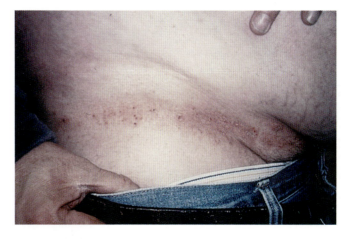

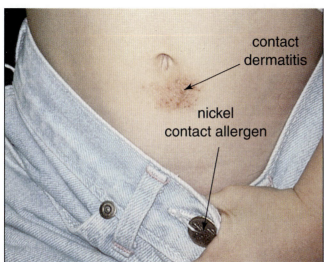

contact
dermatitis

nickel
contact allergen

Plate 18 *(Figure 16-6)*
Allergic contact dermatitis. This 6-year-old girl has dermatitis on the abdomen, caused by contact with a nickel-containing pants snap.
(Courtesy of Peggy R. Cyr.)

Plate 19 *(Figure 16-7)*
Irritant contact dermatitis. This child has severe developmental delay and drools onto his chest. Note the erythematous patches confined to the area of direct contact with chemical action of saliva.
(Photograph by Susan Boiko.)

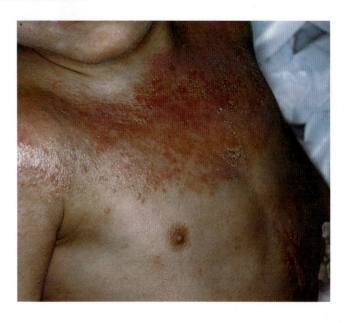

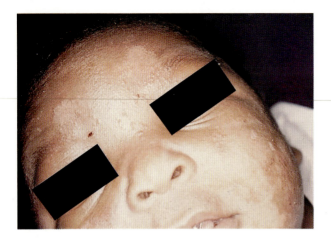

Plate 20 *(Figure 16-8)*
Seborrheic dermatitis in an infant. Note the classic scaling and erythematous rash on the infant's scalp, eyebrows, and eyelids. *(Photograph by Susan Boiko.)*

Plate 21 *(Figure 16-9)*
Nummular eczema. Note the characteristic coin-shaped plaques on the legs. *(Photograph by Susan Boiko.)*

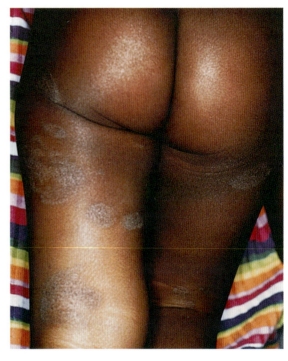

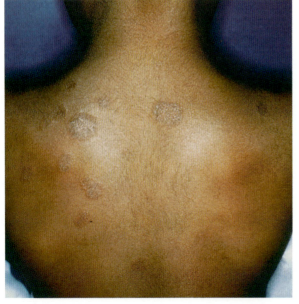

Plate 22 *(Figure 16-10)*
Tinea corporis on the back. This fungal infection invades the epidermis to the level of keratin and produces scaly, erythematous, discoid lesions that resemble the lesions of nummular eczema. *(Photograph by Susan Boiko.)*

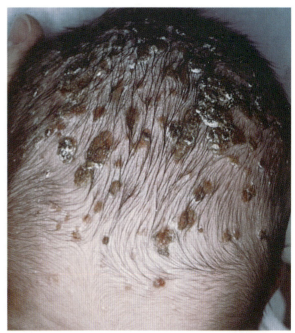

Plate 23 *(Figure 16-11)*
Langerhans cell histiocytosis. This dermatologic condition can appear as "cradle cap" (seborrheic dermatitis) with hemorrhage. Compare it with true seborrheic dermatitis in Plate 24 (Figure 16-12). *(Photograph by Susan Boiko.)*

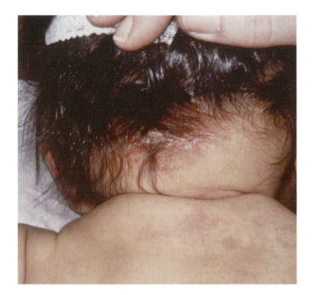

Plate 24 *(Figure 16-12)*
Seborrheic dermatitis. Compare with Langerhans cell histiocytosis in Plate 23 (Figure 16-11). *(Courtesy of Peggy R. Cyr.)*

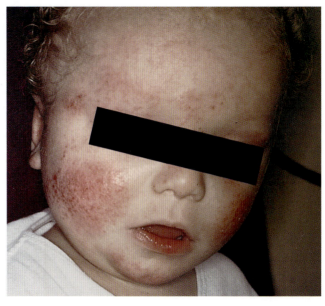

Plate 25 *(Figure 16-13)*
Atopic dermatitis. Atopic dermatitis in young children has its typical location on the face. Note the characteristic dry, scaling lesions. *(Photograph by Susan Boiko.)*

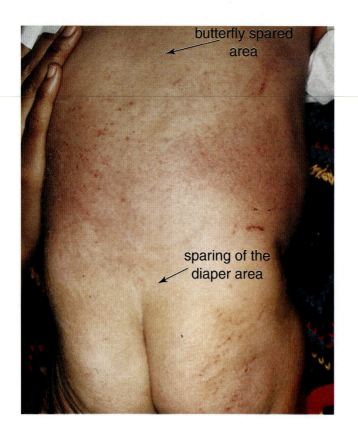

butterfly spared area

sparing of the diaper area

Plate 26 *(Figure 16-14)*
Atopic dermatitis. In atopic dermatitis, there is often relative sparing of skin in the moist diaper area and also relative sparing of skin in areas where the patient is unable to reach and scratch, such as the upper back.
(Photograph by Susan Boiko.)

Plate 27 *(Figure 16-15)*
Atopic dermatitis on the hands. In atopic dermatitis, the lichenified skin lesions (margins indicated by arrows) may appear similar to the plaques of psoriasis.
(Courtesy of Peggy R. Cyr.)

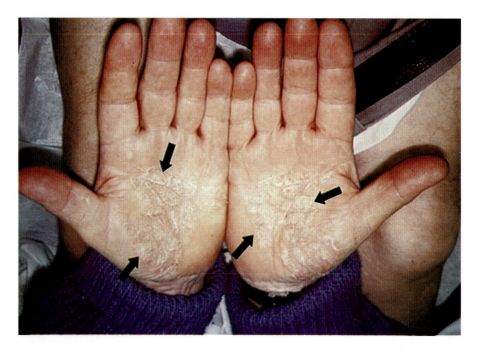

film, to photograph lesions at 13 in or more from the subject. Photographs can be saved in the medical record for future reference to assess the effect of treatment. They also may be presented to a consulting dermatologist for assistance in initial diagnosis or to document the original appearance of the rash, should referral become necessary later in the course of treatment. If the rash is biopsied, the practitioner can compare the biopsy diagnosis with the photograph to improve skill at dermatitis recognition.

Skin Scrapings

SCABIES

The mite of scabies can sometimes be observed with a microscope. To perform this examination, the clinician places a small drop of mineral oil over a suspected burrow hole with a cotton swab. The burrow is then unroofed, and scrapings are obtained and placed on a microscope slide for viewing. Although many clinicians use a scalpel blade for unroofing the burrow and obtaining scrapings, a dermal ring curette can also be used and poses less danger of injury to the patient.

DERMATOPHYTES AND YEAST

Dermatophytes and yeasts can often be identified microscopically. The clinician obtains scrapings using either a sharp ring curette or a no. 15 scalpel blade. The instrument should be wet with water before scraping. The leading edge of the rash is scraped and put on a microscope slide. A drop of 10 to 20% potassium hydroxide is then mixed with the skin scrapings to dissolve the keratin, and a cover slip is applied. Gentle pressure on the cover slip with a pencil eraser and waiting 10 min usually allows the keratin to dissolve. Warming the slide is not necessary, and it may distort the specimen. The sample is examined under a high-power lens for hyphae and spores. If they are seen, the clinician

may safely conclude that a dermatophyte is present in the rash. However, whether the dermatophytes represent a primary etiologic process or a secondary infection of eczema needs to be determined by the patient's history and response to treatment.

Allergen Challenge Tests

FOOD CHALLENGES

Food challenge tests are most helpful for children under the age of 1 year, in whom food antigens are the most likely allergens to cause atopic dermatitis. By the time children reach 2 to 4 years of age, food challenges are less useful because inhalant allergens are the more likely cause of eczema.

Food challenges are the "gold standard" for determining whether atopic dermatitis is caused or exacerbated by certain foods, and they are preferable to food-allergen skin tests and blood testing. This is because virtually all eczema patients have elevated levels of IgE on blood testing, and most have positive skin or radioallergosorbent test (RAST) responses to inhalants and many foods, but these blood test results do not necessarily correlate with clinical symptoms. A negative skin test or RAST response gives 90 percent assurance that there is no food allergy, but a positive test has only a 25 percent positive predictive value, since children may react to a skin test or RAST to a specific food but have no clinical problems from ingesting that food.

Food challenges involve dietary manipulation and are usually reserved for those with nearly daily symptoms that are not responsive to therapy. If symptoms are intermittent, it is difficult to ascertain whether improvement occurs with dietary manipulation. Finally, food challenges are contraindicated for patients with a history of anaphylaxis.

The best approach to food challenge is first to optimize eczema therapy for 2 to 4 weeks, with bathing instructions, topical steroids, and emollients, as outlined later. Documentation of the effect of food challenge usually includes a symptom diary and body chart (Fig. 16-16). Weekly photographs, taken either in the office or at home, to document pre-food challenge dermatitis are helpful. Then, the foods likely to be causing allergy are completely withheld while optimal therapy continues. Foods to be withheld can either be those suspected of causing eczema in the particular patient, or foods that are most likely to cause allergy in the general population (milk, eggs, wheat, fish, and soy).

After 2 to 4 weeks of withholding suspect foods, challenge occurs with reintroduction of no more than one food per day. Specific foods can be introduced with the knowledge of the patient. Alternatively, a blind or double-blind food challenge can be accomplished by dissolving the suspected offending food in juice or using of food capsules from a camping store. A positive response involves dermatitis and itching that develops within 2 h of the challenge in a currently or previously rash-involved area. Photographs of the areas before and after the challenge are helpful. If a positive test response occurs, the food is again eliminated and the patient observed for resolution of eczema. If resolution occurs, exacerbation caused by a second reintroduction confirms the diagnosis.

Another approach to food challenge is to administer an oligo-antigenic diet (described by Binkley) for 2 weeks before challenging the patient with suspected foods. Such a diet consists of baked or broiled chicken, broccoli, cauliflower, sweet potatoes or yams, cooked or canned apples and pears, water, and salt.

CONTACT ALLERGEN DIARIES

Because allergic contact dermatitis can be cured by eliminating the causative antigen, it is useful to identify the antigen. Symptom diaries can help detect contact reactions following such activities as petting or holding a pet, lying on a

Figure 16-16

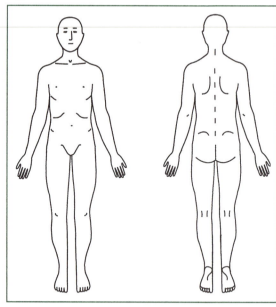

Practitioner's directions:

Use during the first visit and follow-up examinations. Patients can be given a copy to keep at home and record their progress. Black, green, blue, red, and yellow markers or pens are needed.

Patient's directions:

This is a map to see where and how eczema affects your body. Please color your body map as follows:

Yellow: Color all areas yellow where your skin feels dry.

Green: Color skin areas green that are a little red with a small amount of scaling and involve only the very top part of the skin.

Blue: Color areas blue that are red, with scaling and involve deeper skin.

Red: Color areas red that are bright red with a lot of scaling and thickened skin and are very scratched up. If they look infected or have pus or pain, circle them also.

Please rate your itchiness from 0 to 5. Zero means you are not itchy at all, and 5 means you are the most itchy you have ever been. Use black to put the number in the skin areas you have colored.

Body map for assessing pruritus, erythema, exudation, excoriation, and lichenification. *(Adapted with permission from FA Bahmer, J Schafer: Quantification of the extent and severity of atopic dermatitis: The ADASI score. Arch Dermatol 127: 1239, 1991. Copyright 1991 by the American Medical Association. Body drawings from U.S. Department of Health and Human Services, Public Health Service, Agency for Health Care Policy and Research, AHCPR publication no 95-643, 1994.)*

wool rug, or lying on a rug where a pet has been lying. Since the exacerbation of eczema typically occurs 1 to 2 h following exposure, diary entries should specify activities 1 to 2 h before exacerbation.

PATCH TESTING

Some allergens causing an acute allergic contact dermatitis, such as poison ivy or a nickel-plated wrist watch, can be identified by history and physical examination. When the allergen is unknown, however, application of a low concentration of possible antigens to small areas of the skin can sometimes identify the offender. This so-called patch testing is most useful for patients with persistent, lichenified, allergic contact dermatitis who have not responded to treatment. Patch testing can also identify the suitable treatments for dermatitis-prone individuals with histories of rash from topical medications, by identifying preparations that contain allergenic ingredients, thereby permitting selection of an alternative topical agent.

Patch testing is best performed by a trained and experienced practitioner skilled in antigen selection and application. The patch tester must have access to the different chemical and commercial names for the same antigen and be able to correlate patch test results with the patient's clinical condition and environmental exposures. The American Academy of Dermatology standard patch testing tray contains 20 commercially prepared allergens. Although 15 of the most common allergens in the United States are present on the tray, many common allergens must be ordered separately or mixed by the practitioner.

False-positive patch tests results are not uncommon, and various studies indicate that the predictive value of a positive result ranges from 20 to 76 percent. False-positive tests can be due to use of allergens at excessive (irritant) concentrations or to marked dermographism ("excited skin syndrome") from multiple simultaneous tests. Suspected false-positives can usually be clarified by repeating the patch tests individually and/or in lower concentrations.

False-negative patch test results can occur when the skin is exposed to potent topical steroids or oral steroids (at doses over 30 mg/d). Thus, patch testing should be postponed until the patient is off steroids. Oral antihistamines probably do not inhibit patch test responses.

Skin Biopsy

The diagnosis of common dermatitis-eczema conditions is not always obvious following the history and physical examination. Statistically, however, dermatitis is the most likely diagnosis in primary care patients with benign skin disorders that a clinician cannot identify. This fact is supported by a study of over 1000 skin biopsies performed by primary care clinicians to identify lesions not suspected of being cancer; dermatitis was the most common histologic diagnosis.

Atopic dermatitis, seborrheic dermatitis, irritant and allergic contact dermatitis, and nummular eczema all share a common histology. Thus, they cannot be differentiated from one another by biopsy findings. However, skin biopsy of patients with eczematous skin lesions is indicated in two situations. First, dermatitis appearing as a persistent solitary lesion or patch should be biopsied to differentiate it from psoriasis and CTCL. Second, biopsy should be performed when eczematous skin conditions are not responsive to therapy.

Skin biopsies can be performed by scalpel excision or with standard dermatologic punch biopsy instruments. Punch biopsies are usually preferable for large rash areas because they yield a suitable specimen, are easier, and give cosmetically better results. Occasionally, the pathologist cannot make a histopathologic diagnosis on a skin biopsy specimen. Second opinions should be considered in such situations, as well as when the histologic diagnosis is not in concordance with the patient's clinical history or the physician's clinical judgment.

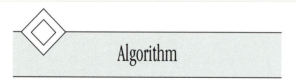

Algorithm

The algorithm in Fig. 16-17 provides a general outline of how to integrate the history, physical examination, and ancillary tests to determine which of the five common types of eczema is present.

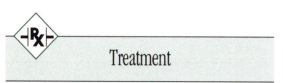

Treatment

General Considerations

One important aspect of treating eczema is to eliminate or avoid factors that aggravate or predispose to eczema in susceptible patients. Thus, irritants and contact allergens, tobacco smoking, and air pollution should all be avoided. As noted, air pollutants such as sulfur dioxide and nitrogen oxide, as well as tobacco smoke, increase IgE synthesis and are associated with increased incidence of eczema. Eczema-prone individuals should also avoid "wet" occupations, since the highest incidence of chronic eczema occurs in food handlers, janitorial workers, construction workers, mechanics, metal workers, horticulturists, hairdressers, nurses, and domestic workers, all of whom are exposed to moist working conditions.

The treatment goal for symptomatic eczema is to control the dryness, itching, and erythema by skin lubrication and appropriate use of topical corticosteroids. Support by the practitioner for initiation and consistent application of treatment is key to successful symptom control and prevention of complications.

Before and during treatment, patients can document the extent of their skin involvement with a body chart such as that shown in Fig. 16-16. Assessment of exacerbating factors and past treatments can be performed using questions from Table 16-4. These questions are especially useful in developing treatment plans for patients with atopic dermatitis. The patient and clinician should discuss treatment goals, and anticipated time frames for results.

Psychological Considerations

Clinicians can be more effective in administering treatments if they understand the severity of and disability caused by their patients' skin problems. Research has shown that significant skin disorders, including eczematous skin conditions, can have a major influence on emotional behavior, social interactions, sleep, rest, work, and recreation. Questionnaires for evaluating the effect of skin disorders on life-style have been developed by Finlay and others. Questions similar to those shown in Table 16-5 can be used for measuring the life-style effects of eczema.

Treatment of Atopic Dermatitis, Seborrheic Dermatitis, and Nummular Eczema

Treatments of atopic dermatitis, nummular eczema, and seborrheic dermatitis are similar. They focus on controlling the key symptoms of xerosis and pruritus, and treating the inflammation of the eczematous process. Treatments include skin moisturizers, behavioral techniques, topical and oral corticosteroids, and antihistamines.

XEROSIS

Appropriate bathing and moisturizing can turn a brittle, dry, and vulnerable stratum corneum into one that is flexible and protective. Most skin treatments use water to hydrate the

Figure 16-17

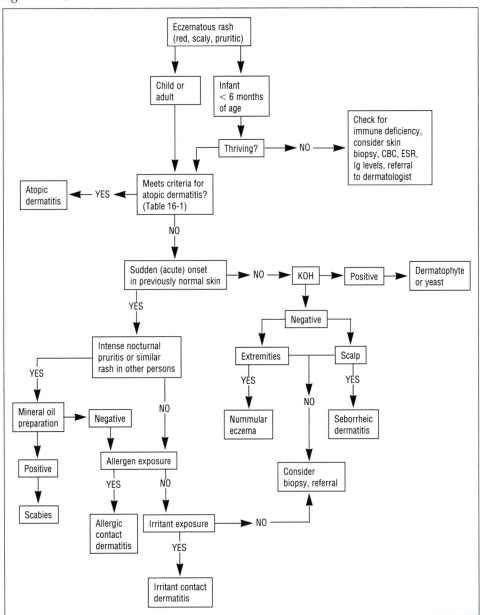

Algorithm for the diagnosis of dermatitis-eczema.

Abbreviations: CBC, complete blood count; ESR, erythrocyte sedimentation rate; Ig, immunoglobulin; KOH, potassium hydroxide.

stratum corneum and moisturizers (emollients) to keep that water in the skin. Individualized modification of bathing and moisturizing routines, based on information gained from questions in Table 16-4, can help resolve and prevent exacerbations.

Generally, bathing adds moisture to the skin, and this moisture can be retained in the skin if moisturizing agents or oils are subsequently applied. One method for doing this is to add a non-irritating, non-allergenic oil (e.g., olive oil) to bath water. This is somewhat hazardous, however, because the oil can cause the tub to be slippery and result in falls. A more common method is to apply the moisturizer to the skin within 3 min after the shower or bath. It is important to "pat," and not rub, the skin dry with a towel. In general, baths (up to twice a day) are appropriate during exacerbations, and showers can be used when skin is in good control.

The choice of a moisturizer depends on the climate, tolerance, and cosmetic needs of the individual patient. Generally, lotions are less effective because they do not keep water in the stratum corneum as well as creams and ointments. Creams are more tolerable for persons living in hot humid climates, whereas ointments may be preferred in cool, low-humidity climates.

The choice of a moisturizer also depends on the degree of skin dryness. Several commercial products are available. For very dry skin, suggested moisturizers include Crisco solid shortening (not butter flavored), Vaseline Intensive Care Cream, Plastibase, or petrolatum. For medium-dry skin, Aquaphor, Albolene, Eucerin Plus, and Neutrogena Norwegian Formula are useful. Nivea or Keri moisture creams are appropriate for mildly dry skin.

Pruritus

Itching is increased with heat, irritants or allergens, wool, xerosis, psychological stress, and inflammation. Reduced pruritus follows limiting exposure to these factors by keeping cool; avoiding soaps, allergens, and irritants; using cotton clothing; skin hydration; stress reduction; and reducing inflammation. The clinician can also use education of the patient, behavioral techniques, and judicious application of topical corticosteroids to decrease itching.

BEHAVIORAL TECHNIQUES   Itching is influenced by psychological factors, and it responds to placebo in about 50 percent of cases. Research evidence indicates that behavior modification therapy can reduce the number of scratching episodes.

One technique for treating patients with severe eczema-related pruritus involves giving them a manual counter (e.g., those used in the laboratory for differential blood counts) and a form on which to record the frequency of scratching and intensity of itching. Over a three-week period, patients record their itching and scratching and describe trigger events or antecedent thoughts or feelings that precede or lead to scratching. Patients also rate the amount of pleasure experienced each time they scratch. In one study by Cole that used this technique, after reviewing their personal records patients reported that events associated with feelings of helplessness, anxiety, anger, or resentment led to scratching. Scratching, in turn, ultimately worsened these feelings. These patients were then taught, with success, to use relaxation techniques just before periods of severe itching (e.g., after work or before bed). They were also successfully trained in avoidance of scratching by trying alternate techniques for managing itching, such as gentle rubbing, slapping, and cold slush mixture.

PHARMACOTHERAPY   Standard pharmacotherapy for itching includes topical glucocorticoids and oral antihistamines. For severe flares, oral steroids and ultraviolet light may be used. Rarely, cyclosporin A and azothioprine may be required.

Topical Corticosteroids   Topical corticosteroids control most acute eczematous flares when used in adequate amounts and with appropriate follow-up. They exert anti-pruritic, anti-inflammatory, and antiproliferative effects. Judicious use involves knowledge of the best potency and vehicle of the topical steroid for the particular rash and site. Follow-up care requires knowledge of adverse reactions from the vehicle and long-term effects of steroids. Clinicians find it useful to become acquainted with the topical steroids on their formulary by identifying the lowest-cost and least allergenic cream and ointment in each of the standard categories of steroid potency. A representative list of topical steroids by potency, dose form, package size, and relative cost, is displayed in Table 16-6.

Potency The choice of steroid potency depends on the severity and site of the eczema. Low-potency preparations are used in mild cases and on the face. The most commonly used low-potency prescription steroid is topical 1% hydrocortisone. Mid-potency steroids are used for general management in chronic eczema not involving the face. Triamcinolone (0.1 to 0.5%) is an often used mid-potency topical steroid. High-potency topical steroids (e.g., fluocinonide and halcinonide) are appropriate for severe or highly lichenified eczema, such as on the palms and soles.

Potent fluorinated corticosteroids are effective for controlling acute flares. However, intertriginous (skin-fold) areas, especially the eyelids, scrotum, and vulva, are very responsive and sensitive to topical corticosteroids. Therefore, low-potency, non-fluorinated steroids are most appropriate for these areas. Smooth skin reacts variably to topical corticosteroids, and the scalp responds best if scale is removed before applying medication.

Vehicle The choice of a vehicle depends on the amount of xerosis, stage of lesions, and site. Creams are appropriate for acute and subacute dermatitis and slightly dry skin in warm, humid environments. Ointments are best for chronic, lichenified, scaling dermatoses and in cooler, low-humidity environments. Lotions,

while readily absorbed, are used infrequently because their chemical contents can sting broken or inflamed skin.

Side Effects Adverse effects of topical steroids can be due to either topical effects or systemic absorption. Infants, children, and the elderly are more susceptible to adverse local and systemic effects.

Corticosteroids interfere with cellular replication, thereby causing epidermal, dermal, and subcutaneous thinning (atrophy). Atrophy occurs most readily in skin-fold areas and on genital and facial skin. As noted, therefore, mid- or high-potency steroids generally should not be used in these areas. In atrophic skin, subcutaneous vessels are visible, and petechiae and ecchymosis from scratching can be observed. Steroid-induced atrophy can also result in development of striae. Atrophy of the skin of hands and feet may cause fissuring. In addition to atrophy, other signs of adverse steroid skin effects are telangiectasia, corticosteroid rosacea, perioral dermatitis, and acne.

In addition to site of application and potency, duration of use also determines the risk of adverse effects from topical steroids. Prolonged use can occur when the steroid has successfully treated the rash, but a new (steroid-induced) rash develops, and the patient continues to use the drug to treat the new rash without seeking appropriate follow-up.

Systemic absorption of topical steroids can occur when the drug is absorbed through eczematous areas because of damage to the skin barrier. Fortunately, after a few days of steroid use, the skin barrier is improved and systemic absorption of the drug is reduced. Systemic absorption is also influenced by daily dosage, duration of administration, extent of body surface covered, potency of steroid, and whether or not occlusion (covering the skin with plastic wrap after applying steroid) is used. For example, only 1 percent of the dose of topically applied plain hydrocortisone is absorbed systemically from normal skin, and adrenal sup-

Table 16-6

Topical Corticosteroids and Their Relative Strengths and Costs

DRUG, STRENGTH*	DOSE FORM	PACKAGE SIZE	RELATIVE COST PER PACKAGE
WEAK POTENCY, NONFLUORINATED			
Hydrocortisone, 0.5%, 1%	Cream or ointment	20 g	2
Hydrocortisone, 0.5% hydrophilic	Lotion	60 mL	2
Hydrocortisone, 1.0% hydrophilic	Lotion	60 mL	5
LOW POTENCY, FLUORINATED			
Fluocinolone, 0.01%	Solution	20 mL	24
Triamcinolone, 0.025%	Lotion	60 mL	7
MID POTENCY, FLUORINATED			
Fluocinolone, 0.01%	Cream	30 g	2
Fluocinolone, 0.025%, 0.01%	Cream or ointment	30 g	2
Desoximetasone 0.05%	Ointment	30 g	18
Desoximetasone 0.05%	Cream	30 g	57
Triamcinolone, 0.025%	Cream	30 g	1
Triamcinolone, 0.1%	Cream	30 g	2
Triamcinolone, 0.025%	Ointment	15 g	1
Triamcinolone, 0.1%	Ointment	30 g	2
Triamcinolone, 0.5%	Ointment	15 g	3
HIGH POTENCY, FLUORINATED			
Halcinonide, 0.1%	Cream or ointment	15 g, 60 g	40
Fluocinonide, 0.05%	Ointment	15 g, 60 g	9
Fluocinonide, 0.05%	Gel	30 g	14
Fluocinonide, 0.05%	Ointment	15 g, 60 g	17
Desoximetasone, 0.25%	Cream	60 g	24
Desoximetasone, 0.25%	Ointment	60 g	65
ULTRA-HIGH POTENCY, FLUORINATED			
Clobetasol, 0.05%	Lotion	25 mL	27
Clobetasol, 0.05%	Cream or ointment	45 g	35

* Drugs are listed in order of potency.
SOURCE: Adapted with permission from Group Health Cooperative of Puget Sound: *Drug Formulary: 1997.* Hudson, OH, Lexi-Comp, Inc.

pression does not occur. Similarly, a 4-week treatment of eczema with topical steroids over 20 percent or greater of children's bodies twice a day for 4 weeks with 2.5% hydrocortisone ointment does not suppress the adrenal gland. On the other hand, the application of low- or medium-potency steroids under occlusion can increase absorption significantly, and adrenal suppression may occur, especially when steroids are applied to large areas of skin.

Mild suppression of adrenal cortical function from topical steroids often has no clinical significance. However, with the newer ultra-high-potency topical corticosteroids (e.g., clobetasol propionate), the risk of significant adrenal suppression is quite real. Adrenal function should be checked if long-term, high- or ultra-high potency corticosteroids have been administered, especially to patients who will be undergoing surgery. Adrenal function usually returns to normal within a week after topical steroids are discontinued.

The vehicle in which the topical steroid is suspended can also cause side effects. The vehicle can be irritating and cause irritant dermatitis. If this problem is suspected, a corticosteroid suspended in petrolatum may be substituted. If the problem persists, there may be an allergy to the corticosteroid itself. This situation can be confirmed with patch testing.

Oral Corticosteroids In extreme cases, oral steroids can be used to control or treat eczema. This is rarely done, however, because rebound flares of eczema occur after short courses of oral steroid, and significant adverse effects may occur if steroids are used chronically.

Oral Antihistamines Oral antihistamines control pruritus and provide a sedative effect that enables patients to fall asleep faster and scratch less during sleep. They are rarely sufficient therapy without concomitant topical corticosteroids.

Elderly patients need to be cautioned about sedation and other anticholinergic side effects of antihistamines. Depending on overall health and concomitant medical conditions, antihistamines may be contraindicated in elderly individuals. The newer non-sedating antihistamines are helpful for itching in some patients but lack the potentially beneficial sedative effect. Topical antihistamines (e.g., diphenhydramine) or anesthetics (e.g., benzocaine) should be avoided because of the risk of sensitizing the already-inflamed skin and inducing allergy to these compounds.

SPECIALIZED TREATMENTS The above-mentioned therapies usually work if used appropriately and consistently. Recalcitrant cases can be referred to dermatologists for consideration of specialized treatments.

One such treatment is ultraviolet (UV) light (both UV-A and UV-B), which increases the itch threshold and decreases histamine release in the skin. Immunosuppressive agents such as cyclosporin or azothioprine can also be used; they block the inflammatory response in eczematous skin. Cyclosporin A is effective in severe refractory atopic dermatitis, but its use is limited by side effects, including nephrotoxicity, hypertension, hepatotoxicity, tremor, and gingival hyperplasia. Azothioprine is also effective in refractory patients. The response usually occurs within 1 month and is associated with less antibiotic use, fewer changes in steroid medication, and lower rates of hospital admissions and outpatient visits.

Patients whose condition is refractory to the aforementioned therapies may be considered for enrollment in research protocols. Alternative medical practitioners may be able to provide treatment for some patients (see "Controversies").

Treatment of Allergic and Irritant Contact Dermatitis

The best approach for irritant and allergic contact dermatitis is to identify the offending agent and eliminate it. Treatment of symptomatic skin eruptions is often necessary, however.

Topical steroids are frequently used in the acute and subacute stages of irritant and acute allergic contact dermatitis. However, in the acute edematous and vesicular stage, topical corticosteroids may not be effective, especially if the rash is extensive. In this situation, a short course of oral steroids is an appropriate form of therapy, assuming no contraindications exist. A regimen such as prednisone [1 (mg/kg)/d for 10 days and then 0.5 (mg/kg)/d for 10 days for children; and 60 mg for 10 days and then reduced to 30 mg and tapered to zero over 10 days for adults] is less expensive than a commercially pre-packaged taper regimen. It may also be more effective because a consistently high dose for the first 10 days may stop the reaction better than the more rapid decrease of a tapered-dose package.

In addition to oral or topical steroids, acute vesicular weeping eruptions may benefit from drying agents, such as compresses of aluminum sulfate and calcium acetate. In the chronic stage of irritant and contact allergic dermatitis, after weeping and swelling have resolved, topical steroids are generally effective.

Treatment Failure

When standard treatments fail to resolve eczematous skin problems, secondary infection with bacteria, fungus, or herpesvirus should be considered as a possible cause. Superinfection can appear to be a treatment failure because it will not respond to hydration and topical corticosteroids. Diagnosis and treatment with antibacterials, antifungals, or antivirals will improve the condition. Generalized infection with herpes simplex virus (eczema herpeticum) requires hospitalization and intravenous antiviral therapy.

In atopic dermatitis, treatment failure can also result from inconsistent skin hydration, or irritation by or allergy to topical medication. It can also occur if topical steroids are applied less frequently than recommended, if steroid potency is inadequate, or if the vehicle is inappropriate.

For allergic contact dermatitis and irritant dermatitis, a person may be cured after eliminating the allergen or irritant and then seem to relapse. Such a treatment failure may result from unwitting re-exposure to the allergen or irritant. It can also occur when a commercial non-allergenic product the patient previously used without difficulty is reformulated to include an allergen or irritant. Patients need to read product labels and learn the various different names for allergens and irritants.

Finally, treatment failures should raise concern that the diagnosis is incorrect. The patient may have one of many conditions discussed under "Principal Diagnoses." The various ancillary tests mentioned above and/or dermatologic consultation may be helpful in identifying such cases.

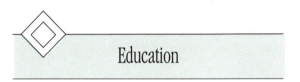

Education

Eczema can cause substantial disability, significant enough to result in exclusion from the military. Nonetheless, eczema sufferers often report that eczema is not taken seriously by medical practitioners. The National Eczema Association for Science and Education (a nonprofit organization) indicates that persons with eczema want clinicians to acknowledge that eczema causes psychological and physical distress. Patients also want to know about the most effective daily routines and about the roles of allergy, stress, and diet in aggravating cutaneous symptoms. They may want the option of referral to a dermatologist.

Education of the patient about atopic dermatitis, seborrheic dermatitis, and nummular eczema should emphasize that these are chronic diseases without quick cures. Patients should be counseled about and offered the varicella (chicken pox) vaccine if they are not immune to varicella, to prevent further skin irritation, scarring, and secondary infection from varicella. Arrangements should be made among the office staff, the clinician, and the patient to facilitate prompt treatment of exacerbations and infections. Clinicians should be open to discussing and reviewing claims of "quick cures," since this helps patients to discern appropriate treatments from potentially ineffective or harmful ones.

Specific, well-written handouts describing eczema's cause, diagnosis, treatment, and expected outcome are helpful to patients. Such literature can be obtained from the organizations listed in the Appendix. These organizations also can provide information about eczema support groups and informational newsletters.

Finally, smoking cessation counseling and information for all patients and family members, especially when the eczematous skin condition is atopic dermatitis, is an important measure. Information about how to reduce exposure to indoor and outdoor air pollution is available from the American Academy of Allergy, Asthma, and Immunology.

Family Approach

Eczema is usually a familial condition, and frequently the family history involves a family member who "outgrew" the eczema. Thus, family dynamics may not change at all with a diagnosis of eczema. However, when the patient is a child whose eczema is doing poorly, the condition may have important ramifications for the child and the family. Any chronic skin disorder has the potential to adversely affect growth and development if it decreases the frequency with which the family handles the infant. Similarly, too much tactile stimulation has been shown to increase atopic dermatitis symptoms.

Excessive scratching and other eczema-related symptoms can cause stress in parents. This can be a problem when children with eczema sleep in their parents' bed, since itching by the child can interfere with parental sleep and cause resentment by the parents, thus increasing anxiety and pruritus in the child. Appropriate counseling can enable the parents of children with eczema to care for the child's skin and set appropriate behavioral limits.

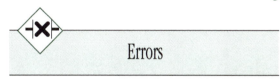

Errors

One important error that occurs in the management of eczema is not recognizing that treatment failure or a treatment-resistant rash might be due to a secondary infection, such as herpes simplex virus. Similarly, severe or treatment-resistant eczema may be a sign of immunodeficiency or other systemic disorder, and this may not be readily identified.

A second error involves the inappropriate use of topical steroids. As noted above, fluorinated topical steroids are generally inappropriate for use on the face or genitals, and their use should be limited on intertriginous skin. In addition, providing unlimited or large-quantity prescription refills for topical steroids increases the likelihood that patients will use the medication for an inappropriately long period of time, even after the skin problem is controlled or resolved. Large-quantity prescriptions also increase the chance that patients will continue using topical steroids if the skin condition does not respond to treatment, instead of seeking re-evaluation by a clinician.

A third error is that clinicians often focus too heavily on treatment with topical steroids and give insufficient weight to other modes of therapy. Treatment results are better if clinicians also emphasize the need for consistent use of moisturizers, appropriate bathing instructions, and other nonpharmacologic treatments.

Finally, research indicates that, when primary care clinicians are unable to identify a benign skin condition by the history and physical examination and so perform a biopsy to identify the condition, the most common diagnosis is allergic contact dermatitis. Thus, the inability to identify allergic contact dermatitis is common, and this diagnosis should be considered when one is faced with an eczematous rash. A careful history will often reveal the identity of offending allergens.

Controversies

Eczema sufferers may seek the help of alternative medicine practitioners who use therapies that are unfamiliar to traditional clinicians. Alternative practitioners may treat eczema with dietary supplements (e.g., lactobacillus), special diets, evening primrose oil, or traditional Chinese herbal therapy.

Dietary Supplements

For a variety of conditions, the dietary supplement most-commonly used by naturopathic practitioners is lactobacillus. The basis for its use in food-associated exacerbation of atopic dermatitis is that food antigens are introduced into the systemic circulation through functional defects in the immunologic defense barrier of the intestinal barrier. Human intestinal lactobacillus is thought to produce an immune response that protects mucosa from these food antigens. A randomized controlled study of daily lactobacillus therapy for atopic dermatitis showed objective improvement of the rash and subjective improvement of pruritus and sleep.

Special Diets

Alternative medicine practitioners may prescribe a vegan diet (i.e., a strict vegetarian diet without any animal products, including milk, cheese, eggs, or fish). In addition, they may suggest that food additives be eliminated from the diet. A vegan diet would, in fact, eliminate the most common food allergens from the diet, but those on vegan regimens must be careful to include all essential nutrients in the diet. Double-blind placebo-controlled studies that challenged patients with preservatives, coloring agents, citric acid, and flavorings have shown that these substances exacerbate atopic dermatitis in about 2 percent of patients. Thus, eliminating these preservatives, colorings, and flavorings from the diet is not likely to help the majority of atopic dermatitis patients.

Evening Primrose Oil

Polyunsaturated fatty acids have been found to be low in the blood of infants at risk for atopic dermatitis. Addition of essential fatty acids via primrose oil has been used to decrease the severity, dryness, and inflammation and erythema of the skin of such individuals. Double-blind and placebo-controlled studies, however, have not shown primrose oil to be effective, and its safety in infants has not been studied extensively.

Chinese Herbal Therapy

Traditional Western medicine is based on the use of purified active ingredients. Traditional Chinese medicine, on the other hand, uses complex mixtures of herbs such as the Traditional Chinese Herbal Therapy (TCHT) for atopic dermatitis. The TCHT is a 10-herb tea, of which approximately 200 mL is consumed each day for treatment of atopic dermatitis. A placebo-controlled crossover study on adults and a blinded trial in children with refractory atopic dermatitis showed that TCHT resulted in statistically significant improvement in erythema and surface skin damage. This improvement persisted during 1 year of TCHT treatment in the majority of patients. The only adverse effect noted was a reversible elevation of serum aspartate aminotransferase in some children. Studies are underway to isolate the pharmacologically active components in TCHT.

Emerging Concepts

New Medications

Recent developments in the treatment of atopic dermatitis involve interventions that modulate the immunoresponsiveness of skin. Perhaps the most intriguing of these treatments are topical immunosuppressants and phosphodiesterase inhibitors.

A prototype topical immunosuppressant is tacrolimus, a medication generally used for prevention of organ transplant rejection. It has an action similar to that of cyclosporin: inhibition of immunoreactive lymphocytes. In topical formulations varying in concentration from 0.03 to 0.1%, tacrolimus is effective in improving edema, pruritus, erythema, oozing, and other symptoms of atopic dermatitis.

Phosphodiesterase inhibitors are another potential future treatment for atopic dermatitis. Their use is based on the fact that c-AMP phosphodiesterase levels are increased in the monocytes of patients with atopic dermatitis, and in the umbilical cord blood of infants of atopic parents. Determination of c-AMP phosphodiesterase levels may prove a useful diagnostic test for atopic dermatitis, and phosphodiesterase inhibitors may subsequently become a useful treatment.

Gene Therapy

As noted earlier in this chapter, the eczema of Wiskott-Aldrich syndrome clears following successful engraftment of bone marrow from a non-atopic individual. This suggests the possibility that, as the genetic basis of common skin disorders is better understood, gene therapy for eczematous skin conditions may one day be possible.

Telemedicine

Finally, advances in video-communications and computer technology will almost certainly influence the way patients, dermatologists, allergists, and primary care clinicians interact with one another. In some current health care systems, interactive video-communications already permit long-distance visual consultations between primary care practitioners and specialists, and remote video diagnosis of skin disorders. This mode of practice is likely to become more common in the future.

Appendix
Useful Resources for Patients with Eczema

Eczema Association for Science and Education: 1221 S.W. Yamhill Street, Suite 303, Portland, OR, 97205; 503-228-4430. This association offers patients' education and information packets for adults, children, and practitioners, written in consultation with a nationally recognized panel of experts. A patients' newsletter shares information about research studies and effective treatments. Pen pals for children with atopic dermatitis are listed.

National Eczema Association: 800-818-SKIN.

American Academy of Allergy and Immunology: 611 E. Wells St.; Milwaukee, WI, 53202; 414-272-6071; info@aaaai.org. This organization provides practitioner education materials and courses for practitioners.

American Academy of Dermatology: 930 N. Meacham Rd., Schaumburg, IL, 60173-4965; 847-330-0230. This organization can locate referral dermatologists and provide continuing medical education seminars and materials.

Epstein, E: *Common Skin Disorders*, 3d ed. Oradell, NJ, Medical Economics Books. This manual has well-organized physician-directed information with accompanying reproducible educational handouts for patients.

Bibliography

Berth-Jones J, Graham-Brown RA: Placebo-controlled trial of essential fatty acid supplementation in atopic dermatitis. *Lancet* 341:1557, 1993.

Binkley KE: Role of food allergy in atopic dermatitis. *Int J Dermatol* 31:611, 1992.

Boiko P, Piepkorn MW: Reliability of skin biopsy pathology. *J Am Board Fam Pract* 7:371, 1994.

Brehler R, Hildebrand A, Luger TA: Recent developments in the treatment of atopic eczema. *J Am Acad Dermatol* 36:983, 1997.

Cohen DF, Brancaccio R, Anderson D, et al: Utility of standard allergen series alone in evaluation of allergic contact dermatitis: A retrospective study of 732 patients. *J Am Acad Dermatol* 36:914, 1997.

Cole WC, Roth HL, Sachs LB: Group psychotherapy as an aid in the medical treatment of eczema. *J Am Acad Dermatol* 18:286, 1998.

Cyr PR: Family practice center-based training in skin disorders: A photographic approach. *Fam Med* 27:109, 1995.

Faergmann J, Maibach HI: The *Pityrosporon* yeasts: Their role as pathogens. *Int J Dermatol* 23:463, 1984.

Finlay AY, Lhan GK, Luscombe DK, et al: Validation of UK sickness impact profile and psoriasis disability index in psoriasis. *Br J Dermatol* 123:751, 1990.

Fitzpatrick TB, Eisen AZ, Wolff K, et al: (eds): *Dermatology in General Medicine*, 4th ed. New York, McGraw-Hill, 1993.

Fuglsang G, Madsen G, Halken S, et al: Adverse reactions to food additives in children with atopic symptoms. *Allergy* 49:31, 1994.

Galli E, Picardo M, Chini L, et al: Analysis of polyunsaturated fatty acids in newborn sera: A screening tool for atopic disease? *Br J Dermatol* 130:752, 1994.

Guin JD, Lowery BJ, Veazey MC, et al: Patch testing for contact dermatitis. *Dermatol Nursing* 9:178, 1997.

Hanifin JM: Atopic dermatitis in infants and children: Pediatric dermatology. *Pediatr Clin North Am* 38:763, 1991.

Hederos, Berg A: Epogam evening primrose oil treatment in atopic dermatitis and asthma. *Arch Dis Child* 75:494, 1996.

Janniger CK, Schwartz RA: Seborrheic dermatitis. *Am Fam Phys* 52:149, 1995.

Jones TP, Boiko PE, Piepkorn MW: Skin biopsy indications in primary care practice. *J Am Board Fam Pract* 9:397, 1996.

Kanny G, Hatahet R, Moneret-Vautrin DA, et al: Allergy and intolerance to flavouring agents in atopic dermatitis in young children. *Allerg Immunol (Paris)* 26:204, 1994.

Krowchuk DP, Bradham DD, Fleischer AB: Dermatologic services provided to children and adolescents by primary care and other physicians in the United States. *Pediatr Dermatol* 11:199, 1994.

Larsen FS, Holm NV, Henningsen K: Atopic dermatitis: A genetic-epidemiologic study in a population-based twin sample. *J Am Acad Dermatolol* 15:487, 1986.

Latchman Y, Whittle B, Rustin M, et al: The efficacy of traditional Chinese herbal therapy in atopic eczema. *Int Arch Allerg Immunol* 104:222, 1994.

Lear JT, English JSC, Jones P, et al: Retrospective review of the use of azothioprine in severe atopic dermatitis. *J Am Acad Dermatol* 35:642, 1996.

Lucky AW, Grote GD, Williams JL, et al: Effect of desonide ointment, 0.05%, on the hypothalamic-pituitary-adrenal axis of children with atopic dermatitis. *Cutis* 59:151, 1997.

Neame RL, Berth-Jones J, Kurinczuk JJ, et al: Prevalence of atopic dermatitis in Leicester: A study of methodology and examination of possible ethnic variation. *Br J Dermatol* 132:772, 1995.

Niwa Y, Iizawa O: Abnormalities in serum lipids and leukocyte superoxide dismutase and associated cataract formation in patients with atopic dermatitis. *Arch Dermatol* 130:1387, 1994.

Ruzicka T, Bieber T, Schopf E, et al: A short-term trial of tacrolimus ointment for atopic dermatitis. *New Engl J Med* 337:816, 1997.

Saurat J-H: Eczema in primary immune deficiencies: Clues to the pathogenesis of atopic dermatitis with special reference to the Wiskott-Aldrich syndrome. *Dermatovenereol (Suppl)* 114:125, 1985.

Schafer T, Dirschedl P, Kunz B, et al: Maternal smoking during pregnancy and lactation increases the risk of atopic eczema in the offspring. *J Am Acad Dermatol* 36:550, 1997.

Schultz Larsen F, Diepgen T, Svensson A: The occurrence of atopic dermatitis in north Europe: An international questionnaire study. *J Am Acad Dermatol* 34:760, 1996.

Sheehan MP, Rustin MH, Atherton DJ, et al: Efficacy of traditional Chinese herbal therapy in adult atopic dermatitis. *Lancet* 340:13, 1992.

Stern RS: Utilization of outpatient care for psoriasis. *J Am Acad Dermatol* 35:543, 1996.

Zug KA, McKay M: Eczematous dermatitis: A practical review. *Am Fam Phys* 54:1243, 1996.

L. Kevin Hamberger
Daniel C. Vinson
Barry D. Weiss

Chapter 17

Hidden Problems

This chapter explores three of the most common problems in primary care practice. These problems warrant special attention because, in nearly all cases, clinicians do not identify them. These three problems—domestic violence, problem alcohol drinking, and low literacy—have prevalence rates ranging from 10 to 50 percent among patients in many primary care practices, making them more common than most of the other problems discussed in this book. However, because clinicians do not identify these problems, they remain hidden from view and hidden from potential treatments and interventions.

DOMESTIC VIOLENCE

L. Kevin Hamberger

How Common Is Domestic Violence?

Domestic violence in adults can be defined as any type of assaultive behavior that functions to dominate, control, or punish another individual who is supposedly in a peer relationship with the perpetrator of the violence. Domestic violence is often referred to as partner violence, battering, or spousal or wife abuse. The various forms of domestic violence are discussed below.

The primary victims of violence are women. Although surveys show that men are assaulted by female partners at rates equal to male assaults of women, the clinical emphasis (and the emphasis in this chapter) has been primarily on female victims because, compared to males, female victims are more likely to be injured and injured more seriously by acts of violence. Female victims are also more likely than males to seek medical care for domestic violence-related issues, including psychological problems, such as depression and anxiety, as well as physical injuries. Finally, female perpetrators are more likely than male perpetrators to use violence for self-defense or retaliation, while male perpetrators are more likely to use violence for dominating or controlling their partners.

Domestic violence occurs in all social, ethnic, and economic groups. Religious affiliation, education, and occupational status are not consistently associated with domestic violence.

Prevalence

Prevalence of domestic violence has generally been studied with representative sample surveys. The most well-known national surveys show that approximately 12 percent of married women report having been physically assaulted in the past year, and more than a quarter of those women reporting an assault tell of severe physical violence.

Among individuals who are not married, the rates of violence are higher. Prevalence rates of violence between dating couples are between 20 to 30 percent, and about one-third of unmarried, cohabiting couples report having been involved in domestic violence. The prevalence of domestic violence in gay and lesbian relationships is similar to that observed in heterosexual populations.

Prevalence of domestic violence in primary care outpatient medical settings roughly mirrors

that in the general population. In family medicine and internal medicine offices, between 12 and 28 percent of adult females report being victims of domestic violence within the past year, and lifetime prevalence rates range between 28 percent and 54 percent. Although domestic violence is not always identified or formally diagnosed in clinical practice, these statistics demonstrate that domestic violence is one of the most common problems of patients of primary care clinicians.

Principal Diagnoses

Domestic violence is a recognized medical diagnosis, with its own *International Classification of Disease*, 9th ed. (ICD-9) code, adult maltreatment syndrome (995.81). There are four basic types of domestic violence: (1) direct, bodily physical aggression; (2) sexual aggression; (3) destruction of property or pets; and (4) psychological battering or terror tactics. Each type of violence comprises a continuum of severity. For example, acts of physical aggression range from restraining and pushing to beating, clubbing, stabbing, and shooting. Sexual aggression ranges from unwanted touching to rape. Property and pet destruction range from punching walls or kicking the family pet to destroying an entire residence by arson or killing the pet. Psychological battering ranges from subtle looks and gestures to stalking or overt threats of homicide.

Interpersonal Dynamics

To effectively diagnose domestic violence, clinicians must have an appreciation of the interpersonal dynamics involved in abusive relationships. These dynamics include fear and terror, inability to secure safety, and traumatic bonding.

FEAR AND TERROR

As noted above, domestic violence functions to control the behavior of another. The chief mechanism of control is the victim's fear that failure to comply with the perpetrator's demands will result in assault or injury. Victims frequently go to great lengths to avoid behaviors that upset their partners, often at great personal cost, such as withdrawal from work, friends, family, and other potential sources of support. This withdrawal can isolate victims from those who might tell them that the violence is wrong or that they need not live with the abusive partner.

SECURING SAFETY

A second dynamic is the difficulty that victims experience in securing safety. Many victims make multiple efforts to escape violent relationships or at least obtain relief from them. However, these efforts to escape are often thwarted by the very individuals who might otherwise provide support and assist the victim's escape. For example, counselors may seek to help the victim "adjust" to her situation. Clergy may recommend against divorce and encourage forgiveness of the perpetrator. Police may not arrest perpetrators, and prosecutors may not press charges. Family members and friends may not want to get involved. Health care professionals may fail to ask about abuse or may not perceive the victim's situation as serious.

Prior efforts to leave the perpetrator may have ended in a return home due to economic hardship or difficulty obtaining housing. In some cases, perpetrators continue to pursue victims after escape, to the point of stalking and further violence. Indeed, the most dangerous time in a battered victim's life is at the point of ending the relationship.

Even victims who manage to escape violence suffer aftereffects. In fact, nearly two-thirds of abuse survivors meet clinical criteria for posttraumatic stress disorder. Hence, merely escaping a violent relationship does not always resolve the emotional burden of battered victims.

TRAUMATIC BONDING

A third important dynamic is the very context of the violence. Unlike violence perpetrated by strangers, victims and perpetrators of domestic violence have a relationship that often involves feelings of affection and affiliation, shared social networks, and possibly children and shared property. Therefore, it is not easy for a victim to simply walk away from the perpetrator, for to do so may mean ending an enduring relationship, loss of home, loss of access to children, and loss or disapproval of friends and family. This combination of strong emotional dependency, together with chronic fear and terror outlined above, develops into what has been referred to as "traumatic bonding." The fear and terror are intolerable, but they conflict with the couple's affiliations and affection. She wants to end the violence, not the relationship.

Typical Presentation

Battered women rarely present to primary care clinicians with a specific complaint of domestic violence. Rather, they typically present with nonspecific somatic or psychological complaints. In particular, the literature suggests that battered women are often diagnosed as having depression or anxiety disorders, including posttraumatic stress disorder. Battered women with children may present to clinicians with concerns about their child's behavior or emotional distress. Finally, one study indicated that abused women seek more treatment for functional bowel disorders, miscarriages, induced abortion, and substance abuse than women with no history of domestic violence.

Some women, however, present with injuries suggesting domestic violence. Such injuries include contusions and bruising of axial portions of the body, including the head, face, breasts, abdomen, and genitals. Abuse-related injuries of the forearms and hands also occur, because the upper extremities can be injured when used for self-defense.

In nonprimary care settings, the presentations are similar. In emergency departments, the vast majority of battered women seek care for complaints other than abuse-related injuries. In psychiatric and mental health practices, the presentation is more likely to be related to depression, anxiety, or relationship problems.

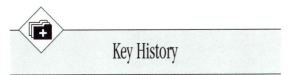

Key History

Despite its frequency, identifying domestic violence is difficult. This difficulty relates to factors concerning both the clinician and the patient. Researchers have identified several clinician barriers to victim identification, including insufficient knowledge and training, time constraints, concern about opening a "Pandora's box" if abuse is identified, and losing control of the clinician-patient relationship. Among barriers on the part of patients are the different concepts held by many women about what constitutes abuse. Recent research indicates that some women define certain behaviors as abusive, while others do not. For example, 3 to 7 percent of women do not consider abuse to include behaviors such as being pushed, having something thrown at them, or being kicked or slapped.

When an abused woman is accompanied to medical examinations by the abusing partner, detection of violence is particularly challenging. The abusing partner often will not leave the woman alone in the examination room. Furthermore, regardless of the reason for a medical office visit, clinicians should be aware that when

women appear to defer to their partners for answering questions or when partners attempt to control the medical interview, this may indicate an abusive relationship.

Screening

Screening for domestic violence by identifying sociodemographic risk factors is not practical, because the only consistently identified risk factors for domestic violence are low socioeconomic status and having witnessed violent relationships between ones' parents. In primary care practices, battered women tend to be younger, report relationships of shorter duration, and are more likely to be separated or divorced than nonbattered women. However, none of these risk factors is sufficiently specific to use for screening. Thus, other approaches are advocated to identify victims of domestic violence. The most widely recommended approach is universal screening. The other is selective case finding.

UNIVERSAL SCREENING

Universal screening involves incorporating questions about domestic violence into the standard medical history for all patients. Typically, this is done by routinely asking about domestic violence along with other behaviors, such as cigarette smoking, alcohol and drug use, sexual activity, and so forth. This screening context reduces perceptions that questions about abuse are being asked in response to some unique characteristic of a patient.

The actual questions about abuse should avoid general terms such as *abuse* or *violence*, since these terms are subject to interpretation and are often emotionally charged. Instead, questions about specific behaviors are preferred, for example, "In my practice, I am concerned about safety and prevention of injuries. Are you currently in a relationship where someone is shoving, hitting, kicking, controlling, or making you feel afraid?" Such inquiries require only simple, yes-no answers, need no interpretation, and are less likely to arouse defensive responses.

CASE FINDING

In case finding, the health care provider observes markers of abuse and asks questions to determine if abuse is present. Hence, upon noticing bruises on a patient's face, the clinician can ask: "In my experience, this type of injury is often caused by other people's actions. Is anyone hurting you or threatening you?" This type of inquiry goes beyond simply asking how the injury happened by proactively asserting the clinician's expertise about injury profiles and placing the inquiry in a specific context. As with screening, patients must only answer yes or no.

Violence History

If screening or case finding identifies a victim of domestic violence, the history is then used to determine the victim's risk of sustaining severe or fatal injury. Violence that is increasing in frequency or severity that is associated with substance abuse poses greater risk to the victim. Risk is also increased if the couple's relationship is characterized by the perpetrator's feeling a sense of ownership over the victim. Finally, if the perpetrator's behavior changes markedly when the victim leaves the relationship (e.g., stalking, threatening, or disobeying court-ordered restraining orders), there is a higher risk of lethal injury. Useful questions for assessing risk of injury are shown in Table 17-1.

The Validity of Victims' Reports

A common question is whether victims exaggerate the true magnitude of violence, but most studies indicate that victims' reports of violence are generally accurate. This fact has relevance to the role of medical records as legal evidence in criminal or civil actions related to domestic violence. Thus, the victim's history must be carefully documented to accurately reflect her report,

Table 17-1

Questions for Determining the Risk of Severe or Lethal Violence

QUESTIONS TO DETERMINE THE PATTERN AND SEVERITY OF VIOLENCE
Is the violence becoming more severe or more frequent over time?
Are violent episodes often accompanied by the perpetrator's use of alcohol or drugs?
Has the perpetrator threatened or committed any type of sexual contact with you?
Have you been injured from the violence?
Has your partner threatened to kill you?
QUESTIONS ABOUT THE NATURE OF THE RELATIONSHIP
Has your partner ever told you he can't live without you?
Is he obsessed with you, in that he can't seem to get by without you?
QUESTIONS ABOUT TERMINATING THE RELATIONSHIP
Since you've left your partner, does he continue to contact you?
Is he showing up at places he knows you are going to be?
Is he threatening you if you don't go back?
Is he violating the restraining order?
Is he threatening to take (or hurt) the children (or anyone else in your life)?

NOTE: A yes response to any of these questions indicates a higher risk of severe or lethal injury.

using direct quotes whenever possible. Specific acts of aggression should be described verbatim, and specific names should be used, including that of the perpetrator.

Physical Examination

Except in cases of overt violent trauma, there are usually few unequivocal signs of domestic violence on physical examination. Nonetheless, the physical examination may be of value because battered women report that they value the examination as a measure of caring if the examination is conducted in a sensitive and gentle manner.

In performing the examination, it is important to look for patterns of injury (e.g., central or truncal injuries) that, as noted above, may be clues to physical assault. Multiple bruises in various stages of healing should also suggest abuse. Finally, any injury or scar that has not been noted previously or that is inconsistent with its reported cause should raise suspicion of domestic violence.

Ancillary Tests

Several questionnaires have been developed to screen for domestic violence. These instruments vary in length, and all involve self-reports by patients, thus making them subject to the limitations of self-report methodologies. Nonetheless, these instruments can aid in the screening process during routine or focused history taking and, if screening suggests abuse, the clinician can conduct a more in-depth interview to confirm the diagnosis.

Long Instruments

The most widely used long instrument is the Conflict Tactics Scales (CTS). The CTS measures many forms of family violence, including partner violence, child and elder abuse, and sibling violence. The CTS also measures verbal reasoning, psychological abuse, and minor and severe physical violence. This instrument is used more often in research than in clinical settings. If used in clinical settings, the CTS is best considered an adjunct to a careful history.

The Index of Spouse Abuse (ISA) was also developed for research on domestic violence, but it is sometimes used in clinical settings. The ISA is

a 30-item, self-report measure that assesses severity of physical and nonphysical partner abuse.

Short Instruments

The Abuse Assessment Screen (AAS) is a five-item structured interview developed for use with pregnant patients that has also been modified for use with women who are not pregnant. The AAS yields results comparable to those of longer, in-depth instruments, making it more suitable for primary care clinical settings.

The Partner Violence Screen (PVS) consists of three questions and is administered as part of a routine medical interview (Table 17-2). Sensitivity of the PVS for detecting domestic violence ranges from 64 to 71 percent. Positive predictive value ranges from 51 to 64 percent, and negative predictive value is around 88 percent. Although originally developed for emergency room settings, it can also be used in primary care practice.

Treatment

Treatment of domestic violence is complex and requires the coordinated efforts of many community resources to support and protect the vic-

Table 17-2

Partner Violence Screen (PVS) for Domestic Violence

The PVS consists of three questions:
  Have you been hit, kicked, punched, or otherwise hurt by someone within the past year? If so, by whom?
  Do you feel safe in your current relationship?
  Is there a partner from a previous relationship who is making you feel unsafe now?

NOTE: A yes response to any of the three questions is to be considered a positive screen for partner violence.

tim. In general, treatment should not be directed at preserving the couple's relationship or teaching perpetrators to discontinue abusing their partners, since such efforts are frequently unsuccessful and, as described below, may violate the victim's confidentiality and further endanger her safety.

Essential Treatment

Treatment should focus on five tasks. The first is emotional support: telling the woman that she is not to blame for the violence and that she deserves to be safe, and providing assurances that what she tells her clinician or social service agencies is confidential from her partner. The second task is ensuring safety, which involves determining the level of danger (Table 17-1), asking if victims feel safe going home, inquiring about childrens' safety, and helping victims develop escape plans in the event of future violence. The third task is to provide information about community resources, including shelters and advocacy, legal, and social services. The fourth is arranging for follow-up appointments to continue advocacy and supportive care. Finally, it is essential to prepare a careful and complete medical record that documents all information collected.

While provision of safety is the most important short-term concern, perhaps the most important factor relating to successful long-term outcomes is referral to women's shelters and advocacy groups. Such agencies possess the requisite understanding of abuse dynamics, together with knowledge of relevant community resources, to provide optimal supportive and restorative care for victims and survivors.

Supplemental Treatments

Counseling, psychotherapy, and/or pharmacotherapy may be indicated if the battered patient also shows evidence of severe depression, anxiety, posttraumatic stress disorder, or other psychological disorder. However, the individual providing this treatment should be knowledgeable about the dynamics of domestic violence because, without such knowledge, inappropriate attention is often paid to dealing with or "fixing" the victim's problems, thus implicitly blaming the victim for her plight.

Legal Responsibilities

In the United States, all 50 states require health care providers to report suspicion of child abuse to government authorities. Thus, when an adult victim has children suspected of being abused, it is necessary to report this concern to appropriate child protective services agencies. A few states also mandate reporting of adult partner abuse to adult protective services, and many states require reporting of suspected elder abuse. Referral to protective agencies should not be viewed as the end point of intervention. Instead, clinicians should continue to provide ongoing care, support, and advocacy to aid victims as they deal with their relationship and with various social service agencies.

Legal interventions include arrest, prosecution, and adjudication of perpetrators for the protection of victims. Although limited in their effectiveness in stopping domestic violence, legal interventions provide a powerful societal message that domestic violence is wrong. Health care providers can inform victims of legal resources for enhancing safety, including criminal prosecution; the family court system for determining restraining orders, child custody, and child visitation; and civil court for tort actions against perpetrators.

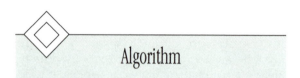

Algorithm

The algorithm in Fig. 17-1 outlines a general method for dealing with domestic violence using the various approaches described above. If violence is detected through case finding or univer-

Figure 17-1

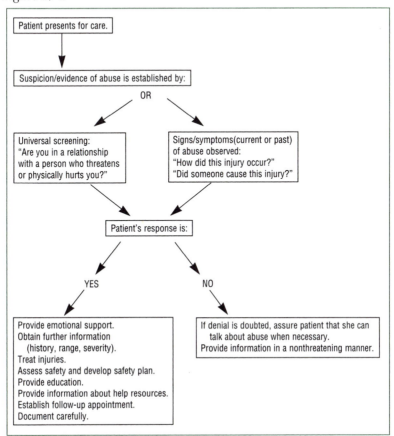

Patient presents for care.

Suspicion/evidence of abuse is established by:

OR

Universal screening:
"Are you in a relationship
with a person who threatens
or physically hurts you?"

Signs/symptoms(current or past)
of abuse observed:
"How did this injury occur?"
"Did someone cause this injury?"

Patient's response is:

YES

NO

Provide emotional support.
Obtain further information
  (history, range, severity).
Treat injuries.
Assess safety and develop safety plan.
Provide education.
Provide information about help resources.
Establish follow-up appointment.
Document carefully.

If denial is doubted, assure patient that she can
  talk about abuse when necessary.
Provide information in a nonthreatening manner.

Domestic violence algorithm.

sal screening, clinicians must treat injuries, provide support for the patient, assist in ensuring her safety, make necessary referrals, and participate in follow-up care.

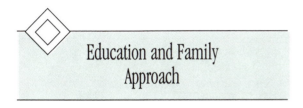

Education and Family Approach

There are three main concepts about which clinicians should educate victims of domestic violence. The first is that violence, in all its forms, is wrong. No one deserves to be abused, regard-

less of shortcomings, and everyone in a household deserves to be safe. Second, there are many community resources to help victims and perpetrators of family violence. Third, family violence poses a danger to all family members and will generally continue if no action is taken. In fact, when followed over a 2-year period, only 7 percent of abusive men completely discontinue violent behavior. The frequency and severity of emotional abuse generally does not decrease at all.

Children are often the unintended victims of partner violence, both emotionally and physically. Although victims and perpetrators may both believe that children are unaware of the violence, a recent study indicated that, in violent families with children, 85 percent of children had witnessed a recent violent episode. It is not surprising, therefore, that, compared to children in nonviolent families, children who observe parental violence exhibit more depression, anxiety, and sleep disorders, and have more problems with behavior, conflict resolution, and school performance. In some cases, children in violent families are physically abused. The abusive parent is usually, but not always, the same parent abusing the spouse. Unfortunately, battered women with children often remain in the violent relationship until the children's physical safety is jeopardized.

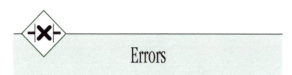

Errors

Clinicians make seven common errors when caring for victims of domestic violence (Table 17-3). First, breaching confidentiality (e.g., by speaking with the perpetrator or other family members) can endanger a victim and should never be done. In fact, it is often inadvisable to speak with the perpetrator or others even if the patient consents to the interaction, because such communication may result in retaliatory violence by the perpetrator. A second error is communicating doubt about the victim's report. Disbelief invalidates the victim's experience and may cause cessation of help-seeking efforts. A third error is

minimizing the effects of violence or implying that the victim may be responsible for the violence. Even nonsevere physical violence or nonviolent abusive behavior can terrify a victim. Furthermore, implying responsibility for abuse reiterates messages the victim has heard from the abuser and creates a dilemma for the patient in that, while she cannot control the abuser's behavior, she feels that she should be able to control his violence.

A fourth, and common, error is expressing outrage at the perpetrator as a way of aligning with the victim. Victims both love and fear perpetrators. If the clinician expresses outrage, it can insult the women's affection for the perpetrator, thereby causing loss of rapport with and trust in the clinician. Fifth, it is inadvisable to instruct patients when and how to leave a relationship. Because victims are at greater risk for injury and death at the time they leave an abusive relationship, leaving should always be the victim's choice, since she is in the best position to judge if and when leaving is appropriate.

The sixth error is that health care providers sometimes disempower victims by taking charge of the situation and doing everything for the victim. Whenever possible, victims should be given choices about how to proceed and then proceed on their own. The final common error is referring victims and their partners for couples counseling to work out the violence problem. Except in very special circumstances, couples counsel-

Table 17-3

Common Errors in Caring for Victims of Spousal Abuse

ERROR	RISK
Breaching confidentiality	Level of (retaliatory) abuse may increase.
Communicating disbelief about violence	Victim may stop seeking help.
Implying the victim is responsible	Sense of powerlessness is increased.
Expressing outrage against perpetrator	Clinician may lose rapport with victim.
Instructing when and how to leave relationship	Leaving increases risk of physical violence.
Doing too much for the victim	Victim may be disempowered.
Referral for couples counseling	Abuse may increase, as with breaching confidentiality.

ing can further endanger victims by creating expectations that information about abuse be disclosed in counseling sessions. This may anger the perpetrator and, without appropriate safety mechanisms, could increase danger to the victim. If and when violence ends, and if both the victim and perpetrator desire to continue in a relationship, conjoint counseling may be indicated at that time.

Controversies

The major current controversy is the role of couples counseling. Many marriage and family therapists believe couples counseling can be effective in treating domestic violence and that claims of danger to victims are overstated. In fact, emerging research suggests that, under tightly controlled conditions with specially trained therapists and carefully selected patients, a couples format for domestic violence counseling can be effective. However, considerable research is still needed to establish parameters for safe use of couples counseling in treating domestic violence.

Emerging Concepts

In recent years, the problem of domestic violence has changed from one that was rarely discussed to one that is now recognized as serious and commonplace. Along with this recognition, there is a growing movement to equip hospitals with policies and procedures, protocols, and training to identify and deal with violence victims. Similarly, outpatient settings will also become a focus of domestic violence interventions, in recognition of the high frequency with which

victims visit outpatient settings. Recommendations for universal screening, perhaps using formal screening questionnaires, are likely to increase. Finally, the approach to domestic violence in the future is likely to see increased collaboration with battered women's resource centers, and domestic violence specialists becoming a regular part of health care teams.

THE PROBLEM DRINKER

Daniel C. Vinson

How Common Is Problem Drinking?

Problem drinking is a spectrum of conditions. At one extreme, the spectrum includes individuals with severe alcohol dependence and its many biomedical complications. At the other extreme are individuals without complications whose drinking places them at risk for developing them. Between the extremes of alcohol dependence and at-risk drinking, there are many individuals who manifest a variety of interpersonal, social, or legal problems related to alcohol consumption. Persons in this intermediate category are often labeled as having alcohol abuse.

The American Psychiatric Association and the National Institute on Alcohol Abuse and Alcoholism have developed formal definitions of *alcohol dependence, alcohol abuse,* and *at-risk drinking*. These definitions are displayed in Tables 17-4, 17-5, and 17-6. Together, alcohol dependence and alcohol abuse constitute alcohol-use disorders.

This section focuses on detection and treatment of problem drinking in outpatient primary care settings, emphasizing at-risk drinking and alcohol abuse. Inpatient treatment and management of specific alcohol-related medical complications (e.g., cirrhosis, gastrointestinal bleeding, etc.) are not discussed.

Prevalence

Throughout its continuum, problem drinking is more prevalent than most clinicians realize. The 1994–1995 Behavioral Risk Factor Surveillance Survey found a past-month prevalence of binge drinking in the United States (defined as five or more drinks on at least one occasion) of nearly 15 percent. The National Longitudinal Alcohol Epidemiologic Survey (NLAES) found a prevalence of alcohol abuse or dependence, defined by the American Psychiatric Association's *Diagnostic and Statistical Manual* (DSM) criteria, of 7.4 percent in the past 23 months. The numbers are similar for adults and adolescents. Based on the NLAES data, 1 in every 7 adults in the United States is an at-risk drinker, and 1 in every 15 has an alcohol-use disorder (i.e., alcohol abuse or dependence).

Because individuals who drink heavily develop a variety of health problems, the rate of problem drinking among patients seen in clinical practice is probably higher than the rate in the general population. Using a conservative estimate of the rate of problem drinking, a primary care clinician seeing 25 patients per day probably sees at least 3 patients in the office each day

Table 17-4

Diagnostic Criteria for Alcohol Dependence

A. A maladaptive pattern of alcohol use leading to clinically significant impairment or distress, as manifested by three or more of the following occurring at any time in the same 12-month period:
1. Need for markedly increased amounts of alcohol to achieve intoxication or desired effect; or markedly diminished effect with continued use of the same amount of alcohol
2. The characteristic withdrawal syndrome for alcohol; or alcohol (or a closely related substance) is taken to relieve or avoid withdrawal symptoms
3. Persistent desire or one or more unsuccessful efforts to cut down or control drinking
4. Drinking in larger amounts or over a longer period than the person intended
5. Important social, occupational, or recreational activities given up or reduced because of drinking
6. A great deal of time spent in activities necessary to obtain alcohol, to drink, or to recover from its effects
7. Continued drinking despite knowledge of having a persistent or recurrent physical or psychological problem that is likely to be caused or exacerbated by alcohol use
B. No duration criterion separately specified. However, three or more dependence criteria must be met within the same year and must occur repeatedly, as specified by duration qualifiers associated with criteria (e.g., "often," "persistent," "continued").
C. Physiological dependence
1 With physiological dependence: Evidence of tolerance or withdrawal (i.e., any of items A1 or A2 above are present).
2. Without physiological dependence: No evidence of tolerance or withdrawal (i.e., none of items A1 or A2 above is present).

Table 17-5

Diagnostic Criteria for Alcohol Abuse

A. A maladaptive pattern of alcohol use leading to clinically significant impairment or
distress, as manifested by one (or more) of
the following occurring within a 12-month
period:
1. Recurrent drinking resulting in a failure to fulfill major role obligations at
work, school, or home
2. Recurrent drinking in situations in
which it is physically hazardous
3. Recurrent alcohol-related legal problems
4. Continued alcohol use despite having
persistent or recurrent social or interpersonal problems caused or exacerbated by the effects of alcohol
B. The symptoms have never met the criteria
for alcohol dependence.

SOURCE: Reprinted with permission from *Diagnostic and Statistical
Manual of Mental Disorders,* 4th ed. Washington, DC, American Psychiatric Association. Copyright 1994.

with a drinking problem. However, since most
patients are not asked about their drinking
habits, clinicians do not identify most of these
problem drinkers. In fact, national surveys indicate that less than 40 percent of individuals who
have visited a health professional during the preceding 2 years report being asked about their
use of alcohol.

Typical Presentation

The presentation of problem drinking in primary
care practice is also a spectrum. At one extreme,
patients may present with severe alcohol dependence accompanied by manifestations of
alcohol-related end-organ damage. These manifestations include alcoholic liver disease (hepatic
failure with jaundice, coagulopathy, and encephalopathy), gastrointestinal bleeding, pancreatitis,
muscle wasting, neurologic and hematologic
complications, and other problems. Other patients have varying degrees of alcohol abuse or
dependence but no overt end-organ damage.
These individuals may present to clinicians for
help with their drinking, be brought to a clinician by their families, or come to a physician's
attention because of behavioral problems, such
as driving while intoxicated. The at-risk drinkers
at the other end of the spectrum, who are far
more numerous than those with alcohol abuse
or dependence, have no apparent alcohol-
related problems and often will not volunteer
information about their drinking habits. While
some patients will deny that they have a drinking problem or even that they drink at all, most
will provide accurate information if asked in
appropriate ways.

Finally, patients with problem drinking may
present with medical problems not obviously
due to drinking. The list is long and includes
problems such as hypertension, depression,

Table 17-6

NIAAA Definition of At-Risk Drinking

MEN	WOMEN
Drinking > 4 drinks on one occasion or Drinking > 14 drinks per week (more than an average of 2 per day).	Drinking > 3 drinks on one occasion or Drinking > 7 drinks per week (more than an average of 1 per day).

ABBREVIATION: NIAAA, National Institute on Alcohol Abuse and Alcoholism.

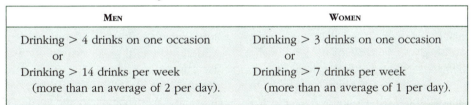

insomnia, accidental injury, chronic abdominal pain, and many others. As noted in Chap. 3, problem drinking may be one of the most frequent causes of secondary, and potentially reversible, hypertension. However, there is no one medical problem that indicates problem drinking with sufficient sensitivity (i.e., most problem drinkers have it) or specificity (i.e., non-problem drinkers and nondrinkers seldom have it) to serve as a clinically useful indicator of alcohol problems. Instead, for detection of alcohol abuse and at-risk drinking, clinicians must ask direct, specific questions about patients' drinking patterns.

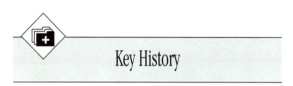

Key History

Detecting Problem Drinking

As with other hidden problems, such as domestic violence, problem drinking can be detected either by selected case finding or by universal screening.

CASE FINDING

When patients present with alcohol-related end-organ problems or medical problems, or when family members bring a patient to the office for help with an alcohol problem, the probability of problem drinking is high and the clinician should directly question the patient about alcohol use. Some of these problem drinkers will deny alcohol use, and they present a special challenge requiring empathy and concern if clinicians are to establish effective communication with these individuals. Research indicates that, with a properly established physician-patient relationship, most patients are willing to discuss their drinking and will provide accurate estimates of the frequency and quantity of alcohol consumption.

UNIVERSAL SCREENING

Because at-risk drinking and alcohol-use disorders are usually hidden problems, many expert groups, including the U.S. Preventive Services Task Force, recommend asking all adolescent and adult patients about their alcohol consumption. While many clinicians do this by asking questions such as, "How much do you usually drink?," this question often yields inaccurate answers. For example, someone who drinks two drinks each weekday and 6 to 8 drinks each weekend day might honestly answer "Two."

More accurate screening for problem drinking can be accomplished using one of several quick screening instruments and questions. Two common screening instruments are the CAGE questions and the Alcohol Use Disorders Identification Test. In addition, recent research has evaluated the accuracy of screening for problem drinking with a single focused question.

CAGE QUESTIONS   The four CAGE questions are widely used, and the small number of questions and ease of administration make the instrument practical for use in office practice (Table 17-7). The CAGE questions effectively identify persons with alcohol dependence and alcohol abuse. They are not, however, effective as a screening test for at-risk drinking and may lack sensitivity for detecting alcohol problems in women.

ALCOHOL USE DISORDERS IDENTIFICATION TEST   The Alcohol Use and Disorders Identification Test (AUDIT), developed by the World Health Organization, screens for at-risk drinking in addition to alcohol dependence and abuse (Table 17-8). Its major limitations are that it is a 10-item written questionnaire that requires time for administration and may not be suitable for use with low-literacy populations, and its sensitivity has varied in several studies to as low as 65 percent. Its advantage, however, is that it has demonstrated clinical utility in a variety of cultural settings, and a Spanish-language version is available.

Table 17-7
The CAGE Questions

> Have you ever felt you should **C**ut down on your drinking?
>
> Have people **A**nnoyed you by criticizing your drinking?
>
> Have you ever felt bad or **G**uilty about your drinking?
>
> Have you ever had a drink first thing in the morning to steady your nerves or to get rid of a hangover (i.e., an **E**ye opener)?

NOTE: Item responses on the CAGE are scored 0 for no answers and 1 for yes answers, with a higher score indicating a greater likelihood of alcohol problems. A total score of 2 or greater suggests alcohol abuse or dependence.
SOURCE: Mayfield D, McLeod G, Hall P: The CAGE questionnaire: Validation of a new alcoholism screening instrument. *Am J Psychiatry* 131:1121, 1974: and Ewing JA: Detecting alcoholism: The CAGE questionnaire. *JAMA* 252:1905, 1984.

SCREENING WITH A SINGLE QUESTION A recent study suggests that screening for problem drinking in primary care practice can also be accomplished by asking the single question, "On any single occasion during the past three months, have you had more than five drinks containing alcohol?" The advantage of this method is that a single question permits screening of all patients in a practice with little expenditure of time. In one published study with this technique, the question's sensitivity for detecting alcohol abuse was about 65 percent, and the specificity was 93 percent.

What to Do If Problem Drinking Is Detected

If a patient screens positive for problem drinking or if there is clinical suspicion of problem drinking based on general history, additional information is needed about the quantity and frequency of drinking and about the effect of alcohol on the patient's social, occupational, or recreational activities.

QUANTITY AND FREQUENCY OF DRINKING

As noted above, the general question, "How much do you drink?" is not generally adequate to quantify alcohol intake. Rather, specific, direct questions about recent consumption are more useful. Appropriate questions include: "When was the last time you drank?," "How much did you drink then?," and "How much do you usually drink on a weekday? On a weekend day?" In addition, engaging patients in a dialogue about alcohol consumption can help generate their interest in doing something about their drinking problem.

EFFECT ON SOCIAL, OCCUPATIONAL, OR RECREATIONAL ACTIVITIES

To determine whether alcohol has had an important effect on a patient's social, occupational, or recreational activities, it is often useful to begin with a question such as, "Have you ever had any problems because of alcohol?" The CAGE questions, if not already used for screening, are also useful. In addition, other open-ended questions may facilitate recall and encourage candid reporting about job and family problems or arrests for driving while intoxicated. The important thing is to engage the patient in an open and reflective dialogue, remembering that primary care clinicians can address alcohol problems over multiple visits, taking advantage of the continuity of relationships that often develop with patients over time.

Physical Examination

Compared to the history, the physical examination has limited value in identifying problem drinking. The primary role of the physical examination is in assessing biomedical complications of heavy alcohol use. While a general physical

Table 17-8

Alcohol Use Disorders Identification Test (AUDIT)

1. How often do you have a drink containing alcohol?
   0. Never
   1. Monthly or less
   2. 2 to 4 times a month
   3. 2 to 3 times a week
   4. 4 or more times a week
2. How many drinks containing alcohol do you have on a typical day when you are drinking?
   0. 0
   0. 1 or 2
   1. 3 or 4
   2. 5 or 6
   3. 7 to 9
   4. 10 or more
3. How often do you have 6 or more drinks on one occasion?
   0. Never
   1. Less than monthly
   2. Monthly
   3. Weekly
   4. Daily or almost daily
4. How often during the last year have you found that you were unable to stop drinking once you had started?
   0. Never
   1. Less than monthly
   2. Monthly
   3. Weekly
   4. Daily or almost daily
5. How often during the last year have you failed to do what was normally expected from you because of drinking?
   0. Never
   1. Less than monthly
   2. Monthly

   3. Weekly
   4. Daily or almost daily
6. How often during the last year have you needed a first drink in the morning to get yourself going after a heavy drinking session?
   0. Never
   1. Less than monthly
   2. Monthly
   3. Weekly
   4. Daily or almost daily
7. How often during the last year have you had a feeling of guilt or remorse after drinking?
   0. Never
   1. Less than monthly
   2. Monthly
   3. Weekly
   4. Daily or almost daily
8. How often during the last year have you been unable to remember what happened the night before because you had been drinking?
   0. Never
   1. Less than monthly
   2. Monthly
   3. Weekly
   4. Daily or almost daily
9. Have you or someone else been injured as a result of your drinking?
   0. No
   2. Yes, but not in the last year
   4. Yes, during the last year
10. Has a relative, friend, doctor, or other health worker been concerned about your drinking or suggested you cut down?
    0. No
    2. Yes, but not in the last year
    4. Yes, during the last year

Note: Numbers to the left of each response represent points, which are totaled. The minimum score (i.e., for nondrinkers) is 0, and the maximum possible score is 40. Scores of 8 or more are usually considered positive for problem drinking. In some situations, lower cut-off points are appropriate.
Source: Adapted with permission from Saunders JB, Aasland OG, Babor TF, et al.

examination is unlikely to reveal abnormalities, except in chronically alcohol-dependent individuals, clinicians should remain alert for such findings as spider angiomas, palmar erythema, hepatomegaly, caput medussae, and scleral icterus, any of which suggest the possibility of chronic alcohol dependence.

Ancillary Tests

As with the physical examination, the primary use of laboratory tests relates to biomedical complications of alcoholism. However, none of these laboratory tests substitutes for direct and empathetic questioning of patients or engaging patients in conversations about dealing with their alcohol problems.

Screening

Results of a variety of blood tests, some of which are included in routine hematologic and chemistry panels, may be abnormal in persons with problem drinking. These tests include determinations of the serum gamma-glutamyl transferase (GGT) level, the mean corpuscular red blood cell volume, serum triglyceride levels, and the serum uric acid level (Table 17-9). Unfortunately, these tests have inadequate sensitivity (30 percent or lower) to be clinically useful in routine screening for problem drinking. Nonetheless, if any of these test results is abnormal in a given patient without other obvious explanation, clinicians should consider the possibility that the laboratory abnormality is due to excessive alcohol intake.

Feedback

There is evidence that the GGT level can be used as an informational feedback tool for prob-

Table 17-9

Blood Tests That May Indicate Problem Drinking

TEST	ABNORMAL VALUE
γ-Glutamyl Transferase	>30 IU
Mean corpuscular red blood cell volume	>96 fL
Serum triglycerides	>180 mg/dL
Uric acid	>7 mg/dL
Carbohydrate-deficient transferrin	>20 g/L

lem drinkers. Specifically, one study showed that men who were regularly given information about their GGT level, along with counseling about drinking, developed fewer alcohol-related problems over 5 years than did control subjects who received no information about GGT.

Confirming Intoxication

Occasionally a problem drinker will be overtly intoxicated at the time of an office visit or alcohol-related injury, or have an obvious breath odor of alcohol. In such instances, measuring breath or blood alcohol levels may be useful. During the episode of intoxication, the patient's ability to recall consumption or discuss problem drinking will usually be limited. The results of the alcohol tests, however, can provide information that can be used later in follow-up discussions with the patient or in referral to alcohol treatment programs.

Monitoring

Elevated serum levels of carbohydrate-deficient transferrin correlate with alcohol consumption above five drinks per day. While not useful in screening for alcohol use because of inadequate sensitivity, it may have value in following patients being treated for alcoholism, since it can be used to verify compliance with treatment.

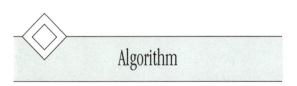

Algorithm

The National Institute on Alcohol Abuse and Alcoholism recommendations for dealing with problem drinking are summarized in the algorithm in Fig. 17-2. The basic approach involves screening patients for problem drinking. Those found to have at-risk or mild to moderate drinking problems should receive brief clinician counseling. When such counseling is not effective or if a patient has a more serious drinking problem, in-depth assessment and specialized treatment are in order.

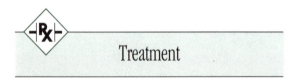

Treatment

A variety of treatments are used for problem drinking. The most common are brief interventions by clinicians and specialized alcohol treatment programs, both of which can be supplemented with administration of medications.

Brief Interventions by Clinicians

There have been more than a dozen randomized controlled clinical trials of brief office-based interventions with at-risk drinkers and patients with alcohol abuse. Most, but not all, of the studies demonstrate the interventions to be successful. On average, about 40 percent of patients in the intervention groups reduce alcohol consumption to safer levels, defined in various studies as three or four drinks per day for men and two or three drinks per day for women. In contrast, this only occurs in about 20 percent of persons who do not receive the intervention. Although these brief interventions do not eliminate the risk of alcohol complications for most drinkers, the rate of success with these interventions is better than the success rate in smoking cessation programs.

Brief office-based interventions involve four basic steps, which are outlined in Table 17-10. It should be noted that brief office-based interventions have not been studied in persons with severe alcohol dependence.

Specialized Treatment

Multiple types of specialized treatments for alcohol-use disorders are available. These include Alcoholics Anonymous and similar programs, motivational enhancement therapy, and cognitive behavioral therapy. Research indicates that these programs are effective, but there is no evidence that one treatment approach works better for most patients. Therefore, if a patient is willing to become involved with a specialized treatment program, the choice of program can be guided by the patient's preferences.

The choice of treatment venue (i.e., inpatient, residential, or outpatient) can also be guided by the patient's preferences, along with the severity of dependence, presence or absence of withdrawal symptoms, availability of social support, and biomedical complications. A reality of current medical practice is that insurance coverage often determines which therapy can be used and where it will be administered.

Medications

Medications can also play a role in helping patients with alcohol problems, including alcohol

Figure 17-2

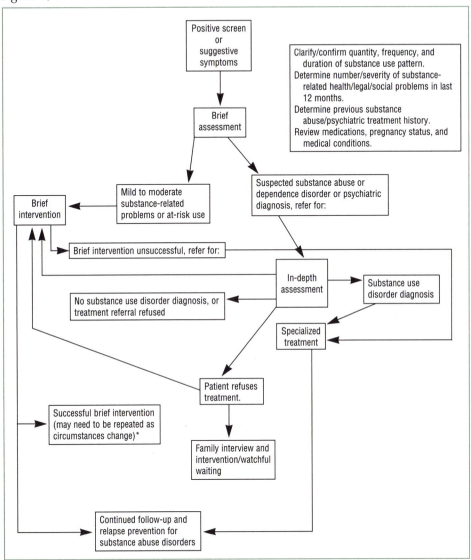

Algorithm for problem drinking, showing patient's flow through primary care and referral. *(Adapted from Brown R, in Fleming MF, Barry KL (eds): Addictive Disorders. St. Louis, Mosby-Year Book 1992.)*
*If situation deteriorates over time, a referral for specialized treatment remains an option.

dependence. The most widely used medications are naltrexone, antidepressants, and disulfram.

NALTREXONE

Naltrexone is an opioid antagonist with no opioid agonist properties. In two independent randomized clinical trials, naltrexone reduced 12-week relapse rates from 54 to 23 percent in one study, and from 80 to 40 percent in the other. While about 6 percent of patients in these clinical trials were unable to take naltrexone because of nausea, it should be considered a

Table 17-10

Four Steps in Brief Office-Based Interventions for Problem Drinking

STEP	ACTION
Ask	Screen all adolescent and adult patients, using screening instruments and interview techniques, to identify at-risk and alcohol-abusing drinkers.
Assess	Patients who screen positive should be asked for more details about the quantity and frequency of their drinking and about alcohol-related problems.
Advise	Provide problem drinkers with specific feedback, helping them understand the connection between their drinking and the problems you identify (e.g., job or marital problems, dyspepsia, hypertension, etc.).
	Tell at-risk drinkers what safe drinking limits are, advise them to reduce consumption to below those limits, and advise those who may have alcohol abuse or dependence to stop drinking completely. Keeping a diary of alcohol consumption may help patients gain an understanding of the quantity of their drinking.
	Give specific advice about steps to take, and negotiate a plan with the patient.
	Be willing to accept intermediate steps. Initially, a patient may only be willing to think about decreasing alcohol consumption.
	Point out that people can change: "You can make some positive changes in your lifestyle."
	At the same time, point out that it is the patient who must change: "It's your responsibility."
Follow-up	Primary care clinicians are in an excellent position to engage problem drinkers in ongoing discussion about alcohol consumption. Patients who are not yet ready to change sometimes make progress over time, even over years.

first-line drug, particularly for patients willing to engage in ongoing inpatient or outpatient therapy for alcohol dependence.

ANTIDEPRESSANTS

For patients who are depressed, treatment with an antidepressant should be initiated. The role of antidepressant therapy is twofold. First, it will help with depression, a therapeutic goal in and of itself. Second, at least with desipramine, it may improve a patient's coping skills and ability to succeed in decreasing alcohol consumption.

DISULFIRAM

Disulfiram is an inhibitor of aldehyde dehydrogenase, an enzyme in the pathway of alcohol metabolism. Inhibition of the enzyme causes accumulation of acetaldehyde if alcohol is consumed, resulting in a toxic acetaldehyde reaction that includes nausea, vomiting, tremor, hypertension, and other autonomic symptoms. Disulfiram is used as an aversion therapy, with patients avoiding alcohol to avoid a disulfram reaction. The drug is only marginally helpful but may be of benefit if given in the context of a social intervention by the patient's family members.

DRUGS FOR ALCOHOL WITHDRAWAL

For acute alcohol withdrawal, benzodiazepines are the drugs of choice, given either orally or parentally. They reduce the symptoms of severe withdrawal, such as hallucinations and seizures. Clonidine and beta blockers can also relieve some of the symptoms of alcohol withdrawal, including tachycardia and hypertension, but they have not been shown to reduce hallucinations or prevent withdrawal-associated seizures.

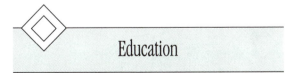

Education

Some patients are offended by what they infer is a diagnosis of alcoholism and object to discussions about the implications of their drinking problems. Furthermore, simply telling patients about the dangers of alcohol is unlikely to benefit problem drinkers or lead to a reduction in alcohol consumption. Nonetheless, an empathetic approach, frankly pointing out the connections between drinking and any medical or social problems the patient is actually experiencing, can sometimes encourage an open discussion of solutions to a patient's problem drinking.

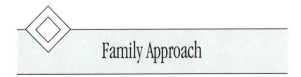

Family Approach

Family members are often greatly affected by a patient's drinking. Simply knowing that an individual's problems may be related to a family member's drinking can lead to discussions about the harm the drinker is causing others. In addition, it is useful to have open discussions involving the problem drinker and affected family members to help each individual understand the effects they have on one another. However, there is no evidence that confrontations or surprising patients with evidence that they have been drinking is of any benefit to problem drinkers.

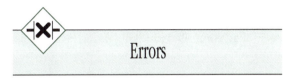

Errors

The most common error made by clinicians is failing to ask patients about drinking. Furthermore, when clinicians do ask about drinking, they are frequently unprepared to deal with an answer that indicates at-risk drinking or alcohol abuse or dependence. These errors stem in part from a misconception that alcohol problems are not present unless a patient manifests evidence of biomedical disease. As outlined in this chapter, however, many individuals have drinking patterns that put them at risk for future biomedical problems, and much can be done to help both at-risk drinkers and alcohol abusers.

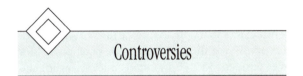

Controversies

Abstinence is the preferred goal for patients with alcohol abuse or dependence, but there is considerable controversy about whether "controlled drinking" is an acceptable alternative. Empirical studies have long demonstrated that aiming for controlled drinking is as effective as aiming for abstinence, at least among some alcoholics.

However, three-fourths of the treatment programs in the United States have abstinence as the only goal of therapy. Some experts feel that, for carefully selected patients with alcohol abuse and dependence, controlled drinking may be an acceptable intermediate goal while seeking to have the patient enter an abstinence-focused specialized treatment program. This approach is not universally accepted, and more research and education are needed to clarify the role of controlled drinking. There is little controversy, however, that controlled drinking is an acceptable approach for at-risk drinkers.

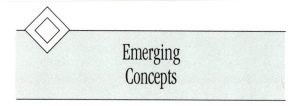

Emerging Concepts

Over the next several decades, there are likely to be several developments in the management of alcohol use problems.

Genetics

Alcohol problems have a strong genetic component, with close relatives of alcoholics having a four-fold risk of developing alcohol abuse problems in comparison to the general population. The basis for this genetic predisposition is not well understood. Continued understanding of the human genome is likely to provide reliable tests for detecting individuals at high risk of alcohol dependence even before they take their first drink. How this information will be incorporated into primary care practice, however, remains to be determined.

Neurochemistry

Developments in neurochemistry will lead to greater understanding of the biochemical basis of alcohol abuse problems. New medications will probably become available in the next few years that affect an individual's desire to consume alcohol. These new drugs, combined with increasing knowledge about behavioral therapies, are likely to lead to more effective treatment strategies.

LOW LITERACY

Barry D. Weiss

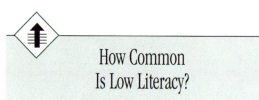

How Common Is Low Literacy?

In 1993, the U.S. Department of Education conducted the National Adult Literacy Survey (NALS), the largest systematic sampling to date of the literacy skills of the adult U.S. population. Based on testing of over 26,000 persons, NALS results estimated that 40 to 44 million people, or nearly 22 percent of the adult U.S. population, are at the lowest level of literacy skill (Table 17-11). These individuals are generally unable to read and understand basic written messages, such as a note from their child's teacher, a bus schedule, or directions for proper use of poisonous household chemicals. Another 27 percent (50 million persons) have only marginal literacy skills, greatly limiting their ability to achieve self-determined social and economic goals.

Low literacy is present in all segments of the population. It is particularly prevalent among older individuals; nearly half of those over 65 scored in the lowest level of the NALS survey. Poor literacy skills are also common among persons of lower socioeconomic status and among immigrants to the United States. However, the majority of persons in the United States with poor literacy skills are white, U.S.-born Americans. Furthermore, NALS data indicate that educational attainment does not predict reading ability, since even 20 percent of high school graduates in the NALS survey scored at the lowest level of literacy.

Table 17-11

Results of the National Adult Literacy Survey—Prose and Document Literacy

SKILL LEVEL	SAMPLE TASKS AT EACH SKILL LEVEL	U.S. ADULTS
1	Sign your name.	22%
	Identify country in a short article.	
	Locate expiration date on driver's license.	
	Locate time of meeting on a form.	
	Locate one piece of information in a sports article.	
2	Locate intersection on street map.	27%
	Locate two features of information in a sports article.	
	Identify and enter background information on applications for a social security card.	
	Interpret instructions from an appliance warranty.	
3	Identify information from a bar graph.	32%
	Write a brief letter explaining error made on a credit card bill.	
	Read a news article and identify a sentence that provides interpretation of a situation.	
	Use bus schedule to determine appropriate bus for a given set of conditions.	
	Enter information into an automobile maintenance record form.	
4	State in writing an argument made in lengthy newspaper article.	16%
	Identify percentage meeting specified conditions from a table of such information.	
	Use information table to determine pattern of oil exports over time.	
	Contrast views expressed in two editorials about technologies available to make fuel-efficient cars.	
5	Use information in table to complete graph including labeled axes.	3%
	Compare approaches stated in a narrative on growing up.	
	Using table comparing two credit cards, identify two categories used, and write two differences between them.	
	Interpret a brief phrase from a lengthy news article.	

SOURCE: From *Adult Literacy in America: A First Look at the Results of the National Adult Literacy Survey*. Washington, National Center for Education Statistics, U.S. Department of Education, 1993.

With NALS data indicating that more than half the U.S. population has low or marginal literacy skills, the problem of low literacy is pervasive in society. The broad demographic characteristics associated with low literacy suggest that, whether they know it or not, most primary care clinicians—indeed most clinicians in any specialty—see patients with poor literacy skills every day, making it one of the most common problems in primary care practice.

Why Is Low Literacy Important?

Poor Health Literacy

Poor reading skills translate into poor "health literacy": the inability to comprehend information necessary to function in health care settings. Many persons with poor literacy skills have difficulty understanding information on appointment slips or prescription medication labels. Persons with poor literacy skills frequently cannot understand educational handouts and informed consent forms because many of these documents are written at difficulty levels requiring advanced (high school level or higher) reading skills.

Patients with poor literacy are also commonly unaware of basic health information. For example, low literacy skills are associated with less frequent use of preventive health services, such as mammography and cervical cancer screening. Many persons with poor literacy skills do not know that high blood pressure can be lowered with weight loss and exercise, and only half of diabetics with low literacy know the symptoms of hypoglycemia. Poor literacy skills correlate with improper use of metered-dose inhalers by patients with asthma and a variety of other less-than optimal health behaviors.

Poor Health Outcomes

Poor literacy skills are associated with poor health outcomes. Research has shown that, as a group, persons with limited literacy skills have poorer physical and psychological health than do those with better reading skills (Fig. 17-3). These relationships are most well established for persons with extremely low reading skills (i.e., grade levels 0 through 3), and they persist even after accounting for covariables such as age, income, employment status, education level, and ethnic background. In fact, several studies have

Figure 17-3

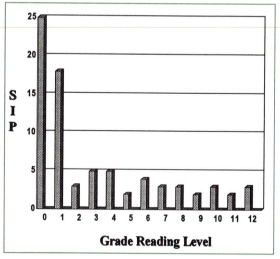

Relationship between reading level and physical illness. The graph shows that persons with lower reading levels have higher levels of physical illness, as measured with the Sickness Impact Profile (SIP). (*Data from Weiss BD, Hart G, McGee D, et al.*)

found literacy to be a stronger correlate of health status than any other sociodemographic variable.

Persons at the lowest level of literacy also use the health care system more frequently than do others. In comparison to those with more well-developed literacy skills, individuals at the lowest level of literacy have twice the likelihood of being hospitalized and make an average of two to three more visits to clinicians each year. In some indigent Medicaid populations, the annual health care bills for individuals with poor literacy skills are four times higher than the bills of enrollees with more highly developed literacy skills (Fig. 17-4). These findings are unaffected by sociodemographic variables and occur even when all subjects in a study are of similar socio-economic status.

The mechanism by which poor literacy translates into poorer health outcomes is unknown. Several theories have been put forth, including suggestions that persons with low literacy skills (1) make more medication or treatment errors, (2) are unable to comply with treatments, (3) fail

Figure 17-4

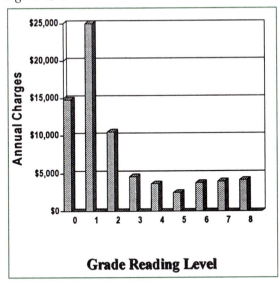

Relationship between reading level and annual health care costs. Among randomly selected patients enrolled in a man-aged-Medicaid program because of medical indigence, persons with very low grade-equivalent reading levels have annual charges for health care that are three to five times higher than those of persons with more well-developed reading skills.

to seek preventive care, and (4) lack the self-empowerment needed to successfully negotiate today's health care system.

Effects on Clinical Tests

Poor literacy skills can affect the results of common clinical tests, such as the Mini-Mental State Examination for detection of dementia. Because several of the items on this test are reading- and language-dependent, nonreaders and individuals with very limited reading may score similarly to patients with dementia. In fact, multiple studies have shown that the correlation of Mini-Mental State Examination scores with literacy level is stronger than the correlation with any other sociodemographic variable, including education.

Literacy skills may also influence the results of other clinical tests. These include intelligence tests, tests to assess patients with aphasia, and screening for a variety of psychological and medical conditions with written screening instruments, such as the depression and anxiety screening instruments discussed in Chaps. 8 and 9.

Medicolegal Implications

Several national health care accreditation organizations have established policies that have a bearing on patients with limited literacy. The National Committee for Quality Assurance has issued guidelines about written materials provided to clientele of managed care organizations. The Joint Commission on Accreditation of Health Care Organizations requires health care organizations to ensure that patients can understand important medical documents, such as consent forms and discharge instructions. Legal experts indicate that these and other published guidelines establish a "standard of care" that requires clinicians to ensure that patients understand information provided to them by health care providers—a standard of care that is not always met.

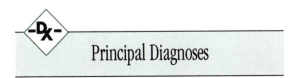

Principal Diagnoses

For practicing clinicians, the most important diagnostic issue is determining whether a patient can understand medical information provided to them. Relatively less emphasis is placed on actually measuring patients' literacy skills or determining why an individual reads poorly.

It is typically assumed that some persons have poor reading skills simply because they grew up in families or social situations that placed little value on acquisition of reading skills and received little reinforcement in their homes to acquire those skills. Poor literacy in such individuals is also commonly attributed to failures of the public education system, with many students being passed from year to year in school without developing grade-appropriate reading skills. Some persons are thought to read poorly because of "disuse;" that is, reading skills may regress if not continually used and reinforced, a phenomenon that may explain poor reading skills in some older individuals. In the case of individuals born in other nations, a growing proportion of the population in many English-speaking countries, it is often assumed that these individuals emigrated from countries with poorly developed education systems or that they read only in languages other than English.

While the above-noted factors contribute to and explain literacy problems in many cases, there is also evidence that, for many poor readers, those factors provide an overly simplistic explanation for their limited literacy skills. Specifically, recent research involving urban populations has revealed that a high percentage, perhaps more than half, of persons with poor reading skills have various neurocognitive disorders (e.g., learning disabilities such as dyslexia). These individuals were not recognized as having learning disabilities during childhood, and their poor academic progress in school was incorrectly attributed to attention deficit disorder, behavior problems, lack of motivation, or low intelligence. Awareness that neurocognitive disorders are common in low-literacy individuals may lead to better identification of learning disabilities in the adult low-literacy population.

Typical Presentation

Low literacy is truly a hidden problem. Most individuals with limited literacy skills do not

readily share this limitation with others. In fact, research indicates that poor literacy is associated with a great deal of shame, and most low-literacy individuals go to great lengths to conceal their reading problems from others, even from family members. Thus, clinicians are rarely aware that patients cannot read or read poorly.

There are clues, however, that may suggest that a patient's literacy skills are poor. These include patients' responses to being given written forms and behaviors noted in the course of clinical interviews and medical care. Some of these clues are listed in Table 17-12.

Table 17-12

Clues That a Patient May Have Poor Literacy Skills

BEHAVIORS WHEN DEALING WITH FORMS, QUESTIONNAIRES, AND OTHER WRITTEN MATERIALS
Registration and other forms filled out incompletely or incorrectly
Forms and other materials handed to relative or other accompanying individual
Patient says: "I will read this at home."
Patient says: "I'd like to bring this home so my daughter (or other relative) can read it."
Patient says: "I can't read this now, I forgot my glasses."
RESPONSES TO THE MEDICAL INTERVIEW
Inappropriate or confusing responses to questions
Aloofness or withdrawal during questioning or explanations
BEHAVIORS IN THE COURSE OF CLINICAL CARE
Frequent noncompliance with treatments
Frequent missed appointments
Failure to obtain recommended consultations or ancillary tests
Medication errors

Key History and Physical Examination

While few experts advocate directly asking patients about their reading skills, it is possible to use the medical history to identify factors increasing the likelihood that a patient has limited literacy. The most basic history questions pertinent to literacy are about educational attainment (i.e., years of school completed) and occupation; such questions should be in the routine medical history for all new patients. As noted earlier, educational attainment and occupation do not translate directly into reading skill, but patients who did not complete high school or who are unemployed or work at unskilled occupations are at higher than average risk of having poor literacy skills.

It is also appropriate to ask patients if they ever have difficulty understanding information given to them by clinicians. An affirmative response to this question may facilitate a dialogue leading to an understanding of patients' reading and health literacy skills.

Physical examination, obviously, offers no direct information about literacy skills. However, careful observation of patient's behaviors and "body language" when presented with written materials or medical explanations may reveal a discomfort or aloofness that might be a sign of limited literacy.

Ancillary Tests

Many testing instruments are available for measuring reading skills (Table 17-13). Use of these instruments is widely advocated in the medical literature. As discussed later, however, the role

and potential benefits of literacy testing in clinical practice are controversial.

Reading assessment instruments include word recognition tests, reading comprehension tests, cloze procedures (see below), and others. Word recognition tests involve presenting patients with a list of words of increasing difficulty and complexity. Patients are asked to pronounce the words out loud, beginning with the simplest word and progressing to more difficult words. The difficulty level at which patients are unable to properly pronounce words translates into an approximate grade-equivalent reading level.

Reading comprehension tests present subjects with text to read and then ask the subject questions about the text. The cloze procedure presents subjects with text from which selected words have been omitted and replaced by blank spaces. Subjects must fill in the blank spaces with appropriate words. Those who understand the text are able to insert appropriate words into the blank spaces because they understand the contextual content of the text. Some reading instruments involve more complex testing techniques, and others use a combination of methods.

In clinical practice, the most widely used instrument is the Rapid Estimate of Adult Literacy in Medicine (REALM), an instrument specifically designed to measure reading skills in clinical settings. The REALM is a word recognition test in which all the words are medical words, and when scored it gives an approximate reading level that is sufficient to guide efforts to educate the patient. The reliability and validity of REALM reading level estimates compare favorably to other, more detailed and sophisticated reading assessment instruments. The REALM test and scoring instructions are shown in Table 17-14.

The only important limitation of the REALM is that it cannot be used to measure literacy skills in languages other than English. Several Spanish-language instruments are available, but they are relatively complex and require substantially more time to administer than does the REALM.

Table 17-13

Instruments for Assessment of Literacy Skills

INSTRUMENT	ACRONYM	COMMENTS
WORD RECOGNITION TESTS		
Rapid Estimate of Adult Literacy in Medicine	REALM	Most widely used in medical settings, uses medical words, requires 2–3 min to administer
Slosson Oral Reading Test	SORT	Generally used for assessing reading skills of children in school settings
Wide-Range Achievement Test	WRAT	Most widely used test in academic settings, better for measuring reading skills at higher levels
READING COMPREHENSION AND CLOZE TESTS		
Test of Functional Health Literacy in Adults	TOFHLA	Tests understanding of medical concepts with reading comprehension and cloze techniques, requires 15–20 min to administer
SPANISH-LANGUAGE TESTS		
Instrumento para Diagnosticar Lecturas	IDL	Bilingual (English-Spanish) reading comprehension test, requires 20–30 min to administer
Test of Functional Health Literacy in Adults—Spanish	TOFHLA-S	Same as English-language TOFLHA, but translated into and validated in Spanish

NOTE: The instruments listed in this table are those most often discussed in the medical literature. Many other reading assessment instruments are available.

Treatment

Adult Literacy Programs

Treatment of literacy, per se, involves special educational techniques that are not within the skills of most clinicians. However, many communities have private or publicly funded adult education programs specifically designed to teach reading skills to adults. Clinicians should familiarize themselves with the availability of these programs and make appropriate referrals when patients are found to have limited literacy. The National Institute for Literacy (phone number 202-632-1500), a federal agency established to coordinate literacy programs throughout the United States, can provide information about state and local programs.

Communicating with Patients Who Have Low Literacy

For clinicians, the most important issue in dealing with low-literacy patients is to establish effective communication, providing patients with essential information about their medical conditions and treatments. This communication can sometimes be achieved with written materials if they are constructed at appropriately low reading levels. For many patients, however, non-written methods of communication may be preferable, including various forms of media

Table 17-14

The Rapid Estimate of Adult Literacy in Medicine (REALM) Test

Instructions: Give REALM instrument to patient. Say, "I want to hear you read as many words as you can from this list. Begin with the first word on list 1 and read out loud. When you come to a word you cannot read, do the best you can or say "blank" and go on to the next word." If the patient takes more than 5 s on a word, say "blank" and have the patient go on to the next word. When patients begin to miss every word, have them say only known words.

List 1	List 2	List 3
Fat	Fatigue	Allergic
Flu	Pelvic	Menstrual
Pill	Jaundice	Testicle
Dose	Infection	Colitis
Eye	Exercise	Emergency
Stress	Behavior	Medication
Smear	Prescription	Occupation
Nerves	Notify	Sexually
Germs	Gallbladder	Alcoholism
Meals	Calories	Irritation
Disease	Depression	Constipation
Cancer	Miscarriage	Gonorrhea
Caffeine	Pregnancy	Inflammatory
Attack	Arthritis	Diabetes
Kidney	Nutrition	Hepatitis
Hormones	Menopause	Antibiotics
Herpes	Appendix	Diagnosis
Seizure	Abnormal	Potassium
Bowel	Syphilis	Anemia
Asthma	Hemorrhoids	Obesity
Rectal	Nausea	Osteoporosis
Incest	Directed	Impetigo

NOTE: *Scoring instructions:* Count the number of correctly pronounced words in each list and add the three numbers together. Determine reading grade level from table below:

Score	Grade Level	Interpretation
0–23	Below 3rd grade	Cannot read even most low-literacy materials
24–44	4th to 6th grade	Will need low-literacy materials
45–59	7th to 8th grade	May struggle with "regular" written materials
60–66	High school	Can read most patient education materials

SOURCE: Copyright Terry Davis. Used with permission.

and/or face-to-face discussion. In all cases, the approach to communication should be specifically tailored to the needs and skills of individual patients.

WRITTEN INFORMATION

When it is essential to use written (text) materials with low-literacy patients, these materials should be written at the lowest reading level possible, generally at the fifth-grade level or lower. Computer-based word processors contain grammar review functions that calculate reading levels of text, based on mathematical formulas that rely on word length and sentence length. In these formulas, low grade-level text typically has simple words of no more than one or two syllables, and short sentences that contain no more than one phrase per sentence. While useful as a general guide to a text's complexity, computer calculations of reading level alone are not sufficient for creating materials that will be understood by a low-literacy audience.

Rather, in addition to using simple words and sentences, written materials for low-literacy populations must also have other characteristics. The vocabulary must avoid medical or technical jargon, and should use words and concepts that are culturally appropriate for the target audience. Use of large type and liberal use of open (unprinted) space is also important to readability. Effective communication with written materials can be further enhanced by the use of pictures to highlight important concepts. Sources of information about creating effective low-literacy written health education materials are listed in Table 17-15.

Table 17-15

Guides to Creating Low-Literacy Educational Materials for Patients

Beyond the Brochure: Alternative Approaches to Effective Health Communication. AMC Cancer Research Center, 1600 Pierce St., Denver, Colorado 80214.

Clear and Simple: Developing Effective Print Materials for Low-Literate Readers, NIH publication no 95-3594. Available from National Cancer Institute, Cancer Information Service; phone 1-800-4-CANCER.

Doak CC, Doak LG, Root J: *Teaching Patients with Low Literacy Skills*, 2d ed. Philadelphia, Lippincott, 1996.

Doak and Doak emphasize three essential components of well-designed educational materials for patients. First, they must be interactive. Materials that engage learners' participation, rather than simply present information, are more effective for adult learners. Second, pictures and other visuals should tell a story, rather than present information or data. In fact, comic strip formats (or picture books or photonovellas) are particularly useful ways to present information. Third, patients should be given the opportunity to review and practice information to enhance the likelihood of retention.

It should also be emphasized that simply giving printed documents to patients, even if written at an easy reading level, does not necessarily constitute effective communication. Instead, effective communication requires clinicians to ensure that patients understand the concepts important to medical care and that pertinent questions have been answered. Furthermore, while short-term comprehension of medical information can be enhanced with low-literacy information, there is only limited evidence that using such materials improves long-term medical outcomes. Research is needed to confirm the value of using low-literacy education materials.

NONWRITTEN INFORMATION

Most individuals report obtaining medical and other information from television and radio, not from written sources. In addition, research indicates that, among non-English-speaking individuals, oral speech (via media or in person) is probably the most widely used form of communication. Thus, it may be appropriate, if not preferable, to use any of several nonwritten modalities to provide patients with important educational information, including anatomic models, audiotapes, and videotapes. Numerous nonprofit and for-profit organizations produce such nonwritten materials, some of which are specifically designed for low-literacy audiences. Several studies have demonstrated improved comprehension when these nonwritten modalities are used for education of patients. However, as with low-literacy written materials, there is little evidence that using nonwritten educational materials has a beneficial effect on long-term disease outcomes.

In the end, the essential objective is to ensure that patients understand information important to treatment and prevention of medical problems. Depending on the patient, the clinical setting, and the resources available to the patient and clinician, any of the abovementioned communication methods, or a variety of them, may be necessary to achieve that objective. These methods also include face-to-face verbal communication and/or referral to patient educators and others who can spend sufficient time with patients to help them learn what they need to know.

Family Approach

When dealing with patients who have poor literacy skills, involvement of families is often critical. Many poor readers, especially older individuals, already rely heavily on family members or friends to read for them or to them, and to interpret information provided by clinicians. If acceptable to patients, involving these family members or friends in medical discussions can enhance communication between health care providers and patients.

Errors

Without doubt, the major error that clinicians make in communicating with low-literacy patients is not recognizing limited literacy and thus presenting information in ways that patients do not understand. This error can easily be avoided if clinicians do not assume that all patients can read and by taking steps to confirm that patients understand what they need to know. This confirmation can often be achieved by simply asking patients to explain concepts of importance. Inability to grasp basic concepts may signal a problem with health literacy and warrant more intensive and personalized educational efforts.

The other common error, often made by well-meaning clinicians who recognize the importance and prevalence of literacy problems, is excessive reliance on computer-scored low-reading-level text. As noted earlier, computer programs assign reading difficulty levels to text based only on mathematical formulas that ignore the format and context of the material being presented. For this reason, educational handouts based solely on computer-scored reading levels are often ineffective in communicating key concepts to patients.

Controversies

Should Clinicians Test Patients' Literacy Skills?

Some experts recommend that individual patients' literacy skills be tested upon entry into a medical practice, as part of routine intake information. As noted above, this can be easily accomplished with instruments such as the REALM. However, the majority of experts in health literacy disagree with the notion of routine testing, since the benefits of routinely identifying the literacy skills of all patients have not been demonstrated.

Instead, many experts recommend testing a sample of patients in a medical practice to determine the approximate or average reading skill level of the practice's clientele. This permits clinicians in the practice to gear educational materials for patients to an appropriate level.

Others suggest that low-literacy educational materials, whether in written or nonwritten forms, are the preferred mode of health education for *all* patients in a practice, regardless of literacy skills. There is considerable evidence that most individuals, even those with advanced levels of education and literacy, prefer simple and easy-to-understand materials to more complex information and are not offended when given information presented at a grade level below their reading skill. Furthermore, comprehension of such documents as consent forms is improved when they are presented in simpler fashion, regardless of the reader's literacy skill.

Is Simplification Desirable?

Some clinicians argue that using low-literacy educational materials represents "dumbing down" of educational material, making it impossible to present information in a sufficiently comprehensive fashion. It is further argued that the appropriate response to the societal problem of low literacy is not to reduce complexity of information but, rather, to improve the population's literacy skills. Most health literacy experts respond to this concern by pointing out that, while improving population literacy is a worthwhile goal, it is not achievable in the short term and certainly not within the skills of the medical profession to do so. Instead, if it is important for patients to understand medical concepts and information pertinent to their care, clinicians should use whatever format and communication method is effective to transmit the necessary information. For a major proportion of the population, this involves simplified presentations of information.

What Is the Value of Using Low-Literacy Materials?

Because of evidence that poor literacy skills are a risk factor for adverse health outcomes and higher health care costs, substantial resources, on both the local and national levels, are devoted to creating low-literacy educational materials for patients. Despite these efforts, there is a paucity of evidence that developing and using educational materials specially designed for low-literacy populations offer any advantage to patients in terms of long-term medical outcomes. Additional research is necessary to determine the benefit of special communication strategies for low-literacy populations.

Emerging Concepts

The rapid development of computer technologies such as CD-ROM and the Internet is creating new opportunities for educating patients. At this time, however, patients with low literacy, who frequently have limited financial resources, have limited access to these technologies. In the future, the decreasing cost of these technologies will make them more accessible to larger percentages of the population, and it is likely that media- and computer-based educational materials will become the predominant form in which clinicians and health educators provide education to patients.

With these technologies, it is possible to create educational materials that are truly interactive. They can involve patients in a hands-on interchange, vary content according to patients' needs and knowledge, and present information with graphics, moving pictures, and sound instead of text. As these technologies develop further, they will be increasingly easy for patients to use.

Several studies have shown that using nonwritten modalities enhances patients' learning, increases their knowledge, decreases their anxiety, and, according to some studies, improves short-term medical outcomes. However, as with written materials, there is not yet evidence that long-term clinical outcomes are improved by using media-based or other nonwritten communication modalities. Ongoing study is necessary to ensure that these increasingly technological methods of communication achieve the desired effect.

Bibliography

Domestic Violence

Abbott J, Johnson R, Koziol-McClain J, et al: Domestic violence against women: Incidence and prevalence in an emergency department population. *JAMA* 273:1763, 1995.

Bergman B, Brismar B: A 5-year follow-up study of 117 battered women. *Am J Public Health* 81:1486, 1991.

Brookoff D, O'Brien KK, Cook CS, et al: Characteristics of participants in domestic violence. *JAMA* 277:1369, 1997.

Elliott BA, Johnson MP: Domestic violence in a primary care setting: Patterns and prevalence. *Arch Fam Med* 4:113, 1994.

Feldhous KM, Koziol-McClain J, Amsbury HL, et al: Accuracy of 3 brief screening questions for detecting partner violence in the emergency department. *JAMA* 277:1357, 1997.

Gleason WJ: Mental disorders in battered women: An empirical study. *Violence and Victims* 8:53, 1993.

Hamberger LK, Ambuel B, Marbella A: Physician interaction with battered women: The women's perspective. *Arch Fam Med* 1998.

Hamberger LK, Lohr JM, Bonge D, et al: An empirical classification of motivations for domestic violence. *Violence against Women* 3:401, 1997.

Hamberger LK, Saunders DG, Hovey M: Prevalence of domestic violence in community practice and rate of physician inquiry. *Fam Med* 24:283, 1992.

Jacobson NS, Gottman JM, Gortner E: Psychological factors in the longitudinal course of battering: When do couples split up? When does the abuse decrease? *Violence and Victims* 11:371, 1996.

Johnson M, Elliott BA: Domestic violence among family practice patients in midsized and rural communities. *J Fam Pract* 44:391, 1997.

McCauley J, Kern DE, Kolonder K, et al: The "Battering syndrome": Prevalence and clinical characteristics of domestic violence in primary care internal medicine practices. *Ann Intern Med* 123:737, 1995.

Saunders DG, Hamberger LK, Hovey M: Indicators of woman abuse based on a chart review at a family practice center. *Arch Fam Med* 2:537, 1993.

Stets JE, Straus MA: The marriage license as a hitting license: A comparison of assaults in dating, cohabiting and married couples. *J Fam Violence* 41:33, 1989.

Straus MA: Measuring intrafamily conflict and violence: The Conflict Tactics (CT) Scales. *J Marr Fam* 41:75, 1979.

Wagner PJ, Mongan PF: Validating the concept of abuse:. Women's perceptions of defining behaviors and the effects of emotional abuse on health indicators. *Arch Fam Med* 7:25, 1998.

Problem Drinking

Bradley KA, Boyd-Wickizer J, Powell SH, et al: Alcohol screening questionnaires in women. A critical review. *JAMA* 280:166, 1998.

Buchsbaum DG, Buchanan RG, Centor RM, et al: Screening for alcohol abuse using CAGE scores and likelihood ratios. *Ann Intern Med* 115:774, 1991.

Deitz D, Rohde F, Bertolucci D, et al: Prevalence of screening for alcohol use by physicians during routine physical examinations. *Alcohol Health Res World* 18:162, 1994.

Fleming MF, Barry KL, Manwell LB, et al: Brief physician advice for problem alcohol drinkers. *JAMA* 277:1039, 1997.

Frazier EL, Okoro CA, Smith C, et al: State- and sex-specific prevalence of selected characteristics: Behavioral Risk Factor Surveillance System, 1994 and 1995. *Morb Mort Week Rep CDC Surv Summ* 46(SS-3):1, 1997.

Grant BF, Harford TC, Dawson DA, et al: Prevalence of DSM-IV alcohol abuse and dependence: United States, 1992. *Alcohol Health Res World* 18:243, 1994.

Litten RZ, Allen JP, Fertig JB: Gamma-glutamyl-transpeptidase and carbohydrate deficient transferrin: Alternative measures of excessive alcohol consumption. *Alcohol Clin Exp Res* 19:1541, 1995.

Mason BJ, Kocsis JH, Ritvo EC, et al: A double-blind, placebo-controlled trial of desipramine for primary alcohol dependence stratified on the presence or absence of major depression. *JAMA* 275:761, 1996.

Mayo-Smith MF: Pharmacological management of alcohol withdrawal: A meta-analysis and evidence-based practice guideline. *JAMA* 278:144, 1997.

National Institute on Alcohol Abuse and Alcoholism: *The Physician's Guide to Helping Patients with Alcohol Problems*. Bethesda, MD, National Institutes of Health, 1995 (available at http://www.niaaa.nih.gov/publications/physicn.htm).

O'Conner PG, Schottenfeld RS: Patients with alcohol problems. *New Engl J Med* 338:592, 1998.

O'Malley SS, Jaffe AJ, Chang G, et al: Naltrexone and coping skills therapy for alcohol dependence: A controlled study. *Arch Gen Psychiatry* 49:881, 1992.

Project MATCH Research Group: Matching alcohol treatments to client heterogeneity: Project MATCH posttreatment drinking outcomes. *J Stud Alcohol* 58:7, 1997.

Rosenberg H, Davis LA: Acceptance of moderate drinking by alcohol treatment services in the United States. *J Stud Alcohol* 55:167, 1994.

Saunders JB, Aasland OG, Babor TF, et al: Development of the Alcohol Use Disorders Identification Test (AUDIT): WHO Collaborative Project on Early Detection of Persons with Harmful Alcohol Consumption—II. *Addiction* 88:791, 1993.

Taj N, Devera-Sales A, Vinson DC: Screening for problem drinking: Does a single question work? *J Fam Pract* 46:328, 1998.

Volpicelli JR, Alterman AI, Hayashida M, et al: Naltrexone in the treatment of alcohol dependence. *Arch Gen Psychiatry* 49:876, 1992.

Wilk AI, Jensen NM, Havighurst TC: Meta-analysis of randomized control trials addressing brief interventions in heavy alcohol drinkers. *J Gen Intern Med* 12:274, 1997.

Low Literacy

Baker DW, Parker RM, Williams MV, et al: The relationship of patient reading ability to self-reported health and use of health services. *Am J Public Health* 87:1027, 1997.

Baker DW, Parker RM, Williams MV, et al: The health care experience of patients with low literacy. *Arch Fam Med* 5:329, 1996.

Brandes WL, Furnas S, McClellan FM: *Literacy, Health, and the Law*. Philadelphia, Health Promotion Council of Southeastern Pennsylvania, 1996.

Davis TC, Long SW, Jackson RH, et al: Rapid estimate of adult literacy in medicine: A shortened screening instrument. *Fam Med* 25:391, 1993.

Davis T, Michielutte R, Askov EN, et al: Practical assessment of adult literacy in health care. *Health Educ Behav* 25:613, 1998.

Doak CC, Doak LG, Root JH: *Teaching Patients with Low Literacy Skills*, 2d ed. Philadelphia, Lippincott, 1996.

Doak LG, Doak CC, Meade CD: Strategies to improve cancer education materials. *Oncol Nurs Forum* 23:1305, 1996.

Gottesman RL, Bennet RE, Nathan RG, et al: Inner-city adults with severe reading difficulties: A closer look. *J Reading Disabil* 29:589, 1996.

Kelly MS, Gottesman RL: Adults with severe reading and learning difficulties: A challenge for the family physician. *J Am Board Fam Pract* 10:199, 1997.

Kirsch I, Jungeblut A, Jenkins L, et al: *Adult Literacy in America: A First Look at the Results of the National Adult Literacy Survey*. Washington, National Center for Education Statistics, U.S. Department of Education, 1993.

Mostenthal PB, Kirsch IS: A new measure for assessing document complexity: The PMOSE/IKIRSCH document readability formula. *J Adolesc Adult Literacy* 41:63, 1998.

Plimpton S, Root J: Materials and strategies that work in low literacy health communication. *Public Health Rep* 109:86, 1994.

Sugarman J, McCrory DC, Hubal RC: Getting meaningful informed consent from older adults: A structured literature review of empirical research. *J Am Geriatr Soc* 46:517, 1998.

Weiss BD, Blanchard JS, McGee DL, et al: Illiteracy among Medicaid recipients and its relationship to health care costs. *J Health Care Poor Underserved* 5:99, 1994.

Weiss BD, Coyne CA: Communicating with patients who cannot read. *New Engl J Med* 337:272, 1997.

Weiss BD, Coyne C, Michielutte R, et al: Communicating with patients who have limited literacy skills: Report of the National Work Group on Literacy and Health. *J Fam Pract* 46:168, 1998.

Weiss BD, Hart G, McGee D, et al: Health status of illiterate adults: Relation between literacy and health status among persons with low-literacy skills. *J Am Board Fam Pract* 5:257, 1992.

Weiss BD, Reed RL, Kligman EW, et al: Literacy and

performance on the Mini-Mental State Examination. *J Am Geriatr Soc* 43:807, 1995.

Williams DM, Counselman FL, Caggiano CD: Emergency department discharge instructions and patient literacy: A problem of disparity. *Am J Emerg Med* 14:19, 1996.

Williams MV, Baker DW, Parker RM, et al: Relationship of functional health literacy to patients' knowledge of their chronic disease: A study of patients with hypertension or diabetes. *Arch Intern Med* 158:166, 1998.

Williams MV, Parker RM, Baker DW, et al: Inadequate functional health literacy among patients at two public hospitals. *JAMA* 274:1677, 1995.

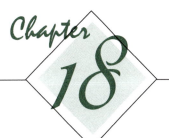

Mark H. Ebell
Henry C. Barry

Chapter 18

Urinary Tract Infection

How Common Are Urinary Tract Infections?

Urinary tract infections (UTIs) are among the most common acute medical problems affecting women. Women in the United States make more than 7 million visits to clinicians each year for management of UTIs, at a cost conservatively estimated to exceed $500 million. Approximately 20 to 30 percent of women will have at least one UTI in their lifetime, and about half of women experiencing one UTI will have another. Thus, it is not surprising that in the National Ambulatory Medical Care Survey, UTI and its symptoms are among the top 20 reasons for seeking care from physicians in the United States. With the exception of prostatitis, UTIs rarely affect men. Thus, this chapter will focus primarily on urinary tract infections in adult women.

Principal Diagnoses

A number of host defenses act in concert to provide natural protection against UTIs. These defense mechanisms include normal voiding, which mechanically flushes bacteria out of the bladder; the acidic pH of urine, which suppresses growth of bacteria; and intrinsic immunologic functions of the bladder mucosa. Despite these protective mechanisms, however, UTIs still occur. They are most common in women, probably because the short length of the female urethra is an insufficient barrier to perineal and perirectal flora entering the bladder.

When UTIs occur, they include a spectrum of conditions ranging from mild infections of the bladder mucosa to severe, complicated infec-

tions of the renal parenchyma. Among women seen in primary care practice, the most common UTIs are acute uncomplicated cystitis, recurrent cystitis, and urethritis. In addition, pyelonephritis and infections classified as complicated, because of underlying conditions, are sufficiently common to warrant discussion.

Acute Uncomplicated Cystitis

The most common urinary tract infection is acute uncomplicated cystitis (infection of the urinary bladder), also referred to as lower UTI. Most acute uncomplicated lower UTIs are caused by ascending infection from the perineal and perianal areas. Therefore, the usual infecting bacteria are fecal organisms, the most common of which is *Escherichia coli*. *Staphylococcus saprophyticus* and enterococci are the next most frequent causes of infection. Other gram-negative bowel flora may also infect the bladder but are uncommon in women with simple uncomplicated cystitis.

Recurrent Cystitis

Recurrent cystitis is usually defined as more than three episodes of cystitis per year. Recurrent infections may represent reappearance of the original infecting bacteria after cessation of antibiotic therapy (relapse) or infection with a new strain after the original bacteria has been eradicated (reinfection). Reinfection accounts for the vast majority of recurrent UTIs. The infecting organisms in recurrent UTIs are usually the same as those causing acute uncomplicated cystitis, but they may also include other species of bacteria, such as *Proteus*, *Klebsiella*, *Pseudomonas*, and others.

Many women with recurrent UTIs have identifiable risk factors that predispose them to recurrence. These factors include pregnancy, prior infections of the upper urinary tract, use of a contraceptive diaphragm, residual urine after voiding, and compromised host defenses due to systemic illness. In some women, sexual activity that is more frequent or vigorous than usual can increase the risk of recurrent UTIs.

Urethritis

In addition to infecting the bladder, lower UTIs usually also involve the urethra. However, some women develop urethritis without cystitis. Isolated urethritis typically occurs in women with sexually transmitted diseases. In such individuals, *Chlamydia trachomatis* is the most common cause of urethritis. *Neisseria gonorrhea* and herpes simplex type II are also common causes of sexually transmitted urethritis.

Pyelonephritis

Pyelonephritis is typically a complication of cystitis resulting from ascent of infecting organisms from the bladder to the kidney. Pyelonephritis can be caused not only by *E. coli* and enterococcus but also by a variety of other gram-negative bacteria, including *Proteus*, *Klebsiella*, and various species of *Pseudomonas*. Pyelonephritis can be a serious, life-threatening condition accompanied by bacteremia and sepsis syndrome. It may also be relatively mild and amenable to outpatient therapy.

Complicated UTIs

Because they are at higher risk of developing pyelonephritis and other complications, women with certain underlying conditions are considered to have "complicated" UTIs, even if they appear to have only simple cystitis. This group of women includes those who are pregnant or who have diabetes, urolithiasis, or structural anomalies of the urinary tract. Urinary infections in such patients can be caused by the same individual organisms that are involved in pyelonephritis, but the infections may also be polymicrobial.

Typical Presentation

In primary care practice, young and middle-aged women with cystitis and urethritis, whether acute or recurrent, usually present with one or more typical symptoms. These symptoms include dysuria, urinary frequency, nocturia, and urinary urgency, but the entire constellation of symptoms is present in only a minority of patients with UTI. In all likelihood, however, most patients present with a complaint of, "I think I have a bladder infection." As described later, more often than not, these patients are exactly right.

In contrast to the situation in young and middle-aged women, geriatric-aged or debilitated women often lack or cannot verbalize the typical symptoms of UTI. Instead, such patients may present with unexplained incontinence, fever, weakness, or changes in mental status. Clinicians must be alert for the possibility of UTI in such patients and rely more heavily on laboratory tests to make the diagnosis.

Finally, the presentation of UTI is somewhat different in urologic practice than it is in primary care practice. Patients presenting to urologists more often have a history of frequent or complicated urinary infections and a greater likelihood of having structural abnormalities in the urinary tract. Therefore, imaging studies and cystoscopy are needed more frequently in urology practice than in primary care settings. Similarly, the higher rate of recurrent infections in patients seen by urologists, and the concomitant likelihood of past exposure to multiple antibiotics results in a greater prevalence of antibiotic-resistant infections in urologic practice. Thus, urine cultures and antibiotic sensitivity testing are often indicated in urology practice, while they are often unnecessary in primary care settings.

Key History

Taking a history in patients with suspected UTI has three main objectives. The first objective is to make a diagnosis of UTI. The second is to detect clues suggesting the possibility of pyelonephritis. The third objective of the history is to identify patients with risk factors for complicated infections and those in need of special evaluation or treatments.

Diagnosis of Urinary Tract Infection

Most patients (70 percent) presenting to a primary care clinician with a suspected UTI have already made a correct self-diagnosis. Soliciting information about dysuria, frequency, and urgency does little to increase the already high likelihood of UTI, and the absence of any of these symptoms does not rule out the diagnosis.

The only important caveat is the need to ask whether the patient has a vaginal discharge. The presence of a vaginal discharge in women with symptoms of UTI is highly suggestive of vaginitis, rather than UTI, and substantially reduces that likelihood that UTI is present. In fact, only about 30 percent of such women have a UTI.

The test characteristics of the symptoms most commonly associated with UTI are summarized in Table 18-1. These test characteristics include the sensitivity, specificity, and likelihood ratios for each symptom, as well as the resulting likelihood that a UTI is present. As shown in the table, the symptoms and history most strongly associated with the presence of UTI are nocturia, dysuria, and previous UTI, although none is as strongly associated as a woman's self-report that she has a UTI. Because most women who think

Table 18-1

Operating Characteristics of History and Physical Examination in Suspected UTI

| | | | | | LIKELIHOOD OF UTI | |
SYMPTOM OR SIGN	SENSITIVITY, %	SPECIFICITY, %	LR+	LR−	WITH SYMPTOM OR SIGN, %	WITHOUT SYMPTOM OR SIGN, %
Nocturia	67	62	1.8	0.6	80	55
Dysuria	75	52	1.6	0.6	79	53
Previous UTI	40	75	1.6	0.6	79	65
Urgency	35	75	1.4	0.7	77	67
Frequency	87	32	1.3	0.4	75	49
Offensive odor of urine	20	85	1.3	0.9	76	69
Combination of dysuria, frequency, and urgency	84	40	1.4	0.4	77	48

NOTE: Data in the table are calculated on the assumption that 70 percent of patients with suspected UTI actually have a UTI. The positive likelihood ratio (LR+) is the percentage of patients with UTI divided by the percentage of patients without UTI among patients with a particular symptom or sign. The negative likelihood ratio (LR−) is the percentage of patients with disease divided by the percentage of patients without disease among patients without a particular symptom or sign. A likelihood ratio > 1 means that disease is more likely with (or without) the sign or symptom, and a likelihood ratio < 1 means that disease is less likely.

they have a UTI actually have one, the presence of any single symptom of UTI makes the likelihood of UTI more than 75 to 80 percent in most primary care settings.

Detecting Pyelonephritis

The classic symptoms of upper UTI (i.e., pyelonephritis) include fever, flank pain, chills, rigors, nausea, vomiting, and headache. The presence of these symptoms should prompt clinicians to consider the possibility of pyelonephritis and undertake appropriate diagnosis and treatment, as described below.

History alone, however, cannot definitively diagnose or exclude pyelonephritis. Some patients with symptoms of pyelonephritis have other conditions, such as pelvic inflammatory disease (PID). Furthermore, while most clinicians will exclude the possibility of upper tract infection in patients without classic pyelonephritis symptoms, substantial evidence indicates that upper tract infection can be present in the absence of these symptoms. For example, research using urine tests for antibody-coated bacteria, which develop in upper UTIs, reveals that antibody-coated bacteria are present in some patients who appear to have only uncomplicated cystitis. The frequency with which this occurs is unknown, because patients with cystitis do not undergo antibody-coated bacteria tests in routine clinical practice. Fortunately, since patients with apparent cystitis shown to have upper tract involvement by antibody-coated bacteria testing generally have an uncomplicated clinical course, failure to detect these "silent" upper tract infections probably has little clinical consequence.

Identifying Risks for Complicated Infections

Certain patients are at a higher risk for complicated UTIs. These patients include individuals with diabetes mellitus, immunodeficiencies, structural urinary tract abnormalities, and a history of frequent or serious UTIs in the recent past. Pregnant women and geriatric-aged women are also at higher risk for complications, including pyelonephritis and sepsis. The indications for further investigation in these groups are discussed under "Ancillary Tests" and special considerations for management in the "Treatment" section.

Physical Examination

The physical examination contributes relatively little to the diagnosis of cystitis. However, it is useful in identifying patients with pyelonephritis and those who have conditions other than UTI, such as vaginitis or PID. The important physical findings are fever, flank and abdominal tenderness, and vaginal discharge.

Fever

Fever is the physical examination finding most strongly associated with pyelonephritis. Unfortunately, it is not a completely dependable indication of pyelonephritis because over half of patients with pyelonephritis are afebrile (Table 18-2), and about 20 percent of patients with simple cystitis have fever. However, patients who are seriously ill with pyelonephritis are often obviously septic, with tachycardia, tachypnea, and temperature over 38°C (100.4°F) or under 36°C (95°F). Nonetheless, even if a patient does not look septic, the presence of fever in combination with typical cystitis symptoms of frequency, dysuria, urgency, or nocturia makes it essential to consider and exclude the possibility of pyelonephritis.

Flank and Abdominal Tenderness

Flank (costovertebral angle) tenderness is classically associated with upper tract involvement,

Table 18-2

Operating Characteristics of History and Physical Examination for Diagnosing Pyelonephritis in Patients with Apparent UTI

SYMPTOM OR SIGN	SENSITIVITY, %	SPECIFICITY, %	LR+	LR−	LIKELIHOOD OF PYELONEPHRITIS	
					WITH SYMPTOM OR SIGN, %	WITHOUT SYMPTOM OR SIGN, %
Chills and rigors	32	87	2.5	0.8	22	8
Fever	44	80	2.2	0.7	20	7
Flank pain	48	67	1.5	0.8	14	8
Nausea/vomiting	24	84	1.5	0.9	14	9

NOTE: Data in the table are calculated on the assumption that 10% of patients with suspected UTI actually have pyelonephritis, rather than simple cystitis. The positive likelihood ratio (LR+) is the percentage of patients with pyelonephritis divided by the percentage of patients without pyelonephritis among patients with a particular symptom or sign. The negative likelihood ratio (LR−) is the percentage of patients with disease divided by the percentage of patients without disease among patients without a particular symptom or sign. A likelihood ratio > 1 means that disease is more likely with (or without) the sign or symptom, and a likelihood ratio < 1 means that disease is less likely.

but it is a non-specific finding. It occurs in pyelonephritis, but also in PID, cholecystitis, and many other intra-abdominal processes. Abdominal tenderness can also occur in both cystitis and pyelonephritis, but it, too, is nonspecific, since it can be found in PID, trichomonas vaginitis, and numerous other intra-abdominal conditions.

Vaginal Discharge

As noted above, if a patient reports vaginal discharge on history, the likelihood of a diagnosis other than UTI increases. In this situation, a pelvic examination should be performed to evaluate the vaginal discharge to detect or exclude vaginal infections and/or PID.

Ancillary Tests

A variety of urine tests are available for evaluating patients with suspected UTI. However, recent evidence suggests that these tests may be overused, since test results often do not change diagnoses, influence management, or provide important prognostic information.

Specific Urine Tests

Proper interpretation of urine tests requires that the urine be collected in a manner that minimizes contamination of the urine by vaginal microbes or skin flora. This translates into the common method of collecting a "clean-catch" urine specimen, in which the labia are separated, the vulva is cleaned, and the urine stream is started. Once the flow is started, a mid-stream sample is collected in a sterile container. Unfortunately, in spite of patients' best efforts, contamination is common, and test results may not be useful in clinical decision making. Thus, when attempts to obtain an uncontaminated specimen fail or when an accurate, uncontaminated specimen is of importance, the urine specimen can be obtained by sterile "in-and-out" catheterization.

The most commonly performed urine tests are dipstick tests, microscopic urinalysis, and urine culture. The operating characteristics of these tests are summarized in Table 18-3.

URINE DIPSTICK

Dipsticks measure many characteristics of and substances in urine, but three substances are particularly relevant to the diagnosis of UTI: leukocyte esterase, nitrites, and blood.

Table 18-3

Characteristics of Common Tests Used for Diagnosis of Suspected UTI

| | | | | | LIKELIHOOD OF UTI | |
| | | | | | WITH | WITH |
TEST	SENSITIVITY, %	SPECIFICITY, %	LR+	LR−	POSITIVE TEST, %	NEGATIVE TEST, %
URINE DIPSTICK						
Nitrites	53	94	8.8	0.5	95	50
Leukocyte esterase	87	68	2.7	0.19	85	28
URINE MICROSCOPY						
≥ 10 bacteria/hpf	85	99	85	0.15	99	23
≥ 1 bacteria/hpf	95	85	6.3	0.06	93	11
≥ 5 RBC/hpf	44	88	3.7	0.60	88	56
≥ 10 WBC/hpf	82	65	2.3	0.28	83	36
≥ 5 WBC/hpf	91	48	1.8	0.19	78	28
URINE CULTURE						
Laboratory culture	96	96	24.0	0.04	98	8
Office culture	93	93	13.3	0.08	96	13

NOTE: Data in the table are calculated on the assumption that about 70% of patients with suspected UTI actually have a UTI. The positive likelihood ratio (LR+) is the percentage of patients with UTI divided by the percentage of patients without UTI among patients with a positive test result. The negative likelihood ratio (LR−) is the percentage of patients with disease divided by the percentage of patients without disease among patients with a negative test. A likelihood ratio > 1 means that disease is more likely with a particular test result, and a likelihood ratio < 1 means that disease is less likely.

ABBREVIATIONS: hpf, high-power field; RBC, red blood cells; WBC, white blood cells

LEUKOCYTE ESTERASE Leukocyte esterase is an enzyme found in white blood cells, which appear in the urine during acute infection. The likelihood of a positive leukocyte esterase test result is directly related to the number of white blood cells in the urine. Thus, patients with UTI who have few white blood cells may have a false-negative test result. Clinical studies indicate that leukocyte esterase is relatively sensitive for detecting UTI, but approximately 1 in 7 women with UTI will have a false-negative leukocyte esterase test result.

NITRITE Gram-negative bacteria convert dietary nitrates in the urine into nitrites, and these nitrites can be detected with dipstick urine tests. Dipstick tests for nitrites are very specific; if nitrites are detected, UTI is likely. However, as nitrates are predominantly the result of meat consumption, vegetarians or those who have not recently eaten meat will have little nitrate in the urine and may have a false-negative nitrite test.

BLOOD Blood appears in the urine of many patients with UTI, and this hematuria can be detected by dipstick tests based on the peroxidase-like activity of hemoglobin in the urine. Not all patients with UTI have hematuria, however, and hematuria can be caused by a variety of conditions other than UTI (e.g., urolithiasis and glomerulonephritis). Unfortunately, no good information is available on the sensitivity, specificity, and predictive values of urine blood testing for diagnosis of UTI.

MICROSCOPIC ANALYSIS OF URINARY SEDIMENT

Properly performed microscopic examination of urine for white blood cells, bacteria, and red blood cells is more sensitive and specific than testing with urine dipsticks. Table 18-3 provides a summary of the test characteristics of urine microscopy.

When interpreting the urine sediment, it is important to understand that some findings are useful for confirming the presence of UTI, while others are useful for excluding UTI. For example, as shown in Table 18-3, the presence of more than 10 rod-shaped bacteria per high-power field on an uncontaminated centrifuged urine specimen provides almost certain confirmation that a UTI is present, and the absence of bacteria excludes the diagnosis. The presence of white blood cells in the urine is somewhat less predictive, however, because white cells can appear in the urine of patients with conditions other than UTI, such as urethritis and vaginitis. More than 10 white cells per high-power field in a patient with symptoms of UTI indicate a probability of 83 percent that the patient actually has a UTI.

URINE CULTURE

Although urine culture is often used as a "gold standard" when evaluating other diagnostic tests for UTI, clinicians should recognize that culture results do not always accurately identify infections. In particular, vaginal contamination and delay in processing culture specimens can reduce the specificity of culture, while inadequate specimen volume or an overly dilute urine sample can reduce the sensitivity of cultures (Table 18-3). As discussed below, urine culture is not routinely indicated in patients with suspected UTI and is only indicated in patients with a history of repeated UTIs, in cases of treatment failure following initial empirical therapy, and for patients with pyelonephritis or risks for a complicated infection.

INDICATIONS FOR URINE EXAMINATION

Given the information outlined above and contained in the tables, specific recommenda-

tions can be made about when to perform laboratory tests on urine (Fig. 18-1). A monogamous, sexually active woman presenting with acute dysuria and no fever, chills, nausea, flank pain, or vaginal discharge has a high probability (nearly 70 percent) of having uncomplicated cystitis. Therefore, little is gained by performing a urine evaluation; positive results only increase the probability that the patient has cystitis by about 15 percent (i.e., to 80 to 90 percent). Furthermore, if results of the urine examination are negative, a patient with typical cystitis symptoms is *still* more likely to have cystitis than any other condition. While some clinicians still perform urine tests on low-risk patients, the strategy of diagnosing cystitis by symptoms alone has been confirmed by a recent cost-effectiveness analysis. If such patients turn out not to have cystitis, there is little harm in delaying treatment of conditions such as vaginitis or urethritis.

When clinical circumstances suggest a relatively low probability of having a UTI (under 30 percent), a complete urine evaluation to guide management is the most cost-effective strategy. In addition, urine testing is appropriate for women who appear acutely ill (i.e., suspected pyelonephritis), have recurrent UTIs, or are at risk for "complicated" infections, as defined above. Women with recurrent UTIs, pyelonephritis, or risk factors for complicated UTIs should have a urine culture before treatment and after completion of therapy.

Additional Testing in Acute Pyelonephritis

Complete blood counts and blood cultures are not required in the routine evaluation of patients with UTI. However, they are appropriate for patients who are acutely ill with suspected pyelonephritis. White blood cell counts in excess of $12,000/\mu L$ or below $4,000/\mu L$ may suggest the possibility of severe infection, but white blood cell counts are not sufficiently sensitive or specific to be relied on as a sole discriminator between ill and not so ill patients; clinical judgement must always prevail. Depending on the

Figure 18-1

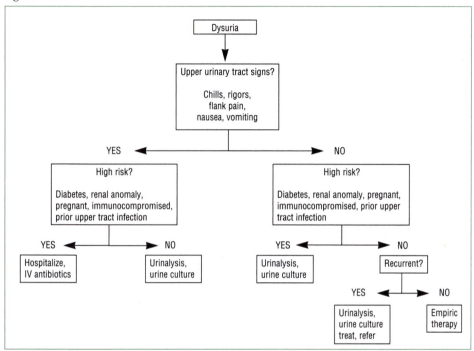

Algorithm for the management of urinary tract infection.

patient's status, other laboratory tests (e.g., renal function tests, serum chemistry tests, imaging studies, etc.) may sometimes be appropriate.

Testing in Patients Following Recurrent Infections or Pyelonephritis

Patients with pyelonephritis or recurrent UTIs should have further investigations in addition to examination of the urine. The purpose of these investigations is to identify structural or functional abnormalities of the urinary tract that may predispose these patients to severe or recurrent infections. In most cases, this investigation will include renal ultrasound studies. If ureteral dilation is identified sonographically, especially in children, a voiding cystourethrogram can be obtained to detect vesicoureteral reflux. Isotope cystograms can also be used to detect reflux, with only a small fraction of the radiation expo-

sure involved in standard voiding cystourethrography. Renal cortical scintigraphy can be used to detect chronic pyelonephritis and renal scarring. Older women with more than three UTIs in a year should undergo cystoscopy to identify such predisposing conditions as urethral diverticuli, bladder cancers, or premalignant lesions such as cystitis cystica.

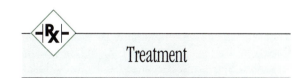

Treatment

Antibiotics are the primary treatment for all UTIs. The choice of antibiotic and the duration of treatment, however, vary for cystitis, recurrent UTIs, UTIs in patients at risk for complications, and pyelonephritis.

Cystitis

For many years, ampicillin (or its congener, amoxicillin) was the antibiotic of choice for treating acute, uncomplicated cystitis. Because of rising rates of resistance to ampicillin, however, trimethoprim-sulfamethoxazole is now considered the preferred antibiotic for treating cystitis. Trimethoprim-sulfamethoxazole is inexpensive and well tolerated, and has clinical and microbiologic cure rates of about 90 percent.

The appropriate duration of antibiotic therapy for cystitis has received much attention in recent years, with recommendations ranging from single-dose therapy to 3-day treatment to 7-day treatment. Due to a high rate of early recurrences following treatment, single-dose therapy is no longer recommended. Three-day therapy is less expensive than 7- or 10-day treatment and is only marginally less effective than the longer treatments. In most cases of uncomplicated cystitis, therefore, 3-day treatment with trimethoprim-sulfamethoxazole is the treatment of choice. For patients allergic to sulfonamides or in communities with high rates of bacterial resistance to trimethoprim-sulfamethoxazole, 3-day treatment with a fluoroquinolone antibiotic is a reasonable alternative.

Recurrent Urinary Tract Infections and High-Risk Patients

Short-duration therapy is not recommended for patients with recurrent cystitis or for those who are at high risk for complicated infections. Such patients should generally be treated for 10 to 14 days. The choice of antibiotic must be individualized, however, especially for patients with recurrent infections, because such individuals have often received many antibiotics and therefore may be infected with microorganisms that are resistant to trimethoprim-sulfamethoxazole. When possible, antibiotic selection is usually based on sensitivity patterns of bacteria isolated from the current or recent infections.

For infections known or thought to be resistant to trimethoprim-sulfamethoxazole, commonly used alternative antibiotics include fluoroquinolones and cephalosporins. The initial antibiotic choice should be reconsidered if the patient fails to respond to treatment or if the results of antibiotic sensitivity testing indicate resistance to the chosen antibiotic.

For patients with frequent recurrent infections, chronic low-dose antibiotic therapy is often recommended. The antibiotic most frequently used for chronic prophylaxis is trimethoprim-sulfamethoxazole, typically prescribed as a once-daily dose. However, any standard oral antibiotic used for treatment of UTI can be used for prophylaxis, typically prescribed in one-quarter to one-half of the usual daily dose.

Pyelonephritis

Patients with pyelonephritis who are only mildly or moderately ill can be treated out of the hospital with oral antibiotics, but treatment should be continued for 2 weeks. Trimethoprim-sulfamethoxazole, fluoroquinolones, or cephalosporins are all reasonable choices for oral outpatient treatment of pyelonephritis.

Acutely ill patients and patients with pyelonephritis who are at risk for complications should be hospitalized and treated with intravenous antibiotics. As with recurrent infections, antibiotic selection must be individualized based on drug sensitivity of the patient's previous infections, local or institutional sensitivity patterns, and the severity of the patient's illness. Seriously ill patients should be treated with multiple broad-spectrum antibiotics, as outlined in various guides and handbooks for treatment of infectious disease.

Recent evidence indicates that pregnant women with pyelonephritis during the first half of gestation (less than 24 weeks) can be safely treated out of the hospital, even if they are febrile. Patients treated in this manner typically receive two 1 g doses of ceftriaxone intramuscularly 24 h apart, followed by 500 mg of oral cephalexin q 6 h to continue until 10 days after fever has resolved. Controlled studies reveal no difference in outcome between this regimen and treatment with intravenous cefazolin or intravenous gentamicin.

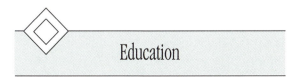

Education

Clinicians should educate women about the causes of and risks for UTIs. The most pertinent information is that infections are caused by entry of bowel flora into the bladder (hence the need for good hygiene), and the relationship of UTI to sexual activity and diaphragm use. Women also should be told about symptoms of upper tract infection (i.e., fever and flank pain) and the need to be evaluated if such symptoms develop.

Women should be told that nearly all patients with simple cystitis experience complete or near-complete resolution of symptoms within 2 to 3 days. Women who are still symptomatic after 3 days of treatment should be re-evaluated for the possibility of antibiotic-resistant infection or undiagnosed risk factors for complications.

Patients should also be told about adjuncts to antibiotic treatment. In particular, maintaining high fluid intake is important. In addition, women should probably avoid sexual intercourse during active UTIs. No special dietary measures are required.

Finally, for women who wish to reduce their risk of recurrent UTI, it may be appropriate to recommend consuming cranberry juice on a regular basis, since cranberry juice has been found to play a role in preventing UTIs. Women with frequent recurrences temporally related to intercourse may benefit from postintercourse antibiotic prophylaxis, such as with a single dose of trimethoprim-sulfamethoxazole. Such women are also often told to urinate before and after intercourse, but there is no evidence that this reduces the rate of recurrent UTI.

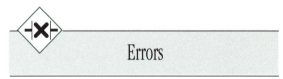

Errors

Clinicians make a variety of errors in the diagnosis and treatment of UTI. Two errors are particularly common. One is obtaining a clean-catch urine specimen for examination instead of a catheterized specimen in circumstances when catheterization is indicated. The second is prescribing inappropriate antibiotic treatment regimens.

Inappropriate Clean-Catch Urine Specimens

When urinalysis or culture is needed and a patient is unable to provide an adequate clean-catch sample, a catheterized urine specimen should be obtained. This typically occurs in women with cognitive dysfunction, significant motor or sensory impairment, or obesity. Failure to obtain adequate specimens can result in cultures that are unsuitable for antimicrobial sensitivity testing or in false diagnoses of UTI, leading to unnecessary antibiotic treatment or even unwarranted hospital admissions. The frequency of this error is such that most clinicians have provided care for patients diagnosed as having multiple recurrent UTIs or admitted to the hospital with a diagnosis of pyelonephritis when, in fact, the diagnosis was based on false-positive cultures of contaminated clean-catch specimens.

Inappropriate Antibiotic Regimens

Two common errors in prescribing antibiotics for UTI are treating for longer than necessary and treating with inappropriate antibiotics. While there is good evidence that short-course (3-day) regimens have approximately equal effectiveness and lower cost when compared to treatment of longer duration, many clinicians still treat simple uncomplicated, nonrecurrent, cystitis with a 10-day course of antibiotics.

The other common error is using inappropriate antibiotics as first-choice therapy for cystitis. For example, many clinicians routinely treat uncomplicated cystitis with new fluoroquinolones or broad-spectrum cephalosporins, when less-broad-spectrum, less-expensive antibiotics (i.e., trimethoprim-sulfamethoxazole) are more appropriate. Finally, some clinicians still treat patients with ampicillin or amoxicillin, when the rate of resistance to these antibiotics is too high to justify using them as first-line treatments.

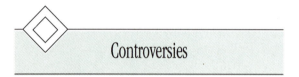

Controversies

Most of the current controversies in diagnosis and management of UTIs in office practice have been mentioned above. These include controversies about the appropriate length of treatment and the need for diagnostic tests. Most experts have now agreed that 3-day treatment is probably the best option for uncomplicated infections, but considerable controversy remains about the need for urine cultures. The result is that, despite evidence that urine cultures are not needed for most patients, many clinicians continue to perform them.

The resolution of the controversy over diagnostic urine testing is not simple. Different perspectives yield different answers. For an individual patient, the difference in cost between one diagnostic approach and another may be small. However, when millions of patients are considered, even small differences in the costs of various testing routines can have substantial financial implications.

A cost-effectiveness study published in 1997 used a population-based decision-analysis technique to evaluate several options for outpatient diagnosis and management of cystitis. The most cost-effective approach was to prescribe empirical antibiotic therapy after making a diagnosis of UTI based on a patient's history (i.e., without laboratory confirmation of infection). The investigators found that, compared to empirical therapy, performing a microscopic urinalysis adds a cost of $30 to each episode of UTI but yields only 0.01 additional quality-adjusted life months for the patient. Performing a dipstick analysis was even less cost effective.

Although empirical therapy is the most cost-effective treatment, some have expressed concern about this approach because it involves treating some patients who do not actually have a UTI, thus contributing unnecessarily to the growing problem of antibiotic resistance. Additional research is needed to clarify the optimal approach to diagnosis and treatment of UTI in primary care practice.

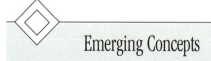

Emerging Concepts

The emerging trend of greatest relevance to treatment of UTIs in primary care practice is the increasing prevalence of bacterial strains that are resistant to common antibiotics. In the last several years, strains of enterococcus have appeared that are resistant to virtually all conventional antibiotics. Because enterococcus is a relatively common cause of UTI, especially in patients with recurrent or complicated infections, the inability to treat such infections has important implications. While continued pharmaceutical research is likely to result in development of new drugs for treating resistant infections, clinicians must exercise caution about prescribing antibiotics or prescribing unnecessarily broad-spectrum antibiotics without proper indication.

The future is also likely to bring advances in the prevention of UTIs. Development of an effective vaccine against antigenic components of *E. coli* will potentially prevent and/or decrease the morbidity of complicated UTIs, thereby mitigating concerns about development of antibiotic resistance.

Bibliography

Avorn J, Monane M, Gurwitz JH, et al: Reduction of bacteriuria and pyuria after ingestion of cranberry juice. *JAMA* 271:751, 1994.

Bailey BL: Urinalysis predictive of urine culture results. *J Fam Pract* 40:45, 1995.

Barry H, Ebell M, Hickner J: Evaluation of suspected UTI in ambulatory women: A cost-utility analysis of office-based strategies. *J Fam Pract* 44:49, 1997.

Blum RN, Wright RA: Detection of pyuria and bacteriuria in symptomatic ambulatory women. *J Gen Intern Med* 7:140, 1992.

Carroll KC, Hale DC, Von Boerum DH, et al: Laboratory evaluation of urinary tract infections in an ambulatory clinic. *Am J Clin Pathol* 101:100, 1994.

Dobbs FF, Fleming DM: A simple scoring system for evaluating symptoms, history and urine dipstick testing in the diagnosis of urinary tract infection. *J R Coll Gen Pract* 37:100, 1987.

Loo SY, Scottolini AG, Luangphinith S, et al: Urine screening strategy employing dipstick analysis and selective culture: An evaluation. *Am J Clin Pathol* 81:634, 1984.

Males BM, Bartholomew WR, Amsterdam D: Leukocyte esterase-nitrite and bioluminescence assays as urine screens. *J Clin Microbiol* 22:531, 1985.

Mills SJ, Ford M, Gould FK, et al: Screening for bacteriuria in urological patients using reagent strips. *Br J Urol* 70:314, 1992.

National Ambulatory Medical Care Survey. Hyattsville, MD, National Center for Health Statistics, 1993.

Osterberg E, Aspevall O, Grillner L, et al: Young women with symptoms of urinary tract infection: Prevalence and diagnosis of chlamydial infection and evaluation of rapid screening of bacteriuria. *Scand J Prim Health Care* 14:43, 1996.

Stamm WE, Hooton TM: Management of urinary tract infections in adults. *New Engl J Med* 329:1328, 1993.

Wigton RS, Hoellerich VL, Ornato JP, et al: Use of clinical findings in the diagnosis of urinary tract infection in women. *Arch Intern Med* 145:2222, 1985.

Wing DA, Hendershott CM, Debuque L, et al: A randomized trial of three antibiotic regimens for the treatment of pyelonephritis in pregnancy. *Obstet Gynecol* 92:249, 1998.

Part 6

Prevention

Doug Campos-Outcalt

Preventive Health Examinations

How Common Are Preventive Health Examinations?

Patient number 1 is a 52-year-old female who presents for her first visit after moving into town from out of state. She is a smoker (35-year history) and has chronic obstructive pulmonary disease. Her last menstrual period was 3 years ago. What should the clinician do in terms of risk reduction, screening, and immunizations for this woman?

Patient number 2 is a 25-year-old male college student who complains of a urethral discharge and dysuria for the past 2 days. In addition to diagnosing and treating the discharge, what preventive measures should the clinician recommend to him?

Patient number 3 is a 24-month-old girl whose mother brings her in for a well-child checkup. The mother receives financial assistance through the Aid for Families with Dependent Children program. What screening tests, immunizations, and health education should the clinician offer?

These three patients illustrate why prevention is *the* most common problem, or issue, faced by primary care clinicians. In addition to the 47 million health care visits per year made specifically for preventive health care—making it the leading cause of visits to clinicians—the reality is that every visit by a patient presents an opportunity to practice preventive care. Preventive interventions should be considered at each encounter with a patient, since any individual visit may be the only chance to address prevention with a particular patient.

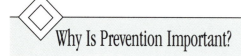

Why Is Prevention Important?

The importance of prevention is illustrated in a study by McGinnis and Foege that demonstrated that 43 percent of deaths in the United States are related to personal behaviors. These behaviors include smoking (400,000 deaths), diet and activity patterns (300,000), alcohol use (100,000), firearms injuries (35,000), sexual activities (30,000), motor vehicle mishaps (25,000), and use of illicit of drugs (20,000). Modifying these behaviors could literally prevent hundreds of thousands of premature deaths and loss of productive lives each year in the United States alone.

Not long ago, most clinicians and patients considered preventive medicine to consist of an annual physical examination along with immunizations and perhaps some advice on exercise and nutrition. The field is now much more complex. Modern preventive medicine has a scientific basis; uses age-, gender-, and risk-specific interventions; and is dependent on proof that these interventions are effective. Unfortunately, however, there are conflicting prevention recommendations from various authoritative groups, and evidence for or against specific interventions changes with time as new research findings become available. Thus, to understand and stay current with recommendations for preventive care, clinicians must understand the basic principles of preventive medicine and put forth some effort to stay abreast of the evolving prevention literature.

The main purpose of this chapter is not to present today's recommendations for preventive care, because those recommendations will inevitably change with time. Instead, the purpose is to review the basic definitions and theories of preventive care, demonstrate how preventive interventions are evaluated, and discuss some evolving concepts in the area of preventive health care.

Definitions and Theory

Primary, Secondary, and Tertiary Prevention

Primary prevention involves preventing illness before it occurs. Examples of primary prevention include immunizations to prevent infectious disease, use of automobile seat belts to prevent injuries, avoiding smoking to prevent lung cancer, and condom use to prevent sexually transmitted diseases.

Secondary prevention involves early detection of an existing disease before it causes harm and implementing interventions to modify its course and improve outcomes. A common example of secondary prevention is detection of early breast cancer by mammography, thus permitting definitive treatment of the cancer before it becomes clinically apparent. Preventing cervical cancer through treatment of abnormalities detected on Pap smear screening is a similar method of secondary prevention. Other examples of secondary prevention include control of hypertension to prevent stroke and controlling blood lipid levels to reduce the risk of heart disease.

Tertiary prevention involves rehabilitation or improving outcomes after a disease has already occurred. For example, prophylactic aspirin therapy or exercise rehabilitation after myocardial infarction can reduce the rate of second infarction and improve physical function. Similarly, laser photocoagulation of established diabetic retinopathy can prevent subsequent visual loss.

Primary prevention, in both theory and practice, is the ideal form of disease prevention and is preferred by experts in preventive medicine. Primary care clinicians, by the nature of the patients and problems they see, practice all three types of prevention simultaneously.

Individual versus Population-Based Prevention

This chapter focuses on preventive efforts for individual patients in primary care practice. While clinical prevention for individual patients is important and should be practiced by all primary care clinicians, it is important to keep these efforts and their resulting benefits in perspective. The most effective prevention interventions have historically been population-based interventions, not efforts aimed at individuals. Such population-based efforts have traditionally been considered the realm of public health professionals, and, while numerous, they are often underappreciated. Examples of some successful population-based preventive interventions are listed in Table 19-1. Clinicians should be aware of these and other public health efforts, most of which represent primary prevention, and should support them through professional organizations and local and national advocacy.

The reality is that individual patient-focused education efforts, while having some benefit, are

Table 19-1

Examples of Successful Public Health Interventions

INTERVENTION	BENEFIT
Potable water	Prevention of enteric infections
Sewage disposal	Prevention of enteric infections
Cigarette taxes	Decreased cardiovascular and respiratory disease
Consumer product safety standards	Decreased home injuries
Air-quality standards	Decreased respiratory disease
Prohibition of smoking in public places	Decreased respiratory disease
Highway safety programs	Decreased automobile injuries
Seat belt laws	Decreased automobile injuries
Iodized salt	Preventing iodine-deficiency goiter
Water fluoridation	Preventing dental caries
School immunization requirements	Preventing childhood infectious disease

not as effective as community-wide public health laws and regulations. Advice to quit smoking is not as effective as raising the price of cigarettes. Cardiopulmonary resuscitation training and drowning prevention classes are not as effective as mandatory swimming pool fences. Advice to keep medications away from children is not as effective as requiring childproof tops on medication bottles. Requiring immunizations for school attendance is better than mailing reminders to parents to have their children immunized. These examples are meant, not to discourage one-on-one prevention interventions with individual patients, but to encourage advocacy of more comprehensive population-based approaches to prevention.

Cost of Prevention

Prevention is frequently advocated as a solution to the problem of escalating health care costs. While effective preventive interventions do reduce morbidity and mortality rates, they do not necessarily reduce costs. In fact, they frequently do not. Expensive interventions, especially if applied to an entire population, can be extraordinarily costly, and the cost may even outweigh the benefit to society if only a few individuals would have suffered from the disease that is prevented. Such lack of cost-effectiveness should not necessarily reduce the desirability of implementing preventive services, since reduction of morbidity and mortality rates are worthwhile goals in and of themselves. However, limitations on a society's economic resources make some preventive efforts more worthwhile to society than others.

Approaches to Prevention

There are four basic approaches to individual, patient-oriented prevention: (1) risk assessment, (2) screening, (3) risk reduction, and (4) immunizations and chemoprophylaxis.

RISK ASSESSMENT

To effectively lower the rates of morbidity and mortality, one must know the conditions for which an individual or population is at risk. This knowledge is achieved through risk assessment.

At the level of individual patients, risk assessment involves examining a patient's medical history, family history, life-style, age, and gender to determine the diseases for which the patient is at highest risk. This assessment requires knowledge of the leading causes of death and disability for various segments of the population. For example, the most common cause of death for a 20 year-old male is a motor vehicle crash, while cancer is the most likely cause of death for a 50-year-old woman. Preventive interventions for each patient would be targeted at different conditions. Table 19-2 lists the leading causes of death for various age and gender groups in the U.S. population. The population-based data in Table 19-2 must be modified for individual patients, based on their personal and family risk factors, underlying medical conditions, socioeconomic status, life-style behaviors, and occupational exposures.

SCREENING TESTS

Screening tests involve questionnaires, laboratory tests, imaging studies, and other methods of detecting either risk factors or asymptomatic disease. Ideally, screening tests are targeted at age and gender risk factors for individual patients or populations. Based on the findings of the screening tests, recommendations can be made for risk reduction, which can include counseling regarding behavioral risk reduction or, in some cases, chemoprophylaxis with medications.

RISK-REDUCTION COUNSELING

Risk reduction involves changing behaviors to reduce the risk of illness or injury. A clinician's role in risk reduction involves counseling patients to make the necessary behavioral

Table 19-2

Leading Causes of Death In the US Population

MALES	**RATE/100,000**	**FEMALES**	**RATE/100,000**
1–4 YEARS			
1. Accidents	19.1	1. Accidents	13.6
Motor vehicle crashes	6.1	Motor vehicle crashes	5.3
Other	13.0	Other	8.3
2. Congenital anomalies	4.8	2. Congenital anomalies	5.4
3. Cancer	3.7	3. Cancer	2.9
4. Homicide	3.4	4. Homicide	2.5
5. Heart disease	2.0	5. Heart disease	1.7
5–14 YEARS			
1. Accidents	11.8	1. Accidents	6.7
Motor vehicle crashes	6.3	Motor vehicle crashes	4.2
Other	5.5	Other	2.5
2. Cancer	3.3	2. Cancer	2.6
3. Homicide	2.2	3. Homicide	1.4
4. Congenital anomalies	1.4	4. Congenital anomalies	1.2
5. Suicide	1.2	5. Heart disease	0.9
15–24 YEARS			
1. Accidents	57.6	1. Accidents	19.1
Motor vehicle crashes	41.8	Motor vehicle crashes	16.0
Other	15.8	Other	3.1
2. Homicide	39.2	2. Homicide	6.9
3. Suicide	22.4	3. Suicide	4.1
4. Cancer	5.5	4. Cancer	4.1
5. Heart disease	3.4	5. Heart disease	2.0
25–44 YEARS			
1. HIV Infection	57.0	1. Cancer	28.1
2. Accidents	51.2	2. Accidents	15.0
Motor vehicle crashes	25.4	Motor vehicle crashes	9.3
Other	25.8	Other	5.7
3. Heart disease	29.0	3. Heart disease	11.4
4. Cancer	24.7	4. HIV infection	9.1
5. Suicide	24.4	5. Homicide	6.4
45–64 YEARS			
1. Heart disease	308.2	1. Cancer	240.1
2. Cancer	298.7	2. Heart disease	120.7
3. Accidents	42.9	3. Stroke	26.2
Motor vehicle crashes	18.9	4. COPD	23.6
Other	24.0	5. Diabetes	20.4
4. Stroke	33.3		
5. HIV infection	31.2		
65 AND OVER			
1. Heart disease	2111.8	1. Heart disease	1740.6
2. Cancer	1473.9	2. Cancer	901.9
3. Stroke	369.1	3. Stroke	423.4
4. COPD	350.2	4. Pneumonia/influenza	211.8
5. Pneumonia/influenza	245.2	5. COPD	204.8
INFANTS (BOTH SEXES)			
1. Congenital anomalies	178.2		
2. Sudden infant death syndrome	116.7		
3. Prematurity and low birth weight	107.7		
4. Respiratory distress syndrome	45.4		
5. Maternal complications of pregnancy	33.6		

ABBREVIATIONS: COPD, chronic obstructive pulmonary disease; HIV, human immunodeficiency virus.
SOURCE: *Month Vital Stat Rep* 44S, 1996.

changes. The efficacy of counseling in improving health outcomes is an area of controversy, as is the relative efficacy of different types of counseling. Further research is needed to clarify the benefits of risk reduction counseling.

Based on current knowledge, the United States Preventive Services Task Force (USPSTF) has made the following ten recommendations regarding education of patients about risk reduction: (1) try to frame education to fit with patients' belief systems; (2) tell patients clearly what they can expect if they adopt the recommendations and when they can expect it; (3) recommend small changes rather than large ones; (4) make specific, rather than general, recommendations; (5) use the authority of the medical profession; (6) link new behaviors to old ones; (7) get patients to make explicit commitments to behavior change; (8) make use of a wide array of written materials, classes, educational aids, and community resources that have been checked for accuracy; (9) involve office staff; and (10) refer for specialized counseling when more assistance or time is needed than the clinician can provide.

IMMUNIZATIONS AND CHEMOPROPHYLAXIS

Immunizations include vaccines and immunoglobulins directed at preventing infectious diseases. Chemoprophylaxis refers to the use of medications to reduce the risk of disease. A common example of chemoprophylaxis is administration of antituberculosis medication to prevent tuberculosis in patients who have a positive tuberculin skin test result but no evidence of clinical tuberculosis disease. Other common forms of chemoprophylaxis are listed in Table 19-3.

Evaluating Preventive Interventions

Most clinicians find it challenging to decide what to do in the areas of risk assessment, screening, risk reduction counseling, and immunizations and chemoprophylaxis. Recommendations from government agencies; nonprofit limited-interest

associations; medical specialty organizations; and other scientific groups often conflict with one another. In addition, some recommendations change frequently. The reason for the heterogeneity of recommendations is that, in many cases, recommendations are more often made from a perspective of advocacy and special interest than based on proof of efficacy. While advocacy and special interest are often well motivated, clinicians need to view these recommendations cautiously, seeking those based on solid scientific evidence.

Probably the least controversial recommendations relate to immunizations and chemoprophylaxis. Two organizations that regularly issue recommendations for applying these two preventive techniques are the Centers for Disease Control and Prevention (CDC) and the American Academy of Pediatrics (AAP). The CDC issues recommendations periodically in the *Morbidity and Mortality Weekly Report (MMWR)*. The AAP compiles its recommendations in the *Red Book*. The CDC and AAP recommendations are usually in agreement, differing only in minor aspects.

The most controversial areas of prevention are those related to screening and counseling. Recommendations from different organizations frequently vary and are often based on the opinions of experts and consensus panels, rather than on the well-defined criteria that have been developed to measure the utility of screening tests.

U.S. PREVENTIVE SERVICES TASK FORCE

Busy clinicians do not have time to evaluate the available data for every possible screening test. Fortunately, there are professional and government advisory groups that conduct such evaluations and publish recommendations based on those evaluations. The most widely accepted and authoritative group is the USPSTF, which publishes its evaluations and recommendations in the *Guide to Clinical Preventive Services*. The USPSTF is a government-sponsored agency that evaluates the research literature on hundreds of

Table 19-3

Commonly Used Methods of Chemoprophylaxis

CHEMOPROPHYLAXIS	CONDITION PREVENTED
Ocular prophylaxis of newborns with tetracycline, erythromycin, or silver nitrate	Gonococcal ophthalmia neonatorum
Folic acid 0.4–0.8 mg/d starting at least 1 month prior to conception through the first trimester (4 mg/d for women who have previously had a pregnancy affected by neural tube defect)	Neural tube defects
Estrogen for postmenopausal women	Osteoporosis, cardiovascular disease
Isoniazide (INH) for tuberculosis skin test converters	Active tuberculosis
Rifampin for family members of those who are infected with *Haemophilus influenzae* type B or *Neisseria meningitidis*	*H. influenzae* B and meningococcal disease and carrier state
Penicillin for group A, beta-hemolytic streptococcal pharyngitis	Rheumatic fever and subsequent valvular heart disease
Coumadin for atrial fibrillation	Cerebral and other systemic emboli and cerebral vascular ischemia
Heparin for deep-vein thrombosis	Pulmonary embolism
Subcutaneous heparin for bed-ridden patients	Venous thrombosis, pulmonary embolism
Antibiotics before and during surgery	Postoperative infection
Antibiotics before invasive procedures in patients with artificial heart valves	Endocarditis

preventive services and ranks the quality of evidence available to support the effectiveness of each service. The highest ranking is given to evidence obtained from at least one randomized controlled trial. The lowest ranking is given to services for which the only available support is the opinions of experts, descriptive studies, case reports, and reports of consensus committees.

In each chapter of the *Guide to Clinical Preventive Services*, the USPSTF reviews the scientific data, explains its recommendations, and describes what other groups recommend. Tables 19-4 through 19-7 provide broad summaries of the USPSTF recommendations for various age groups in the U.S. population. In the sections that follow, the criteria used by the USPSTF are described, and they are applied to several widely practiced preventive health recommendations.

EVALUATING COUNSELING FOR RISK REDUCTION   Several criteria should be considered in determining whether to incorporate a specific risk reduction counseling intervention into clinical practice. The first is whether the behavior at which counseling is directed is clearly linked to increased rates of morbidity or mortality from a particular disease or injury. The second is whether there is evidence that the risk of morbidity or mortality can be reduced by the advocated intervention. The third is whether counseling is effective in achieving the desired risk reduction behavior. If the answer to any of these questions is no, then

Table 19-4

U.S. Preventive Services Task Force Recommendations for Children Ages 0–10 Years

IMMUNIZATIONS*
Diphtheria-tetanus-pertussis
Poliovirus
Measles-mumps-rubella
Haemophilus influenzae type B
Hepatitis B
Varicella

SCREENING†
Height and weight
Blood pressure
Vision screen (age 3–4 years)

COUNSELING
Child safety car seats (age <5 years)
Lap/shoulder belts (age ≥5 years)
Bicycle helmet, bicycle safety
Smoke detector
Flame retardant sleepwear
Hot water temperature <120–130°F
Window and stair guards, pool fence
Safe storage of medication, guns, matches, toxic substances
Ipecac, poison control phone number
Cardiopulmonary resuscitation training for parents and caretakers
Limit fat in diet; emphasize fruits, vegetables, grains
Regular physical exercise
Avoid tobacco use and effects of passive smoking
Regular dental visits
Floss and brush with fluoride toothpaste daily

*Refer to *MMWR* 47:8–12 or to most recent CDC recommendations for detailed information on immunization schedules and types of vaccines.
†Does not include recommendations for newborn metabolic screening.
SOURCE: Adapted with permission from U.S. Preventive Services Task Force: *Guide to Clinical Preventive Services*, 2d ed. Baltimore, Williams & Wilkins, 1996.

the rationale for counseling patients about a particular intervention is weak.

In addition, it is also necessary to consider a fourth criterion, the cost of the risk reduction behavior changes. Finally, a fifth pertinent criterion is whether there are any risks to changing the behavior. Depending on the nature and magnitude of the costs and risks, counseling may or may not be desirable, even if the condition at which efforts are directed causes substantial morbidity and mortality.

Not all counseling interventions have been rigorously evaluated according these criteria. In many cases, therefore, the effectiveness of widely recommend risk reduction counseling is unknown.

Evaluation of a Common Counseling Intervention

The five criteria outlined above can be used to evaluate counseling for smoking cessation, one of the most widely provided forms of risk reduction counseling. The problem of cigarette smoking meets the first criterion for counseling interventions because it is clearly linked to an increased risk of significant health problems. Smoking causes or contributes to about 20 percent of all deaths in the United States, accounting for 5 million years of potential life lost each year. Smoking is clearly linked to cancer of the lung, trachea, bronchus, larynx, pharynx, mouth, and esophagus. It also contributes to cancer of the pancreas, kidney, bladder, and cervix. Smoking causes atherosclerosis and its sequelae of myocardial infarction, strokes, and peripheral vascular disease. It also causes chronic obstructive pulmonary disease and contributes to death from pneumonia. Smoking in pregnancy causes increased rates of low birth weight, preterm deliveries, fetal growth retardation, and perinatal deaths.

There is also substantial evidence that smoking-related morbidity and mortality can be reduced by smoking cessation, even in those with a lifetime of smoking exposure. Thus, smoking cessation counseling meets criterion 2.

Table 19-5

U.S. Preventive Services Task Force Recommendations for Ages 11–24 Years

IMMUNIZATIONS
Tetanus-diphtheria boosters (11–16 years) Hepatitis B (if not previously administered) Measles-mumps-rubella (11–12 years if no prior second dose) Varicella (if susceptible to chickenpox) Rubella (females >12 year, unless positive by serologic testing or history of vaccination)
SCREENING
Height and weight Blood pressure Pap smear (females when sexually active or at age 18 if unreliable history) Chlamydia (females <20 years if sexually active) Rubella serology or vaccine history (females >12 years) Assess for problem drinking
COUNSELING
Lap/shoulder belts Motorcycle/bicycle helmets Smoke detector Safe storage/removal of guns Avoid tobacco, underage drinking, illicit drugs Avoid alcohol and drug use while driving, swimming, boating Sexually transmitted disease prevention. Abstinence, condoms, avoiding high-risk behavior Unintended pregnancy; contraception Limit fat and cholesterol intake; emphasize fruits, vegetables, grains Adequate calcium intake Regular physical activity Regular dental visits Floss and brush teeth with fluoride daily
CHEMOPROPHYLAXIS
Multivitamin with folic acid (females)

SOURCE: Adapted with permission from U.S. Preventive Services Task Force: *Guide to Clinical Preventive Services*, 2d ed. Baltimore, Williams & Wilkins, 1996.

In addition, smoking cessation counseling meets the third criterion because it is effective in convincing patients to quit smoking, particularly if patients are scheduled for follow-up visits, provided with self-help educational materials, referred to smoking cessation support groups, and prescribed nicotine replacement therapy.

There are costs involved with smoking cessation, but they are minimal compared to the lifetime costs of cigarettes and their related health problems; thus, the fourth criterion is met.

Table 19-6

U.S. Preventive Services Task Force Recommendations for Adults Ages 25–64

IMMUNIZATIONS
Tetanus-diphtheria boosters every 10 years Rubella vaccination in women of child-bearing age with no history of vaccination, or negative results on rubella serologic testing

SCREENING
Blood pressure Height and weight Total cholesterol (men ages 35–64, women ages 45–64) Pap smear (women) Fecal occult blood test and/or sigmoidoscopy (ages >50) Mammograms ± clinical breast examination (women 50–69 years) Assess for problem drinking Rubella vaccination history in women of child-bearing age

COUNSELING
Tobacco cessation Avoid alcohol and drug use while driving, swimming, boating Limit fat and cholesterol intake: emphasize fruits, vegetables, grains Adequate calcium intake (women) Regular physical activity Lap/shoulder belts in cars Motorcycle/bicycle helmets Smoke detector in home Safe storage/removal of guns Sexually transmitted disease prevention: condoms, avoiding high-risk behavior Contraception Regular dental examinations Floss and brush teeth with fluoride daily

CHEMOPROPHYLAXIS
Multivitamin with folic acid (women planning pregnancy) Discuss estrogen replacement (postmenopausal women)

SOURCE: Adapted with permission from U.S. Preventive Services Task Force: *Guide to Clinical Preventive Services*, 2d ed. Baltimore, Williams & Wilkins, 1996.

Finally, there are no known hazards of smoking cessation, except possibly weight gain, and thus the fifth criterion is satisfied.

Therefore, smoking cessation receives the highest level recommendation from the USPSTF. Smoking cessation is also strongly advocated by every major health care organization in the United States.

EVALUATING SCREENING TESTS To evaluate the utility of a screening test, eight criteria are typically used. Tests that meet each of the criteria are con-

Table 19-7

U.S. Preventive Services Task Force Recommendations for Adults Ages 65 and Older

IMMUNIZATIONS
Pneumococcal vaccine Influenza vaccine: annually Tetanus/diphtheria (Td) boosters: every 10 years
SCREENING
Blood pressure, height, and weight Fecal occult blood test and/or sigmoidoscopy Mammograms ± clinical breast exam (women through age 69) Pap smear (for women with a cervix, consider discontinuation after age 65 if previous regular screening always had normal results) Assess for vision and hearing impairment Assess for problem drinking
COUNSELING
Tobacco cessation Avoid alcohol and drug use while driving, swimming and boating Limit fat and cholesterol intake: emphasize fruits, vegetables, grains Adequate calcium intake Regular physical activity Lap/shoulder belts Motorcycle/bicycle helmets Fall prevention Safe storage/removal of guns Smoke detector Set hot water heater to 120°–130°F Cardiopulmonary resuscitation training for household Regular dental visits, floss and brush teeth with fluoride daily Sexually transmitted disease prevention—condoms, avoid high risk behavior
CHEMOPROPHYLAXIS
Discuss estrogen replacement(women)

SOURCE: Adapted with permission from U.S. Preventive Services Task Force: *Guide to Clinical Preventive Services*, 2d ed. Baltimore, Williams & Wilkins, 1996.

sidered appropriate for clinical implementation. Those that do not meet the criteria may be inappropriate screening tests.

Criterion 1: The Condition Should Be Sufficiently Serious It is generally accepted that screening should be undertaken only for conditions that

cause significant mortality or morbidity, whether measured as disability, suffering, or decreased quality of life.

Criterion 2: The Condition Should Be Sufficiently Prevalent In most cases, screening the population for very rare conditions is not appropriate.

Entire populations would be screened to detect a condition that affects only a few individuals.

Criterion 3: The Condition Should Have an Asymptomatic or Preclinical Period The goal of screening is to detect conditions at a sufficiently early stage to permit interventions that delay or prevent the onset of complications. For diseases with symptoms that appear de novo without a substantial presymptomatic period, there is no opportunity to detect the disease and institute preventive measures before symptoms occur. In this situation, screening lacks rationale.

Criterion 4: If Identified, the Condition Should Be Preventable or Treatable Obviously, if no interventions are available to prevent or treat the condition, there is no point in detecting it with a screening test.

Criterion 5: The Screening Test Should Be Sufficiently Accurate To be clinically useful, a screening test must be accurate. There are several ways to examine accuracy. These methods include measures of sensitivity, specificity, and positive and negative predictive values.

Sensitivity Sensitivity is a measure of the proportion of persons with a disease that is detected by the test (true-positive results in the numerator, and true-positive plus false-negative results in the denominator). If a test detects every patient with a disease, it has perfect sensitivity (i.e., the sensitivity is 100 percent).

Specificity Specificity is a measure of the proportion of persons without a disease that tests negative (true-negative results in the numerator, and true-negative plus false-positive results in the denominator). If everyone without the disease tests negative, then the test is highly specific for the disease (i.e., the specificity is 100 percent).

Sensitivity and specificity are test characteristics that change depending on how precisely and accurately the test is performed. They also vary

inversely with each other: as sensitivity increases, specificity decreases, and vice versa.

Positive Predictive Value Positive predictive value is the probability of actually having a disease if the test result is positive (true-positive results in the numerator, true-positive plus false-positive results in the denominator). The positive predictive value is the most useful statistic for clinicians counseling patients, since patients usually want to know what a positive test result means for them. Positive predictive value is affected by the accuracy of the test, but, most important, it varies with the prevalence of the disease in the population being tested.

This concept is easily illustrated with screening tests for HIV infection (Fig. 19-1). If the population being tested is at low risk (e.g., married, monogamous, middle-class couples with no prior sexual partners or drug-use histories), HIV infection will be rare in that population (e.g., 1/10,000). In this scenario, even if the test has a sensitivity of 99 percent and a specificity of 99 percent, a positive test result indicates only a 1-percent chance that HIV infection is really present.

However, the positive predictive value of an HIV test is quite different when applied to a high-risk population (e.g., urban intravenous drug users with a disease prevalence of 25 percent). In this population, a positive test result indicates a 97-percent chance that the tested individual really has HIV infection. Thus, the significance of a positive result differs substantially depending on the probability that patients might actually have the condition being tested.

Negative Predictive Value Negative predictive value is the probability of *not* having the disease if the test result is negative (true-negative results in the numerator, and true-negative plus false-negative results in the denominator). Using the HIV example again, a negative HIV test result for a person unlikely to have HIV infection most likely indicates that HIV infection is absent (i.e., high negative predictive value). A negative

Figure 19-1

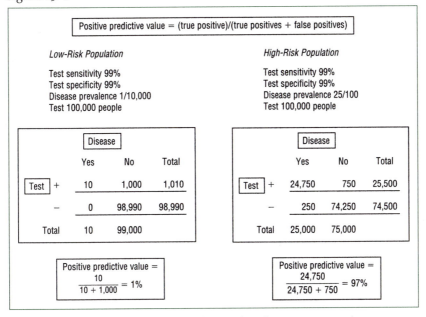

Predictive valve of screening tests. The predictive value of a positive test result can vary considerably depending on the underlying frequency of disease in the population being tested. The example above uses a test for HIV that has 99-percent sensitivity and 99-percent specificity. In the low-risk population, with a disease frequency of 1 in 10,000, a positive test result indicates only a 1-percent chance that a patient actually has HIV infection. In a high-risk population, however, with a disease prevalence of 25 per 100, a positive result on the same test indicates a 97-percent chance that the patient actually has HIV infection.

HIV test result in urban intravenous drug users who share needles and have unprotected sexual intercourse is more likely to represent a false-negative result than in a low-risk population.

Criterion 6: The Cost of the Screening Test Should Be Affordable Less expensive tests are obviously more desirable than more costly tests. Some tests can be prohibitively expensive for mass population screening, even if they are extremely accurate and could diminish the morbidity and mortality associated with a common or lethal condition (e.g., mass screening with magnetic resonance imaging to detect a common cancer).

Criterion 7: Risks of the Screening Test Should Be Acceptable Risks of screening tests are measured both in terms of the physical and emotional risks to the patients undergoing the test and in terms of the risks of subsequent tests or procedures that will be undertaken if the screening test is positive.

Criterion 8: Discovery and Treatment of the Disease Should Improve Outcomes If screening detects the disease in the asymptomatic period and treatment is begun at that time, the outcome should be better than waiting to treat the disease after symptoms appear spontaneously. This criterion is extremely important, yet it is frequently overlooked or not evaluated. Often, tests appear to be effective in improving outcomes, when they really are not. These apparent improvements in outcomes are frequently due to "lead-time" or "length" bias.

Lead-Time Bias   Sometimes a screening test will discover an asymptomatic disease early in the course of the disease process. Instituting treatment at this point, however, may have results no different than if treatment were begun when symptoms appeared later in the course of the disease. In this situation, starting treatment at the time of early detection will make it appear that survival with the disease has been prolonged, but all that has really occurred is that the disease was detected earlier in an asymptomatic period. This "lead-time bias" will make screening and treatment appear to be beneficial, when they actually are not.

Length Bias   Similarly, screening may permit detection of less severe, less symptomatic cases of a disease, for which survival is naturally longer. For example, prostate cancer in some patients is a rapidly progressive, fatal illness. In others, prostate cancer is a relatively indolent condition in which patients survive for many years (i.e., a longer "length" of illness) and die of other causes. Detection and treatment of such indolent cases will inevitably have good outcomes, since the survival time would have been long even without treatment. However, the outcomes only seem better because less severe cases with inherently longer survival times have been detected and treated, an effect known as "length bias."

Because of lead-time and length biases, many studies demonstrating the effectiveness of screening tests are flawed. To avoid these biases, a controlled trial with randomization of subjects to screening and non-screening groups, and outcome measures including death and disability, is the preferred way to evaluate the effectiveness of a screening test. For most screening tests, however, such randomized controlled trials are prohibitively expensive and rarely available to guide clinical decisions. Thus, many commonly recommended preventive services have never been adequately tested for effectiveness.

An Evaluation of Common Screening Tests   Use of the principles and criteria described above can

be illustrated by systematically evaluating benefits of tests commonly used to screen for colon and prostate cancer.

Colon Cancer Screening   About 130,000 new cases of colorectal cancer were diagnosed in 1998. In the same year, there were 57,000 deaths due to this disease. Thus, colon cancer is not only common, but it also entails substantial mortality rates (criteria 1 and 2). There is also a long asymptomatic period (criterion 3), estimated to be as long as 10 to 15 years, during which 5 to 40 percent of initially benign adenomatous polyps develop into cancer. Furthermore, there is an effective treatment (criterion 4) if polyps are detected in this precancerous stage, since polypectomy appears to prevent polyps from undergoing malignant transformation. Based on these four criteria, there is justification to screen for colon cancer.

Next, one must consider the fifth criterion: accuracy of the screening test. Two screening tests are currently advocated for colon cancer screening: sigmoidoscopy and fecal occult blood tests (FOBT). Sigmoidoscopy has a sensitivity of 50 to 55 percent for detecting polyps and an unknown specificity. Various studies have found FOBT to have a sensitivity of 30 to 90 percent and a specificity of 90 to 99 percent, with a positive predictive value of 2 to 11 percent for cancer and 20 to 30 percent for adenomas. That is, a person with a positive FOBT result has a 2- to 11-percent chance of actually having cancer and a 20- to 30-percent chance of having an adenoma. It should be noted that the accuracy of FOBT depends on whether the test is conducted properly. Specifically, research that established the accuracy of FOBT used samples of three consecutive daily stools with two specimens from each stool, along with avoidance of certain foods (e.g., rare meats) and medications (e.g., aspirin and vitamin C) for several days prior to the test. Performing FOBT without these precautions will decrease the accuracy of the test. Thus, a rectal examination with testing of stool smeared on a Hemocult card is not a proper FOBT, and its accuracy has not been subjected to study.

The sixth and seventh criteria to consider are risk and cost. Screening sigmoidoscopy costs $100 to $200 and carries a small (less than 1:1000) risk of bowel perforation. There is little risk or expense in performing a FOBT, although subsequent evaluation of patients with positive test results, which requires colonoscopy, is costly and carries risk of bowel perforation and risks from sedating medications.

Finally, satisfying the eighth criterion requires evidence that screening with FOBT and/or sigmoidoscopy can reduce the mortality rate due to colorectal cancer. There is, in fact, evidence, that this is the case. However, there is no good evidence as to the best age to start screening, how long to continue, or the best frequency for sigmoidoscopy.

Based on this information, the USPSTF recommends screening for all persons age 50 and over with sigmoidoscopy, annual FOBT, or both. The recommended frequency of sigmoidoscopy screening is not stated, but it is mentioned that every 10 years might be as effective as every 3 to 5 years. The USPSTF does not recommend screening for colon cancer with digital rectal examination, barium enema, or colonoscopy because of a lack of proof of efficacy. The American Cancer Society, on the other hand, recommends annual digital rectal examinations starting at age 40, annual FOBTs starting at age 50, and sigmoidoscopy or colonoscopy every 3 to 5 years starting at age 50.

Prostate Cancer Screening   In recent years, use of the serum marker prostate-specific antigen (PSA), as a screening test for prostate cancer has become widespread. Screening for PSA is considerably more controversial than is colon cancer screening.

Prostate cancer is the most common cancer and the second leading cause of cancer deaths in American men, with close to 250,000 new cases and 40,000 deaths each year. Thus, prostate cancer screening meets criteria 1 and 2. The natural history of prostate cancer is not well understood because there are both aggressive and indolent forms of the disease. Both forms, however,

appear to have an asymptomatic period during which screening might be effective. This observation satisfies criterion number 3.

Criterion 4 requires evidence that effective treatments are available for prostate cancer. Prostate cancer treatment options include radical prostatectomy, radiation therapy, and hormonal treatment. The efficacy of these treatments is less than certain, being based on uncontrolled trials subject to length and lead-time bias related to detection of early indolent cancers that may never have become symptomatic or caused clinically apparent disease.

Criterion 5 examines the accuracy of PSA testing. The sensitivity of PSA for detecting prostate cancer has been reported as anywhere between 29 and 80 percent, and the positive predictive value is between 28 and 35 percent. However, a large proportion of tumors discovered with PSA testing are the indolent prostate cancers that are unlikely ever to become clinically significant. In fact, it is known that only a small subset of men with prostate cancer will have clinically significant disease, and most men with prostate cancer die of other causes. Therefore, not all prostate cancers detected by screening require treatment because PSA is not accurate for distinguishing prostate cancers that will cause death from those that will never become symptomatic. Thus, prostate cancer screening with PSA does not pass criterion 5.

The cost (criterion 6) of a PSA test is small, but the cost of working up false-positive results is considerable. It has been estimated that mass PSA screening in the United States could cost $12 to $28 billion annually. There is also risk associated with PSA screening (criterion 7) because prostate needle biopsy, the test usually used to evaluate patients with abnormal PSA test results, can cause infection (0.3 to 5 percent), septicemia (0.6 percent), and bleeding (0.1 percent). Radical prostatectomy, one of the principal treatments for prostate cancer, has an operative mortality rate of close to 1 percent and results in impotence in 20 to 80 percent of cases. It can also cause urinary incontinence (2 to 27 percent) and urethral stricture (10 to 18 percent).

Prostate-specific antigen screening also fails criterion 8 because at this time there is no solid evidence that PSA screening improves the outcome of prostate cancer. Large clinical trials to determine whether PSA screening improves outcomes are in progress, but results are not expected until after the year 2000.

Based on the foregoing analysis, the most recent USPSTF recommendations do not include screening for prostate cancer with PSA. However, the American Cancer Society believes that the potential benefits outweigh the risks, and, not being willing to wait for the results of controlled trials, recommends annual PSA testing starting at age 50. The American Urological Association makes the same recommendation as the American Cancer Society.

Providing Preventive Care in Clinical Practice

It has been stated that prevention is like the weather: everyone discusses it, but no one does much about it. Several reasons are cited for not providing preventive services. These reasons include a perceived lack of time, lack of a systematic approach to delivering preventive services, resistance on the part of patients, difficulty staying current on recommendations that change frequently, and inadequate financial reimbursement for providing preventive services.

It may be that these are rationalizations rather than legitimate reasons for not practicing prevention, since a systematic approach to preventive services can substantially improve performance. This approach includes the use of prevention flow sheets, health education booklets, and prevention routines, and the involvement of office staff in preventive services. If such an approach is adopted and preventive interventions are lim-

ited to those with proven efficacy, prevention can be addressed with most patients in a reasonable amount of time and with adequate reimbursement. Furthermore, provision of preventive services is rapidly becoming a quality standard used by health care organizations to determine clinicians' performance, and satisfactory performance in this area is likely to be required for clinicians to maintain enrollment as a provider in these organizations.

Nonetheless, the large number of recommended preventive services (Tables 19-4 through 19-7) makes it unrealistic to provide them all to individual patients during a single office visit, even if the visit is explicitly for the purpose of obtaining preventive care. Instead, most clinicians who are successful providing preventive care organize their practices so that one or more aspects of prevention are addressed at each office visit, with the goal of providing comprehensive preventive care during a series of office visits over time.

Publications and action kits have been developed to assist clinicians in organizing their practices for efficient provision of preventive services. In particular, the widely available Put Prevention into Practice (PPIP) Education and Action Kit consists of tools including patient-reminder post cards, patient-care flow sheets, chart stickers, self-sticking removable reminder notes, prevention prescription pads, and mini-records for patients to keep in their possession. Adoption of PPIP or similar aids can increase the rate with which preventive services are provided.

Errors

The most common errors in office-based preventive health care are not providing preventive care, errors related to immunization practices, and performing inappropriate screening tests.

Not Providing Preventive Care

Citing the reasons described above, clinicians frequently miss opportunities to provide preventive services when patients are in their offices. This occurs even for simple interventions, such as immunizations. For example, the CDC reports that clinicians administer influenza vaccine to fewer than 30 percent of the 32 million persons over 65 who should receive it each year, even though most of these individuals are seen in the health care system and could be immunized. Rates for pneumococcal immunizations in older individuals are also low. As a result, more than 20,000 potentially preventable deaths occur during influenza epidemic years, nearly all of which are directly attributable to influenza or complicating pneumonia.

Similarly, clinicians frequently fail to ask patients about their tetanus immunization status. Again, older individuals tend to be those who are not adequately immunized. The result is that, in the United States, most cases of tetanus (an entirely preventable disease) occur in the geriatric population.

Withholding Childhood Immunizations

Perhaps one of the most important errors clinicians make is to inappropriately delay or postpone scheduled childhood immunizations. This most often occurs because of a misconception that immunizations should not be given to children who have colds, earaches, gastroenteritis, or similar mild infections of childhood. Withholding immunizations in these circumstances results in many children's falling behind on, or perhaps never receiving, scheduled immunizations. Recommendations from the CDC and other national organizations are that routine childhood immunizations be withheld for serious febrile illnesses but not for otherwise-uncomplicated common childhood infections. Children who are only mildly ill with simple colds, sore throats, earaches, and so on can safely receive routine immunizations, even if the infection is accompanied by low-grade fever.

Administration of Immunizations at the Wrong Site

Another error is the administration of immunizations into the wrong site. Some immunizations, notably hepatitis B vaccine, have diminished effectiveness if not administered intramuscularly. Administration of such vaccines into the buttocks of adults frequently results in deposition of the immunizing material into the gluteal fat, rather than into the muscle, because needles used for routine injections are not sufficiently long to reach through the gluteal fat. For this reason, hepatitis B vaccine should be administered only into the deltoid muscle, which is easily entered with standard-sized immunization needles.

Performing Inappropriate Screening Tests

Clinicians frequently order and perform screening tests and examinations that are not indicated. For example, there is no evidence that "annual physical examinations" or "complete physicals" are necessary for any U.S. adults. Instead, screening examinations should be targeted at age- and gender-specific risks, as outlined in Table 19-2 and Tables 19-4 through 19-7. Complete head-to-toe physicals rarely yield benefit other than that which would accrue from focused risk-related screening.

Similarly, clinicians frequently order screening blood tests, such as complete blood counts and chemistry panels, as "screening tests" in patients with no indications for these tests. Time and effort would be more effectively spent performing age- and gender-appropriate screening tests and providing indicated immunizations and other preventive care.

Emerging Concepts

Over the next 1 to 2 decades, clinicians are likely to see many changes in the way preventive services are provided. There will be an emphasis on services for which effectiveness has been clearly demonstrated. The aging of the U.S. population will focus more preventive resources on maintaining the health and independence of the geriatric-aged population. Research in behavioral science holds the promise of finding ways of more effectively changing human behavior toward healthier life-styles. In addition, several technological advances, outlined below, are likely to influence the types and delivery of preventive services available in the United States.

New Immunizations

Basic and applied scientific research will lead to an expanding number of available immunizations and development of immunizations against microorganisms such as HIV, group B streptococci, *Escherichia coli*, rotavirus, human papillomavirus, and others. It is likely that some of these immunizations will be available within the next 1 to 2 decades.

Genetics

As research on the human genome progresses, it will be possible to conduct more sophisticated risk assessments that identify conditions to which specific individuals are genetically predisposed. Then, screening might focus only on individuals at genetic risk for certain diseases. This approach to screening has already begun with the discovery of the BRCA-1 and BRCA-2 genes, which serve as markers for an increased risk of breast and ovarian cancer. Similarly, basic research is likely to reveal the genetic basis of chronic diseases ranging from diabetes to

Alzheimer's disease. Novel genetics-based treatments and interventions are likely to be developed and applied to persons at risk for these conditions, making it productive to screen for these conditions.

Computerized Medical Records

As the number of conditions for which screening and prevention is available increases, these advances will tax the ability of clinicians to keep abreast of current screening and treatment recommendations. With the advent of computerized medical records and diagnostic systems, new recommendations for prevention will be incorporated into the computerized systems. Thus, rather than clinicians' having to remember large numbers of ever-changing preventive health recommendations, computer systems will prompt clinicians to provide indicated preventive services at appropriate times for individual patients.

Bibliography

Advance report of final mortality statistics 1993. *Month Vital Stat Rep* 44 S, February 29, 1996.

American Academy of Pediatrics: *1997 Red Book: Report of the Committee on Infectious Diseases*, 24th ed. Chicago. American Academy of Pediatrics, 1997.

American Cancer Society: *Guidelines for the Cancer-Related Checkup: An Update.* Atlanta, American Cancer Society, 1993.

American Urological Association: *Executive Committee Report.* Baltimore, American Urological Association, January 1992.

Cancer statistics 1998. *Ca Cancer J Clin* 48:6, 1998.

Centers for Disease Control and Prevention: Cigarette smoking: Attributable mortality and years of potential life lost—United States, 1990. *MMWR* 42:645, 1993.

Dickey LL, Kamerow DB: Seven steps to delivering preventive care. *Fam Pract Manage* 1:32, 1994.

Dietrich AJ, Woodruff CB, Carney PA: Changing office routines to enhance preventive care: The preventive gaps approach. *Arch Fam Med* 3:176, 1994.

Gnauck R, Macrae FA, Fleisher M: How to perform the fecal occult blood test. *Ca Cancer J Clin* 34:134, 1984.

Lorig K: Patient education and counseling for prevention, in U.S. Preventive Services Task Force: *Guide to Clinical Preventive Services, 2d ed*. Baltimore, Williams & Wilkins, 1996, pp lxxv–lxxxiii.

Lowes, R: Implementing and measuring clinical preventive services, in *Vital Signs*, vol 5. Kansas City, American Academy of Family Physicians, 1997.

McGinnis JM, Foege WH: Actual causes of death in the United States. *JAMA* 270:2207, 1993.

Morson BC: The evolution of colorectal carcinoma. *Clin Radiol* 35:425, 1984.

Muto T, Bussey HJR, Morson BC: The evolution of cancer of the colon and rectum. *Cancer* 36:2251, 1975.

Optenberg SA, Thompson IM: Economics of screening for carcinoma of the prostate. *Urol Clin North Am* 17:719, 1990.

Recommended childhood immunization schedule: United States, 1998. *MMWR* 47:8, 1998.

Schappert SM: *National Ambulatory Medical Care Survey: 1991 Summary*. Vital and Health Statistics series 13, no 116, May 1994.

Trepka MJ, DiGuiseppi C: Counseling to prevent tobacco use, in *Guide to Clinical Preventive Services*, 2d ed. Baltimore, Williams & Wilkens, 1996, pp 597–609.

Woolf SH: Screening for colorectal cancer, in *Guide to Clinical Preventive Services: Report of the U.S. Preventive Services Task Force*, 2d ed. Baltimore, Williams & Wilkins, 1996, pp 89–103.

Woolf SH: Screening for prostate cancer, in *Guide to Clinical Preventive Services: Report of the U.S. Preventive Services Task Force*, 2d ed. Baltimore, Williams & Wilkins, 1996, pp 119–134.

Mindy A. Smith
Jill Larkin

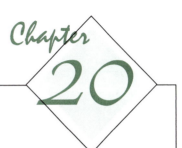

Chapter

20

Birth Control

How Common Are Office Visits for Contraception?

According to the National Ambulatory Medical Care Survey (NAMCS), approximately 18 percent of all women's contacts with physicians focus on reproductive health, and 7 percent (12.6 million) of visits by women aged 15 to 44 are specifically for contraception. This places reproductive health and contraception among the most common reasons why women seek medical care in the United States. Most of this care is rendered in primary care settings.

Despite these statistics, many women in the United States are not using contraception. Be-

tween 50 and 60 percent of pregnancies in the United States are unplanned, and the average sexually active adolescent has intercourse for 23 months before seeking contraceptive counseling. Data published in 1995 indicate that the percentage of sexually active women aged 15 to 44 who do not use contraception had increased since 1988 (from 7 to 12 percent), and 22 percent of women aged 15 to 19 were sexually active in the past month without using contraception.

Without contraception, 85 percent of women engaging in intercourse over the course of 1 year will become pregnant. Nonetheless, many women express concerns about potential health risks and side effects from the use of contraceptives and therefore do not use them. In fact, in one study of women with unintended pregnancies, the most frequent reason cited for not using two of the most effective contraceptive methods (oral contraceptives and intrauterine devices) was concern about side effects.

Even among women who use contraception, compliance is poor. In the 1990 National Survey of Family Growth, only 42 percent of women using barrier methods such as condoms and diaphragms reported using the method with each act of intercourse.

Given that more than half of pregnancies in the United States are unintended and that many sexually active individuals do not use effective, or any, contraceptive methods, prescribing and counseling about contraception is one of the most important preventive interventions that clinicians can make. To be successful in this preventive effort, primary care clinicians must take an active role in assessing patients' needs for birth control and be prepared to provide information, counseling, and prescriptions for contraceptive methods.

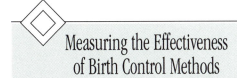

Measuring the Effectiveness of Birth Control Methods

The effectiveness of the various methods of birth control is important in any discussion of contraception. Unfortunately, optimal statistical methods for reporting effectiveness (i.e., prevention of unintended pregnancy) have yet to be developed. The most frequently used methods for measuring effectiveness are the Pearl index, user and method failure rates, and life-table analysis.

Pearl Index

The Pearl index, used in much of the older literature, reports rates of unintended pregnancy per woman-year of use. The Pearl index is not particularly effective, however, in measuring pregnancies that occur with the passage of time. That is, it is unable to distinguish between a small number of women followed for long periods of time and larger numbers of women followed for shorter periods of time.

User and Method Failure Rates

Failure rates are a simple calculation of the number of failures divided by the number of users. User failure rates include both those individuals who use a method properly and those who do not. Method (theoretical) failure rates assume perfect use and, therefore, are calculated after excluding failures (i.e., pregnancies) that occur due to imperfect use of a method. The calculations of method failure rates are often inappropriately high because few investigators successfully exclude all women who become pregnant from imperfect use.

Life-Table Analysis

Life-table analysis computes the probability of unintended pregnancy within a particular time frame. The method has been criticized for its lack of precision in identifying variations in effectiveness with differing patterns of use. For example, life-table analysis assumes that most initial users of a method are continuous users and that use of a particular method is uninterrupted over the time period under study. These assumptions frequently do not reflect the real-life use of contraceptive methods. While some studies attempt to account for these problems using statistical adjustments, the validity of life-table methods for measuring contraceptive effectiveness is unclear.

Despite these limitations, life-table analyses are widely used and avoid some of the weaknesses of the Pearl index and method and user failure rates. Whenever possible, this chapter uses life-table data to report the effectiveness of contraceptive methods, based on reports from the literature. These data are summarized in Table 20-1.

Table 20-1

Failure Rates among Typical Users and Potential Advantages and Side Effects of Birth Control Methods

Method	Failure Rate, % in First Year	Annual Cost $*	Advantages	Common or Serious Adverse Effects
Female sterilization	0.4–1.8	1200–2500[†]	Permanent, safe, decreased rate ovarian cancer	Ectopic pregnancy, menstrual disorders, dysmenorrhea, regret
Male sterilization	0.5–1.6	500[†]	Permanent, safe	Hematoma, epididymitis, orchalgia, sperm granuloma
Oral contraceptives	3.0	200–325	Fewer STDs, decreased rate of ovarian and endometrial cancer, less menstrual pain and bleeding	Cardiovascular complications, nausea, dizziness, headache, spotting, weight gain, breast tenderness, chloasma
Depo-Provera (medroxyprogesterone MDPA)	0.3	140	Less PID, decreased ovarian and endometrial cancer, easy to use	Irregular bleeding, weight gain, headaches
Norplant	0.1	170[‡]	Less PID, less menstrual pain and bleeding, effective for 5 years	Complications of insertion and removal, irregular bleeding
Female condom	15–21	250	Fewer STDs, nonprescription	Awkward to use
Male condom	4–12	50	Fewer STDs, reduced cervical cancer, easy, inexpensive, non-prescription, delays premature ejaculation	Discomfort, reduced sensitivity, latex allergy, reduced spontaneity
Diaphragm	3–18	155–235	Fewer STDs, decreased cervical neoplasia	Latex or spermicide allergy, bladder infection, bacterial or yeast vaginitis, toxic shock syndrome
Cervical cap	8–19	155–235	Fewer STDs, can remain in vagina longer than diaphragm	Odor, cervical erosion or laceration, other side effects same as diaphragm
Spermicide (alone)	21	85	Low cost, nonprescription, fewer STDs	Allergy, irritation
IUD (copper)	0.6–0.8	180[‡]	Not user dependent, effective for 10 years	PID, perforation of uterus, increased menstrual pain and bleeding, possibly increased ectopic pregnancy
IUD (progestin)	1.5	320[‡]	Not user dependent, effective for 1 year, less menstrual bleeding	Similar to copper IUD
Natural family planning		0	No chemicals or devices needed	No STD protection, unforgiving of imperfect use, requires highly motivated user
Perfect use	1–3			
Imperfect use	19–38			
Lactation	0.5–2	0	Promotes breast-feeding	Only reliable for 4–6 months
Withdrawal	7–19	0	Readily available	No STD protection

*Cost figures from Hatcher RA, Trussell J, Stewart F, et al. †Costs for sterilization calculated as a one-time expense. ‡Assumes retention for 5 years for Norplant, 1 year for prog-estin IUD, and 8 years for copper IUD. ABBREVIATIONS: IUD, intrauterine device; PID, pelvic inflammatory disease; STD, sexually transmitted disease.

Principal Methods of Birth Control

In 1990, 59 percent of U.S. women 15 to 44 years of age (34.5 million women) were using a birth control method. It is estimated that 95 percent of sexually active women use contraception at some time in their lives and that the average woman who uses contraception will use up to three different methods.

Among the available birth control options, sterilization is the most commonly used method worldwide. Sterilization is chosen by 36 percent of couples in the United States. Of these couples, about 60 percent choose female sterilization.

Oral contraceptives (estrogen/progestin combination pills and progestin-only pills) are the next most frequently prescribed method. Oral contraceptives are used by over 10 million (17 percent) U.S. women between 15 and 44 years of age.

Several surveys of U.S. women have reported that condoms are the next most-frequently used method of birth control (6.1 million, 10.5 percent), followed by spermicide use alone (1.2 million, 2 percent). Natural family planning methods are used by about 1 million ever-married women, or between 2 and 3 percent of currently married couples. The diaphragm (1 million, 1.7 percent) and periodic abstinence (0.9 million, 1.6 percent) are next most common methods, followed by intrauterine devices (0.5 million, 0.8 percent) and withdrawal (0.3 million, 0.6 percent). Progestin implants and douching are reported as the least common methods of birth control in the U.S.

It is interesting to note that primary care clinicians and obstetrician-gynecologists tend to differ in the contraceptive methods they prescribe. In contrast to primary care clinicians, obstetrician-gynecologists are far more likely to perform sterilization procedures and far less likely to prescribe barrier methods of contraception. These differences can probably be traced to differences in exposure to and experience with contraceptive methods during residency training.

Sterilization

About 1 million sterilization procedures are performed yearly in the United States. Female sterilization involves occlusion or transection of the fallopian tubes, commonly referred to as "tubal ligation." Male sterilization is performed by vasectomy. Among U.S. women, 33 percent of those aged 30 to 35 and 50 percent of those over age 40 have been sterilized. Vasectomy is used for contraception by approximately 11 to 12 percent of U.S. couples.

FEMALE STERILIZATION

The majority of female sterilization procedures are performed either immediately postpartum or as an elective outpatient surgical procedure using a laparoscope. In either setting, general or regional anesthesia can be used.

Tubal ligation is performed using one of three basic methods. One method is open partial salpingectomy, often performed in the immediate postpartum period. It is performed using an abdominal incision through which a portion of each fallopian tube is cut and the ends are tied off. A common procedure for open partial salpingectomy is the Pomeroy method, in which a small loop of each fallopian tube is tied and the top segment of the loop is excised.

A second method involves electrical current to cauterize and thereby occlude the fallopian tubes. Cauterization procedures are generally performed through a laparoscope, and tubal occlusion is achieved with either unipolar or bipolar electrocauterization. Bipolar current is preferred because unipolar cauterization causes considerably more tubal damage, including the possibility of bowel burns. The more extensive tissue damage with unipolar cauterization also makes it more difficult to reverse tubal occlusion in the future, should reversal be desired.

The third method involves placing an occluding device over the tubes, usually a silicone band or spring clip, such as the Hulka or Filshie device. The devices are generally applied through a laparoscope. Because the occluding device causes minimal tubal damage, this type of tubal ligation may be more easily reversible. The Hulka clip is most often used in the United States. The Filshie clip is the most popular technique of tubal ligation in Canada.

FAILURE RATES   The failure rate typically reported for tubal ligation is 0.4 percent in the first year following the procedure (Table 20-1). However, a recent collaborative prospective study of 10,685 women found a higher cumulative failure rate of 18.5 pregnancies per 1,000 procedures over 10 years. In that study, younger women (aged 18 to 27), African-American women, and those undergoing bipolar or spring-clip occlusion methods had the highest failure rates.

COMPLICATIONS   Complications of tubal ligation in the perioperative period are uncommon but include reactions to anesthesia (rare, but can be severe), bleeding (1 percent), and infection (less than 1 percent). Some investigators report that, over the long term, women who have undergone tubal ligation have higher rates of dysmenorrhea and abnormal menstrual cycles than do control groups of women. These findings, however, are not consistent and may be due to differences in follow-up methods.

MALE STERILIZATION

Male sterilization, or vasectomy, involves occlusion of the vas deferens, thereby preventing passage of sperm into the ejaculate. Because the seminal vesicles and prostate gland provide 90 to 95 percent of the fluid volume discharged during ejaculation, the quantity and composition of the ejaculate (except for sperm content) remain virtually unchanged after vasectomy. As with tubal ligation, the methods of occlusion include ligation, cautery, clips, and combinations of these

approaches. Ligation is the most commonly reported method. Virtually all vasectomies are performed under local anesthesia, either alone or with sedation, and the majority are performed in clinicians' offices.

With the conventional vasectomy technique, a single incisions or bilateral incision are made high in the scrotum along the median raphe. Then the vas deferens is identified, cut (usually removing a 1-cm segment), and tied, cauterized, and/or clipped. Percutaneous ("no-scalpel") vasectomy, a technique recently introduced in the United States, eliminates the need for a scalpel by using a sharp, curved hemostat to puncture the scrotal skin and deliver the vas deferens to the exterior. This technique is reported to reduce surgery time to 10 min and to significantly decrease the incidence of infection and hematoma.

FAILURE RATES AND COMPLICATIONS   Failure rates with vasectomy are reported to be between 0.5 and 1.5 percent. Short-term complications include hematoma (1 percent), epididymitis (less than 0.5 percent), and, rarely, chronic testicular pain (1/10,000). The later is believed due to high intraepididymal pressures proximal to the occlusion.

Several concerns have been raised about long-term effects of vasectomy on the immune system. In particular, there were concerns that the antisperm antibodies that routinely develop after vasectomy might cross-react with coronary artery antigens and predispose to coronary artery disease. However, these concerns have not been borne out in epidemiological studies.

SELECTION AND COUNSELING OF PATIENTS

It is essential to emphasize that sterilization should be considered permanent. While reversal methods exist, success rates resulting in a pregnancy are only 70 to 80 percent for reversal of tubal ligation and about 50 percent for vasectomy reversal. Differences in rates of successful reversal appear to be based on the sterilization procedure performed (less success with electrocautery methods for women and with removal of long segments of the vas deferens for men), time since surgery (inversely related to success), and other factors, including older age.

Regret about sterilization and requests for reversal occur in 2 to 7 percent of individuals. Regret is higher among young patients, those who express a desire for more children before they undergo sterilization, and those who suffer the loss of a child or divorce following the procedure. These issues should be discussed. If individuals or couples express uncertainty, alternative contraceptive methods should be recommended.

Combined Oral Contraceptives

The U.S. Food and Drug Administration first approved a combined estrogen-progestin oral contraceptive pill (OCP) in 1960. Since that time, OCP manufacturers have progressively lowered the dose of estrogen, which has reduced adverse effects without compromising contraceptive ef-

ficacy. In addition, newer OCPs contain progestins that are less androgenic than those in older preparations, thereby reducing androgenic side effects (e.g., acne) and adverse effects on blood lipid profiles. Because of the lower estrogen levels and safer progestins in current OCPs, this method of birth control can be used by a broader group of women than before and often can be continued until menopause.

MECHANISMS OF ACTION

Estrogens and progestins in combined OCPs act both synergistically and independently to prevent pregnancy, primarily by suppressing ovulation. The principal contraceptive effects of estrogen and progestins are shown in Table 20-2. With these multiple methods of action, it is not surprising that OCPs are highly effective at preventing pregnancy. The pregnancy rate in typical OCP users is about 3 percent. The most common cause of OCP failure is thought to be forgetting to take the pills.

Table 20-2

Effects of Estrogen and Progestin in Oral Contraceptive Pills

EFFECT	RESULT
ESTROGEN	
Suppression of follicle-stimulating hormone (FSH)	Impairs maturation of ovarian follicle, which prevents ovulation
Impaired ovum transport	Prevents fertilization
Altered endometrial secretions and cellularity	Prevents implantation
Accelerated luteolysis	More rapid degeneration of corpus luteum
PROGESTIN	
Suppression of luteinizing hormone (LH)	Prevents ovulation
Thickening of cervical mucus	Inhibits sperm transport
Inhibits capacitation (activation of enzymes that facilitate sperm penetration of the ovum)	Prevents fertilization
Altered fallopian tube secretions	Impairs ovum transport
Decidualized endometrium with atrophied glands	Prevents implantation

ESTROGEN   Currently, OCPs used in the United States contain one of two estrogens: ethinyl estradiol or mestranol (Tables 20-3 and 20-4). Ethinyl estradiol is pharmacologically active, while mestranol becomes pharmacologically active after conversion by the liver to ethinyl estradiol. Current doses of ethinyl estradiol in OCPs range from 20 to 50 µg. The lowest mestranol dose available in OCPs in the United States is 50 µg (roughly equivalent to 30 to 35 µg of ethinyl estradiol).

Table 20-3

Monophasic Combined Oral Contraceptives

ESTROGEN	PROGESTIN, µG	BRAND NAME
50-µG PREPARATIONS		
Mestranol	Norethindrone, 1.0	Genora 1/50 Nelova 1/50 Norethin 1/50 Norinyl 1 + 50 Ortho-Novum 1/50
Ethinyl estradiol	Ethynodiol diacetate, 1.0	Demulen 1/50
Ethinyl estradiol	Norethindrone, 1.0	Norlestrin 1/50 Ovcon-50
Ethinyl estradiol	Norethindrone, 2.5	Norlestrin 2.5/50
Ethinyl estradiol	Norgestrel, 0.5	Ovral
35-µG PREPARATIONS		
Ethinyl estradiol	Ethynodiol diacetate	Demulen 1/35
Ethinyl estradiol	Norethindrone, 1.0	Ortho-Novum 1/35 Norinyl 1/35
Ethinyl estradiol	Norethindrone, 0.4	Ovcon-35
Ethinyl estradiol	Norethindrone, 0.5	Modicon Brevicon Genora 0.5/35 Nelova 0.5/35
Ethinyl estradiol	Norgestimate, 0.25	Ortho Tri-Cyclen
30-µG PREPARATIONS		
Ethinyl estradiol	Norgestrel, 0.3	Lo-Ovral
Ethinyl estradiol	Levonorgestrel, 0.15	Nordette Levlen
Ethinyl estradiol	Norethindrone, 1.5	Loestrin 1.5/30
Ethinyl estradiol	Desogestrel, 0.15	Ortho-Cept Desogen
20-µG PREPARATIONS		
Ethinyl estradiol	Norethindrone, 1.0	Loestrin 1/20
Ethinyl estradiol	Levonorgestrel, 0.1	Alesse

Table 20-4

Multiphasic Combined Oral Contraceptives

ESTROGEN µG	PROGESTIN, µG	BRAND NAME
	BIPHASIC PREPARATIONS	
Ethinyl estradiol, 35	Norethindrone, 0.5 × 10 days, 1.0 × 11 days	Ortho-Novum 10/11
	Norethindrone, 0.5 × 7 days, 1.0 × 14 days	Jenest
	TRIPHASIC PREPARATIONS	
Ethinyl estradiol, 35	Norethindrone, 0.5 × 7 days, 0.75 × 7 days, 1.0 × 7 days	Ortho-Novum 7/7/7
Ethinyl estradiol, 35	Norethindrone, 0.5 × 7 days, 1.0 × 7 days, 0.5 × 7 days	Tri-Norinyl
Ethinyl estradiol, 35	Norgestimate, 0.18 × 7 days, 0.215 × 7 days, 0.25 × 7 days	Ortho Tri-Cyclen
Ethinyl estradiol 20 × 5 days, 30 × 7 days, 35 × 9 days	Norethindrone, 1	Estrostep
Ethinyl estradiol 30 × 6 days, 40 × 5 days, 30 × 10 days	Levonorgestral, 0.05 × 6 days, 0.075 × 5 days, 0.125 × 10 days	Triphasil Tri-Levlen

PROGESTIN Numerous progestins are used in OCPs (Tables 20-3 and 20-4). They are norethindrone, norethindrone acetate, ethynodiol diacetate, norgestrel, levonorgestrel, norethynodrel, desogestrel, norgestimate, and gestodene. Comparing the various progestins is difficult because each has variable progestational, androgenic, and endometrial properties. However, the clinical effects of the various progestins (Table 20-2) in the current low-dose OCPs are relatively similar because they are all used in biologically equivalent doses.

SELECTION OF PATIENTS

The clinician's role in prescribing OCPs is to counsel women about their suitability for OCPs, screen for contraindications, review side effects, and determine the most appropriate OCP for an individual patient.

SUITABILITY CHARACTERISTICS The most important suitability characteristic for OCPs is that they are only appropriate for women who can remember to take pills daily. In addition, some women will derive beneficial results over and above the contraceptive effect of OCPs, making these women particularly good candidates for OCP contraception. For example, combined OCPs generally improve acne, anovulatory or irregular periods, endometriosis, and heavy or painful menses. They also reduce the likelihood of recurrent ovarian cysts and lower the risk of ovarian cancer (important for patients with a family history of ovarian cancer).

CONTRAINDICATIONS   Clinicians should screen patients for overt contraindications to OCPs. These are shown in Table 20-5. Hypertension is not a contraindication if the patient is under the age of 35 and does not smoke, and the hypertension is well controlled.

Some women may not be good OCP candidates even if they do not have overt contraindications. For example, women who have demonstrated poor medication compliance or who have previously become pregnant while using OCPs may not be good candidates for OCPs. Similarly, OCPs may not be advisable for women taking long-term medications known to interfere with the effectiveness of OCPs. These drugs include barbiturates, carbamazepine, rifampin, primadone, phenytoin, and possibly penicillins and tetracyclines.

PRESCRIBING

Combined OCPs are available in monophasic, biphasic, and triphasic forms. Monophasic OCPs (Table 20-3) use the same dose of estrogen and progestin for the entire cycle. Biphasic and triphasic formulations (Table 20-4) vary the concentrations of these hormones into two or three

phases, respectively. Biphasic and triphasic OCPs were developed primarily to address the problem of mid-cycle spotting that occurs in monophasic pills, in which low estrogen doses are maintained throughout the month.

Packets of OCPs can be prescribed in 28- and 21-day regimens. The 28-day regimen has 21 active OCPs and 7 placebo pills, allowing pills to be taken every day with no interruptions between packets (Fig. 20-1). The 21-day regimen does not contain placebo pills, and users take a 7-day break after completing each 21-day packet.

There are many pill choices available in the United States. The process of selecting an OCP

Table 20-5

Contraindications to Estrogen-Progestin Oral Contraceptive Pills

History of thromboembolic disease
History of cerebrovascular accident
History of coronary artery disease
Impaired liver function
Cigarette smoking (if >35 years old)
Hypertension (if >35, blood pressure not well controlled, or smokes cigarettes)
Sickle cell disease
Active gallbladder disease
Known or suspected breast cancer
Irregular vaginal bleeding for which a cause has not been determined

Figure 20-1

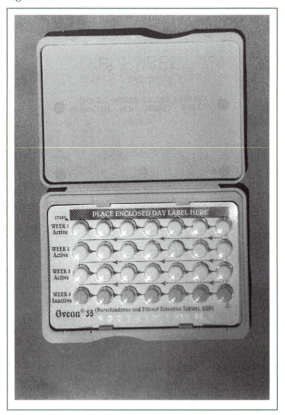

Birth control pills. A 28-day pill packet of combined estrogen-progestin contraceptives contains 21 active pills (top three rows) and 7 inactive pills (fourth row).

begins by determining whether a woman can safely use estrogen by excluding contraindications (Table 20-5). Then, one must consider the appropriate dose of estrogen, the cost of various OCP preparations, and whether any particular side-effect profile would be of importance to an individual patient. For safety reasons, it is best to start with an OCP containing less than 50 μg (usually 35 μg) of estrogen. If cost is of concern, generic preparations may be preferable.

STARTING ORAL CONTRACEPTIVE PILLS Options for starting OCPs include beginning on the first day of the menstrual period, the first Sunday after the menstrual period begins, or immediately after visiting the clinician. All are reasonable options, but beginning on or after the menstrual period decreases the likelihood of starting OCPs by a woman who is pregnant.

For women in the postpartum period, OCPs should be not be started until at least 2 to 3 weeks after delivery to avoid problems with immediate-postpartum hypercoagulability and resultant thromboembolic complications. Starting OCPs before that time can also interfere with the initiation of breast feeding. However, OCPs can be safely used once lactation is established, since no adverse effects on infant growth and development have been reported. Some authorities recommend waiting longer than 2 to 3 weeks to start OCPs for women who exclusively breast feed. This recommendation is based on the fact that ovulation, and the possibility of pregnancy, rarely occurs before the third postpartum month because lactating women are protected from pregnancy by the contraceptive effect of lactational amenorrhea. In addition, studies indicate that starting OCPs is associated with a decreased duration of breast feeding.

For postpartum women who are not lactating, OCPs should be started no later than the third week after delivery because ovulation resumes on average around 45 days after giving birth. After an abortion, OCPs may be started immediately.

The OCP should be taken at about the same time every day. Suggesting that the woman asso-

ciate taking the pill with another activity carried out at the same time each day (e.g., brushing teeth or removing contact lenses) may be helpful. A 3-month supply of OCPs should be given initially, with a follow-up visit scheduled before the last pack is finished. Although women who begin the pill by the fifth day of the menstrual cycle are probably fully protected against pregnancy, many clinicians suggest use of a back-up method in the first month of use.

SIDE EFFECTS AND COMPLICATIONS

Common side effects of OCPs are summarized in Table 20-1. The most serious side effects are related to the enhanced coagulation effects of estrogen. These include thrombophlebitis, thromboembolic disease, and, rarely, cerebrovascular accidents or myocardial infarction. The risk of cerebrovascular accidents and myocardial infarction is primarily among women who smoke cigarettes. While OCP formulations using the new progestins may demonstrate favorable lipid changes, thereby lowering cardiovascular risk, it will be many years before outcome studies can confirm the safety of these preparations for older women who smoke.

Although OCPs protect against endometrial and ovarian cancer, estrogen may stimulate breast neoplasia. Studies have yielded conflicting results, but it appears that OCPs may increase the risk of breast cancer slightly in younger women (under age 35). Thus, OCPs are generally considered to be contraindicated in women with a personal history of breast cancer or with breast lumps until cancer has been ruled out. However, some research suggests that OCPs can be prescribed safely to women who have had breast cancer. Thus, more data are required before definitive statements can be made about the safety of OCPs in women with breast cancer.

Hypertension is a rare complication of OCP use. One large study of over 2500 African-American women in the southeastern United States did not find blood pressure changes in pill users that differed significantly from changes in nonusers. When blood pressure elevations do occur, they are usually mild and resolve within a few weeks of discontinuing the pills.

Progestin-Only Contraceptives

Progestin-only contraceptives include implants, long-acting injectable preparations, and progestin-only pills. The prototype implant is the Norplant system, a series of small subdermally implanted silicone rods that contain the progestin steroid levonorgestrel. The system provides 5 years of highly effective, reversible contraception. Injectable progestins are given in the form of Depo-Provera, a long-acting form of medroxyprogesterone acetate (MDPA). The MDPA is administered by intramuscular injection at 3-month intervals. Progestin-only pills, sometimes referred to as the "mini-pill," contain a small amount of progestin and are taken daily.

MECHANISMS OF ACTION

Progestin-only contraceptives prevent pregnancy via several mechanisms that differ by type of method. While inhibition of ovulation, primarily through suppression of luteinizing hormone (LH), occurs consistently with MDPA, about 30 to 40 percent of women using either Norplant or the progesterone-only pills continue to ovulate. The latter two methods have additional mechanisms of action, however, including thickening of the cervical mucus to impede sperm penetration and thinning and atrophy of the endometrium to prevent implantation. The endometrial effect appears less important for women using Norplant because fertilization has not been detected in Norplant users. Premature involution of the corpus luteum may be an additional mechanism of progestin-only pills.

NORPLANT   The Norplant system acts by diffusing levonorgestrel through six tubular silicone capsules that are surgically implanted beneath the skin of the upper arm (Fig. 20-2) and remain in

Figure 20-2

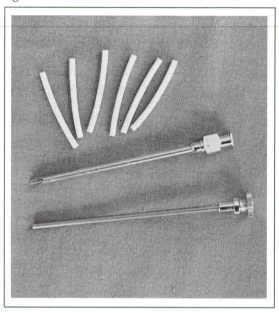

Norplant. The Norplant system consists of six progestin-impregnated rods that are inserted under the skin of the upper arm in a fan-shaped distribution. The trocar apparatus used for insertion consists of a hollow-bore insertion needle and a stylet.

place for up to 5 years. Each capsule contains 36 mg of levonorgestrel. The release rate of the progestin during the first 6 to 18 months averages 50 to 80 μg/d (similar to the levonorgestrel in progestin-only pills). After this time, the rate of release declines to 25 to 30 μg/d and remains at that level for the remainder of the 5 years. At the end of 5 years, the implants are removed through a small incision under local anesthesia. Replacement capsules may then be implanted. The system is completely reversible, with blood levels of levonorgestrel returning to normal within 96 h after removal and ovulatory cycles resuming within 7 weeks.

DEPO-PROVERA   Depo-Provera is an aqueous suspension of MDPA microcrystals. A deep intramuscular injection of 150 mg of MDPA is given every 3 months. The microcrystals dissolve slowly and release the progestin. A delay in conception of about 9 months is observed after discontinuing injections; by 18 months, 90 percent of users attempting pregnancy will become pregnant.

PROGESTIN-ONLY PILLS Progestin-only pills contain a small amount of a progestin and are taken every day with no pill-free interval. While various brands contain various progestins, there is no evidence of clinically significant differences among the various progestin-only pills.

EFFECTIVENESS

The published failure rates for Norplant range from 0.04 to 0.2 pregnancies per hundred women in the first year of use, with a cumulative pregnancy rate of 3.7 percent over 5 years. There has been some concern about an increased failure rate among obese women, but the extent of the problem is unclear.

Injectable MDPA has a probability of failure of 0.3 percent. While effectiveness depends on patients' receiving their injections in timely fashion, the 3-month recommended interval provides some margin of safety, since the duration of protection following injection is actually closer to 4 months.

Progestin-only pills are generally less effective than other progestin-only methods and also less effective than standard combination OCPs. In the first year of use, between 1.1 and 13.2 percent of users will become pregnant. In lactating women, however, progestin-only pills are nearly 100 percent effective.

SELECTION OF PATIENTS

User acceptance of any contraceptive method is related to the quality of pre-use counseling. Couples and individuals must be informed about each method's effectiveness, complications, advantages, and disadvantages (see Table 20-1).

Progestin-only contraceptives share many advantages. They all lack estrogen side effects. They also have the noncontraceptive benefits of causing scanty or absent menses in many patients, along with decreased frequency of anemia and menstrual cramping. In addition, use of progestin-only contraceptives is associated with a decreased risk of developing endometrial and ovarian cancer and a lower incidence of pelvic inflammatory disease. These agents can also be useful in managing pain associated with endometriosis.

Norplant and MDPA are excellent options for women who have difficulty remembering to take pills. In addition, MDPA is a good option for women taking antibiotics or enzyme-inducing drugs, such as anticonvulsants, on a chronic basis because, in contrast to OCPs, Norplant, and progestin-only pills, there is no interaction between MDPA and these medications. In addition, use of MDPA in women with seizure disorders has been shown to decrease the frequency of seizures. Absolute contraindications to Norplant and MDPA are active thrombophlebitis, undiagnosed genital bleeding, acute liver disease or liver tumors, and breast cancer.

Progestin-only pills are appropriate for women who have relative contraindications to combined OCPs. They can also be used for lactating women, since some studies suggest that, in contrast to the effect of combined OCPs, milk volume may actually increase in progestin-only pill users, and no deleterious effects on infant growth or development have been documented. A short course of progestin-only pills may also be used as a trial to assess how patients might be affected by progesterone side effects prior to insertion of Norplant. Finally, progestin-only pills should not be used in women taking acitretin (a topical retinoid for treatment of psoriasis), since this drug can interfere with contraceptive effectiveness.

PRESCRIBING AND SIDE EFFECTS

NORPLANT Norplant should be inserted either within the first 7 days of the menstrual cycle or immediately after an abortion or delivery. Proper timing will avoid insertion of the device in women with undetected pregnancy. If inserted at the proper time, contraceptive protection is immediate. If inserted at other times, a backup contraceptive is recommended for the first month, particularly for intercourse that occurs within 24 h after insertion.

Norplant insertion is a minor surgical procedure performed under local anesthesia. To insert Norplant, the clinician uses a trocar and places the six implant rods subdermally on the inside of a woman's upper arm in a fanlike configuration. Each Norplant kit comes with detailed step-by-step instructions for insertion. The manufacturer also produces instructional videotapes for patients and clinicians, both available at no cost. The physicians' videotape provides visual and graphic instructions for inserting the device.

Side Effects   Patients should be informed about possible side effects of Norplant, which are listed in Table 20-1. Menstrual irregularities are common. If menstrual irregularities are bothersome, bleeding patterns can temporarily be improved by the administration of oral contraceptives, oral estrogens, nonsteroidal anti-inflammatory drugs, or a combination of these agents.

DEPO-PROVERA   MDPA is packaged in unit-dose vials of 150 mg/mL. Deep intramuscular injections are made into the deltoid or gluteus maximus muscles; the deltoid injections are somewhat more painful. A 21- to 23-gauge needle, 2.5 to 4 cm in length, should be used to ensure delivery of the drug into the muscle and not into subcutaneous tissue. The area of injection should not be massaged because massage may lower the effectiveness of MDPA. Injections are scheduled every 3 months but may be given up to 2 weeks late.

Side Effects   As with implants, menstrual irregularity is common with MDPA, occurring in up to 70 percent of women. Satisfaction with MDPA may be increased if patients are told to anticipate menstrual irregularity, especially during the first

year of use. After the first year, irregular bleeding decreases, and there is an increasing likelihood of amenorrhea in subsequent years, occurring in about 80 percent of users by 5 years. Weight gain is often reported and is probably due to a progesterone-induced increase in appetite, rather than fluid retention.

Occasionally, women question the use of MDPA because of concerns about early research that demonstrated an increased risk of breast cancer in beagle dogs receiving MDPA. It was for this reason that the U.S. Food and Drug Administration did not approve MDPA for contraceptive use in the United States until 1992, even though it had been used worldwide for over 30 years. Clinical and epidemiologic studies in humans have demonstrated no cancer risk from using MDPA for contraception.

PROGESTIN-ONLY PILLS   Progestin-only pills should be started during the first 5 days of the menstrual cycle or immediately postabortion or postpartum. The pill is taken every day (at 24-h intervals) for 28 days, at which time a new pack of 28 pills is started. It is critically important for optimal contraceptive efficacy that progestin-only pills are taken at the same time every day. If a woman is more than 3 h late in taking her pill, an alternative contraceptive method should be used for at least 48 h.

Side Effects   The main side effects of progestin-only pills are acne and irregular bleeding. The most common abnormal menstrual pattern in users of this method is short, irregular cycles, which occur in about 40 percent of women. An additional 20 percent of women may have no apparent cycles and only experience irregular bleeding, spotting, or amenorrhea. The remaining 40 percent of users may have regular, ovulatory cycles. Protection against pregnancy in this group of women depends on the non-ovulation-inhibiting effects of progestin, such as altering the cervical mucus. The incidence of side effects other than bleeding irregularities is low.

Barrier Methods

All barrier methods work by blocking the access of sperm to the cervical canal. Male condoms are the most commonly used barrier contraceptives, and a female condom was recently marketed. Other barrier methods include diaphragms and cervical caps. A contraceptive sponge has also been available, but at the time of this publication, it had been removed from the commercial market because of problems with the production process.

In addition to pregnancy prevention, some barrier methods offer protection against sexually transmitted diseases (STDs). The decreased risk of STDs that accompanies barrier contraception results in less pelvic inflammatory disease and less subsequent fallopian tube scarring, possibly decreasing the rate of tubal pregnancy in users of these methods. This effect is most well demonstrated for condoms.

However, the effectiveness of barrier contraception for preventing both pregnancy and STDs is highly user-dependent. Failures occur, mostly in the first year of use, often because of inconsistent or improper use. Only about half of barrier contraceptive users continue to use them after 1 year.

Other advantages and disadvantages of barrier methods, along with their effectiveness rates, are listed in Table 20-1. While no systemic side effects are noted for any of the barrier methods, vaginal barrier methods (diaphragm and cervical cap) carry a risk of toxic shock syndrome, which occurs in 2 to 3 per 100,000 vaginal barrier users each year.

MALE CONDOMS

Male condoms prevent pregnancy by blocking sperm from entering the vagina and protect against disease by preventing direct contact between mucosal surfaces during intercourse. Some male condoms are prelubricated with spermicide. It is not known whether the addition of spermicide improves efficacy, and an increased frequency of urinary tract infections in women has been associated with spermicide-coated condoms.

Male condoms have been used for centuries. They were initially made from animal skins, but most modern condoms are made from latex or polyurethane. Skin or natural-membrane condoms are still available commercially but are not recommended for use because they contain small pores, and thus provide insufficient protection against STDs, particularly HIV.

FAILURE RATE   The failure rate of the male condom is typically in the range of 4 to 12 percent (Table 20-1). Failure is often attributed to slippage and breakage, but these events are relatively uncommon (approximately 2 to 3 percent for breakage and 1 to 6 percent for slippage). Higher failure rates are associated with age (25 to 34 years old), 5 years or more of sexual activity, use of a condom for less than 5 years, and high frequency of sexual intercourse. Use of a condom with water-based lubricant has been reported to decrease failure rates.

INSTRUCTIONS FOR USE   The male condom is applied over the erect penis. Before applying it to the penis, however, the condom should be unrolled a short distance to be certain it is unrolling properly and to create a half-inch of empty space at the tip of the condom to hold the ejaculate. The last step is unnecessary with reservoir condoms (Fig. 20-3). The condom is then rolled down the shaft to the base of the penis.

Additional lubrication (natural or artificial) is recommended before insertion because condoms are more likely to tear if the vagina or anus is dry. Suggested water-based lubricants include K-Y jelly, Astroglide, Replens, Gyne-Moistrin, or spermicide. After ejaculation, the penis should be withdrawn while still erect, with the rim of the condom held against the base of the penis to prevent slippage. When the penis is away from the partner's genitals, the condom is removed

Figure 20-3

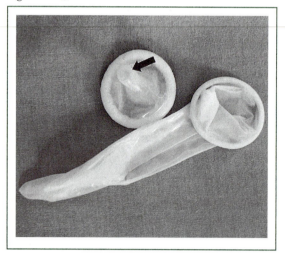

Male condom. Male condoms are rolled when removed from their package and must be unrolled onto the erect penis. Note the "reservoir" at the tip of the rolled condom (arrow), which will collect the ejaculate. The reservoir must remain loose, rather than rolled tightly onto the penis.

without spilling the semen, checked for visible damage, and discarded.

FEMALE CONDOMS

The Reality female condom, available without a prescription, is a thin polyurethane sheath that is 7.8 cm in diameter and 17 cm long (Fig. 20-4). The sheath is prelubricated on the inside and contains two flexible polyurethane rings. One ring lies inside the sheath attached to the closed end. It is used for insertion and sits inside the vagina, positioned similarly to a diaphragm. The other ring forms the external opening of the device. It remains outside the vagina, covering part of the perineum and providing protection to the labia and base of the penis during intercourse.

FAILURE RATE   Female and male condoms appear to offer similar protection against STDs. Experience with the female condom is somewhat limited, but it has a higher reported failure rate than the male condom (Table 20-1).

Figure 20-4

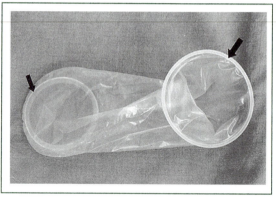

Female condom. The sheath of the female condom is 7.8 cm in diameter and 17 cm long, and contains two flexible polyurethane rings. One ring lies inside the sheath, attached to the closed end of the condom (small arrow). It is used for insertion and sits in the posterior vagina. The other ring (large arrow) remains outside of the vagina and serves as the external opening of the device.

INSTRUCTIONS FOR USE   The female condom is inserted into the vagina by pinching together the inner ring, introducing the device into the vagina, and then pushing it into place with the first finger inserted inside the condom to ensure placement over the cervix (similar to the diaphragm). The external ring is then positioned around the vaginal orifice. Some women find the female condom awkward to use, and problems with slippage have been reported, including slippage of the entire condom into the vagina. Female condoms should not be used simultaneously with a male latex condom because doing so may increase the risk of slippage and breakage. Female condoms cost more than male condoms.

DIAPHRAGMS AND CERVICAL CAPS

The contraceptive effectiveness of diaphragms and cervical caps is due to their action as physical barriers to sperm. Both devices are intended for use with spermicidal cream or jelly, which adds a second mechanism of contraceptive action. Some data indicate a nearly twofold difference in pregnancy rates for diaphragms used without spermicide. However, several studies of the cap found no differences in accidental pregnancy rate for women consistently using spermicide compared to those who did not.

The reported effectiveness of diaphragms and cervical caps is similar (Table 20-1). However, the cervical cap appears to be less effective when used by parous women, in whom accidental pregnancy rates may be as high as 26 to 36 percent. Both the diaphragm and cervical cap require fitting by an experienced health care provider.

DIAPHRAGMS   The standard contraceptive diaphragm is a circular latex cup that is inserted into the vagina (Fig. 20-5). Diaphragms come in three types, "arching," "coil," and "flat spring," referring to the construction of the rim of the cup. Most clinicians prescribe the arching-spring rim type (Allflex by Ortho, Koroflex by Holland-Rantos, and Ramses-Bendex by Schmid). Standard commercially available diaphragms range

in size from 50 to 95 mm (diameter of the rim), but larger sizes can be specially ordered from some manufacturers. Most women are fitted with a size between 60 and 85 mm.

One-size-fits-all 60-mm ("fit-free") diaphragms were recently introduced, but an early report on their efficacy was disappointing. Despite self-reports by over 85 percent of users that the device was in place with every act of intercourse, the 12-month life-table accidental pregnancy rate was 24.1 per 100 women (29.5 per 100 women without female barrier experience and 17.9 per 100 women with barrier experience).

Fitting a Diaphragm   In the vagina, the dome of the diaphragm should cover the cervix. The posterior part of the diaphragm's circular rim is positioned in the posterior fornix. The ring then extends forward to 1 to 2 cm behind the pubic bone, where the anterior rim fits snugly in place. An estimate of the correct size can be obtained during pelvic examination by measuring the distance along the examiner's index finger from the posterior vaginal fornix to about 1 cm posterior to the inside of the pubic arch. This distance corresponds to the approximate diameter of the diaphragm rim.

The diaphragm is inserted by pinching the sides together and gently inserting it into the vagina with a small amount of lubricant on the leading edge. Once inserted, it should cover the cervix and fit snugly with the rim in contact with the posterior and lateral vaginal walls, and the anterior edge about one finger-breadth behind the pubic arch. The diaphragm should be comfortable; in fact, most women will not feel a properly fitted diaphragm when it is within the vagina. Diaphragms should also be easily removed by hooking the anterior rim with the examiner's index finger and gently pulling the device out of the vagina. If the diaphragm is too small it will be very easy to remove and will sit well back from the symphysis; it will also be more likely to become dislodged during intercourse. If it is too large it may cause discomfort and may bow or extend beyond or below the pubic symphysis.

Figure 20-5

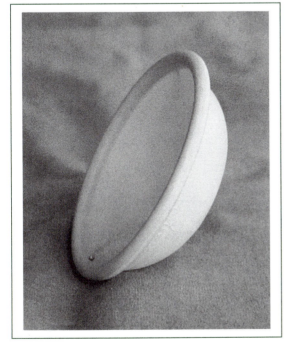

Diaphragm. The photograph shows an arching-spring rim-type contraceptive diaphragm.

Insertion by the Patient Women and/or their partners should be encouraged to practice inserting and removing the device in the clinician's office, after the initial fitting, until they are comfortable with the procedure. Diaphragms can be inserted while the woman is standing, squatting, or lying down. The woman's sex partner can also insert the diaphragm. Women usually find it easiest to insert the diaphragm by pinching it between the thumb and third finger of their dominant hand, introducing the device into the introitus and using the first finger (or the opposite hand) to push the back edge inside the vagina. The direction of insertion is similar to that of a menstrual tampon.

The device should slide easily in place but may spring out of a woman's hand on initial attempts; she should be warned that this may happen so as not to be discouraged. A plastic inserter or introducer can be used to insert the coil and flat-spring types of diaphragms. Removal by the patient is accomplished by inserting the first finger under the rim and pushing forward, or by rotating the wrist (so that the knuckles of the hand are visible), allowing the device to be hooked by the index finger and pulled out of the vagina.

Instructions for Use When the diaphragm is used for contraception, spermicidal cream or jelly should be applied to the inside of the diaphragm. The quantity is not precise and is often described as being a "glob" about the size of a quarter. The device may be inserted 15 to 30 min prior to intercourse. If intercourse does not take place soon after insertion or if more than one episode of intercourse occurs, the diaphragm should not be removed. Instead, additional spermicide should be inserted into the vagina before intercourse. The diaphragm should be left in place for approximately 6 to 8 h after intercourse but should be removed within 24 h because toxic shock syndrome, other infections, or vaginal injury may develop with devices left in the vagina for prolonged periods of time.

Side Effects and Contraindications Diaphragms have few side effects. Some patients experience allergy either to spermicide or to the latex of the diaphragm. Diaphragms also increase the risk of urinary tract infection, presumably because they come in contact with the posterior surface of the urethra. Diaphragms are contraindicated for patients with allergy to latex or spermicide, a history of toxic shock syndrome, recurrent urinary tract infections, uterine prolapse, or inability of the woman to place and remove it correctly.

CERVICAL CAP The Prentif cavity-rim cervical cap, the only FDA-approved cervical cap available in the United States, is a small latex rubber cup that fits directly over the cervix. It is available in four sizes, measured by the inside diameter of the rim of the cap: 22, 25, 28, and 31 mm (Fig. 20-6). Cervical caps must be ordered from the manufacturer/distributor (Cervical Cap, Ltd.,

Figure 20-6

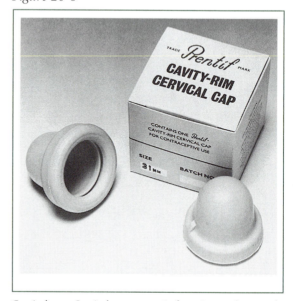

Cervical cap. Cervical caps come in four sizes and are packaged individually. They must be ordered directly from the manufacturer (phone 408-395-2100). (*Courtesy of Cervical Cap, Ltd.*)

Los Gatos, CA, phone 408-395-2100) and dispensed directly to patients by a clinician.

Fitting a Cervical Cap   The cap is inserted over the cervix and held in place by the suction that forms between the rim of the cap and the sides of the cervix. When fitting a patient for a cervical cap, the approximate size is assessed by estimating the diameter of the cervix during bimanual examination. Nulliparous women usually take the smaller sizes (22 or 25 mm).

To insert a cervical cap, the rim of the cap is folded, and the dome is compressed. The cap is then introduced into the vagina and placed over the cervix. Compressing the dome during insertion is important because, after the cap is placed over the cervix, the dome is released and expands to create suction on the cervix.

When the cap is properly fit, it should completely cover the cervix. The rim of the cap should be snug against the cervix and tucked into the vaginal fornices. The examiner should check around the entire 360° circumference of the rim to be sure that no gaps are detected between the rim and the cervix or fornix. The cap should not become dislodged with gentle attempts at pushing forward and downward with the examining fingers, and when the dome is gently pinched, it should remain slightly collapsed and resist tugging. The cap is removed by probing the rim with the index finger, tipping the cap to break the seal, and gently removing the device.

Using this procedure, between 50 to 70 percent of women will be successfully fitted for a cervical cap. For the remainder, identifying a suitable fit is not possible, and these women cannot use a cervical cap.

Instructions for Use   The procedure for insertion of a cervical cap by patients is identical to the fitting procedure described above. As with the diaphragm, a cervical cap can be inserted while lying down, squatting, or standing (usually with one foot on a chair or bed). Prior to insertion, sufficient spermicidal cream or jelly should be applied to fill the lower one- to two-thirds of the inside of the dome of the cap. Additional spermicide may be inserted into the vagina if repeat episodes of intercourse are to take place, but the cap should not be removed when additional spermicide is added. As with diaphragms, cervical caps should be left in place for approximately 6 to 8 h after intercourse. However, in contrast with diaphragms, cervical caps can be left in the vagina for a maximum of 48 h from the time of insertion to the time of removal (with at least 6 h from the time of last intercourse to removal). Leaving a cervical cap in place for longer than the recommended time creates risk of cervical and vaginal injury and infections, including toxic shock syndrome.

Because some patients have difficulty inserting or removing a cervical cap, it is important to have the patient demonstrate insertion and removal before relying on the device for contraceptive protection. Some clinicians do this by having patients return to the office with their cap in place so that proper positioning can be checked. Others have the patient insert and remove the device while still in the office.

Side Effects and Contraindications   Cervical caps have few side effects other than allergic reactions to latex or spermicide; a history of such allergies is a contraindication to using the cervical cap. Other contraindications include a history of toxic shock syndrome, uterine prolapse, and inability to place and remove it correctly. Because cervical caps interfere with egress of blood from the cervix, they should not be used for at least 6 weeks postpartum or postabortion, nor should they be used during menstruation.

Cervical caps are also contraindicated in patients who have had abnormal cervical cytologic test results, exposure to diethylstilbestrol, or a history of cervical cryosurgery, cauterization, or conization of the cervix. These contraindications stem from a controversy over whether the cap induces cervical dysplasia. In 1986, the final report of the FDA on cap safety and efficacy indicated that a higher percentage of cap users than of diaphragm users developed abnormal cervical cytologic characteristics (4 versus 2 percent). While subsequent studies have not shown higher rates of cervical dysplasia among cap users, these contraindications remain.

Spermicides

Spermicides can be used as a primary birth control method or, more commonly, as an adjunct to the barrier methods described above. Spermicides are also important as an emergency method of contraception if a condom breaks or as a backup contraceptive when first beginning other methods, such as oral contraceptives or MDPA.

Spermicides act by killing or inhibiting the mobility of sperm. In addition, spermicides have a number of advantages, listed in Table 20-1. It should be noted that spermicidal chemicals provide protection against STDs and possibly AIDS.

Spermicides contain an active spermicidal chemical mixed in an inert delivery vehicle. All commercially available spermicides contain nonoxynol-9 or a similar agent as the active ingredient. However, there are a variety of delivery vehicles, including foams, jellies, creams, suppositories, tablets, and films (a thin sheet impregnated with spermicide that is placed into the vagina). Spermicidal foams, jellies, and creams act immediately, while suppositories, tablets, and films are active 10 to 15 minutes after insertion.

FAILURE RATES

Used alone as the sole birth control method, the contraceptive protection of spermicides lasts about 1 h. When used with a cap or diaphragm, the jellies and creams last 6 to 8 h. Spermicide used as a sole method has a reported accidental pregnancy rate of 21 percent. Effectiveness probably relates to timing of use, since spermicides offer the best protection when inserted into the vagina shortly before intercourse. When spermicide is used 15 to 30 min prior to intercourse, only 0 to 2 percent of sperm remain mobile. With longer intervals between spermicide application and intercourse, less inhibition of sperm motility is noted. Women with abnormal vaginal anatomy (e.g., septum or prolapse) may have difficulty delivering spermicides properly into the vagina and therefore may have a higher pregnancy rate when relying on spermicides for birth control.

SIDE EFFECTS

Side effects of spermicide include skin irritation and the rare possibility of allergy. There appear to be no systemic adverse effects, even if accidentally used during pregnancy. There is some concern, however, that skin irritation from spermicides can result in subclinical vulvovaginal microabrasions. These microabrasions damage the integrity of the vaginal mucosa or skin. Thus, despite the supposed anti-HIV action of spermicidal chemicals, spermicide-induced microabrasions may actually increase the risk of acquiring HIV infection. Further research is needed to clarify whether spermicides increase or decrease the risk of HIV infection.

Intrauterine Device

Intrauterine devices (IUDs) have long been an important method of birth control and, in many countries, such as China, are the most commonly used contraceptive method. During the mid 1980s, many IUDs were taken off the U.S. market for a number of reasons, including lack of profitability and lawsuits charging that IUDs were responsible for injuries to their users. Despite the fact that most of the cases that went to trial found no fault with the IUDs, legal fees and insurance costs led to withdrawal of many IUDs from the U.S. market. Today, only two IUDs are available in the United States: the TCu-380A (Paragard) and the Progestasert Intrauterine Progesterone Contraceptive System (Progestasert).

Paragard

The Paragard is a T-shaped device made of polyethylene with barium sulfate added for visibility on x-rays. The polyethylene T has copper wire wound around the vertical stem and on each transverse arm (total surface area 380 mm^2), and two monofilament threads attached to the base of the T; the threads are used for removal. The Paragard is currently approved for 10 years of continuous use.

MECHANISM OF ACTION The copper IUD does not affect ovulation. Rather, it prevents pregnancy primarily by preventing fertilization. Using human chorionic gonadotropin (hCG) assays, fertilization is detected in less than 1 percent of menstrual cycles in copper IUD users. Fertilization is prevented by a copper-induced sterile inflammatory reaction (foreign-body response) in the endometrium that prevents sperm from reaching the fallopian tubes. This is important information to provide to patients, since, in the past, some women objected to the use of the IUD when it was believed to function primarily as an abortifacient, preventing implantation of the fertilized egg. The copper is not absorbed systemically to any significant degree, and the amount of copper released each day is less than the amount consumed daily in a regular diet.

FAILURE RATES The Paragard is highly effective. Rates of accidental pregnancy are between 0.5 and 1.5 percent, the latter figure occurring after 7 years of use. Continuation rates are high for the IUD, with most studies indicating that about 70 percent of IUD users are still using the device at the end of 1 year. This may be compared to a rate of about 40 percent among users of oral contraceptives.

Progestasert The Progestasert is also a T-shaped device, but it contains progestin instead of copper. The Progestasert IUD is made of ethylene-vinyl acetate copolymer containing a reservoir of 38 mg of progesterone, along with barium sulfate for visibility on x-ray, in a silicone oil base. The Progestasert must be replaced yearly. While not yet available in the United States, there is an IUD available elsewhere that uses the more-potent progesterone levonorgestrel, which is effective for 5 years.

MECHANISM OF ACTION The progesterone contained in the Progestasert, released at 65 μg/d, acts primarily by thickening cervical mucus and impeding sperm penetration, plus a decidual reaction that results in endometrial atrophy. These actions, in addition to the local foreign-body response, prevent implantation.

FAILURE RATES The effectiveness of the progesterone IUD is slightly lower than that of the Paragard. About 1.5 percent of women experience accidental pregnancies in the first year of use.

How to Prescribe an IUD

The clinician's role in prescribing an IUD is to screen interested women for risk factors and review important information about the device. If a patient decides to use an IUD for contraception, the clinician must obtain written informed consent for insertion, perform insertion under sterile conditions, and arrange for regular follow-up and access to medical care if complications occur.

Identifying women who are suitable candidates for an IUD is the most important step in reducing IUD-related complications. The best candidates for IUDs are women at low risk for STDs (such as those in mutually faithful, monogamous relationships) and who have had children and do not want more in the near future. An IUD should not be placed in a woman with active or recurrent pelvic infection. A prior history of pelvic inflammatory disease (PID) or current risk factors for PID (e.g., prior STDs, multiple partners, and impaired response to infection, such as from chronic steroid use or AIDS) are relative contraindications to IUD insertion. Women with a history of ectopic pregnancy are not candidates for the Progestasert because it increases the risk of ectopic pregnancy. Some clinicians feel that women with a history of ectopic pregnancy may use the Paragard because of its protective effect against ectopic pregnancy and infrequent need for replacement. Women with menorrhagia or anemia who desire an IUD should consider the Progestasert because bleeding may be less than with copper IUDs.

How to Insert an IUD

An IUD may be placed immediately postpartum or after a first-trimester abortion. Advantages of immediate postpartum placement include lower cost, less pain and bleeding, and certainty of no pregnancy. Disadvantages include higher expulsion rates and higher rates of "missing" strings. Since spontaneous expulsion rates are much higher after second-trimester abortions, IUD placement should be deferred in these cases. For other women, IUDs are often inserted during menses, taking advantage of the increased size of the cervical os and lower likelihood of pregnancy during menses. Expulsion rates, however, are higher when IUDs are inserted during menses.

Many clinicians prescribe antibiotic prophylaxis against infectious endocarditis before inserting or removing an IUD in patients with valvular heart disease, including mitral valve prolapse with regurgitation, prosthetic heart valves, congenital heart disease, and hypertrophic cardiomyopathy. However, recently published guidelines from the American Heart Association do not recommend endocarditis prophylaxis with IUD placements or for removals in the absence of infection.

Once all questions are answered and written informed consent has been obtained, insertion of the IUD should be performed under sterile conditions (with the clinician wearing sterile gloves and using sterile instruments). A nonsteroidal anti-inflammatory agent (e.g., 600 mg

ibuprofen) given prior to insertion is helpful for preventing uterine cramping for some women.

Instructions for IUD insertion are included in the package inserts that come with the device. The IUD package is opened and placed on a sterile tray, but the IUD and inserter device, which consists of a barrel with a solid rod (Fig. 20-7), are not removed from their sterile plastic covering. A bimanual examination is performed to determine the position of the uterus and presence of any abnormalities. After a sterile speculum has been placed in the vagina, the cervix is cleaned with iodine solution (or chlorhexidine if the patient is allergic to iodine) using circular motions beginning at the os and moving outward. At this point, some clinicians place a paracervical anesthetic block, but this procedure is not essential, especially postpartum or during menses, when the os is relatively open.

Next, a single-toothed tenaculum is placed on the anterior lip of the cervix (if the uterus is anteverted) or the posterior lip of the cervix (if the uterus is retroverted). The patient should be warned about a pinching sensation as the tenaculum is put in place. Gentle traction is then applied with the tenaculum to control and straighten the uterus. The patient also should be warned about a cramping sensation as a uterine sound, curved to conform to the uterine shape, is passed through the os until resistance is felt

Figure 20-7

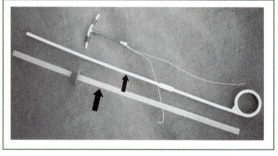

Intrauterine device. The photograph shows a copper IUD, along with the inserter device. The inserter device consists of a hollow barrel (large arrow) and a solid rod (small arrow).

when the sound tip hits the uterine fundus. The sound is then removed and the depth of the uterine cavity noted.

The IUD should then be loaded into its insertion tube under strict sterile conditions. To avoid contamination of the IUD, most clinicians load the IUD without removing it from the protective plastic cover. The thumb and index fingers are placed on the horizontal arms, which are folded down alongside the stem of the T. The stem and two arms of the folded IUD are inserted into the end of the insertion tube (Fig. 20-8).

Once loaded into the insertion tube, the IUD should be placed within 5 min. If more time elapses, the plastic of the IUD may lose its "memory" and fail to revert to its normal T shape after insertion is complete. The movable flange (Fig. 20-8) on the hollow barrel should be moved so that it rests at the same distance from the tip of the folded IUD as the uterine depth measured with the sound. The horizontal arms of the IUD should be in the same horizontal plane as the long axis of the flange so that, upon insertion, the arms of the IUD open in the horizontal plane.

The patient is warned that she may experience cramping as the inserter is introduced through the os until the depth marked by the flange is reached. The IUD is then deposited into the uterine cavity by drawing back on the inserter tube barrel while the rod is held in place. Once the barrel reaches the loop end of the rod and can be withdrawn no further, the barrel and rod are removed from the cervix. The string is cut with a scissors, leaving approximately 2 to 3 cm of string outside of the os. The tenaculum and speculum are removed. Some providers then perform a bimanual examination to note any uterine tenderness that might indicate perforation of the IUD through the uterine wall. Women should be encouraged to feel the string before leaving the examining room.

SIDE EFFECTS AND COMPLICATIONS

The complications associated with IUD use and their management are shown in Table 20-6.

Figure 20-8

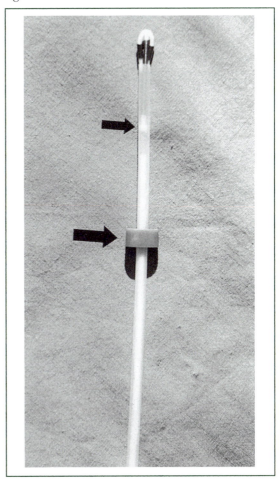

Intrauterine device loaded for insertion. The arms of the copper IUD are folded and inserted into the end of the hollow barrel. The moveable flange (large arrow) is positioned on the shaft of the hollow barrel, at a distance from the tip of the barrel equal to the depth of the uterine sounding. The solid rod is positioned inside of the hollow barrel, with the tip near the bottom end (small arrow) of the IUD.

Some of the more important complications are described below.

PERFORATION One important IUD complication is perforation of the uterus, which most commonly occurs at the time of insertion. Fortunately, this complication is rare (approximately 1.2 per 1,000 insertions); it is thought to be more

Table 20-6

Management Strategies for Selected IUD-Related Complications

COMPLICATION	COMMENTS	SUGGESTED MANAGEMENT STRATEGY
Heavy periods	Usually decreases over time; if persistent, consider pathologic causes, e.g., fibroids, cervicitis, cancer	Monitor hemoglobin; provide iron supplements; try ibuprofen (400–600 mg tid) during the first few days of each cycle
Severe cramping/pain soon after insertion	Consider uterine perforation.	If strings are present, remove IUD and treat for presumptive PID; if strings are absent, ultrasound or x-ray to locate IUD
Severe cramping/pain, occurring distant from insertion	Consider pregnancy or infection.	If fever, purulent discharge, or cervical motion or uterine tenderness present and pregnancy test result negative, remove IUD and treat for presumptive PID
Vaginal bleeding with pain	Must exclude ectopic pregnancy	Examination for PID or adnexal mass; pregnancy test
Pregnancy	Discuss patient's desires for continuation versus abortion; warn about risk of miscarriage.	If string present, remove IUD, assess for ectopic, refer for prenatal care or abortion (per patient decision) if intrauterine; if strings absent, ultrasound, watch for infection, recover IUD at delivery; if infection occurs, refer or manage with uterine evacuation and antibiotic treatment.
Expulsion (partial)	Check for pregnancy.	Remove IUD; may reinsert giving doxycycline (100 mg q 12h for 5–7 days)
Expulsion (complete)	Ultrasound or x-ray to exclude perforation	May reinsert if desired
String too long	Partner may report discomfort.	Exclude partial expulsion; sound cervix to check for presence of IUD in cervix instead of in uterus; if IUD in cervix, treat as partial expulsion; if in uterus, cut string shorter and record length.
String too short	Partner reports discomfort.	Remove and replace IUD if necessary.
String missing	Exclude pregnancy or expulsion.	Ultrasound or x-ray to locate IUD, or examine during next menses; use IUD hook to determine if string is within cervical canal; if yes, bring through os; if no, explore cervix and uterus with IUD hook or alligator forceps

likely when IUDs are inserted by inexperienced clinicians.

INFECTION The other major complication of IUD use is PID. A transient increased risk of PID is seen in the first 4 months after insertion, probably due to the introduction of bacteria into the uterine cavity during the insertion procedure. The risk is fourfold greater in the first month after insertion, returning to baseline by 5 months.

In addition to PID following insertion, there is also a risk of developing infection with long-term use of IUDs. A number of factors influence the risk of developing PID, including exposure to STDs and age; younger women have higher infection rates, probably because they are less likely to be monogamous. A further risk factor is the duration of use of an IUD. The risk of contracting severe PID requiring hospitalization increases after 5 years of use to about five times the risk in nonusers of IUDs. These late infections are often caused by actinomyces.

Finally, IUDs appear to alter the vaginal flora. There are significantly more anaerobic bacteria isolated from the vaginas of IUD users than from users of barrier methods (who maintain a lactobacilli-dominated flora). These microbial changes may contribute to the risk of infection, but the extent of contribution is uncertain.

To reduce the incidence of infections, careful selection of patients is essential, since women without the aforementioned risk factors have a very low risk of infection. In addition, many authorities advocate the use of prophylactic antibiotics just prior to IUD insertion. Typical antibiotic regimens are either a single 200-mg oral dose of doxycycline, or 500 mg of erythromycin in women who are breast feeding or allergic to tetracyclines. Studies of prophylactic antibiotics have shown as much as a 31 percent decrease in the incidence of infection among IUD users, but the number of women who actually develop PID in these studies is too small to provide clear evidence of the benefits of prophylactic antibiotics.

BLEEDING AND ANEMIA A disadvantage of the Paragard is the increased volume of bleeding per cycle. This bleeding can be double the amount experienced with normal menses and may result in anemia. Excessive bleeding is a reason why 4 to 15 percent of women discontinue IUD use. Higher rates of IUD removal are seen in younger women, who may be less tolerant of this side effect. Progestasert IUDs, on the other hand, have the advantage of decreasing menstrual blood flow by as much as 40 percent. However, the number of days on which bleeding occurs (although it may only be light spotting) may be increased.

UTERINE CRAMPING Increased uterine cramping is common in IUD users, particularly in the hours and days after insertion. In addition, some IUD users report more severe menstrual cramps on a long-term basis. Nonsteroidal anti-inflammatory drugs can be used to decrease the quantity and severity of uterine cramps.

ECTOPIC PREGNANCY Progestasert users have a rate of ectopic pregnancy that is 50 to 80 percent higher than in women using no birth control method. Possible causes of the higher ectopic pregnancy rate include higher rates of PID-related fallopian tube scarring and abnormalities of implantation.

Copper IUDs, however, actually lower the risk of ectopic pregnancy by about 50 to 90 percent compared to women using no contraception. However, if pregnancy occurs, there is an increased risk that the pregnancy will be ectopic.

Natural Family Planning

Natural family planning methods have been used for many years, with increasing use since the 1950s. Historically, the earliest of these natural family planning techniques was the calendar method, which determined periods of fertility based on the length of menstrual cycles. With the calendar method, fertile days were determined by subtracting 18 days from the length of the shortest cycle during the last year to determine the first fertile day. Eleven days were then subtracted from the longest cycle to determine the last fertile day. For example, if the shortest cycle during the last year was 22 days, the fertile period was assumed to begin on day 4 (22 minus 18) of each cycle. If the longest cycle was 33 days, the fertile period was assumed to end on day 22 (33 minus 11) of each cycle. Thus, intercourse was to be avoided between day 4 and 22 of each cycle. Unfortunately, the effectiveness of the calendar method is unpredictable because of variability in individual women's cycle length.

Other older natural family planning techniques included the temperature method and the ovulation method. The temperature method involved daily monitoring of body temperature to detect the temperature rise that occurs just after ovulation (0.4 to 1.0°F). The ovulation method monitored the cervical mucus to detect changes (from thick and dry to clear, thin, and sticky) to predict ovulation. Intercourse was avoided during the presumed fertile period.

Today, a combination of these techniques is used. It is known as the "symptothermal method."

MECHANISM OF ACTION

The symptothermal method is based on female reproductive anatomy and physiology. A variable number of days after the onset of menses, an estrogen surge occurs, followed by a surge of LH, which triggers ovulation. The estrogen surge changes the character of cervical mucus by causing the columnar cells of the endocervical crypts to increase the water content of cervical mucus, thereby producing a clear, thin, stretchy mucus (type E, estrogenic) instead of the thick, dry mucus that is secreted earlier in the cycle. Type E mucus, which forms a fern pattern when dried on a microscope slide, allows increased sperm penetration and longer sperm survival (3 to 5 days versus only a few hours), and filters out morphologically defective sperm.

Several studies have shown that detection of type E mucus externally at the vaginal introitus correlates closely with the time of ovulation. By 3 days following peak production of type E mucus, ovulation has occurred in nearly all women.

Following ovulation, progesterone becomes the dominant hormone. Progesterone is thermogenic and thus causes the body temperature to rise. In addition, progesterone secreted following ovulation changes the cervical mucus to an opaque, thick, sticky consistency (type G, gestagenic).

The symptothermal method monitors the cervical mucus and body temperature. The possibility of ovulation is assumed to exist when type E mucus is detected. Ovulation is then assumed to have occured when body temperature rises and type G mucus is detected. Following ovulation, the average length of the menstrual cycle is 13.7 days (range 9 to 17 days, but usually consistent each month in a given woman).

FAILURE RATES

Reported efficacy rates for this method vary greatly, as shown in Table 20-1. A variety of factors may explain these differences, including differences in instructors, variations in how consistently a couple uses the method, and differences in whether studies classify pregnancies as accidental or intended (ovulation methods are also used to monitor fertility as a means of achieving conception). In addition, the precise method used to monitor cervical mucus and body temperature may vary among studies, and some studies may use older methods of natural family planning.

HOW TO PRESCRIBE

Couples need careful instruction in this method, often over several sessions, by a trained instructor to achieve optimal efficacy. In addition to instruction, careful charting of temperatures and mucus changes appears to be an important part of using this method effectively.

Body temperature may be measured orally, rectally, or vaginally, usually upon awakening, before rising from bed. Special basal body temperature thermometers are available that have graduated measurement scales suitable for detecting the small changes in temperature that occur with ovulation.

Monitoring of cervical mucus should begin immediately following menses, focusing on detecting the onset of clear, thin, stretchy or sticky mucus (Table 20-7). When this mucus is detected, intercourse should be avoided. When the mucus changes to "slippery," resembling raw egg white, a woman is entering her most fertile period, which continues until 3 days after the last day that the slippery mucus is detected.

In addition to changes in body temperature and cervical mucus, women may be aware of other symptoms indicative of ovulation. These symptoms include the adnexal pain of ovulation (Mittelschmertz), low backache, abdominal bloating, vulvar swelling, and ovulation-associated spotting. Women who perform internal self-examination may notice a widening of the cervical os.

Finally, the reliability of natural family planning can be improved by using commercially available kits to detect ovulation. These kits detect the LH surge that precedes ovulation. Unfortunately, use of these kits adds greatly to the expense of natural family planning methods, but it also adds certainty about the time of ovulation. After the third day following the LH peak,

couples may resume intercourse until onset of the menses. Intercourse should also be avoided during menses, because women with short cycles may enter their fertile period during the last days of bleeding.

Clinicians must stress that absolute compliance with all aspects of the method is vital. Trussel and Grummer-Strawn noted that the probability of pregnancy increased from 0.2 to 28 percent per cycle when women broke either or both of the following rules: (1) no intercourse during mucus days and (2) no intercourse within 3 days after the peak day. A summary of the rules for the natural family planning method is shown in Table 20-7.

Lactational Amenorrhea Method

The lactational amenorrhea method takes advantage of the postpartum infertility that occurs naturally in association with lactation.

MECHANISM OF ACTION

The precise mechanism by which lactation causes infertility is unknown. Teleologically, lactational infertility prevents a second pregnancy while the woman is involved in feeding and nurturing a new infant, thereby preserving maternal nutritional resources for the current infant. Physiologically, suckling is believed to have a direct

Table 20-7

Key Events and Rules for Symptothermal Method of Natural Family Planning

CYCLE EVENT	DAYS	SIGNS	INTERCOURSE PERMITTED
Menstruation	1–5	Bleeding	No
Safe (dry) days	6–9	No cervical mucus	Yes
Fertile period begins	10	Sticky or stretchy mucus begins	No
Peak fertility	16	Last day of slippery mucus	No
Fertility ends	20	4 days after peak fertility	Next day
Safe days	20–29	Until menses begin	Yes

SOURCE: Adapted with permission from Hatcher RA, Trussell J, and Stewart F, et al.

effect on the hypothalamus, perhaps through oxytocin secretion, that reduces the pulsatile secretion of gonadotropin-releasing hormone, which, in turn, suppresses LH release and ovulation.

Women who exclusively breast-feed their infants (i.e., no bottle or solid-food supplements), who do not have a return of menstruation, and who rely on lactational amenorrhea for contraception have failure rates of only 0.5 to 2 percent. Unfortunately, ovulation may resume prior to the first menses, rendering the woman potentially fertile without her awareness. The probability that this will happen increases with time, from 33 to 45 percent during the first 3 months postpartum to 64 to 71 percent during the next 9 months. The majority of these early ovulations, however, will not result in pregnancy due to a luteal defect that occurs in the first postpartum ovulations.

How to Prescribe

Women using lactational amenorrhea as a birth control method should be advised to breast-feed on demand, avoid bottle feeding or other food supplements, and begin using another method of birth control upon return of menses or by 6 months postpartum, whichever occurs first.

Withdrawal (Coitus Interruptus)

In the withdrawal method, also known as coitus interruptus, the man withdraws his penis from the vagina prior to ejaculation. This method of contraception works by preventing introduction of semen into the vagina, thereby avoiding contact between the sperm and ovum.

Some authorities have expressed concern that, even if the penis is withdrawn before ejaculation, pregnancy may still occur because of sperm in the "preejaculate." The preejaculate consists of lubricating secretions from the Cow-

per's glands that are released prior to ejaculation. However, several small studies have found no sperm in the preejaculate, except in HIV-positive men.

Although the withdrawal method is often criticized as ineffective, it actually provides contraceptive benefit similar to that of the vaginal barrier methods. The accidental pregnancy rate with withdrawal is probably about 19 percent, although failure rates as low as 7 percent have been reported.

How to Prescribe

To effectively use the withdrawal method, a man must be able to determine when he is about to ejaculate and remove his penis from the vagina before ejaculation occurs. Inability to sense impending ejaculation renders the withdrawal method inappropriate.

In addition, as noted above, sperm have been detected in the preejaculates of HIV-positive men. Thus, HIV-positive couples probably should not use this method. Finally, because withdrawal provides no protection against spread of HIV and other STDs, withdrawal is also an inappropriate method for HIV-infected men with HIV-negative partners.

Typical Presentation

Routine Health Care

The most common reason for an office visit at which contraception is discussed or prescribed is typically something other than contraception. Data from NAMCS show that only a minority of women and men whose visits were related to contraception stated that this was the main reason for their visit; fully 81 percent of women and 64 percent of men gave a reason other than contraception. Most often, contraception care occurs when patients are visiting a clinician for general medical or gynecologic examinations.

Care for Contraception and/or Side Effects

Some patients, of course, seek care specifically for prescription of a contraceptive method. Others seek care for contraception-related side effects or difficulties using their current method of birth control.

Postpartum Care

A third common scenario in which contraception care occurs is at a postpartum visit, which usually occurs 6 to 8 weeks after delivery. Unfortunately, however, many women do not begin a contraceptive method until this postpartum visit, even though they resume sexual intercourse shortly after delivery. In fact, nearly 90 percent of U.S. women report being sexually active by 8 weeks postpartum. Ideally, a woman's need for contraception should be addressed before the postpartum visit, such as prior to hospital discharge and/or at the 1- to 2-week newborn examination. For women who are not breast-feeding and therefore at risk for ovulation before the traditional 6-week postpartum visit, a 3-week postpartum visit should be considered if a contraceptive method has not yet been started by that time.

Possible Pregnancy

Some women do not seek a birth control method until they think they might be pregnant. Any visit for possible pregnancy should be viewed as an opportunity to discuss birth control needs (if the patient is not, in fact, pregnant). If the patient is pregnant and plans to seek an abortion, it is imperative that a follow-up visit be planned after

the abortion to discuss and choose a birth control method.

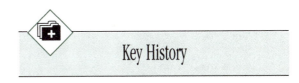

Key History

The history relating to contraception is targeted at determining a patient's need for a birth control method and, if one is needed, deciding which method is most suitable. The first step is to directly solicit information about a patient's sexual activity and contraceptive practices. Questions such as those shown in Table 20-8 are typically the most useful.

The second step is to ask about aspects of the medical, menstrual, and sexual history that are important in selecting a birth control method. These factors include the length of time for which contraception will be needed, identification of contraindications to individual methods, the need for protection against STDs, and menstrual irregularities that might benefit from certain forms of contraception. Figure 20-9 incorporates many of these questions in an algorithm (see "Algorithm," below).

Special Considerations with Adolescents

Special consideration must be given to history-taking with adolescents. Above all, it is essential to create opportunities to speak privately, without parents present, to assess the current needs and understanding of sexual activity and birth control.

For adolescents who are not sexually active, it is important to encourage them not to be urged into early sexual activity. In addition, clinicians should emphasize the need to seek guidance on birth control before engaging in sexual activity, and the fact that abstinence from intercourse does not preclude other types of sexual expres-

Table 20-8

Key History in Patients Being Evaluated for Contraception

Intent of Question	Suggested Phraseology of Question
Determine the patient's level of sexual activity.	Are you currently sexually active?
Determine the type and number of sexual partner.	Are your partners men, women, or both? Do you currently have one partner or more than one?
Determine contraceptive needs and practices.	Do you have need for birth control? Do you need any information on birth control methods?
Identify any sexual or contraceptive problems.	Are you having any problems with sex? Is intercourse painful for you? Are you having any problems with birth control?
If already using contraception, determine satisfaction with current method.	Are you satisfied with your current method of birth control? Are you having any side effects from your birth control method? Do you have any trouble using or remembering to use your birth control method? Do you want to continue the current method, or have you thought about switching?

sion that may be gratifying but safer, such as touching, kissing, massage, and mutual masturbation. It is often useful to provide non-sexually-active teenagers with basic information about how and when conception occurs. Statements such as, "Many of my patients seem confused about how pregnancy occurs. Do you mind if we take some time to talk about this?" or "When, if ever, do you imagine yourself having children? How do you plan to keep (yourself or your partner) from getting pregnant until then?" may be helpful in introducing these topics.

For adolescents who are sexually active, clinicians should ask questions similar to those in Table 20-8 and also provide information about conception and methods of birth control. Asking questions about their enjoyment of sex or worries about pregnancy may lead to more in-depth discussions. The chosen method of birth control should be discussed with respect to safety and efficacy and available alternatives. All ado-

lescents should be asked about coercive sex or sexual abuse; if sexual abuse is discovered, immediate plans for safety (including hospitalization, if appropriate) must be made, along with notification of the proper authorities.

Physical Examination

All sexually active women and men should undergo periodic health examinations for primary and secondary prevention, screening, and counseling. With respect to evaluating patients for birth control methods, several parts of the physical examination are particularly important.

Specifically, a blood pressure measurement should be performed to identify hypertension, a potential contraindication to estrogen-containing

OCPs in older women. Similarly, a breast examination should be performed to detect any breast masses, which may also be a contraindication to OCPs. Certain disabling conditions may also influence the choice of a birth control method. For example, severe arthritis of the hands might make it difficult to insert vaginal barrier devices.

A male genital or female pelvic examination is performed to detect evidence of STD on the skin, penis, vulva, or cervix (Table 20-9). A bimanual examination should be performed on women to detect abnormalities of the vagina and uterus, such as a vaginal septum, cervical abnormalities, uterine fibroids, and bicornuate uterus. Vaginal barrier contraceptives and IUDs are less appropriate contraceptive choices for women with these abnormalities. In addition, IUDs generally cannot be inserted in women with cervical stenosis.

As with the history, the physical examination may also require special considerations for adolescents. In particular, it may be important to start a method of contraception and defer the pelvic examination until another time if the pa-

tient objects to the examination. That is, the clinician should not permit the examination itself to be an impediment to prescribing contraception to teenagers. The examination may be performed at a subsequent office visit, once the adolescent is more comfortable with the clinician.

Ancillary Tests

The principal role of laboratory tests in prescribing a contraceptive method involves detecting STDs and cervical neoplasia. In some situations, metabolic tests are also appropriate.

Detecting STDs and Cervical Neoplasia

Testing for STDs is important because patients requiring contraception are, by definition, sexually active and capable of transmitting STDs. Thus, identification and eradication of infec-

Table 20-9

Physical Examination Findings of Sexually Transmitted Diseases

EXAMINATION FINDING	SEXUALLY TRANSMITTED DISEASE
Maculopapular skin rash	Secondary syphilis
Pharyngitis	Gonorrhea
Vesicles or ulcers on penis, anus, mouth, labia, or cervix; may be associated with lymphadenopathy	Painless: primary syphilis or granuloma inguinale Painful: genital herpes or chancroid
Warts (flesh-colored or brownish exophytic, hyperkeratotic papules) on genital or perianal skin or mucosa	Human papillomavirus
Vaginal discharge	Nonpurulent: primary genital herpes Frothy: trichomoniasis Purulent: gonorrhea, chlamydia
Penile discharge	Gonorrhea, chlamydia
Inflamed cervix that bleeds easily	Gonorrhea, chlamydia
Tender uterus or adnexa, or adnexal mass	PID (polymicrobial)
Rectal tenderness or bleeding	Gonorrhea

tion is desirable, if possible. If eradication is not possible, such as with viral STDs (e.g., human papillomavirus or herpesvirus infections), the presence of infection makes it important to use a contraceptive method that protects against transmitting the infection (e.g., condom with spermicide). Identification of STDs is important if IUDs are being considered, because STDs preclude the use of IUDs.

To test for STDs, cultures for gonorrhea and tests or cultures for chlamydia should routinely be performed unless the sexual history makes such testing unreasonable or inappropriate. In addition, many experts encourage patients in nonexclusive relationships to be tested for HIV, particularly if the history suggests behaviors that put the patient at risk for HIV infection. A Pap smear also should be performed, since it may yield evidence of human papillomavirus or other infections, or may reveal intraepithelial lesions (dysplasia) requiring treatment and contraindicating use of a cervical cap.

If the results of any of the abovementioned STD tests are positive or if the patient's history suggests risk for STD, further laboratory evaluation is in order. This evaluation should include serologic tests for syphilis and liver function or hepatitis screening. In addition, HIV testing should be strongly encouraged if it has not already been done.

Metabolic Tests

Some experts recommend a lipid profile before prescribing OCPs to women over 35, women whose cardiac risk factors are not known, or women who have a family history of hyperlipidemia or a first-degree relative with a history of myocardial infarction before age 50. Kjos and associates, however, found no significant adverse metabolic markers (lipids or carbohydrates) in women over the age of 35 who were long-term users of combined OCPs. Most clinicians do not routinely check lipids levels, obtain hemograms, or perform other metabolic tests before prescribing OCPs.

Algorithm

The algorithm presented in Fig. 20-9 can be used to assist couples or individuals in selecting a method of birth control. Condoms should be strongly encouraged for new partnerships, teenagers, patients with a history of STDs, and couples in which one partner has a viral STD and the other partner is not infected. When maximal pregnancy protection also is needed, patients should combine condoms with a hormonal method such as OCPs or MDPA.

For couples in stable relationships who desire maximal protection from pregnancy, sterilization can be considered. For a maximally protective reversible method, the IUD and Norplant are most useful if long-term contraception is needed. Women who engage in frequent intercourse and desire short-term maximal protection should consider OCPs or MDPA. For those who have less frequent intercourse and are highly motivated (or when patients have contraindications to hormonal contraception), vaginal barrier methods or natural family planning may be appropriate. The cervical cap, however, is less effective than the diaphragm for parous women, and thus the diaphragm should be encouraged in this group. For less-motivated couples or individuals, MDPA may be optimal. Finally, progesterone-only pills are an option for women with contraindications to estrogen.

Education

Education of the patient is an essential part of prescribing contraception. As described earlier, for some methods, such as condoms, education can make a major contribution to the frequency, consistency, and correctness with which patients use the method.

Figure 20-9

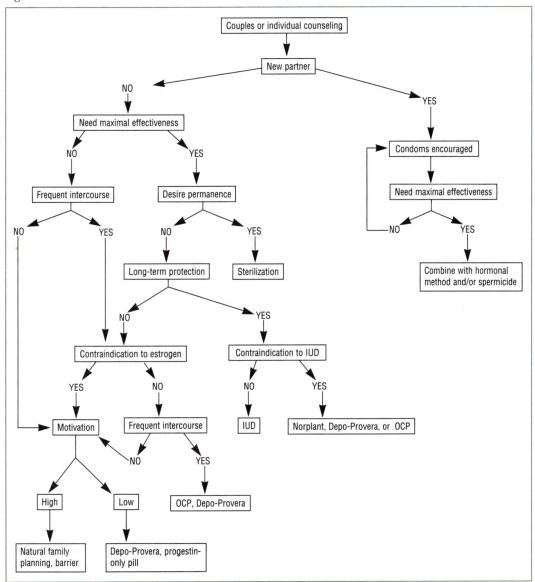

Algorithm providing a guide to the overall selection of a contraceptive method. IUD, intrauterine device; OCP, combined oral contraceptive pills.

General Counseling

In discussing the efficacy of the patient's chosen method of contraception, patients should understand that all methods may fail and that, for most methods, failure is directly related to consistency of use. Thus, clinicians should spend time exploring the patient's motivation and potential barriers to correctly using a contraceptive method. In this regard, peer counselors, particularly for adolescent patients, are helpful in improving compliance.

STD Protection

All sexually active patients, regardless of birth control method, should be advised to use a male or female latex condom with every act of intercourse to prevent STDs (including HIV infection), unless they are in a stable, long-term, mutually monogamous relationship. For added protection against condom breakage, two male condoms can be used simultaneously. However, as noted earlier, male and female condoms should not be used together.

Mouth-to-penis contact can transmit most STDs, including hepatitis B, but few cases of HIV transmission have been reported following oral-genital contact. To protect against oral-genital transmission of STDs, condoms (nonlubricated and non-spermicide-containing) can be used during oral-penile contact. However, for mouth-to-vulva contact, female condoms may not provide sufficient barrier protection against STDs. Plastic wrap is sometimes used to create a barrier for mouth-to-vulva contact, but this method has not been tested for efficacy.

If a condom is not available, a vaginal spermicide will offer some protection against bacterial infections. However, spermicide alone will not provide sufficient protection against HIV. In addition, as noted earlier, spermicides may cause tissue microabrasions that can increase HIV transmission risk. Because any genital lesion will increase susceptibility to HIV, intercourse should be avoided until such a lesion is healed.

Emergency Contraception

Information on emergency (postcoital) contraception should be provided to all patients, but it is particularly important for those using barrier methods because of the possibility of method failure due to breakage or dislodgment. Multiple studies have found emergency contraception to be effective in preventing unwanted pregnancy, whether given at the time of the emergency or prescribed in advance to be used when necessary. The latter method is most cost-effective.

Typical emergency contraceptive regimens involve administration of 0.05 mg ethinyl estradiol and 0.5 mg levonorgestrel, one dose within 72 h of intercourse and a second dose 12 h later. Products containing this dose and specifically packaged for emergency contraception are marketed in Western Europe and as Preven in the United States. However, the appropriate amount of estrogen and progestin can also be achieved with standard OCPs, such as with two tablets of Ovral or four tablets of Lo-Ovral or Levlen.

It must be emphasized that emergency contraception should be initiated within 72 h after unprotected intercourse. This method will reduce the risk of pregnancy by at least 75 percent. The effectiveness of taking the medication longer than 72 h after intercourse is not known.

Method-Specific Education

Information on how to prescribe and use the various contraceptive methods appears earlier in this chapter. Additional information that should be provided to users of each contraceptive method is described below.

STERILIZATION

TUBAL LIGATION   Following tubal ligation, women should be informed that recovery from the procedure averages about 4 days. They should plan to rest for the first 24 h and may resume activities gradually over the first week. Bathing may resume after 2 days and intercourse after 1 week.

Women should be made aware that, should pregnancy occur following tubal ligation, the risk of that pregnancy being ectopic (usually in the fallopian tube) is high, approaching 50 percent. Thus, women undergoing tubal ligation should know the symptoms of ectopic pregnancy, such as pelvic pain and/or vaginal bleeding following a period of absent menses.

VASECTOMY   Following vasectomy, men should keep an ice pack on the scrotum for at least 4 h and wear a scrotal support for the first 2 to 3 days. Strenuous activity may resume in 1 week.

While intercourse may be resumed after 2 to 3 days, men should be aware that they are not sterile immediately after a vasectomy because sperm remaining in the distal vas deferens after the procedure are still viable and able to fertilize an ovum. Thus, couples should abstain from unprotected intercourse until analysis of ejaculated semen demonstrates absence of sperm (azoospermia). The first semen analysis is usually obtained 6 weeks after vasectomy. If sperm are still present, semen analyses are repeated monthly until azoospermia is documented. Following vasectomy, about 80 to 90 percent of men will have azoospermic semen after 12 to 15 ejaculations or by 6 weeks, regardless of ejaculatory frequency.

COMBINED ORAL CONTRACEPTIVES

Women should be instructed on what to do if they miss a pill, since missing a pill is fairly common. If one pill is missed, the missed pill should be taken immediately upon recognition that a pill has been omitted, and a back-up method of contraception should be used for 48 h if the time between doses was more than 27 h. If 2 days of OCPs are missed, the woman should take two pills daily for 2 days in a row, then continue taking one pill per day for the remainder of the cycle, and use a back-up method immediately and for the remainder of the cycle.

For progesterone-only pills, missed doses are of greater concern. As noted earlier, progesterone-only pills must be taken at the same time each day. If more than 3 h have elapsed since a pill was due, contraceptive protection is lost and a back-up method should be used for at least 48 h.

BARRIER METHODS

The importance of providing patients with verbal and written instructions about proper use of barrier methods cannot be overemphasized. Some products, such as the female condom, come with package inserts that provide directions for insertion. The effect of counseling to enhance knowledge and use of barrier methods has been demonstrated in a number of studies. The counseling need not be extensive. For example, a study using brief interventions in waiting areas of public health clinics demonstrated a significant improvement in the consistency with which women used spermicide and condoms. In that study, the best predictor of consistent use was knowledge about how to use the contraceptive method correctly. Notably, fear of acquiring STDs or HIV infection predicted correct or consistent use of the method.

CONDOMS   Because the effectiveness of the condom is highly user-dependent, motivation to use condoms should be increased by relating its use to prevention of pregnancy and STDs. In addition, use of condoms by adolescents is associated with the following beliefs: (1) condoms enable one to have sex on the spur of the moment; (2) condoms are easy to use; (3) condoms are clean; (4) they are popular with peers; and (5) they provide a way for males to participate/have responsibility for using contraception.

Some men complain of pain or discomfort when using condoms. Men who experience this problem should consider the use of polyurethane condoms. These condoms were reported in a recent review of premarketing studies to be preferred over latex in appearance, lack of smell, comfort, sensitivity, and natural look and feel. No significant differences in slippage and breakage rates between latex and polyurethane condoms were noted.

Patients should also be informed that exposure to heat, inappropriate storage (e.g., long periods of time in a wallet), use with oil-based lubricants (mineral oil, shortening, massage oil, etc.), and exposure to vaginal antifungal preparations can reduce the reliability of condoms by increasing the likelihood of breakage.

If a condom has torn or slipped off during use, spermicidal foam or gel should be inserted into the vagina immediately. If such products are not available, the penis (for STD protection) and the vagina (for STD protection and pregnancy prevention) should be washed with soap and water. Postcoital (emergency) contraception should be considered.

DIAPHRAGM AND CERVICAL CAP   To prevent odor and deterioration, these devices should be cleaned after each use with a mild soap or detergent (avoiding deodorant or perfumed soap) and stored in a clean, cool place. Women should be advised to inspect the device before each use for thin spots or tears and to replace it if these problems are identified. The device should also be replaced if odor is detected. As with condoms, contact with oil-based lubricants can cause deterioration. Thus, water-based lubricants are suggested if additional lubrication is needed for intercourse. Women selecting a vaginal barrier method should be advised to use the device every time they have intercourse.

Sign and symptoms of toxic shock syndrome should be reviewed. They include sudden high fever, vomiting and diarrhea, dizziness, faintness or weakness, sunburn-like rash, and aching muscles or joints. Symptoms of urinary tract infections may also be discussed, since they occur with increased frequency in diaphragm users.

INTRAUTERINE DEVICE

Following IUD insertion, women should be instructed to check periodically to be sure they can feel the IUD string coming out of the cervix into the vagina. This is particularly important during the first few menstrual cycles following insertion, since that is when spontaneous expulsion of an IUD is most likely to occur. Expulsion of the IUD occurs in between 1 and 10 per 100 women in the first year after insertion. It is more common among younger women and those who have never been pregnant.

The date for scheduled removal or change of the IUD should be noted and provided to the patient in writing. Changing IUDs more frequently than necessary should be avoided because most complications, including perforation, expulsion, and infection, occur just after insertion.

If pregnancy should occur with the IUD in place, women should be advised to have the IUD removed immediately. Removal of the IUD may precipitate a spontaneous abortion, but the risk of this complication is less than if the IUD is left in place. When the IUD is left in place, spontaneous abortion occurs in 50 to 60 percent of intrauterine pregnancies, and the risk of a septic abortion is 26 times greater than if the IUD is removed.

Because IUDs increase the risk of pelvic infection and ectopic pregnancy, women should be counseled to report any symptoms of pelvic pain, bleeding, odorous discharge, fever, or a missed period. Table 20-6 reviews common problems with the IUD and recommended management strategies.

NATURAL FAMILY PLANNING

Educational efforts are particularly important for couples selecting natural family planning methods. Referral of couples to local natural family planning educational resources and the provision of written materials are often the best way to provide instruction and support. Planned Parenthood agencies can often direct patients to these resources.

Family Approach

By its very nature, contraception is a process that involves couples and families. In addition, other family and social influences, such as religion and culture, play a role in contraception choices and use.

Partners and Parents

When the patient is part of a couple, both partners should be encouraged to come together for counseling and decision-making about contraceptive methods. There is ample evidence about the importance of partner support in compliance with contraceptives, especially for adolescents and young adults.

For adolescents, family involvement is also important. Investigators for the National Survey of Family Growth found that the family may be effective in increasing adolescents' use of contraceptives and in influencing whether a pregnant adolescent selects abortion or adoption as an alternative to parenthood. Others have shown that the presence of a father in the household (i.e., the father of the sexually active woman) has a positive effect on preventing adolescent pregnancy. Furthermore, survey data and anthropologic studies show that family disapproval of contraception is related to nonuse by young women. When appropriate, therefore, encouraging parents to take an active role in communicating with and advising their children about sexual activity and contraception may be important in avoiding unintended pregnancy.

Culture and Religion

In addition to families and partners, religion and cultural affiliation also influence contraceptive practices. Within the Roman Catholic church, where procreation is perceived to be the main purpose of sexual activity, natural family planning and abstinence are the only permissible forms of birth control. Less restrictive positions are held by Protestant and Anglican churches, in which other forms of contraception for medical indications are accepted. In orthodox Judaism, sexual relationships within marriage have two roles: procreation and fulfillment of a woman's sexual needs. Men are duty-bound to propagate, but women are not. Therefore, prohibitions exist for the use of male contraception, including withdrawal, condom use, abstinence, and vasectomy. However, female-dependent contraceptive methods are acceptable.

With the many new immigrant groups now part of U.S. society, heterogeneous cultural and religious beliefs play an important role in prescribing contraception. While Islam, Hinduism, and Buddhism allow contraceptive use, women of these faiths may not be comfortable with certain forms of birth control for cultural reasons. For example, Muslim, Hindu, and Sikh women, brought up to be shy and modest, may have great difficulty submitting to vaginal examinations or using methods that involve self-insertion of a device into the vagina. For these women, condoms, OCPs, and MDPA may be the best choice. Understanding these various cultural and religious constraints will make clinicians more effective in working with patients to prescribe contraceptive methods.

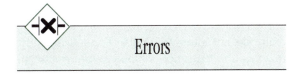

Errors

One of the more common errors clinicians make is not discussing contraception with patients at risk for pregnancy. This is a particular problem in relation to adolescents, especially for physicians who see adolescents infrequently.

Another common error is failure to describe a patient's chosen contraceptive method to the patient in detail, including an actual demonstration or practice with that method in the office. For barrier methods in particular, lack of adequate instruction increases the chance of noncompliance or discontinuation of the method.

A third common error is failure to schedule a follow-up visit to review a patient's progress after a new birth control method is selected. Most clinicians are unaware of their patients' experience with contraceptive methods, for which difficulties with use and compliance are the rule and not the exception. Many potential problems can be averted if patients are reassessed after an initial month or two of experience with a particular method.

Controversies

A number of controversies surround the use of certain contraceptive methods. Some of these controversies relate to conflicts with religious principles, and these will not be discussed here. Other controversies, however, relate to medical uses and indications for contraceptive interventions, including emergency contraception and the new drug mefepristone (RU-486).

Emergency Contraception

Nearly one-half of women with unintended pregnancies report that they would have considered emergency contraception if they had known it was available. However, clinicians generally do not inform patients of the availability, or even the existence, of postcoital contraceptive methods. Some clinicians argue that widespread awareness and availability of postcoital contraception could lead to excessive use of this method and decreased use of conventional contraceptive methods, and this is seen as undesirable. Recent research suggests, however, that ready availability of emergency contraception, including self-administration by patients on an as-needed basis, does not increase the frequency of use of this method in comparison to requiring patients to seek medical care when they need emergency contraception. Huge numbers of unintended pregnancies could be prevented if women knew and took advantage of this form of contraception.

Several methods of postcoital contraception are available. Preven and OCPs are the most widely used methods, as described earlier. Other hormonal methods include progestin alone or danazol, an antigonadotropin. Although used in other parts of the world, neither of these methods has undergone extensive testing, and neither is approved by the FDA for postcoital contraception.

Inserting a copper IUD within 5 to 7 days after ovulation in a cycle during which unprotected intercourse occurred is also effective for preventing pregnancy. The inserted IUD probably works by preventing implantation. The insertion of an IUD for postcoital contraception is used much less frequently than hormonal treatment and is not approved by the FDA for emergency contraception. However, it is an excellent method for women who are suitable IUD candidates and might consider using an IUD for long-term contraception.

The most controversial method, however, is RU-486, the progesterone antagonist used in other countries for elective pregnancy termination. By interfering with the action of progesterone, RU-486 blocks ovulation if it has not occurred and blocks implantation if ovulation has already taken place. A single 600-mg dose of RU-486 given within 72 h after unprotected intercourse is highly effective as a postcoital contraceptive, and it has few side effects. Because the drug is also used as an abortifacient, however, its use for any purpose, including postcoital pregnancy prevention, is controversial in the United States. Nonetheless, in some parts of the world (e.g., China), RU-486 is the most widely used postcoital contraceptive.

Emerging Concepts

A variety of new contraceptive methods are under development. They include new barrier methods, spermicides, hormonal methods, and vaccines.

Barrier Methods

A variety of new barrier methods are under development. The Lea's shield, for example, is currently awaiting approval by the FDA. The

Lea's shield is a bowl-shaped diaphragmlike device that is 55 mm in diameter and thicker posteriorly (to fill the posterior fornix of the vagina). Because it is made of silicone instead of latex, the device is resistant to degrading effects of petroleum-based lubricants, does not absorb odors, and does not cause allergic reactions in users with latex sensitivity. The Lea's shield has an anterior loop for ease of removal and a one-way flutter valve to prevent pressure build-up over the cervix. In a phase I trial, no motile sperm were found in the cervical mucus in any cycle in which Lea's shield was used with spermicide. In a phase II trial, 6-month life-table pregnancy rates among the 185 women who used the shield with spermicide were 5.6 per 100 users.

Spermicides

New spermicides are also being developed. Unlike nonoxynol-9, which acts as a detergent that degrades sperm as well as some of the natural protective vaginal microorganisms, the new agents are more "sperm-specific." The new spermicides have multiple actions that prevent maturation of sperm. They impede release of cholesterol from the plasma membrane of the sperm head, thereby preventing membrane maturation. They block calcium channels in the sperm membrane, thus preventing release of acrosomal enzymes that facilitate penetration of the ovum. They also prevent protein binding between the sperm and the zona pellucida of the ovum. These new spermicides should be more effective than currently available agents and will probably be safer.

Hormonal Methods

Several new hormonal methods are under development. They include methods for both men and women.

Hormonal methods being developed for men include long-acting (3-months duration) intramuscular injections of testosterone and progestin. In addition, researchers are also developing an injection of non-peptide inhibitors of gonadotropin-releasing hormone that will impair fertility by decreasing sperm production.

For women, progestin-releasing vaginal devices, with or without estrogen, are undergoing testing. In addition, dual-rod Norplantlike devices are being developed. These dual-rod devices offer the advantage of easier insertion, and some may be biodegradable, thus eliminating the need for removal.

A new levonorgestrel-releasing IUD is awaiting approval. As with Progestasert, progesterone-induced endometrial atrophy with the new device results in low rates of irregular bleeding. In fact, 83 percent of users in one study had no bleeding or spotting after 1 year of use.

Vaccines

Finally, "antipregnancy" vaccines for men and women (immunocontraceptives) are undergoing phase I and II trials. These vaccines induce antibodies against selected hormones and proteins involved in reproduction. These hormones and proteins include follicle-stimulating and luteinizing-hormone-releasing hormone for men, and hCG and sperm antigens for women. Before these immunocontraceptives will be available for use, testing must demonstrate that their effects on fertility are reversible. In addition, testing must demonstrate safety, particularly with respect to inducing unwanted immune responses against other tissue antigens that might cross-react with the vaccine antigen.

Bibliography

Alexander NJ: Future contraceptives. *Sci Am* 273:136, 1995.

Blumenstein BA, Douglas MB, Hall WD: Blood pressure changes and oral contraceptive use: A study of 2,676 black women in the southeastern United States. *Am J Epidemiol* 112:539, 1980.

Casper LM: Does family interaction prevent adolescent pregnancy? *Fam Plan Perspect* 22:109, 1990.

Cohen D, Reardon K, Alleyne D, et al: Influencing spermicide use among low-income minority women. *J Am Med Wom Assoc* 50:11, 1995.

Fihn SD, Boyko EJ, Normand EH, et al: Association between use of spermicide-coated condoms and *Escherichia coli* urinary tract infection in young women. *Am J Epidemiol* 144:512, 1996.

Forrest JD, Fordyce RR: U.S. women's contraceptive attitudes and practice: How have they changed in the 1980's? *Fam Plan Perspect* 20:112, 1988.

Forrest JD, Frost JJ: The family planning attitudes and experiences of low-income women. *Fam Plan Perspect* 28:246, 1996.

Geerling JH: Natural family planning. *Am Fam Phys* 52:1749, 1995.

Glasier A: Emergency postcoital contraception. *New Engl J Med* 337:1058, 1997.

Glasier A, Baird D: The effect of self-administered emergency contraception. *New Engl J Med* 339:1, 1998.

Gollub EL, French P, Latka M, et al: The women's safer sex hierarchy: Initial responses to counseling on women's methods of STD/HIV prevention at an STD clinic. *Proceed Int Conf AIDS* 11:52 (abstr) 1996.

Hatcher RA, Trussell J, Stewart F, et al: *Contraceptive Technology*, 16th ed. New York, Irvington, 1994.

IUDs—a new look. *Population Reports—Series B. Intrauterine Devices* 5:17, 1988.

Jarow JP, Budin RE, Dym M, et al: Quantitative pathologic changes in the human testis after vasectomy. *New Engl J Med* 313:1252, 1985.

Kegeles SM, Adler NE, Irwin CE: Adolescents and condoms: Associations of beliefs with intentions to use. *Am J Dis Child* 143:911, 1989.

Kjos SL, Gregory K, Henry OA, Collins C: Evaluation of routine diabetes and lipid screening after age 35 in candidates for or current users of oral contraceptives. *Obstet Gynecol* 82:925, 1993.

Landry DJ, Forrest JD: Private physicians' provision of contraceptive services. *Fam Plan Perspect* 28:203, 1996.

Lauersen NH, Wilson KH, Graves ZR, et al: The cervical cap: Effectiveness, safety, and acceptability as a barrier contraceptive. *Mt Sinai J Med* 53:233, 1996.

Mauck C, Glover LH, Miller E, et al: Lea's shield: A study of the safety and efficacy of a new vaginal barrier contraceptive used with and without spermicide. *Contraception* 53:329, 1996.

McCann MF, Moggia AV, Higgins JE, et al: The effects of a progestin-only oral contraceptive (levonorgestrel 0.03 mg) on breast-feeding. *Contraception* 40:635, 1989.

Peterson HB, Xia Z, Hughes JM, et al: The risk of pregnancy after tubal sterilization: Findings from the U.S. Collaborative Review of Sterilization. *Am J Obstet Gynecol* 174:1161, 1996.

Peterson LS: Contraceptive use in the United States: 1982–90. *Adv Data* 260:1, 1995.

Sangi-Haghpeykar H, Poindexter AN 3d, Levine H: Sperm transport and survival post-application of a new spermicide contraceptive: Advantage 24 Study Group. *Contraception* 53:353, 1996.

Savonius H, Pakarinen P, Sjoberg L, et al: Reasons for pregnancy termination: Negligence or failure of contraception? *Acta Obstet Gynecol Scand* 74:818, 1995.

Schenker JG, Rabenou V: Family planning: Cultural and religious perspectives. *Hum Reprod* 8:969, 1993.

Smith C, Farr G, Feldblum PJ, et al: Effectiveness of the non-spermicidal fit-free diaphragm. *Contraception* 51:289, 1995.

Speroff L, Darney PD: *A clinical guide for contraception*, 2d ed. Baltimore, Williams & Wilkins, 1996.

Trussell J, Grummer-Strawn L: Contraceptive failure of the ovulation method of periodic abstinence. *Fam Plan Perspect* 16:5, 1990.

Trussell J, Koenig J, Ellertson C, et al: Preventing unintended pregnancy: The cost-effectiveness of three methods of emergency contraception. *Am J Public Health* 87:932, 1997.

Weiss BD, Bassford T, Davis TL: The cervical cap. *Am Fam Physician* 43:517, 1991.

Index

Page numbers followed by the letters *f* and *t* indicate figures and tables, respectively.

ISBN 0-07-069609-8